Recommended Dietary Allowances (RDA), 1980*

Age (years)	Weight (kg)	Weight (lbs)	Height (cm)	Height (in)	Protein (g)	(RE) Vitamin A	(µg) Vitamin D	(mg) Vitamin E	(mg) Vitamin C	(mg) Thiamin	(mg) Riboflavin	(mg equiv.) Niacin	(mg) Vitamin B$_6$	(µg) Folacin	(µg) Vitamin B$_{12}$	(mg) Calcium	(mg) Phosphorus	(mg) Magnesium	(mg) Iron	(mg) Zinc	(µg) Iodine
Infants																					
0.0–0.5	6	13	60	24	kg × 2.2	420	10	3	35	0.3	0.4	6	0.3	30	0.5	360	240	50	10	3	40
0.5–1.0	9	20	71	28	kg × 2.0	400	10	4	35	0.5	0.6	8	0.6	45	1.5	540	360	70	15	5	50
Children																					
1–3	13	29	90	35	23	400	10	5	45	0.7	0.8	9	0.9	100	2.0	800	800	150	15	10	70
4–6	20	44	112	44	30	500	10	6	45	0.9	1.0	11	1.3	200	2.5	800	800	200	10	10	90
7–10	28	62	132	52	34	700	10	7	45	1.2	1.4	16	1.6	300	3.0	800	800	250	10	10	120
Males																					
11–14	45	99	157	62	45	1,000	10	8	50	1.4	1.6	18	1.8	400	3.0	1,200	1,200	350	18	15	150
15–18	66	145	176	69	56	1,000	10	10	60	1.4	1.7	18	2.0	400	3.0	1,200	1,200	400	18	15	150
19–22	70	154	177	70	56	1,000	7.5	10	60	1.5	1.7	19	2.2	400	3.0	800	800	350	10	15	150
23–50	70	154	178	70	56	1,000	5	10	60	1.4	1.6	18	2.2	400	3.0	800	800	350	10	15	150
51+	70	154	178	70	56	1,000	5	10	60	1.2	1.4	16	2.2	400	3.0	800	800	350	10	15	150
Females																					
11–14	46	101	157	62	46	800	10	8	50	1.1	1.3	15	1.8	400	3.0	1,200	1,200	300	18	15	150
15–18	55	120	163	64	46	800	10	8	60	1.1	1.3	14	2.0	400	3.0	1,200	1,200	300	18	15	150
19–22	55	120	163	64	44	800	7.5	8	60	1.1	1.3	14	2.0	400	3.0	800	800	300	18	15	150
23–50	55	120	163	64	44	800	5	8	60	1.0	1.2	13	2.0	400	3.0	800	800	300	18	15	150
51+	55	120	163	64	44	800	5	8	60	1.0	1.2	13	2.0	400	3.0	800	800	300	10	15	150
Pregnant					+30	+200	+5	+2	+20	+0.4	+0.3	+2	+0.6	+400	+1.0	+400	+400	+150	†	+5	+25
Lactating					+20	+400	+5	+3	+40	+0.5	+0.5	+5	+0.5	+100	+1.0	+400	+400	+150	†	+10	+50

*The allowances are intended to provide for individual variations among most normal, healthy people in the United States under usual environmental stresses. They were designed for the maintenance of good nutrition. Diets should be based on a variety of common foods in order to provide other nutrients for which human requirements have been less well defined. See the text for a more detailed discussion of the RDA and of nutrients not tabulated.

The Committee on RDA has published a separate table showing energy allowances in ranges for each age-sex group and another table for vitamins and minerals not previously covered by the recommendations. These tables appear in Appendix O. The FDA has published a special table of selected RDA values for use on food labels: these, the U.S. RDA, appear on p. 441.

Reproduced from *Recommended Dietary Allowances*, 9th ed. (1980), with the permission of the National Academy of Sciences, Washington, D.C.

†Supplemental iron is recommended.

UNDERSTANDING NUTRITION

UNDERSTANDING NUTRITION

Eleanor Noss Whitney　　　　　　**Eva May Nunnelley Hamilton**

Second Edition

West Publishing Company
St. Paul　　New York　　Los Angeles　　San Francisco

Library of Congress Cataloging in Publication Data

Whitney, Eleanor Noss.
  Understanding nutrition.

  Bibliography: p.
  Includes index.
  1. Nutrition.   2. Metabolism.   I. Hamilton,
Eva May Nunnelley, joint author.   II. Title.
QP141.W46   1981   641.1   80−25784
  ISBN 0−8299−0419−0
1st Reprint—1981

Copy editing: Rebecca Smith
Design: Janet Bollow
Text illustration: Barbara Hack, Brenda Booth
Cartoons: Barbara Clark
Production coordination: Janet Bollow Associates
Composition: Innographics

PHOTO CREDITS

Cover: A microscopic photograph of pantothenic acid.
Tore Johnson/ANA/Woodfin Camp.

58 © Jane Schen/Icon; **130** UNICEF photo; **276** Spring-Daytona, Stock, Boston,
Inc.; **324** Jim Garretson; **388** Ron Alexander, Stock, Boston, Inc.; **394** Jim
Garretson; **420** Courtesy of Gjon Mili; **494** Anestis Diakopoulous, Stock, Boston,
Inc.; **526** Courtesy of Landrum B. Shettles; **534, 541** George Malave, Stock,
Boston, Inc.; **545** Elizabeth Crews/Icon; **576** Lorraine Rorke/Icon; **591** © Kent
Reno, Jeroboam; **606** Frank Siteman, Stock, Boston, Inc.

To the memory of Sam, who gave me the courage to begin to write about nutrition as I love to do, and to my children, Lynn, Russell, and Kara, whose love and understanding sustains me between times of inspiration.

ELLIE WHITNEY

To my late husband, Marshall, who throughout our marriage supported me in my academic ventures, and to our daughters, Gayle, Nancy, and Bonnie, who have sustained me with their joy in my varied activities.

MAY HAMILTON

Acknowledgments

Thank you to our colleagues at The Florida State University for their support; to Jean Burkhart Crozier and Sonthe Bokas for their conscientious help with library research; to Christian's Literature Service for the hours of midnight xeroxing; and to the magnificent staff at West.

Thank you, too, to our most cooperative and helpful reviewers: Sarah E. Burroughs, Wen Chiu, Dorothy Coltrin, Elizabeth A. Donald, Sondra L. King, Joseph Leichter, Dennis Savianno, Ralph G. Somes, Jr., Mary Taylor, Joan Howe Walsh, William Weir, Billie H. Wood, and especially to Stanley Winter whose painstaking critique of our teaching of chemistry has greatly enhanced the book's lucidity.

Finally, thank you to our students, whose probing questions keep making us dig deeper for understanding.

We also appreciate the good work of Gordon and Lorraine Bailey on the Student Study Guide and of Virginia Hillers and Joan Howe Walsh on the Instructor's Manual.

About the Authors

Eleanor Noss Whitney is an associate professor of nutrition at The Florida State University. She received her B.A. in Biology and English from Radcliffe College in 1960 and her Ph.D. in biology in 1970 from Washington University in St. Louis and is a member of the American Dietetic Association. She has done research in nutrition as it relates to growth and development, alcoholism, and cancer and has published articles in *Science, Journal of Nutrition, Genetics,* and other journals.

Eva May Nunnelley Hamilton is an adjunct faculty with The Florida State University. She received her B.S. in nutrition from the University of Kentucky in 1940 and her M.S. in nutrition from The Florida State University in 1975. She has been associated with science and nutrition education for over 35 years.

CONTENTS

APPENDIXES

PREFACE TO THE SECOND EDITION

We wrote *Understanding Nutrition* primarily for ourselves and our students. It was to be the textbook we needed, and nothing like it was available at the time. We had no idea when it went to press that so many other teachers and students of nutrition would find in it what they, too, were looking for. We are gratified by the multitude of enthusiastic responses we have received and are happy to know that our effort at communicating the excitement and importance of nutrition has been successful.

In this, the second edition, we have amplified the sections that we felt were thin in the first. The chapters on vitamins and minerals and nutrition throughout the life cycle have been greatly expanded and updated. A discussion of fiber in the diet has been added to Chapter 1; the lipoproteins and their significance are explained in Chapter 6. New Highlights have been added to help the reader understand the relation of fat to cancer and the role of nutrition in stress.

The U.S. Dietary Goals were published just after the first edition of *Understanding Nutrition* came out, and they have had a trememdous impact on the public. We have presented them and the subsequent USDA Guidelines at intervals throughout this edition.

To help readers apply the information in the chapters, we have supplied a series of Self-Study sections that, taken together, constitute a complete diet analysis and revision. We have also greatly expanded the appendixes so that they now include information on sugar, sodium, fiber, fast foods, the Four Food Group Plan, the Canadian Dietary Standard, and many other items. As in the first edition, the index is as complete as we can make it; if you find anything missing, let us know.

We have made many other changes as well. In fact this is a completely rewritten book and we have put as much effort into it as we did into the first edition. But our primary aim has not changed, and we hope that through this book you will find the study of nutrition as fresh, lively, and enjoyable as we do.

NOTE TO THE STUDENT

You may have some questions in mind as you approach the study of nutrition. In getting to know students over the years, we have some idea of what your concerns may be.

I Keep Hearing Exciting News about Nutrition. How Can I Tell What to Believe?   This is the commonest complaint we hear from students. Because of it, we have designed this book not to be just a book of facts but also a book of principles that you can use to assess the nutrition information you encounter elsewhere. Today's nutrition science stands firmly on the principles of chemistry and molecular biology. This book is based on those principles.

Even with the principles clearly in mind, however, it is sometimes hard to tell whether a statement made in the marketplace is a valid fact or a myth. Some major controversies currently raging in our field concern sugar, fiber, cholesterol, vitamin C and cancer, additives, and many other issues. It would not be fair to present these issues to you in textbook fashion as if they were settled, but it makes the study of our lively science needlessly dull to omit them. Our decision has been to reserve the **chapters** mostly for solid information, on which the experts in our field largely agree, and to present separate **Highlights** on the current issues, for more speculative material. The Highlights alternate with the chapters and are printed on colored pages to remind you that they convey more tentative information.

Even though we are scientists, in some cases we have no facts. Researchers in nutrition are earnestly endeavoring to learn more, but there are many areas where we are still in the dark. Students can be infuriated when a teacher seems to weasel: "I want the facts, and you are hedging. Give me the answer, straight and simple." It is frustrating to ask why and have a cautious scientist reply, "Well, we know this, and this, and . . ." but leave your question dangling. It is insulting to be told, "It's too complicated to understand," which sounds suspiciously like what mother used to say: "Wait until you are older, dear." But the truth of the matter is that there are a great many things we do not understand. One of the most exciting, as well as frustrating, experiences for students can be the dawning realization that they are approaching the outer bounds of human knowledge. The answers are simply not all in yet; no one knows what they all are; no one ever has. In nutrition, this is true in many areas. Nutrition is a growing, young science. Although its questions are immensely important and fascinating, that is all they are—questions. We have tried to be honest in this respect: to show you what we do know (with a high probability) and to admit what we don't.

In attempting to present a fair picture of current nutrition research in the Highlights, we have found ourselves at times confused, frustrated, angered, and amused. If you too respond this way in reading the maybes and probablys of today's nutrition issues, then be assured that you are close to the reality of our science. Any book that claims at this time to present absolute answers to all questions is actually only presenting one person's prejudices. The writer may be proved right in years to come, but some of the winners have not yet been declared. If you wish to be informed on the current issues, you will have to accept the ambiguities and contradictions in the evidence and the dis-agreements among the experts as an intrinsic part of scientific research in progress.

But Then How Can I Choose What to Believe?   In the absence of all the facts, we still have to live and make decisions. Should you eat polyunsaturated fats? Avoid tuna? Beef? Sugar? It would not be fair to answer simply "We don't know" to all these questions. Where the answers are uncertain today, we owe it to you to help in developing the skill to evaluate new information as it appears tomorrow. Our field is beset with claims and appeals, and all of us as consumers need to be equipped to deal with them.

There are some guidelines that would help you discriminate between reliable information and false advertising. It seems to us that a separate chapter devoted to this subject would not serve the purpose. You need continuous, repeated exposure to the kinds of claims made to consumers, and you need practice in assessing them. We offer frequent opportunities, by way of **Digressions** throughout the text, for you to examine such sources of nutrition information and to assess their reliability against the criteria of accurate scientific reporting.

In these digressions we have identified the most common charac-teristics of fraudulent advertising with **flag signs** that will help you to recognize spurious claims; the most common misunderstandings that arise from reading about nutrition research are identified with **caution signs**.

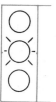

The Digressions are set off with color; if they prove too distracting you can skip them and possibly come back to them later. But they constitute a theme that runs throughout the book.

In some cases we have clear-cut evidence that a claim being made on the marketplace is fraudulent. We feel obligated to explain and elaborate these cases. It is not enough to tell you these are myths and provide nothing to replace them. But there is another problem: It seems to us that it is also not enough to say "That is a myth, and this is a fact." After all, aren't "they" saying their myth is a fact? Confronted with a choice between what "they" say and what "we" (in a nutrition text) say, you are in the bind of having to choose whom to believe, with nothing further to go on. We hope, by providing relevant information, to show you that what we say is more probably true than the myth you might otherwise believe. You will understand why the low-carbohydrate diet is ill advised when you know that carbohydrate is needed to metabolize fat in the body and how the body may be damaged when carbohydrate is not available. You will understand why taking large doses of vitamin C may be harmful when you know what can happen to people who indulge in that practice.

In using some of our space to deal with current issues, consumer questions, and health food myths, we have elected not to present an encyclopedic book of all the important knowledge that has been accumulated in our rapidly expanding field. Instead, we have stressed concepts, using selected facts to illustrate the principles on which they are based. Information in the chapters is, however, amplified by abundant additional information in the **appendixes**. We hope you will explore them and find them useful. We believe it is important to gain an acquaintance with the general principles of nutrition, as well as to develop the incentive and ability to identify reliable nutrition information on your own. Armed with this skill, you can continually gather and apply the information that is relevant to your own particular concerns.

I Have Heard Some Very Scary Rumors about Foods. Am I Right to Worry about What I May Be Doing to Myself with My Diet?   Under a wide range of conditions, the body cares beautifully for itself. To indicate this, we have emphasized physiology more heavily than most textbooks do. Only when people understand and appreciate natural health can they use their knowledge to enhance it. Still, there are circumstances in which physiology becomes abnormal and diseases arise. Cardiovascular disease, cancer, diabetes, and alcoholism are among the major diseases in the developed countries. Nutritional factors and carcinogens found in foods have an influence on the incidence and severity of all these diseases. The relationship between nutrition and disease does not traditionally fall within the province of a beginning textbook, but we feel that it is important to show how nutritional status and food choices may affect susceptibility to these diseases and so have devoted a few pages to each of them.

We also invite you to study your own diet and to compare its characteristics with the recommendations of nutrition authorities. The Self-Studies that appear at the end of most Highlights will help you evaluate your nutritional lifestyle.

I Hate Eating What's Good for Me. Are You Going to Tell Me I Shouldn't Have the Foods I Like?   Absolutely not. There is no one right way to eat and no food that must be included to make a diet healthful—not liver, not carrots, not even orange juice. Eating is primarily a pleasure for most people, and people choose foods mostly on the basis of their own personal taste preferences. But if you wish to make knowledgeable choices so that you can both enjoy and benefit from the foods you eat, this book will help you to do so.

But Your Science Scares Me. Do I Have to Learn Chemistry to Understand Nutrition? Yes. This is the hard part and the most rewarding. We make no apologies: This is a science book, a book that presents the realities as they are understood, as they really are. We are not privileged to change those realities for your convenience or our own. Our approach is biochemical. However, we believe that it is not necessary to have studied chemistry and biology extensively before embarking on the study of nutrition. We have assumed only a high school background in these sciences. The background chemistry is reviewed and explained in Appendix B to provide a refresher course. Further concepts that underlie nutrition are presented gradually in a logical sequence as they are needed; they are fully explained. Detailed diagrams of biochemical structures in Appendix C give you the option for further study of this aspect of nutrition.

In mastering the chemical concepts, you may find it helpful first to read each chapter for the general ideas involved and then to study the marginal **definitions**, which explain the chemistry in words. We have also employed verbal analogies wherever possible, comparing enzymes to machines, the process of digestion to a disassembly line, and nutrient molecules to Tinker Toys whose sticks are the electrons. These are not intended to insult you; if they seem too simple-minded for you (and they may be, especially if you have studied chemistry before), please be patient and allow us to indulge in what for us is the enjoyable and harmless practice of playing with words and ideas.

The rewards of understanding nutrition at the molecular level are as great as the effort needed to gain that understanding. When you have struggled with an unfamiliar system, picked it apart, looked at it from every angle, and finally put it back together again, you'll find that suddenly everything falls into place. The experience of grasping a whole new concept in chemistry is an "Aha!" experience that can generate tremendous excitement and pleasure. Once understood, these concepts will not slip away. When you learned to read (through effort), to play the piano (with practice), to ride a bicycle (with painful falls), these skills stayed with you. So will nutritional chemistry once you learn it. It too will stay with you, giving you a skill and a new dimension of understanding that can be used again and again to see deeper into things.

In our introduction we state that human beings are a collection of molecules that move. To say this is not to say that human beings are nothing more than molecules. Do not be affronted at what may seem to be a mechanistic view of humankind. We are sharing with you this way of seeing things, not because it is "the" reality but because it is a part of reality, a way of seeing that can deepen and enhance your understanding of yourself. We find the chief reward of our study of nutrition to be that it enhances our lives, our understanding, and our effectiveness as human beings.

UNDERSTANDING NUTRITION

PART ONE

THE ENERGY NUTRIENTS:
Carbohydrate, Fat, and Protein

INTRODUCTION

CONTENTS

MOLECULES: The Unseen Actors

All things are in process and nothing stays still.... You would not step twice into the same river.

HERACLITUS

You are a collection of molecules that move. All these moving parts are arranged into patterns of extraordinary complexity and order—cells, tissues, and organs. The arrangement is constant, but its parts are continuously being replaced. Your skin, which has reliably covered you from the time you were born, is not the same skin that covered you seven years ago; it is made entirely of new cells. The fat beneath your skin is not the same fat that was there a year ago. Your oldest red blood cell is only 120 days old, and the entire lining of your digestive tract is renewed every three days. To maintain your "self," you must continually replace the pieces you lose.

All of these pieces have come from your food: You are made entirely of what you have eaten. This is not meant to imply, of course, that if you ate spaghetti last night, you are made of spaghetti now! Some complex events take place between your eating of food and its becoming "you." A bowl of spaghetti or a piece of apple pie must be entirely taken apart and

food: nutritive material taken into the body to keep it alive and to enable it to grow (**nutritive:** containing nutrients).

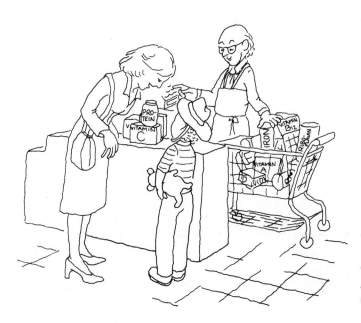

"Darling, would you go back to aisle 6 and get us another 40 milligrams of iron?"

nutrient: a substance obtained from food and used in the body to promote growth, maintenance, and/or repair.

adequate diet: a diet providing all the needed nutrients in the right total amounts. Such a diet is ideally also **balanced,** providing nutrients in the proportions that best meet the body's needs.

science of nutrition: the study of nutrients and of their digestion, absorption, transport, metabolism, interaction, storage, and excretion. A broader definition includes the study of the environment and of human behavior as it relates to nutrition.

Atoms, molecules, and compounds: Appendix B summarizes basic chemistry facts and provides definitions.

Organic: see the following pages.

Additives, including pesticides and possible carcinogens, are the subject of Highlight 13.

ash: minerals that remain after a food is completely burned (oxidized).

rearranged before its pieces can be used to make the structures of your eye, brain, or skin. You eat foods, but what you obtain from them is nutrients, and these undergo many transformations and rearrangements in your body. If the spaghetti and the apple pie, together with the other foods you choose to eat, do not contain the nutrients you need, you lose a little. For optimum nutrition you need an adequate diet.

The science of nutrition is the study of the nutrients in food and the body's handling of these nutrients.

The Nutrients

Almost any food you eat is composed of dozens or even hundreds of different kinds of materials, tinier by far than the smallest things that can be seen with the most powerful microscope; they are atoms and molecules. The complete chemical analysis of a food such as spinach shows that it is composed mostly of water (95 percent) and that most of the solid materials are organic compounds: carbohydrate, fat, and protein. If you could remove these materials, you would find a tiny residue of minerals, vitamins, and other organic materials. Water, carbohydrate, fat, protein, vitamins, and some of the minerals are nutrients. Some of the other organic materials and minerals are not.

The six classes of nutrients:

carbohydrate	vitamins
fat	minerals
protein	water

A complete chemical analysis of your body would show that it is made of very similar materials. If you weigh 150 pounds, your body contains about 90 pounds of water and (if 150 pounds is the proper weight for you) about 30 pounds of fat. The other 30 pounds are mostly protein, carbohydrate, and related organic compounds made from them, and the major minerals of your bones: calcium and phosphorus. Vitamins, other minerals, and incidental extras constitute a fraction of a pound. Thus you, like spinach, are composed largely of nutrients.

(This book is devoted mostly to the nutrients, but you should be aware that other constituents are found in foods and in your body—organic additives, both intentional and incidental, and trace minerals—of no recognized positive value to humans. Some may even be harmful. Later sections of the book focus on these and their significance.)

If you burn a food like spinach in air, it disappears. The water evaporates, and all of the organic compounds are oxidized to gas (carbon dioxide) and water vapor, leaving only a residue of ash. This leads us to a definition of the word *organic*.

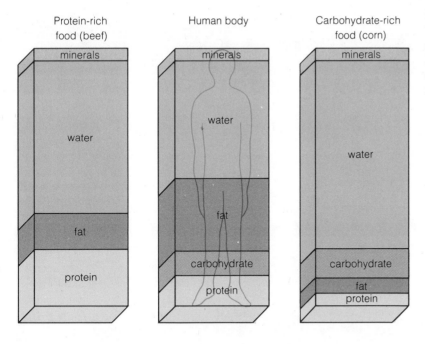

Protein-rich food (beef)

Human body

Carbohydrate-rich food (corn)

Figure 1 Food and the human body are made of the same classes of chemicals. (Vitamins are not shown because the amount is too small to be seen in a picture this size.)

The Meaning of Organic An organic compound is one that contains carbon atoms. The first organic compounds known were natural products synthesized by plants or animals; indeed, it used to be thought that only living things contributed organic compounds to our world. The term has since been expanded to include all carbon compounds, whatever their origin. Actually, in a sense, all organic compounds are produced by living things. Some of them, like petroleum (which comes from the remains of microorganisms, plants, and animals that grew in prehistoric times), began life millions of years ago. Others are produced by plants and animals alive today. Still others come from the laboratories where chemists (who are also "living things") produce them in the test tube.

organic: containing carbon or, more strictly, containing carbon and hydrogen or carbon-carbon bonds. This definition excludes coal (which has no defined bonds); a few carbon-containing compounds, such as carbon dioxide (which contains only a single carbon and no hydrogen); and salts such as calcium carbonate ($CaCO_3$), magnesium carbonate ($MgCO_3$), and sodium cyanide ($NaCN$).

Labels on food products sometimes make the claim that the product is "organic," implying that it is therefore somehow superior to a chemically fertilized food. By the definition given above, any carbon compound is organic, even a synthetic vitamin preparation from the laboratory of a pharmaceutical company. Is there any reason to believe that "organic" or "natural" foods or nutrient preparations sold in "health food" stores are superior to grocery store foods or synthetic vitamins? Let us take vitamin C as an example.

Vitamin C, or ascorbic acid, is an organic compound with a certain chemical structure (see Chapter 10). Regardless of its source, it always has the same structure. One carbon atom (or hydrogen atom or oxygen atom) is exactly like all the others. They have no individuality; all molecules with this structure are identical. When a molecule of vitamin C enters your bloodstream, your body cannot tell where it came from. Hence the vitamin C from a chemist's lab is no different from the vitamin C in an orange fresh from a Florida citrus grove. An important point made by the American Dietetic Association is that:

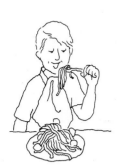

All foods are "organic," because they are all composed of organic compounds containing carbon.[1]

However, the orange may still be better for you, because the orange also contains carbohydrate, calcium, potassium, and other nutrients, as well as beneficial nonnutrient fiber. The pill contains only vitamin C—nothing more. In other words:

There is no advantage to eating an organic nutrient from one source as opposed to another, but there may be fringe benefits to eating that nutrient in a food as opposed to a purified nutrient preparation.

To interpret what you read on food labels you need two kinds of information. First, of course, you need to know the meanings of the terms that are used (an acquaintance with the definitions given throughout this book will help). Second—and this is especially important with "health food" products—you must be aware that a technical term may be misused by an industry to imply an inflated importance or value. The word *organic* is an example. As used on health food labels it is intended to imply superiority to ordinary foods. The product labeled organic has merely been organically grown; that is, in soil to which no "chemical fertilizer" has been added (only "natural fertilizer," such as manure and compost) and without the use of any insecticide sprays, such as DDT. The term *health food* is another example, implying that the food has extraordinary power to promote health. Actually, a food promotes health depending solely on the amounts and balance of nutrients it contains and on the response to it of the person who eats it.

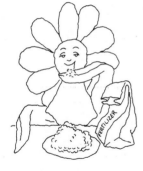

Your choice of what foods to buy is a personal choice. Insofar as it is based on your knowledge of the nutritional value of the foods, the information in this book may help you to choose wisely. The subject is a big one, and different aspects of it will be taken up in the series of

[1]Position paper on food and nutrition misinformation on selected topics, *Journal of the American Dietetic Association* 66 (1975):277-280.

digressions that follow. For the present, let us content ourselves with one additional important point—about fertilizers.

Plants take up minerals from the soil (including those from fertilizers) depending not on what is present in the soil but on what the plant needs. A tomato grown on synthetic fertilizer achieves the same chemical composition as one grown on decomposed organic material, such as compost. To put it most simply, the composition of a plant depends more on the plant than on the soil. Nutritionally, therefore, an "organically grown" plant is not superior to a "chemically fertilized" one, and a label that implies otherwise is misleading. All fertilizers are composed of chemicals.

A FLAG SIGN OF A SPURIOUS CLAIM IS THE USE
OF THESE WORDS:

organic
health food

spurious: false, fraudulent.

Pending legislation proposes forbidding the use of these words on labels.

Of course, if a needed element is absolutely lacking in the soil, the plant cannot select it. Plants grown on soil that lacks iodine, for example, will be iodine-poor. *Any* poorly (inadequately) fertilized soil is inferior to adequately fertilized soil. There are good and poor "organic" fertilizers, as well as good and poor "chemical" fertilizers. By the same token, there may be fringe benefits from the use of natural fertilizers like compost. For example, such a fertilizer has a beneficial effect on the structure (tilth) of the soil, which most chemical fertilizers do not have. This is not a nutritional but a mechanical advantage to the plant.

An "adequate diet" for a plant might be defined as any plant food (fertilizer) that supplies all the needed nutrients for the plant.

The only unequivocal statement about the nutritive quality of a fertilizer is a statement of the specific chemicals it contains and the amount of each; their source is irrelevant. The only unequivocal statement about the nutritive quality of a food is a statement of the specific nutrients it contains and the amount of each; their source is also irrelevant.

unequivocal: clear, unambiguous, leaving no doubt.

The Principal Actors: The Energy Nutrients

The organic nutrients:

carbohydrate   protein
fat   vitamins

The distinction between organic and inorganic nutrients is important for several reasons. For one thing, in cooking foods you need to be aware that some organic nutrients are sensitive to and can be altered or destroyed by chemical and physical agents such as acids, air, heat, and light. This is especially important with respect to the vitamins. The minerals, however, are simple elements that cannot be destroyed.

Moreover, when organic nutrients are metabolized, waste materials (such as carbon dioxide) are produced. Everything has to go somewhere, and the metabolism of certain organic nutrients obligates the body to excrete these wastes.

Furthermore, organic nutrients can release heat or other kinds of energy. When oxidized, they break down; that is, their carbon atoms and others come apart and are combined with oxygen. If you burn a potful of food on the range, the same thing happens. Heat is released together with carbon dioxide and water vapor, and you are left with a ruined pot, blackened with the carbon and mineral residue from the food. But when you oxidize food in your body, the energy is not all released as heat. Some is transferred into other compounds (including fat) that compose the structures of your body cells, and some of the energy that holds the atoms of the energy nutrients together is used to power your activities, enabling you to move.

At the outset we stated that you are a collection of molecules that move. Now you can see a little more clearly what this means. Human beings are made of atoms taken from some of the molecules of food and rearranged into the molecules of their bodies. You move thanks to the energy released when other food molecules are taken apart.

You can metabolize all four classes of organic nutrients, but only three yield energy for the body's use. These three are the energy nutrients.

> The energy nutrients:
> carbohydrate
> fat
> protein

The amount of energy they release can be measured in "calories" (or more properly, kilocalories), which no doubt are familiar to you as those things that make foods "fattening." The calorie content of a food thus depends on how much carbohydrate, fat, and protein it contains. If not used immediately, these nutrients and the energy contained in them are rearranged, mostly into body fat, and then stored. Thus an excess intake of any of the three energy nutrients can lead to overweight. Too much

Metabolism, the set of processes by which nutrients are rearranged into body structures or broken down to yield energy, is defined on page 221.

oxidation: a reaction in which atoms from a molecule are combined with oxygen, usually with the release of energy. Chemical oxidation of nutrients differs from oxidative combustion (burning) in that the energy released is largely chemical and mechanical, rather than heat and light energy. A further explanation is given in Appendix B.

calorie: a unit in which energy is measured. Technically, a calorie is the amount of heat necessary to raise the temperature of a gram of water one degree Centigrade. Food energy is measured in **kilocalories** (thousands of calories), abbreviated **kcalories** or **kcal,** or capitalized: **Calories.** Most people, even nutritionists, speak of these units simply as calories, but on paper they should be prefaced by a k. (The pronunciation of "kcalories" ignores the k.) We will use this convention throughout this book.[2]

[2] Food energy can also be measured in kilojoules (kJ): A kilojoule is the amount of energy expended when a kilogram is moved one meter by a force of one newton. One kcalorie equals 4.2 kJ. The kilojoule is now the international unit of energy, and the United States and Canada will slowly be switching to it over the next decades, but it is not in popular use as yet. This book does not use the kilojoule.

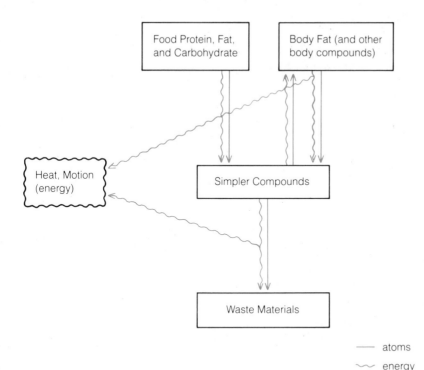

Food Protein, Fat, and Carbohydrate

Body Fat (and other body compounds)

Heat, Motion (energy)

Simpler Compounds

Waste Materials

—— atoms

~~ energy

Figure 2 Metabolism of the energy nutrients. The atoms in a molecule are held together by energy in the form of chemical bonds. When a large molecule, such as a carbohydrate molecule, is broken apart, some of the chemical bonds are broken and energy is released. The atoms themselves are never broken apart in chemical reactions, only regrouped.

(We will use the convention throughout this book that arrows pointing downwards represent reactions in which molecules [groups of atoms] are being broken into smaller molecules and energy is being released. Arrows pointing upwards represent reactions in which larger molecules are being built with energy used for the bonding.)

meat (a protein-rich food) is just as fattening as too many potatoes (a carbohydrate-rich food).

It is important not to forget the organic compound found in alcoholic beverages: alcohol. This compound is not properly called a nutrient by the definition given on page 4, but it shares several characteristics with the energy nutrients. Like them, it is metabolized in the body to yield energy. When taken in excess of energy need, it, too, is converted to body fat and stored. But when alcohol contributes a substantial portion of the energy in a person's diet, its effects are damaging. (Highlight 9 is devoted to this compound.)

Practically all foods contain mixtures of all three energy nutrients, although they are sometimes classified by the predominant nutrient. Thus it is not correct to speak of meat as a protein or of bread as a carbohydrate; they are foods rich in these nutrients. A protein-rich food like beef actually contains a lot of fat as well as protein; a carbohydrate-rich food like corn also contains fat and protein, as shown in Figure 1. Only a few foods are exceptions to this rule, the common ones being sugar (which is pure carbohydrate) and oil (which is almost pure fat).

The energy nutrients are the principal actors in the drama of nutrition and are the subject of Part One of this book. Figure 2 outlines very simply the flow of the energy nutrients into and through the body. The vitamins and the inorganic nutrients—minerals and water—serve functions other than providing energy and the direct building of body compounds; they are the subject of Part Two.

Summing Up

The six classes of nutrients found in foods are carbohydrate, fat, protein, vitamins, minerals, and water. The first four are organic compounds, the last two inorganic. The first three of these, the energy nutrients, are the subject of Part One.

After entering the body, the energy nutrients are metabolized to simpler compounds that may be reassembled into body compounds or may be oxidized, releasing energy. The energy they release may be used to help construct other body compounds, to move body parts, or to generate heat. The final products, after complete oxidation, are excreted from the body.

To Explore Further

People interested in nutrition often want to know where, in their own town or county, they can find reliable nutrition information. One place you are not likely to find it is the local library, where fad diet books sit side by side on the shelf with books of facts. However, wherever you live, there are several sources you can turn to:

● The Department of Health may have a nutrition expert.

● The local extension agent is often an expert.

● The food editor of your local paper may be well informed.

● The dietitian at the local hospital had to fulfill a set of qualifications before he or she became an R.D. (Registered Dietitian).

● There may be knowledgeable professors of nutrition or biochemistry at a nearby college or university.

In addition, you might want to begin to accumulate a small library of your own. The references suggested below are of a general nature, related to many topics covered in this book.

Nutrition Reviews' Present Knowledge in Nutrition, 4th ed. (Washington, D.C.: Nutrition Foundation, 1976), 605 pages (paperback) will bring you up to date on 53 topics, including energy, obesity, 29 nutrients, diabetes, coronary heart disease, fiber, renal disease, parenteral nutrition, malnutrition, growth and its assessment, brain development, immunity, alcohol, fiber, milk intolerances, dental health, drugs, and toxins. The only major omissions seem to be nutrition and food intake and nutrition status in the United States and Canada.

Goodhart, R. S., and Shils, M. E., eds., *Modern Nutrition in Health and Disease*, 6th ed. (Philadelphia: Lea and Febiger, 1979), 1370 pages, is a major technical reference book on nutrition topics, containing 40 encyclopedic articles on the nutrients, foods, the diet, metabolism, malnutrition, age-related needs, and nutrition in disease, with 36 appendixes.

Lagua, R. T., V. S. Claudio and V. F. Thiele's *Reference Dictionary*, 2nd ed. (St. Louis: Mosby, 1974), 330 pages, is a dictionary of nutrition terminology with 38 appendixes, including dietary standards of other countries, food grouping systems, biochemical pathways, agencies, research methods, weights and measures, and others.

Many students also like to have a separate copy of the Table of Food Composition (Appendix H in this book), which is available in softcover from the U.S. Government Printing Office (address in Appendix J).

Another more comprehensive book of food composition, which also gives foods in household measures, is:

Church, C. F., and Church, H. N., *Bowes and Church's Food Values of Portions Commonly Used*, 12th ed. (Philadelphia: Lippincott, 1975).

There are also many excellent publications on the important subject of food faddism and misinformation. A whole issue of *Nutrition Reviews* was devoted to this topic, and it includes a list of suggested readings to help the reader identify faddists, quacks, and promoters:

Nutrition Reviews/Supplement: Nutrition Misinformation and Food Faddism, July 1974.

R. Deutsch has recently revised his entertaining and revealing book on food faddism:

Deutsch, R. *The New Nuts among the Berries: How Nutrition Nonsense Captured America* (Palo Alto, Calif.: Bull Publishing, 1977).

A helpful pamphlet by S. Margolius, *Health Foods: Facts and Fakes*, PAP no. 498, is available from Public Affairs Pamphlets, 381 Park Avenue South, New York, NY 10016.

The FDA, through the *FDA Consumer*, published *Nutrition Sense and Nonsense* in 1972, DHEW publication no. (FDA) 73-2009, available from the U.S. Government Printing Office (address in Appendix J).

The syndicated column on nutrition by J. Mayer and J. Dwyer, which appears in many newspapers, presents well-researched, reliable answers to current questions, as does the column by R. Alfin-Slater and E. F. P. Jelliffe. Mayer's book is also a useful reference:

Mayer, J. *A Diet for Living* (New York: Pocket Books, 1977).

For the athlete we recommend:

Smith, N. J. *Food For Sport* (Palo Alto, Calif.: Bull Publishing, 1977).

And for the vegetarian:

Lappé, F. M. *Diet for a Small Planet*, rev. ed. (New York: Ballantine Books, 1975).

One of the most readable, entertaining, and relevant books of readings on nutrition to come out in recent years:

Hofmann, L., ed., *The Great American Nutrition Hassle* (Palo Alto, Calif.: Mayfield, 1978) would make good supplementary reading for a nutrition course in which *Understanding Nutrition* is assigned. *Hassle* includes articles by recognized authorities on the RDAs, fast foods, additives, infant nutrition, fad diets, sugar, alcohol, and most of the other topics treated in this book's Highlights.

Another book that you may wish to add to your library is the latest edition of *Recommended Dietary Allowances*, available from the National Academy of Sciences (address in Appendix J).

We also recommend our own book, E. M. N. Hamilton and E. N. Whitney, *Nutrition: Concepts and Controversies* (St. Paul: West, 1979), which offers an approach to nutrition for the nonmajor who has never studied chemistry and presents 20 nutrition controversies, not all of which are treated in this book.

Some readers like to subscribe to journals and to receive nutrition information from organizations such as the American Dietetic Association. A listing of journals and addresses for further information is given in Appendix J.

This is the first of a series of exercises you will find at the ends of the chapters throughout this book. Our purpose in including them is to encourage you to study your own diet. Doing these exercises as you read presents advantages and disadvantages. The bad news about them is that they will slow you down, and filling out all the forms is tedious. Like income tax returns, they have to be done carefully, with frequent checking of arithmetic and tidy handwriting, so that they will be accurate and meaningful.

The advantages, however, may well outweigh these drawbacks. Most students who do them with thoughtful attention report that they are intriguing, informative, and often reassuring. In further contrast to income tax returns, these exercises will reward you in direct proportion to your honesty.

In this exercise you are to make a record of your typical food intake and analyze it for the nutrients it contains. It may seem premature to undertake this analysis before you have learned very much about the nutrients, but having this Self-Study in front of you as you read will make the information more meaningful to you. As you read about each nutrient, you will want to ask yourself, "How much of this nutrient do I consume?" The answer will already be in front of

you if you follow the procedure suggested here.

The first step is to use Form 1 to record all the foods you eat for a three-day period. If, like most people, you eat differently on weekdays and weekends, then you should probably record for two weekdays and one weekend day to get a true average (or record your food intake for a week). As you record each food, make careful note of the measure. Estimate the amounts of each food to the nearest ounce, quarter-cup, tablespoon, or other common measure. In guessing at the sizes of meat portions, it helps to know that a piece of meat the size of the palm of your hand weighs about 3 or 4 oz. If you are unable to estimate serving sizes in cups, tablespoons, or teaspoons, try measuring out half-cup-, tablespoon-, and teaspoon-size servings onto a plate or into a bowl to see how they look. It also helps to know that a slice of cheese (like the sliced "American" cheese) or a 1 1/2-inch cube of cheese weighs about 1 oz.

You may have to break down mixed dishes to their ingredients. However, many

mixed dishes, including soups, are listed in Appendix H, in the miscellaneous section at the end; the nutrient contents of some "fast foods" appear in Appendix N. Other mixtures are simple to analyze. A ham and cheese sandwich, for example, can be listed as two slices of bread, 1 tbsp mayonnaise, 2 oz ham, 1 oz cheese, and so on. If you can't discover all the ingredients, estimate the amounts of only the major ones, like the beef, tomatoes, and potatoes in a beef-vegetable soup.

You will of course make errors in estimating amounts, but errors are expected and tolerated. You can expect your calculations to be off by as much as 20 percent, or even more. Still, you will have a rough approximation that will enable you to compare your nutrient intakes with the recommended ones.

The next step is to calculate for each day your total intakes of kcalories, protein, fat, fatty acids (saturated, oleic, and linoleic), carbohydrate, calcium, iron, vitamin A, thiamin, riboflavin, niacin, and vitamin C. If the foods you have eaten are not included in Appendixes H and N, read the label on the package or use your ingenuity to guess their composition, using the most similar food you can find as a guide. (For example, if you ate halibut, which is not listed, you would not be far

Form 1. Nutrient Intakes (use one form for each day)

Food	Approximate measure or weight	Energy* (kcal)	Protein‡ (g)	Fat‡ (g)	Fatty acids†(g) Saturated (total)	Fatty acids†(g) Oleic	Fatty acids†(g) Linoleic	Carbo-hydrate† (g)	Cal-cium* (mg)	Iron‡ (mg)	Vitamin A* (IU)	Thia-min‡ (mg)	Ribo-flavin‡ (mg)	Niacin‡ (mg)	Vitamin C† (mg)
Total															

*Compute these values to the nearest whole number.
†Compute these values to one decimal place.
‡Compute these values to two decimal places.

wrong in using the values for haddock or perch. If you ate garbanzo beans, you might substitute the values for navy beans.)

Be careful in recording the nutrient amounts in odd-size portions. For example, if you used 1/4 c milk, then you will have to record a fourth of the amount of every nutrient listed for 1 c milk. And note the units the nutrients are measured in:

● *Energy* is measured in kcalories as explained on page 8.

● *Protein, fat, fatty acids, and carbohydrate* are measured in grams (g). A gram is the weight of a cubic centimeter (cc) or milliliter (ml) of water under defined conditions of temperature and pressure. For example, 1 tsp salt weighs about 5 g.

● *Calcium, iron, thiamin, niacin, riboflavin, and vitamin C* are measured in milligrams (mg). A milligram is 1/1,000 of a gram (0.001 g).

A microgram (mcg or μg) is a thousandth of a milligram or a millionth of a gram (0.001 mg or 0.000001 g).

● *Vitamin A* is measured in international units (IU). An international unit is an arbitrary unit that investigators used for the fat-soluble vitamins before they had been chemically purified and measured. Vitamin A values can also be expressed in RE (retinol equivalents); 1 RE equals 5 IU. (For further details, see Chapter 11.)

Now total the amount of each nutrient you've consumed for each day, and transfer your totals to Form 2. Form 2 provides a convenient means of deriving and keeping on record an average intake for each nutrient.

As a final step, enter your average intakes on Form 3 for future reference. For comparison, enter the intakes recommended for a person of your age and sex, using either the Recommended Dietary Allowances (the U.S. rec-

ommendations shown on the inside front cover) or the Canadian Dietary Standard (in Appendix O), whichever you prefer. Note that no recommendations are made for intakes of fat or carbohydrate. Guidelines for these nutrients—and for others, like cholesterol and fiber—will be presented and discussed in the chapters to come. Succeeding Self-Studies will guide you in focusing on each of the nutrients provided by your diet.

Suspend judgment about the adequacy of your diet for the moment. You have much to learn about your individuality, about the nutrients, and about the recommendations before you can reach any reasonable conclusions. Exercises to help you, using the information you have collected here, are presented at the ends of Chapters 1 to 3 and 7 to 13.

Form 2. Average Daily Energy and Nutrient Intakes

Day	Energy (kcal)	Protein (g)	Fat (g)	Fatty acids (g)			Carbo-hydrate (g)	Cal-cium (mg)	Iron (mg)	Vitamin A (IU)	Thia-min (mg)	Ribo-flavin (mg)	Niacin (mg)	Vitamin C (mg)
				Saturated (total)	Oleic	Linoleic								
1														
2														
3														
Total														
Average daily intake (divide 3-day total by 3)														

Form 3.   Comparison with a Standard Intake

Day	Energy (kcal)	Protein (g)	Fat (g)	Fatty acids (g) Saturated (total)	Oleic	Linoleic	Carbo-hydrate (g)	Cal-cium (mg)	Iron (mg)	Vitamin A (IU)	Thia-min (mg)	Ribo-flavin (mg)	Niacin (mg)	Vitamin C (mg)
Average daily intake (from Form 2)														
*Standard**														
Intake as percentage of standard†														

*Taken from RDA tables (inside front cover) or Canadian Dietary Standard (Appendix O).

†For example, if your intake of protein was 50 g and the standard for a person your age and sex was 46 g, then you consumed $(50 \div 46) \times 100$, or 109 percent of the standard.

CHAPTER 1

CONTENTS

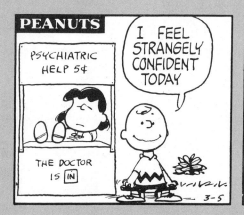
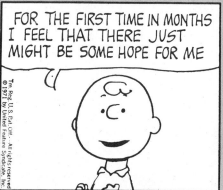
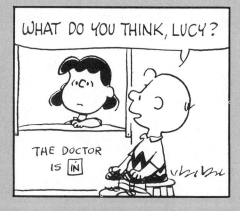
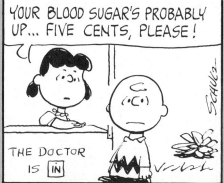

THE CARBOHYDRATES: Sugar, Starch, and Fiber

The Universe is not only queerer than we imagine—it is queerer than we can imagine.

J.B.S. HALDANE

Most of us would like to feel good all the time. The enjoyment available in a day, no matter what the day may bring, can be tremendous if your body and mind are tuned for it. The feeling of well-being that comes from being full of energy, alert, clear-thinking, and confident is so rewarding that if you know how to produce it, you will probably make the effort required.

It would be an exaggeration to say that good eating habits alone produce this feeling of well-being. If you try to think of what makes you feel good, you can come up with several answers. Being in love, for example, is certainly one. Facing and solving a personal problem is another. Being well rested helps too; when you wake up after a good night's sleep, you may feel bright-eyed and bushy-tailed, ready to take on the world, without having eaten a thing for 12 hours or more. Exercise helps too; the feeling of being physically tired after climbing a mountain or running a mile is a "good tired." Being clean is still another; a cold shower after heavy work or exercise can be bracing and exhilarating. Sparkling weather, clean air, beautiful scenery, pleasant company—all these play a part.

Even among the best of these pleasures, however, some limits are set by your nutritional state. You can feel really good only when your blood sugar (glucose) level is right. If that condition isn't met, neither the most beautiful mountaintop nor the most stimulating companion can compensate.

The health and functioning of every cell in your body depend on blood sugar to a greater or lesser extent. Ordinarily the cells of your brain and nervous system depend *solely* on this sugar for their energy. The brain cells are continually active, even while you're asleep, so they are continually drawing on the supply of sugar in the fluid surrounding them. They oxidize it for the energy they need to perform their functions. To maintain the supply, a continuous flow of blood moves past these cells, replenishing the sugar as the cells use it up.

Because your brain and other nerves ordinarily cannot make use of any other energy source, they are especially vulnerable to a temporary deficit in the blood sugar supply. This is why sugar is sometimes known

Glucose, a simple sugar, is often called blood sugar, because it is the principal carbohydrate found in mammalian blood (see also p. 28).

For the exception to this rule—ketosis—see p. 234.

Oxidation: see p. 8.

19

as brain food. When your brain is deprived of energy, your mental processes are affected. You may be unable to think clearly. Your brain controls your muscles, so you may feel weak and shaky. You are likely to miscalculate—perhaps by making an error in balancing your checkbook or by tripping while walking downstairs. Your mind resides in your brain, and so your attitude toward life, the world, and other people may also be distorted. You may become anxious, easily upset, depressed, or irritable. Your head may ache; you may feel dizzy or even nauseated. These are the signs of hypoglycemia, or too little glucose in the blood.

The body has an amazing ability to adapt to changing conditions by altering its own chemistry to maintain an internal balance. For example, when you get too hot, your blood circulation is routed closer to the skin surface so that the blood can be cooled; you perspire, and the evaporation of the secreted moisture cools you still further. When you are too cold, your circulation is rerouted inward so that heat will not be lost by exposure of the blood to the outside air. In the same way, when your blood sugar concentration rises too high or falls too low, your body makes internal adjustments to bring it back to normal. Still, human folly can defeat the body's best efforts to keep in balance. An awareness and understanding of how blood sugar is regulated can enable you to cooperate with your body in the best interest of both of you. The following paragraphs show how the body maintains its blood glucose level and what can be done to help.

The Constancy of the Blood Glucose Level

When you wake up in the morning, your blood probably contains between 80 and 120 milligrams (mg) of glucose in each 100 milliliters (ml) of blood (about half a cup). This range, which is known as the fasting blood glucose concentration, is normal and is accompanied by a feeling of alertness and wellbeing (provided that nothing else is wrong, of course—that you don't have the flu, for example). If you don't eat, the blood glucose level gradually falls as your cells draw on the supply. At 70 mg/100 ml, the low end of the normal range, a feeling of hunger is often experienced. The normal response to this sensation is to eat. If the meal includes some carbohydrate, your blood sugar level soon rises again.

If your meal has been unusually high in carbohydrate, and especially if it has consisted mostly of simple carbohydrate (ordinary, granulated sugar or syrup), your blood sugar concentration may threaten to rise too high. This too is an undesirable condition, known as hyperglycemia. A simple way for the body to contend with this imbalance would be to excrete the excess sugar in the urine. But the body is conservative; it stores the excess against a possible future need. The first organ to respond is the pancreas, which detects the excess and puts out a message about it; then liver, muscle, and fat cells receive the message, remove the sugar from the blood, and store it.

hypoglycemia (HIGH-po-gligh-SEEM-ee-uh): an abnormally low blood glucose concentration. Hypoglycemia is a symptom of a number of disease conditions.

hypo = too little
glyce = glucose
emia = in the blood

normoglycemia (NOR-mo-gligh-SEEM-ee-uh): a normal blood glucose concentration—80 to 120 mg/100 ml.

normo = normal

Milligrams and milliliters are metric measures of weight and volume. For definitions of these terms, see Appendix D.

hyperglycemia (HIGH-per-gligh-SEEM-ee-uh): an abnormally high blood glucose concentration.

hyper = too much

Chapter 5 describes some of the functions of the pancreas and liver. Their anatomical relationship to the digestive system is shown in Figure 1 in that chapter.

Special cells of the pancreas are sensitive to the blood glucose concentration. When it rises, they respond by secreting more of the hormone insulin into the blood. As the circulating insulin bathes the liver cells, they take up sugar from the blood, just as all cells in the body do. Within the liver cells, the small glucose units are assembled into long chains of glycogen and stored. Muscle and fat cells also participate in bringing blood glucose down to normal. In muscle, as in the liver, the glucose is stored as glycogen. In fat cells the glucose is used to make fat.

After you have eaten, then, your blood glucose level has returned to normal, and any excess glucose has been put in storage. During the hours that follow, before you eat again, the stored glycogen (but not the fat) can replenish the glucose supply as the brain and other body cells use it to meet their energy needs. Only glycogen from the liver, not from muscle, can return glucose units to the blood.

These special cells are the **beta cells** (BAY-tuh): one of the four types of cells in the pancreas. The beta cells secrete insulin in response to increased blood glucose concentration.

Hormone: see p. 165.

insulin (IN-suh-lin): a hormone secreted by the pancreas in response to increased blood glucose concentration.

glycogen (GLIGH-co-gen): a storage form of glucose in liver and muscle (see also p. 38).

glyco = glucose
gen = gives rise to

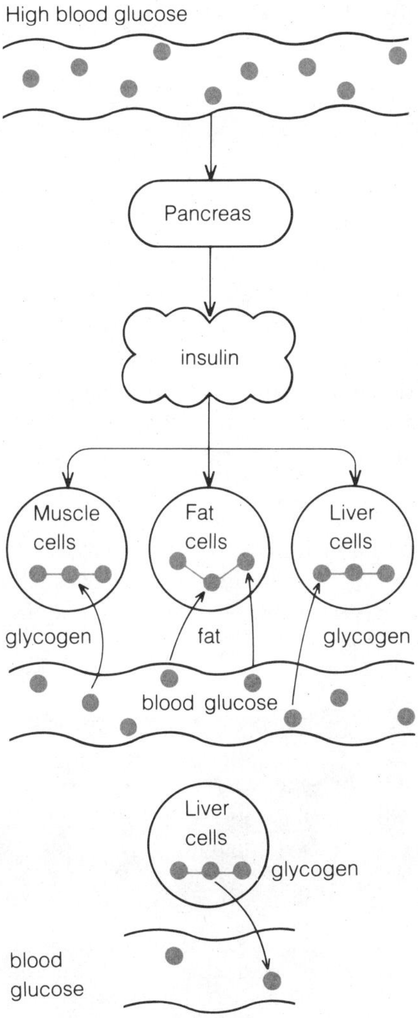

High blood glucose

1. High blood glucose stimulates pancreas to release insulin.

Pancreas

insulin

Muscle cells   Fat cells   Liver cells

glycogen   fat   glycogen

blood glucose

2. Insulin stimulates the uptake of glucose into cells and its storage as liver and muscle glycogen and as fat.

Liver cells

glycogen

3. Later, low blood glucose is raised by reconverting liver glycogen to glucose and releasing it into the blood. (Other hormones are involved but not shown.)

blood glucose

epinephrine (epp-ih-NEF-rin): a hormone secreted by the adrenal glands in response to stress. Epinephrine used to be called **adrenaline** (uh-DREN-uh-lin).

adrenal glands: two small glands located on top of the kidneys.

ad = on
renal = kidney

One of the hormones that can call glucose out of the liver cells is the famous "fight-or-flight" hormone, epinephrine. Epinephrine is produced quickly when you are under stress, insuring that all your body cells have energy fuel in emergencies. At ordinary times other hormones guarantee that liver glycogen returns glucose to the blood whenever it is needed for maintenance.

Muscle glycogen, too, can be dismantled to glucose, but this glucose is used primarily within the muscle cells themselves, where it serves as an important fuel for muscle action. Long-distance runners know that adequate stores of muscle glycogen can make a crucial difference in their endurance toward the end of a race. Before an event, the athlete is well advised to eat a meal high in carbohydrate (see "Nutrition for Athletes," Chapter 16). If there is an extraordinary need for blood glucose and the liver supply has run low, muscle glycogen can break down to an intermediate product, lactate, which can enter the blood. The liver can pick it up, convert it to glucose, and release it once again. Thus muscle glycogen can contribute indirectly to the blood glucose supply if necessary.

The maintenance of a normal blood glucose level thus depends on two types of safeguards. When the level gets too low, it can be replenished quickly either from liver glycogen stores or from a food source of glucose. When the level gets too high, insulin is secreted to siphon the excess into storage. (There is more to this story; insulin performs other roles too. This description is intended only to give you a sense of how the body maintains balance.)

If your blood glucose level reaches 70 mg/100 ml and you don't eat, the level may fall further still as the glycogen reserves are used up. Then you feel the undesirable symptoms associated with hypoglycemia. In addition to those already mentioned (weakness, mental confusion, dizziness), you may experience a craving for sweets. Some people succumb to this craving and eat a quick-energy food, such as a coke or a candy bar—and this is maladaptive behavior. The blood glucose level shoots up rapidly in response to pure simple carbohydrate of this type, and an insulin overreaction may occur. Then blood glucose rebounds to a too-low level, and hypoglycemia once again sets in. This alternation between extremes upsets the system, destroying the normal state of well-being.

maladaptive behavior: behavior intended to help an organism meet its needs that is not actually in its best interest.

reactive hypoglycemia: a temporary hypoglycemia that may be experienced by any normal person in response to an overload of sugar. Also called functional or **postprandial** hypoglycemia.

post = after
prandial = a meal

The hypoglycemia described here is the symptom of a temporary imbalance and is known as reactive hypoglycemia. It may be experienced briefly by any normal person. It has been reported, for example, in one out of every five women under the age of 45.[1]

[1]Y. Jung, R. C. Khurana, D. G. Corredor, A. Hastillo, R. F. Lain, D. Patrick, P. Turkeltaub, and T. S. Danowski, Reactive hypoglycemia in women: Results of a health survey, *Diabetes* 20 (June 1971): 428-434.

Spontaneous hypoglycemia, on the other hand, is an extremely rare disease condition in which the pancreas chronically oversecretes insulin, so that the person's blood glucose is constantly too low. Such a person must eat high-protein foods frequently and must exclude simple carbohydrates altogether. Among the quarter-million or so patients seen annually at the Mayo Clinic, fewer than a hundred have true, spontaneous hypoglycemia.[2]

The symptoms of anxiety, dizziness, weakness, and the rest can be caused by a number of conditions other than hypoglycemia, such as oxygen deprivation to the brain. In fact, eating concentrated sweets sometimes attracts large volumes of fluid from the bloodstream into the digestive tract, thus lowering the blood volume and causing reduced blood flow to the brain. The same symptoms may also be caused psychologically, by an anxiety state. Even such a serious condition as multiple sclerosis can be mistaken for hypoglycemia by the unwary diagnostician. Thus we laypersons, who are not trained in the diagnosis of conditions that present similar symptoms, are extremely unwise if we try to diagnose ourselves.

spontaneous hypoglycemia: a rare chronic hypoglycemia seen in people with abnormal carbohydrate metabolism; requires diagnosis, medical treatment, and a special diet.

CAUTION:

A little knowledge is a dangerous thing.
Don't self-diagnose.

For maximum well-being, you need to eat in such a way as to avoid either extreme. This primarily means doing two things. First, when you are hungry you should eat, without waiting until you are famished. For most people, hunger is a reliable indicator of the appropriate time to eat (although in some—notably the intractably obese and diabetics—hunger is not necessarily a sign of physiological need for food). Second, when you do eat, you should eat a balanced meal, including some protein and fat as well as complex carbohydrate. The fat slows down the digestion and absorption of carbohydrate, so that it trickles gradually into the blood rather than flooding the system all at once. The protein elicits the secretion of a hormone antagonistic to insulin that damps its effect. The protein also provides a more slowly digested, alternative source of blood glucose for use in case the glycogen reserves are exhausted.

Hunger and appetite: see p. 283.

The hormone antagonistic to insulin is **glucagon** (GLOO-kuh-gon), produced by the alpha cells of the pancreas.

For a discussion of how fat slows down digestion and the absorption of carbohydrate, see Chapter 5. Chapter 6 tells how protein yields glucose.

[2] F. J. Service, Hypoglycemia, *Contemporary Nutrition* 2 (July 1977).

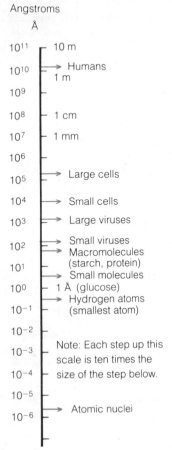

Angstroms

Å

Relative sizes of atoms, cells, and organisms.

Compound and chemical formula: for basic chemistry, see Appendix B.

The Chemist's View of Sugars

Those who work with atoms and molecules—chemists, physicists, and other scientists—are people whose curiosity has impelled them to ask questions about everything. The answers they seek are explanations of substances in terms of the next smaller units of which they are made. These scientists also explain you in this way; that is, you are a bundle of a great many atoms (perhaps 3,000,000,000,000,000,000,000,000,000,000, give or take 1,000,000,000,000,000,000,000,000,000), held together and moved about by virtue of their associated energy.

If your mind boggles at such a thought, don't be dismayed. It staggers anyone's imagination to contemplate the ultimate realities of our universe. If you willingly go along with the chemists, all the way down to the atoms of which the carbohydrates are made, you may feel a little bit out of your depth, but you stand to gain much insight. An understanding of how energy is contained in glucose molecules and of how it is released when these molecules are metabolized in the body will help you achieve some desirable ends—to acquire the energy you need from your food at a minimum dollar cost, for example, or to balance your food energy sources for maximum health and efficiency without weight gain.

To promote an understanding of the carbohydrates, the remainder of this section is devoted to a discussion of the structures of glucose and the other single sugars (monosaccharides) and of the reactions by which glucose and similar molecules are put together to make the larger sugars (disaccharides). (The release of energy from glucose and the ways the body uses this energy are the subjects of Highlight 7.)

Glucose A chemist views a glucose molecule as a compound composed of 24 atoms: 6 carbon, 12 hydrogen, and 6 oxygen atoms. These atoms are symbolized by the letters C, H, and O. Thus the chemical formula for glucose, which reflects the number of atoms it contains, is $C_6H_{12}O_6$.

Each type of atom has a characteristic amount of energy available for forming chemical bonds with other atoms. A carbon atom can form four such bonds; an oxygen atom two; and a hydrogen atom only one. One way to represent the number of bonds associated with each type of atom is to use lines radiating from the letters. The bond of a hydrogen atom is represented by one line radiating from the H; the bonds of an oxygen atom are represented by two such lines; and those of a carbon atom by four:

$$H- \qquad -O- \qquad -\underset{|}{\overset{}{N}}- \qquad -\overset{|}{\underset{|}{C}}-$$

$$1 \qquad\quad 2 \qquad\quad 3 \qquad\quad 4$$

(Nitrogen—N—is included here because it comes up later.)

C, H, and O atoms may be put together in any way that satisfies their bonding requirements. The following drawing of the active ingredient of alcoholic beverages shows that each atom's bonding capabilities are fully used in its structure:

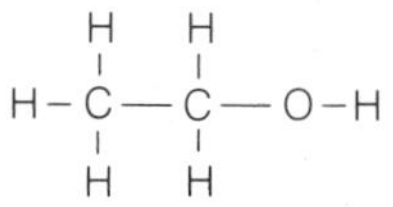

Chemical structure of ethyl alcohol.

The carbons both have four lines (bonds), the oxygen has two, and the hydrogens each have one to connect them to other atoms. In any drawing of a chemical structure these conditions must be met, not because a fussy scientist made up these rules but because this represents the way nature demands it.

Glucose is a larger and more complicated molecule than alcohol, but it obeys the same rules—as do all chemical compounds. The complete structure of a glucose molecule is:

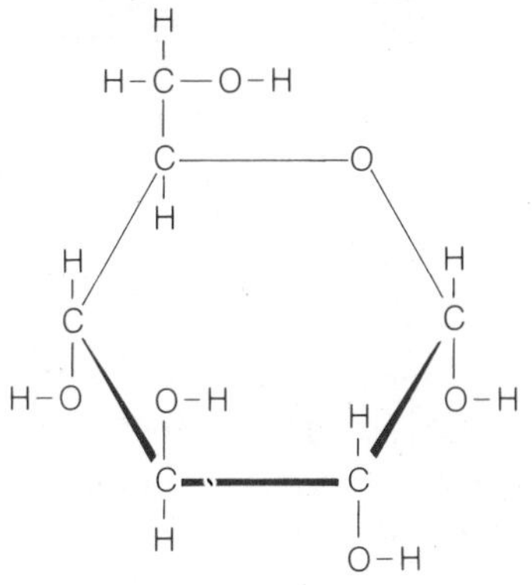

Chemical structure of glucose. On paper, it has to be drawn flat, but in nature the ring is on a plane and the attached structures extend above and below.

Again, each carbon atom has four bonds, each oxygen two, and each hydrogen one bond connecting it to other atoms.

The diagram of a glucose molecule may look formidable, but it shows all the relationships between the parts and proves simple on examination. Since you will be viewing other complex structures (not necessarily to memorize them but rather to understand certain things about them), let us adopt a simpler way to depict them—one that shows fewer details. In the following drawing, the corners where lines intersect represent carbon atoms; thus many of the bonds need not be shown. Wherever a carbon atom needs Hs to complete its four bonds, the Hs can be dropped from the diagram and can be assumed to be present. Knowing the rules of chemical structure, it is possible to reconstruct the complete structure, with all its details, from such a picture:

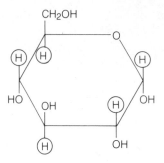

Future drawings of the glucose structure
will be made simpler still, by omitting the circled Hs:

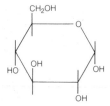

Another way to look at glucose
is to notice that its six carbon atoms
are all connected:

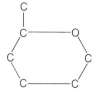

In the simplest diagrams of all,
when the number of carbon atoms
is the only concern,
glucose is symbolized this way:

$$C-C-C-C-C-C$$

carbohydrate: a compound composed of carbon, hydrogen, and oxygen, arranged as monosaccharides or multiples of monosaccharides.

carbo = carbon (C)
hydrate = water (H_2O)

monosaccharide (mon-oh-SACK-uh-ride): a carbohydrate of the general formula $C_nH_{2n}O_n$; *n* may be any number, but the monosaccharides important in nutrition are all **hexoses** (monosaccharides containing 6 carbon atoms—$C_6H_{12}O_6$).

mono = one
saccharide, ose = sugar
hex = six

disaccharide: a pair of monosaccharides bonded together.

di = two

All carbohydrates are composed of glucose and other C-H-O compounds very much like glucose in structure. They come in three main sizes: single molecules, like glucose; pairs (for example, two glucose molecules bonded together); and chains (for example, 300 glucose molecules strung in a line). The chemist's terms for these three types of carbohydrates are mono-, di-, and polysaccharides.

With this information, the chemist's terms defining the carbohydrates are understandable, and the common terms we use to describe them—sugars and starches—can be understood more precisely. The sugars are the mono- and disaccharides; starch, glycogen, and some fibers are the polysaccharides. Store-bought cane or beet sugar is one of the disaccharides.

It remains to be seen how these units are put together and taken apart in the continuous flow of matter and energy through living things.

Making and Breaking Pairs: Chemical Reactions When a disaccharide is formed from two monosaccharides, a chemical reaction known as a condensation reaction takes place. In a condensation reaction, a hydrogen atom is removed from one monosaccharide and an oxygen-hydrogen (OH) group is removed from the other, leaving the two molecules bonded by a single O:

polysaccharide: many monosaccharides bonded together.

poly = many

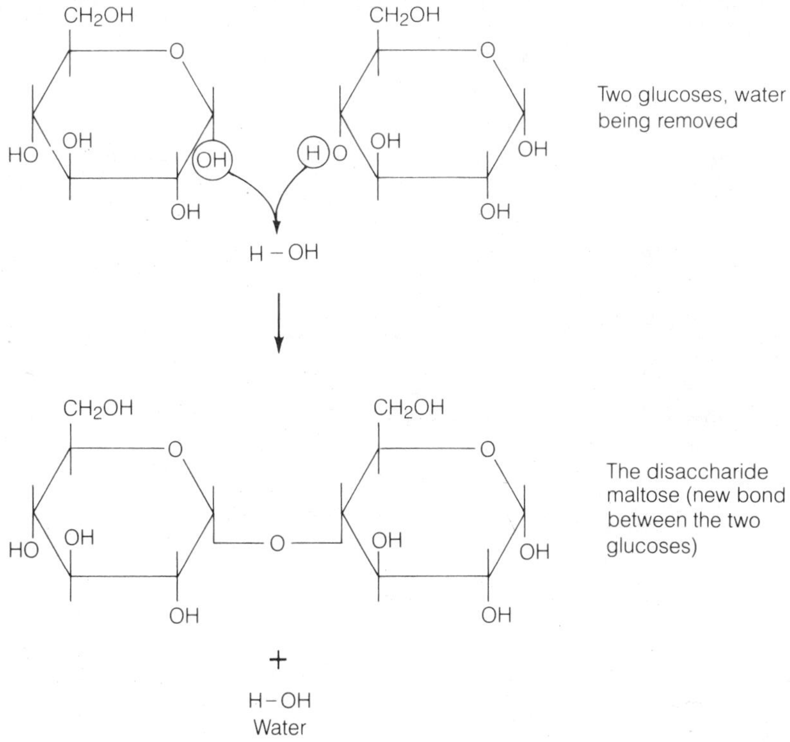
CH2OH
O
HO
OH
OH
OH
H
H – OH
OH
Two glucoses, water being removed
The disaccharide maltose (new bond between the two glucoses)
+
H–OH
Water

Chemical reaction: See Appendix B.

Condensation.

The H and OH that were removed from the monosaccharides in this reaction also bond to form a molecule of water (H_2O).

When a disaccharide is taken apart to form two monosaccharides again, as during digestion in the human body, a molecule of water participates in the reaction. H is added to one monosaccharide and OH to the other to reform the original structures. This reaction is called a hydrolysis reaction:

condensation: a chemical reaction in which two reactants combine to yield a major product, with the elimination of water or a similar small molecule.

hydrolysis (high-DROL-uh-sis): a chemical reaction in which a major reactant is split into two products, with the addition of H to one and OH to the other (from water).

hydro = water
lysis = breaking

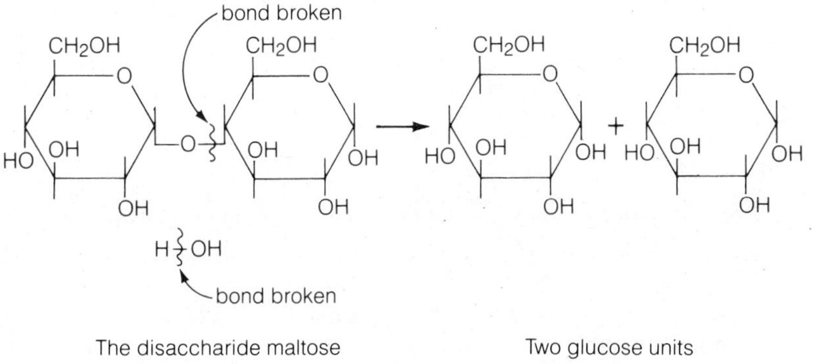
bond broken
CH2OH
O
HO
OH
H–OH
bond broken
+
The disaccharide maltose
Two glucose units

Hydrolysis.

It is by condensation and hydrolysis reactions that all of the carbohydrates are put together and taken apart. For this reason among many others, water is of tremendous importance to living things like yourself; without it, literally nothing would happen. (Chapter 14 is devoted to this extraordinary substance.) As you read, notice that water is involved in every process that is described.

Enzyme: see also p. 101.

The enzymes, the facilitators of condensation and hydrolysis reactions, are also of great importance. (They are described fully in Chapter 3.) For the moment, however, let us adopt a simple definition: An enzyme is a giant molecule (about the size of a molecule of starch) that provides a surface on which other molecules (such as glucose) may come together and react with one another. Since the making and breaking of chemical bonds tells the whole story of growth, mainenance, and change in living creatures, the enzymes that facilitate these reactions are indispensable to life.

But enough about chemical bonds. You know now that glucose is the predominant energy source for all the body's cells and can appreciate the importance of having a constant energy supply if you are to feel well. So let's return to the more familiar chemical mixtures called foods, which are the sources of glucose in the diet.

The Sugars in Foods

One exception: Alcohol also contributes energy (kcalories). See Highlight 9.

Practically all your energy comes from the food you eat, about half from carbohydrate and half from fat and protein. In fact, one of the principal roles of carbohydrate in the diet is to supply energy in the form of blood glucose. A look at the carbohydrates found in foods and at the way they are put together will show why this is so.

complex carbohydrates: the polysaccharides (starch, glycogen, and cellulose).

simple carbohydrates: the monosaccharides (glucose, fructose, and galactose) and the disaccharides (sucrose, lactose, and maltose); also called the sugars.

The carbohydrates are conveniently divided into two classes: the complex carbohydrates, of which starch is the most familiar example, and the simple carbohydrates, exemplified by ordinary table sugar. All carbohydrates are composed of monosaccharides, and by far the most common is glucose. Starch is the most significant contributor of glucose to people's diets, but let us first consider the simple carbohydrates. There are actually six common sugars found in foods: glucose, fructose, galactose, sucrose, lactose, and maltose.

glucose: a monosaccharide; sometimes known as blood sugar, sometimes as grape sugar; also called **dextrose.**

Glucose This monosaccharide is one of the sugars. Glucose is not especially sweet tasting; a pinch of the purified sugar on your tongue gives only the faintest taste sensation. However, it is absorbed with extraordinary rapidity into the bloodstream. If a diabetic has gone into a hypoglycemic coma (for example, from an overdose of insulin), a quick way to supply the needed blood glucose is to tip his head to one side and to drip a water solution of glucose into his cheek pocket. The glucose will be absorbed directly into his bloodstream.

● = glucose

Fructose   When you bite into a ripe peach or plum and savor the natural sweetness of its juice, the sugar you are enjoying is fructose. Curiously, fructose has exactly the same chemical formula as glucose—$C_6H_{12}O_6$—but its structure is quite different:

fructose: a monosaccharide; sometimes known as fruit sugar.

▲ = fructose

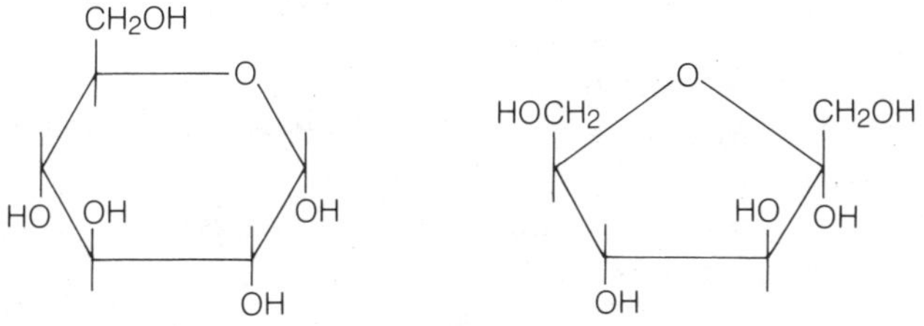

CH₂OH

Glucose   Fructose

(If you learned the rules on p. 26, you will be able to "see" 6 Cs, 12 Hs, and 6 Os in both these compounds.)

The different arrangements of the atoms in these two sugars stimulate the taste buds on your tongue in different ways. The next time you sit down to a plate of pancakes dripping with pure Vermont maple syrup, give thanks to the way nature has arranged the carbon, hydrogen, and oxygen atoms in fructose to make it the sweetest of the sugars.

Fructose can be absorbed directly into your bloodstream. When the blood circulates past the liver, the fructose is taken up into the liver cells, where enzymes rearrange the C, H, and O atoms to make compounds indistinguishable from those derived from glucose and sometimes glucose itself. Thus the effect of fructose on the body is very similar to the effect of glucose.

Food chemists have studied the exact arrangement of the atoms in sweet-tasting substances, such as fructose, and have identified the structures in them that stimulate your sweetness taste buds. They have developed a number of artificial, nonnutritive sweeteners, such as saccharin and the cyclamates, that stimulate your taste receptors in the same way but cannot be oxidized by the body to yield energy. Thus they are noncaloric.

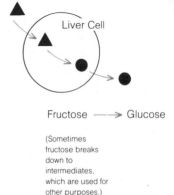

Fructose ⟶ Glucose

(Sometimes fructose breaks down to intermediates, which are used for other purposes.)

For the advantages and disadvantages of these additives, see Highlight 13.

Galactose   Glucose and fructose are the only two monosaccharides of importance in foods; a third, galactose, is seldom found free in nature but is instead found as part of the disaccharide lactose. Like glucose and fructose, galactose is a hexose with the formula $C_6H_{12}O_6$. It is shown here beside a molecule of glucose for comparison:

galactose: a monosaccharide; part of the disaccharide lactose.

■ = galactose

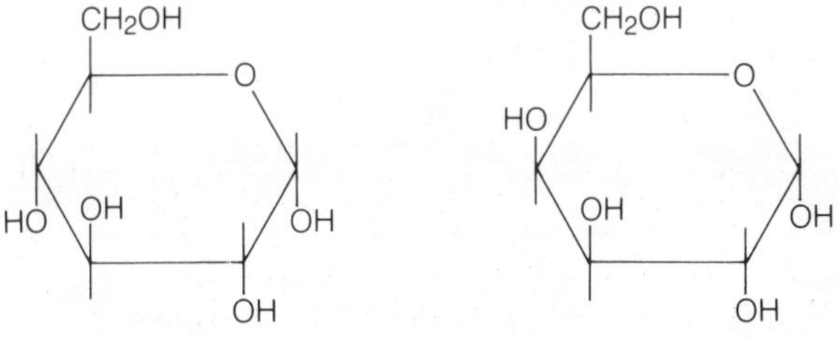

CH₂OH   CH₂OH

(Can you see
the difference?)

Glucose   Galactose

sucrose: a disaccharide composed of glucose and fructose; commonly known as table sugar, beet sugar, or cane sugar.

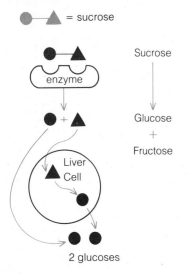

Digestion of sucrose.

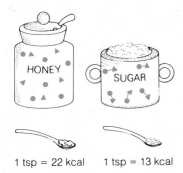

1 tsp = 22 kcal   1 tsp = 13 kcal

Sucrose   The other three common sugars are disaccharides—pairs of monosaccharides linked together. Glucose is found in all three; the second member of the pair is either fructose, galactose, or another glucose.

Sucrose (*sucro* means sugar)—table sugar—is the most familiar of the disaccharides. It is the sugar found in sugar cane and sugar beets; it is purified and granulated to various extents to provide the brown, white, and powdered sugars available in the supermarket. Because it contains fructose, it is a very sweet sugar.

When you eat a food containing sucrose, enzymes in your digestive tract hydrolyze the sucrose to yield glucose and fructose. These monosaccharides are absorbed, and the fructose may be converted to glucose in the liver. (Alternatively, the fructose may be broken down to smaller compounds identical to those derived from glucose.) Thus one molecule of sucrose can ultimately yield two of glucose.

You can see from this description that it makes no difference whether you eat these monosaccharides hitched together as table sugar or already broken apart. In either case they will end up as monosaccharides in the body. People who think that the "natural sugar," honey, is somehow superior to purified table sugar fail to understand this point.

It so happens that honey, like table sugar, contains glucose and fructose. Like table sugar, honey is concentrated to the point where it contains very few impurities, even such desirable ones as vitamins and minerals. In fact, being a liquid, honey is more dense than its crystalline sister and so contains more kcalories per spoonful. Table 1 shows that honey is not significantly more nutritious than sugar:

Table 1.   Vitamins and Minerals Supplied by Sugar Sources

Sugar source (1 tbsp)	Calcium (mg)	Iron (mg)	Vitamin A (IU)	Thiamin (mg)	Riboflavin (mg)	Vitamin C (mg)
Sugar (white granulated)	0	trace*	0	0	0	0
Honey (strained or extracted)	1	0.1	0	trace*	0.01	trace*
Possible daily nutrient need†	1,000	18	5,000	1.5	1.7	60

*A trace is an amount large enough to be detectable in chemical analysis but too small to be significant in comparison to the amounts recorded in these tables.

†These are amounts that an adult might typically need in a day. Not all the vitamins and minerals are listed.

To say that honey is no more nutritious than sugar, however, is not to say that there are no differences among sugar sources. Consider a piece of fruit, like an orange. From the fruit you would receive the same monosaccharides and the same kcalories as from the sugar. But the packaging is different. The fruit's sugars are diluted in a large volume of water which contains valuable trace minerals and vitamins, and the flesh and skin of the fruit are supported by fibers that also offer health value.

From these two comparisons, you may see that the really significant difference between sugar sources is not between "natural" and "purified" sugar but between concentrated sweets and the dilute, naturally occurring sugars that sweeten nutritious foods.

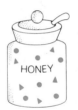

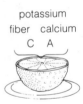

potassium
fiber calcium
C   A

1 tsp = 22 kcal

1 tsp = 2 kcal
with vitamins,
minerals,
and fiber

> A FLAG SIGN OF A SPURIOUS CLAIM
> IS THE ASSERTION THAT:
>
> Added honey makes a product more nutritious.

A newcomer on the fad diet scene is the fructose diet, whose advocates claim that it is a wonderfully effective means of losing weight. Purified fructose, they say, is a "natural sugar" that gives you energy without accumulating as body fat. The diet plan requires that you buy bottles of purified fructose and use this sugar in place of the "unnatural sugar," sucrose, which causes ugly weight gain. In light of what has just been said about honey, it should be clear that there is nothing more natural about purified, crystalline fructose sold in bottles than about its cousin, sucrose.

> A FLAG SIGN OF A SPURIOUS CLAIM
> IS THE ASSERTION THAT:
>
> Fructose (purified) is more natural than any other refined sugar.

Sucrose is the principal energy-nutrient ingredient of carbonated beverages, candy, cakes, frostings, cookies, and other concentrated sweets. Highlight 1 (at the end of this chapter) addresses the questions of whether sucrose is necessary in the diet at all and whether it may be, in fact, a threat to health.

Lactose Lactose is the principal carbohydrate found in milk, comprising about 5 percent of its weight. A human baby is born with the digestive enzymes necessary to hydrolyze lactose into its two

lactose: a disaccharide composed of glucose and galactose; commonly known as milk sugar.

 = lactose

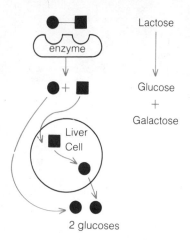

Digestion of lactose.

lactose intolerance: inherited or acquired inability to digest lactose, due to failure to produce the enzyme lactase. Lactose intolerance is prevalent in the majority of adult human population groups.[3]

maltose: a disaccharide composed of two glucose units; sometimes known as malt sugar.

●━━● = maltose

fermentation: the breakdown of sugar in the absence of oxygen, yielding alcohol.

monosaccharide parts, glucose and galactose, so that they can be absorbed. The galactose is then converted to glucose in the liver, so each molecule of lactose yields two molecules of glucose to supply energy for the baby's growth and activity. Babies can digest lactose at birth, but they don't develop the ability to digest starch until they are several months old. This is one of the many reasons why milk is such a good food for babies; it provides a simple, easily digested carbohydrate in the right amount to supply energy to meet their needs.

Some individuals lose the ability to digest lactose as they grow older and become lactose-intolerant. They react badly to large doses of milk, feeling nauseated and sometimes having diarrhea when they drink it. Lactose intolerance arises at about the age of four and is especially common among American Indians, Orientals, and the black races; it is less frequently found in whites. It is not the same as the commonly observed milk allergy, which is caused by certain babies' hypersensitivity to the protein in cow's milk and sometimes to that in other milks.[4]

Maltose The third disaccharide is found at only one stage in the life of a plant. When the seed is formed, it is packed with starch—stored glucose—to be used as fuel for the germination process. When the seed begins to sprout, an enzyme cleaves the starch into maltose units. Another enzyme splits the maltose units into glucose units. Other enzymes degrade the units still further, releasing energy for the sprouting of the shoot and root of the plant. By the time the young plant is established and growing, all the starch in the seed has been used up, and the plant is able to capture the sun's light in its leaves. The plant then uses this light energy to put new molecules of glucose together and to elaborate chains of starch, cellulose, and other plant constituents from them. Thus the sugar maltose is present briefly during the early germination process, as the starch is being broken down. The malt found in beer contains maltose formed as the grains germinate (the alcohol is produced by yeast in a process known as fermentation).

As you might predict, when you eat or drink a food source of maltose, your digestive enzymes hydrolyze the maltose into two glucose units, which are then absorbed into the blood.

In summary, then, the simple carbohydrates or sugars are:

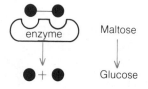

Digestion of maltose.

Monosaccharides		Disaccharides	
glucose	●	maltose	●━━●
fructose	▲	sucrose	●━━▲
galactose	■	lactose	●━━■
(found only in lactose)			

[3]N. Kretchmer, Lactose and lactase, *Scientific American* 227 (1972): 70-78.
[4]Kretchmer, 1972.

All of these are derived from a variety of plants except for lactose, which is the sugar of mammalian milk, and galactose, which is part of the lactose molecule.

Sugar, Starch, Fiber, and Your Health

For years people have learned that carbohydrates were "bad" for them. Sugar and starch have been accused of being fattening, and protein-rich foods like meat have been praised as being nutritious and nonfattening. It now comes as a surprise to learn that carbohydrate is not only not "bad" but is also the ideal fuel for most body functions. The educated consumer would probably choose carbohydrate as the principal kcalorie source in the diet. To convey this idea means trying to confront beliefs as deeply ingrained as people's religious faith. To persuade a person to act on it may be harder still, for food prejudices linger in the mouth.

Before this theme is developed further, the use of words like *good* and *bad* deserves a brief comment. Nutrition is a science, and science cannot make value judgments; only people can. Science involves finding out what happens under different sets of circumstances and experimenting to see how things happen. It can show, for example, that people with artery disease or cancer more often have diets high in fat or protein than diets high in carbohydrate. But science cannot pronounce these nutrients "bad" and certainly cannot prove that it is morally wrong to eat them, even though they may entail health disadvantages.

In this book we never mean to imply moral judgments, but we do have a prejudice in favor of health. When we say that something is "good" or "bad," we mean that it is "health-promoting" or "harmful to health." We use these terms because they are in common use and save space, but we have put them in quotation marks wherever they appear to remind you of what we really mean.

During the 1970s, public interest in nutrition grew tremendously. Earlier surveys in both the United States and Canada had shown that some people in these developed countries were inadequately nourished, despite the countries' wealth. Public and governmental inquiry into the significance of nutrition for health led to the development of programs to remedy nutritional deficiencies. Some of these programs are described in later chapters.

The concerns of the 1970s evolved into an interest in overnutrition—the consumption of too much food. Among the agencies inquiring into the consequences of being overfed was a committee of the United States Senate: the Select Committee on Nutrition and Human Needs. In 1977 this committee published a document titled *Dietary Goals for the United States*.

The publication of the *Dietary Goals* kicked up a whirlwind of conflicting opinions. Their proponents hailed them as long overdue and only regretted that they were understated and conservative. Their opponents criticized them as premature, exaggerated, and inappropriate for dissemination to the public. One of the objections to the *Goals* was that they had come out under the auspices of a political body—a powerful Senate committee—rather than a group of scientists. This criticism, among others, led to the disbanding of the Senate committee at the end of 1977, and the distribution of its responsibilities to two government departments whose charges include matters of nutrition and health: the Department of Agriculture (USDA) and the Department of Health, Education, and Welfare (USDHEW).

In 1979, after much more discussion and disagreement, representatives of these two departments produced a document entitled *Dietary Guidelines for Americans*, which included seven guidelines similar to the *Goals* but less specific and less controversial (see box).

Dietary Guidelines for Americans and Suggestions for Food Choices*

1. *Eat a Variety of Foods Daily.* Include these foods every day: fruits and vegetables; whole grain and enriched breads and cereals; milk and milk products; meats, fish, poultry and eggs; dried peas and beans.

2. *Maintain Ideal Weight.* Increase physical activity; reduce kcalories by eating fewer fatty foods and sweets and less sugar, and by avoiding too much alcohol; lose weight gradually.

3. *Avoid Too Much Fat, Saturated Fat, and Cholesterol.* Choose low-fat protein sources such as lean meats, fish, poultry, dry peas and beans; use eggs and organ meats in moderation; limit intake of fats on and in foods; trim fats from meats; broil, bake or boil—don't fry; read food labels for fat contents.

4. *Eat Foods with Adequate Starch and Fiber.* Substitute starches for fats and sugars; select whole grain breads and cereal, fruits and vegetables, dried beans and peas, and nuts to increase fiber and starch intake.

5. *Avoid Too Much Sugar.* Use less sugar, syrup, and honey; reduce concentrated sweets like candy, soft drinks, cookies, etc.; select fresh fruits or fruits canned in light syrup or their own juices; read food labels—sucrose, glucose, dextrose, maltose, lactose, fructose, syrups, and honey are all sugars; eat sugar less often to reduce dental caries.

6. *Avoid Too Much Sodium.* Reduce salt in cooking; add little or no salt at the table; limit salty foods like potato chips, pretzels, salted nuts; popcorn, condiments, cheese, pickled foods, and cured meats; read food labels for sodium or salt contents especially in processed and snack foods.

7. *If You Drink Alcohol, Do So in Moderation.* For individuals who drink—limit all alcoholic beverages (including wine, beer, liquors, etc.) to one or two drinks per day. NOTE: use of alcoholic beverages during pregnancy can result in the development of birth defects and mental retardation called Fetal Alcohol Syndrome.

*USDA, USDHEW, 1979

The publication of these two sets of recommendations—the *Goals* and *Guidelines*—so close together in time reveals the nation's increased interest in nutrition and especially its concern about overnutrition. Whichever document you look at, you will see the same general principles stressed: the *Goals* state them in terms of nutrients, the *Guidelines* translate them into foods.

Altogether the Select Committee listed seven goals.[5] The first was to avoid excess weight by consuming only as many kcalories as expended or to lose weight, if necessary, by reducing kcalorie intake and increasing energy expenditure. The next two Goals dealt with carbohydrate. According to the Select Committee, people should

● Increase the consumption of complex carbohydrates and "naturally occurring" sugars (mainly those from fruits).

● Reduce the consumption of refined and processed sugars.

In terms of foods, these Goals translate into the practical recommendations of Guidelines 4 and 5.

● Increase consumption of fruits and vegetables and whole grains.

● Decrease consumption of refined and other processed sugars and of foods high in such sugars.

[5]U.S. Senate, Select Committee on Nutrition and Human Needs, *Dietary Goals for the United States*, 2nd ed. (Washington, D.C.: Government Printing Office, December 1977).

The recommended changes in the diet are shown in Figure 1. The bottom part of each column deals with carbohydrate. As you can see, the Select Committee advised that we cut sugar intake in half and more than double the intake of complex carbohydrate and naturally occurring sugars.

This was startling news. It meant eating not only more fruits and vegetables but also more bread, pasta (spaghetti, macaroni, noodles, and the like), rice, and potatoes. How could you do this without getting fat?

The secret is that carbohydrates by themselves are really not so fattening. A 3 1/2-oz baked potato is only about 90 kcal, far less than a

For the definition of kcalories, see p. 8.

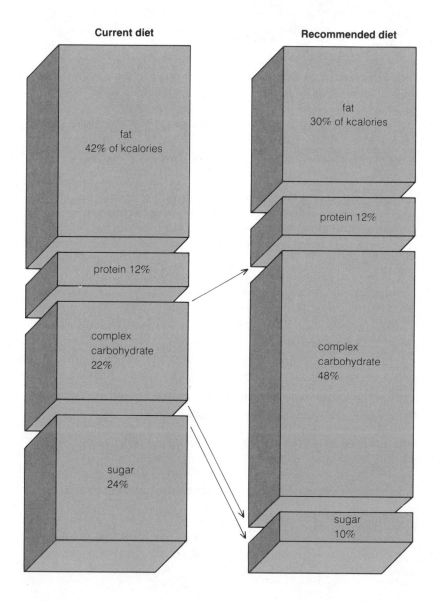

Current diet

Recommended diet

fat
42% of kcalories

fat
30% of kcalories

protein 12%

protein 12%

complex
carbohydrate
22%

complex
carbohydrate
48%

sugar
24%

sugar
10%

Figure 1 The U.S. Dietary Goals.

3 1/2-oz hamburger (about 285 kcal). What adds kcalories to starchy foods is not the starch itself so much as the fat—butter, margarine, sour cream, and so forth—that is often served with them. With two pats of butter, the 90-kcal potato becomes a 160-kcal potato. With a heaping tablespoon of sour cream on top of that, it becomes a 210-kcal potato. Butter and sour cream are fats, and fats are a much more concentrated source of kcalories than are carbohydrates. As you might expect, several of the Dietary Goals recommend reduced intake of fats (see Chapter 2). If you do cut back on fats, you can easily afford the extra kcalories you gain by eating more starchy foods.

For the composition of foods from which these numbers are calculated, see Appendix H.

The evidence that shows that complex carbohydrates and naturally occurring sugars are "good" for you is not presented here but will emerge at intervals throughout the book. But now it is time to deal with the complex carbohydrates. You should recall that these are polysaccharides—and the most important among them are starch, glycogen, and cellulose.

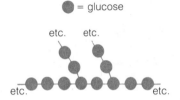

Portion of a starch molecule.

The Chemist's View of Complex Carbohydrates

Now that you know something about the structure and role of carbohydrates in the diet, you have a basis for understanding the importance of the complex carbohydrates—starch, glycogen, and cellulose.

starch: a plant polysaccharide composed of glucose and digestible by humans.

Starch   As the chemist sees it, starch is a branched chain of dozens of glucose units connected together. These units would have to be magnified more than 10 million times to appear at the size shown on this page. However, as molecules go, starches are rather large. A single starch molecule may contain from 300 to 1,000 or more glucose units linked together. These giant molecules are packed side by side in the rice grain or potato root—as many as a million in a cubic inch of food.

In the plant, starch serves a function similar to that of the glycogen in your liver. It is a storage form of glucose needed for the plant's first growth. (When you eat the plant, of course, you get the glucose to use for your own purposes.)

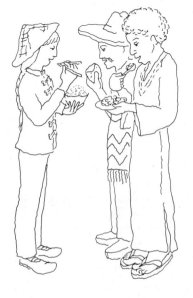

All starchy foods are in fact plant foods. Seeds are the richest food source; 70 percent of their weight is starch. Many human societies have a staple grain from which 50 to 80 percent of their food energy is derived. Rice is the staple grain of the Orient. In Canada, the United States, and Europe the staple grain is wheat. If you consider all the food products made from wheat—bread (and other baked goods made from wheat flour), cereals, and pasta—you will realize how all-pervasive this grain is in the food supply. Corn is the staple grain of much of South America and of the southern United States; the Mexicans use corn in their tacos and tortillas. The staple grains of other peoples include millet, rye, barley, and oats. In each society a bread, meal, or flour is made from the grain, which is then used for many purposes.

A second important source of starch is the bean and pea family, including such dry beans found in the supermarket as lima beans, kidney beans, "baked" beans, black-eyed peas (cowpeas), chickpeas (garbanzo beans), and soybeans. These vegetables are about 40 percent starch by weight and also contain a significant amount of protein. A third major source of starch is the tubers such as the potato, yam, and cassava. One of these may serve as the primary starch source in many non-Western societies.

Starch can be broken down to shorter chains of glucose units known as **dextrins**. These can be used as thickening agents in foods; the word sometimes appears on labels.

When you eat any of these foods, the starch molecules are taken apart by enzymes in your mouth and intestine. The enzymes hydrolyze the starch molecules to yield glucose units, which are absorbed across the intestinal wall into the blood. One to four hours after a meal, all the starch has been digested and is circulating to the cells as glucose.

glycogen (GLIGH-co-gen): an animal polysaccharide composed of glucose, manufactured in the body, and stored in liver and muscle.

Glycogen   Glycogen is not found in plants and is stored in animal meats only to a limited extent. It is not, therefore, of major importance as a nutrient, although it performs an important role in the metabolism of carbohydrates in the body, as already described. Glycogen is more complex and more highly branched in structure than starch.

cellulose (CELL-yoo-lose): a plant polysaccharide composed of glucose and indigestible by humans.

Cellulose   The third polysaccharide of importance in nutrition is cellulose. Cellulose, like starch, is found abundantly in plants and is composed of glucose units connected in long chains. However, the bonds holding its glucose units together are different. This difference is of major importance for humans, because each type of bond requires a different enzyme to hydrolyze it. The human digestive tract is supplied with abundant enzymes to hydrolyze the bonds in starch but has none that can attack the bonds in cellulose. As a result, starch is digestible for humans and cellulose is not. Cellulose passes through the digestive tract largely unchanged, which explains the different roles of these two major plant polysaccharides: Starch is the most abundant energy source in the staple foods of the world, whereas cellulose provides no energy for humans at all.

Cellulose is, however, one of the fibers, and these are as important to health as the energy nutrients are. During the last decade, cellulose and other plant fibers have received increasing attention as the public has learned of their health value. Researchers are still very actively trying to determine what they do and do not do, and there is much disagreement. But because some of the fibers are polysaccharides, it seems appropriate to present here the most important facts about the fibers as a group.

fiber: a loose term denoting the indigestible substances in plant food. It would be best for this term to disappear from common use, to be replaced by the terms *crude fiber* and *dietary fiber*, which are more clearly defined (see p. 40).

pectin and **hemicellulose:** carbohydrates found in plant foods. Like cellulose, they are indigestible.

Besides cellulose, two other carbohydrates—pectin and hemicellulose—provide indigestible residue in the human digestive tract and so are classified as fiber. Another material classified as fiber because it is

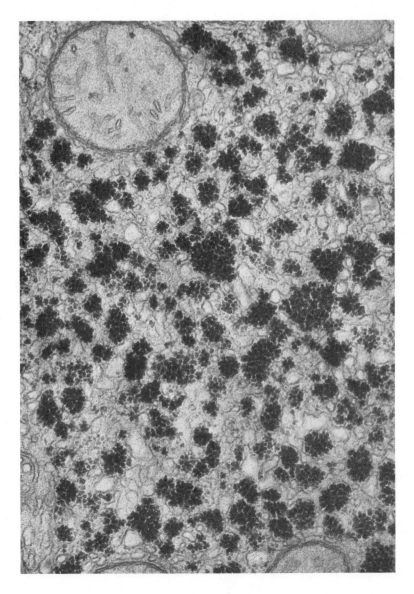

Glycogen in a liver cell. The black "rosettes" are aggregates of glycogen granules. The circular membrane-bound bodies, such as the one in the upper-left corner, are subcellular energy-producing organelles known as mitochondria. This cell was photographed under an electron microscope at a magnification of 65,000X.

From D. W. Fawcett, *An Atlas of Fine Structure* (Philadelphia: Saunders, 1966), Fig. 161. Courtesy of the author and publisher.

indigestible is lignin, a noncarbohydrate. Still others are the gums and mucilages often used as thickening agents in prepared foods.

Some of these food fibers may have beneficial effects on long- or short-term health, including:

- To attract water into the digestive tract, thus softening the stools and preventing constipation.
- To exercise the muscles of the digestive tract so that they retain their health and tone and resist bulging out into the pouches characteristic of diverticulosis.

lignin: a noncarbohydrate fiber that occurs in plant foods.

Constipation: see also Chapter 5.

Diverticulosis: see p. 121.

● To speed up the passage of food materials through the digestive tract, thus shortening the "transit time" and helping to prevent exposure of the tissue to cancer-causing agents in food.

● To bind lipids such as cholesterol and carry them out of the body with the feces so that the blood lipid concentrations are lowered and possibly the risk of artery and heart disease as well.

bran: the fiber of wheat.

However, not all the fibers have similar effects. For example, the fiber of wheat—bran, which is composed mostly of cellulose—has no cholesterol-lowering effect, whereas the fiber of apples—pectin—does lower blood cholesterol. On the other hand, bran seems to be one of the most effective stool-softening fibers, especially if a certain particle size is used.

crude fiber (CF): the residue of plant food remaining after extraction with dilute acid followed by dilute alkali in a laboratory procedure.

Another problem for people trying to sort out the effects of fiber is that the amounts of fiber in food are hard to estimate. Food can be analyzed for fiber content in the laboratory by digesting it with acids and bases. Whatever remains is called crude fiber. But if you eat the same food, subjecting it to the action of your own enzymes, the undigested residue will be greater, because the body's enzymes are less harsh than the laboratory treatment. What we really need to know is how much fiber remains in the body after the normal human digestive process, but how can we measure that? One imprecise and unpleasant procedure involves collecting all the stools excreted over a 24-hour period and then drying and weighing them.

dietary fiber (DF): the residue of plant food resistant to hydrolysis by human digestive enzymes.

The fiber that remains in the human digestive tract after the body's normal action on food is known as dietary fiber. For every gram of crude fiber in a food, there are probably about 2 or 3 grams of dietary fiber.

Diets in the United States presently provide about 4 g of crude fiber a day, as compared with about 6 g in 1900. If foods such as fruits, vegetables, and whole-grain breads and cereals are used as the fiber sources, then 6 g is probably a safe intake. The wholesale addition of purified fiber (for example, bran) to foods is probably ill-advised, however, because it can cause dehydration and siphon off needed minerals with the lost water. (Appendix K presents what is known about the fiber contents of foods.)

Food Groups and the Carbohydrates

Most authorities agree that dietary carbohydrate is essential as a source of glucose. You must have some every day—but how much? One authority recommends intakes considerably above a minimum level of 50 to 100 grams a day,[6] so you might aim for at least 125 g carbohydrate a day for yourself. At 4 kcal per gram, that would be not less than 500 kcal. How can you be sure that you get at least that amount?

[6] Recommended Dietary Allowances, 9th ed. (Washington, D.C.: National Academy of Sciences, 1980), p. 33.

The number and variety of different foods that people eat is staggering. Appendix H lists 615 of the most common ones, and no two are exactly alike in nutritional value. Must you memorize the nutrient composition of all these foods in order to plan and assess your diet properly? This would be a formidable task. To avoid such a tedious undertaking, experts have devised various systems of grouping foods together. The two most useful kinds are exchange systems and food group systems. Some understanding of both will help you to get a feel for the composition of foods.

Exchange Systems   In an exchange system, foods are grouped so that their carbohydrate, fat, protein, and kcalorie contents are similar. For example, a slice of bread is similar to a small potato because both contain about 15 g carbohydrate, 2 g protein, and negligible fat. Both provide about 70 kcal of energy. A slice of bread could be exchanged (traded) for a potato without altering the amount of carbohydrate or protein or the number of kcalories served.

Exchange systems emphasize carbohydrate, fat, protein, and kcalories.

A typical exchange system divides foods into six classes, as shown in Table 2.

Foods containing carbohydrate:

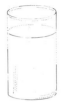

12 g in 1 c milk

Table 2.   The Six Exchange Groups*

Exchange group	Serving size	Carbohydrate (g)	Protein (g)	Fat (g)	Energy (kcal)
(1) **Skim milk**	1 c	12	8	0	80
(2) **Vegetables**	1/2 c	5	2	0	25
(3) **Fruit**	varies†	10	0	0	40
(4) **Bread**	1 slice	15	2	0	70
(5) Lean meat	1 oz	0	7	3	55
(6) Fat	1 tsp	0	0	5	45

*Taken from the ADA Exchange System (see Appendix L).

†Serving sizes for fruits vary (see Appendix L).

(The variable amounts of fat in milk exchanges are explained fully in Chapter 2.)

5 g in 1/2 c vegetables

Carbohydrate is found in four of the six types of food listed: milk, vegetables, fruits, and breads.

> 1 c skim milk (or any other serving of food in the milk list) provides 12 g carbohydrate as lactose, a naturally occurring sugar. Cheeses have negligible carbohydrate and so are not included with milk in this system.

> 1/2 c green beans (or any other serving of food on the vegetable list) provides 5 g carbohydrate, mostly as naturally occurring sugars. Starchy vegetables are not included on this list.

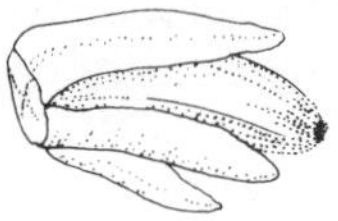

10 g in one fruit exchange

> 1 serving of fruit (serving sizes are shown on the fruit list) provides 10 g carbohydrate as naturally occurring sugars.

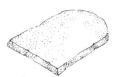

15 g in one slice bread

> 1 slice of bread (or any other serving of food on the bread list) provides 15 g carbohydrate, mostly in the form of starch. All grain foods, such as cereal and pasta, and such starchy vegetables as corn, lima beans, and potatoes are included on this list.

Exchange systems do not include sugary foods like candy, jam, and soft drinks, because they are not considered desirable in diet plans. But people do consume them. To estimate an accurate total of the carbohydrate you may consume, you may need a "sugar list," and we have invented one for the purpose:

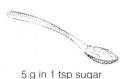

5 g in 1 tsp sugar

> 1 tsp white sugar (or any other concentrated sweet) provides 5 g carbohydrate.

Among the other concentrated sweets treated as equivalent to 1 tsp of white sugar are:

- 1 tsp brown sugar
- 1 tsp molasses
- 1 tsp corn syrup
- 1 tsp maple syrup
- 1 tsp honey
- 1 tsp jam
- 1 tsp jelly
- 1 tsp candy

1 tbsp catsup = 1 tsp sugar

8-oz can cola
  beverage = 6 tsp sugar

For a person who uses catsup (ketchup) liberally, it may help to remember that 1 tbsp catsup supplies about 1 tsp sugar. An 8-oz can of a cola beverage contains about 6 tsp sugar, or 30 g carbohydrate.

To sum up, all of the foods containing carbohydrate have been identified in these five boxes. A familiarity with the gram amounts gives you a command of the total carbohydrate content of any diet.

You can translate carbohydrate grams into kcalories if you multiply by 4. That is, a gram of any carbohydrate—sugar or starch—yields 4 kcal in the body. (A gram of protein also yields 4 kcal, but a gram of fat yields 9 kcal.) A study of Table 2 will reveal that the kcalorie amounts for each group of foods have been derived from these numbers and then rounded off. For example, a slice of bread contains 15 g carbohydrate (that's 60 kcal) and 2 g protein (that's another 8 kcal), or about 70 kcal

1 g carbohydrate = 4 kcal
1 g fat   = 9 kcal
1 g protein   = 4 kcal

in all. A half-cup of vegetables (not including starchy vegetables) contains 5 g carbohydrate (20 kcal) and 2 g protein (8 more) and has been rounded *down* to 25 kcal. (This slight understatement of the energy value of vegetables is probably intended to encourage people to use them in abundance. At 25 kcal a serving, you could consume eight servings of vegetables for less than the kcalorie cost of a single hamburger patty.)

The complete exchange systems used in the United States and Canada are presented in Appendix L. If you familiarize yourself with the specific foods in each list, you can become quite proficient at diet planning or diet evaluation.

Suppose that one day's meals consisted of the menus illustrated here. That day's meals contain the following carbohydrate exchanges:

Breakfast:	1 bread
Lunch:	2 bread
	2 tsp sugar[7]
	1 milk
Dinner:	2 bread[8]
	1 vegetable[9]
Snack:[10]	1 bread
	1 fruit
	6 tsp sugar

Thus your total carbohydrate consumption for the day is:

6 bread	= 90	g carbohydrate
8 tsp sugar	= 40	
1 milk	= 12	
1 vegetable	= 5	
1 fruit	= 10	
Total:	157	g carbohydrate

This is more than the recommended 125 g and so is adequate in carbohydrate.

This kind of calculation provides only an estimate but is close enough for most purposes. A more accurate way to determine the carbohydrate composition of foods is to refer to Appendix H, which lists individual foods rather than food groups. Adding the carbohydrate values obtained from Appendix H yields 138 g carbohydrate.

[7]The sandwich contains 2 tsp jelly.

[8]This is a 1 c serving of mashed potato.

[9]This is a 1/2 c serving of green beans.

[10]This is a 2-inch diameter biscuit with 3/4 c strawberries, 1 tbsp heavy cream, and 6 tsp sugar added in preparation.

Complete lists of the foods in each group appear in Appendix L.

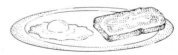

Breakfast:
fried egg
toast with margarine

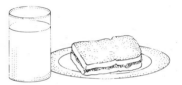

Lunch:
peanut butter and jelly sandwich
milk

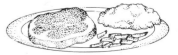

Dinner:
6-oz steak
green beans
mashed potato with margarine

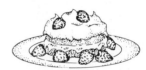

Evening snack:
strawberry shortcake
whipped cream

The difference between the 157-g estimate and the 138-g amount obtained by the more accurate calculation may be disconcerting. Rough estimates are often more valuable than close calculations, however, because of the time saved and because often only a "ballpark" figure is needed. In this example, we know that 50 g carbohydrate would be too little, but 260 would be more than twice the recommended amount (125 g). The numbers 157 and 138 both fall between these extremes; the difference between them becomes insignificant from this perspective.

Most estimates of the nutrient contents of foods are rough but serviceable approximations. In this book we refer repeatedly to a "90-kcal potato"; you should understand this to mean "90 plus-or-minus-about-20-percent," which makes it not significantly different from a 100-kcal potato. In general, for most purposes, a variation of about 20 percent is tolerable.

It takes only one or two calculations of this kind to get a feel for the carbohydrate content of your diet. Once you are aware of the major carbohydrate-contributing foods you eat, you can return to thinking in terms of these foods alone, developing a sense of how much of each is enough.

Food groups emphasize protein, vitamins, and minerals.

Food Group Plans   Food group plans emphasize the protein, vitamin, and mineral contents of foods and are quite inexact with respect to carbohydrate, fat, and kcalories. Still, they have their uses. The most familiar of them is the Four Food Group Plan. This plan separates nutritious foods into the four groups shown in Table 3. For an adequate diet, an adult should select a 2-2-4-4 pattern each day: two servings from the milk group, two from the meat group, four from the fruit/vegetable group, and four from the bread/cereal group.

This pattern ensures diet adequacy for several important nutrients. Two servings of milk or milk products (including cheese) provide some of the protein and most of the calcium needed by an adult in a day. Two servings of meat or meat substitutes complete the protein requirement and make a substantial contribution of iron. Four servings of fruits and vegetables (including starchy vegetables), if properly chosen, will meet the needs for vitamin A and vitamin C. These three groups also contribute B vitamins. Four servings of grain products (breads and cereals) add additional B vitamins and iron.

A complete presentation of the Four Food Group Plan, with its uses and limitations, is presented in Appendix M. For the remainder of Part

Table 3. Servings in the Four Food Group Plan*

Food group	Recommended number of servings (adult)	Serving size
Meat and meat substitutes	2	2-3 oz cooked meat, fish, or chicken; 1 c cooked legumes
Milk and milk products	2[†]	1 c (8 oz) milk; 1-2 oz cheese
Fruits and vegetables	4[‡]	1/2 c fruit, vegetable, or juice
Grains (bread and cereal products)	4[§]	1 slice bread; 1/2 c cooked cereal; 1 c ready-to-eat cereal

*For further details, see Appendix M.

†For children up to 9, 2-3 c; for children 9 to 12, 3-4 c; for teenagers and pregnant women, 3-4 c; for nursing mothers, 4 c or more.

‡One should be rich in vitamin C; at least one every other day should be rich in vitamin A.

§Enriched or whole-grain products only.

One, which deals with carbohydrate, fat, protein, and kcalories, the exchange system will be emphasized. In Part Two the uses of the Four Food Group Plan will become more apparent. With practice, you can use both to great advantage.

Before leaving this subject, however, you might look back at the day's meals just presented and ask whether they meet the recommendations of the Four Food Group Plan. Inspection will show that the foods chosen fall short because they include only one milk serving and poor choices in the fruit/vegetable group. A complete analysis would show that as a consequence the day's intakes of calcium and vitamin A were less than ideal.

This chapter began by showing you how important glucose is for the functioning of the brain and the body's other tissues. Then it went on to demonstrate how the body can derive glucose from all carbohydrates. Finally, it showed where the carbohydrates are in foods. Armed with this information, you can explode some of the myths perpetrated by television commercials advertising sweets. Sugar is brain food? True, but which sugar are we talking about? Not sucrose! When you need quick energy, what is the best source? A candy bar? A coke? No. Carbohydrate-containing *foods* are a better choice, for many reasons.

Summing Up

The world's people derive 50 to 80 percent of their food energy from carbohydrate, most of it from starch, although sugar (sucrose) can make a large contribution to their diet. The carbohydrates can be grouped into complex carbohydrates—the polysaccharides—and simple carbohydrates—the mono- and disaccharides.

Of the monosaccharides, fructose, or fruit sugar, is the sweetest; it gives honey, syrup, and many fruits their sweet flavor. Both fructose and glucose are found free in these and other plant foods. All three monosaccharides—glucose, fructose, and galactose—share the chemical formula $C_6H_{12}O_6$, but they differ in the arrangement of their atoms. This difference in arrangement gives each its particular character.

Each of the three disaccharides contains a molecule of glucose paired with another monosaccharide. The two disaccharides of importance in nutrition are lactose and sucrose. Lactose is the simple carbohydrate of milk. It is very digestible, except by those who lack the digestive enzyme to hydrolyze lactose and thus are lactose-intolerant. Sucrose, or table sugar, is the sugar of candies, sweets, and confections. (It is featured in Highlight 1.) Nutritionists are attempting to decide whether sucrose is innocent or guilty-as-charged in the rising incidence of diabetes and heart disease.

Of the polysaccharides, starch and cellulose are found in plants. Starch is found predominantly in grains and starchy vegetables; cellulose is found in all plants, especially as the bran in wheat. Cellulose, being an indigestible carbohydrate, provides the diet with fiber. Other fibers occurring in plant foods are pectin, hemicellulose, and lignin (a noncarbohydrate). Glycogen, or animal starch, is the polysaccharide synthesized in animal liver and muscle from temporary excess glucose. All three polysaccharides are chains of glucose units strung together. Cellulose is indigestible because of a difference in the character of the bonds holding the glucose units together.

People need about 125 grams of carbohydrate or more each day, preferably mostly as complex carbohydrate. Food grouping systems enable consumers to estimate the amounts of nutrients in foods; for carbohydrate the most useful system is the exchange system. The exchange system groups foods according to their carbohydrate, fat, and protein content and includes four groups of food containing carbohydrate: milk (12 g per cup), vegetable (5 g per half-cup serving), fruit (10 g per serving), and bread (15 g per serving). In addition to these four groups, a category that might be called the sugar group contributes 5 g per teaspoon; an 8-oz cola beverage contains 6 tsp. These five groups of food constitute a complete list of the carbohydrate-containing foods in the diet.

The more familiar Four Food Group Plan is not so useful for estimating carbohydrate and fat intakes as for estimating protein, vitamin, and mineral intakes, but it is introduced here for later use. The food groups and recommended servings are shown in Table 3.

Sugar: Is It "Bad" for You?

Rabbit said, "Honey or condensed milk with your bread?" [Pooh] was so excited that he said, "Both," and then, so as not to seem greedy, he added, "But don't bother about the bread, please."

A. A. MILNE, *Winnie the Pooh*

A heated argument over sugar is presently in progress in the nutrition literature. The questions being debated are: (1) How much sugar do North Americans consume? (2) Is the consumption of refined sugar a causative factor in the rising incidence of diabetes and cardiovascular diseases? (3) Is sugar a physiologically worthless substance, a contributor of empty kcalories? The answers to these questions are often contradictory.

It is important to understand the term *sugar* in the context of this discussion. *Sugar in the United States or Canadian diet* includes all the sugars that occur naturally in foods, such as lactose in milk or fructose in fruits, as well as sugar that is provided by caloric sweeteners. The major caloric sweeteners are refined sugar, corn syrup, and corn sugar; others include honey, maple syrup, sorghum, and molasses. About 98 percent of the sweeteners consumed in the United States are white, granulated table sugar; brown sugar or packaged raw sugar; pancake syrups; or sugar used in preparation of such food products as cakes, pies, cookies, candy, cola beverages, and alcohol.[1] These sweeteners, and not the naturally occurring

sugars in foods, are the subject of this Highlight.

Some areas of agreement on the dietary role of sugar appear in the literature. For one thing, it is known that obesity correlates with both diabetes and cardiovascular diseases. Obesity has become a prime health problem in this country, largely because we are exercising less than previous generations. Excess energy intake from any energy source, including sugar, can only exacerbate this problem. One 12-oz fruit-flavored carbonated drink, for instance, contributes about 170 kcal (see Appendix H). Any time a person consumes about 3,500 kcal in excess of need, a pound of fat is produced. In other words, if you drink one 12-oz orange soda a day in excess of your energy need, you will gain a pound about every 20 days.

Another concern that nutritionists share is that in

some individuals kcalories from sugar may be replacing kcalories from other carbohydrate sources, which would contribute vitamins, minerals, protein, complex carbohydrates, and fiber in addition to the kcalories. You may know someone who says, "I can't eat that baked potato because I have to count my kcalories," and then drinks a cola beverage without giving a thought to its kcaloric content. Yet a baked potato of medium size has only about 90 kcal and gives the body at the same time 3 g protein, 21 g complex carbohydrates, 9 mg calcium, and 20 mg vitamin C. (Notice that nothing has been said about the kcalories from the butter or sour cream that may be on that potato.) Table 1 compares the nutrients contributed by 100-kcal portions of several supposedly high-kcalorie foods with 100-kcal portions of table sugar and cola beverage.

Another thing that nutritionists agree on is the role of sweeteners in the development of dental caries. Of all the carbohydrates we eat, sucrose is the one most readily used by mouth bacteria for producing acid and is the most consistently damaging to the teeth. The longer the acid is allowed to remain in contact with the enamel, the greater the damage. Eventually the enamel is broken down, and a cavity forms. The American Dental Association recommends that you

[1]L. Page and B. Friend, Level of use of sugars in the United States, in *Sugars in Nutrition*, ed. H. L. Sipple and K. W. McNutt (New York: Academic Press, 1974), p. 99.

Table 1. Nutrient Composition of Selected Foods

Food	Size of 100-kcal portion	Percentage of U.S.RDA*							
		Pro-tein	Cal-cium	Iron	Vita-min A	Thia-min	Ribo-flavin	Nia-cin	Vita-min C
Bread, whole wheat	1 1/2 slices	7	4	7	—	9	3	6	—
Cereal, enriched 40% bran	1 c	6	3	68	0	9	4	11	0
Cola beverage	1 c	0	0	0	0	0	0	0	0
Lima beans	1/2 c	10	4	12	5	10	5	6	25
Milk, partly skim 2% fat	3/4 c	17	26	—	3	5	23	—	3
Sugar, white	2 1/2 tsp	0	0	0	0	0	0	0	0
Sweet potatoes	2/3 potato (5" × 2")	2	3	4	118	4	3	2	26

*Percentages are rounded to nearest whole number. A dash means the percentage has not been determined and is insignificant. The U.S. RDAs are explained on pp. 440-441.

select foods and snacks that are lower in sucrose content—for example, more milk and less chocolate milk, more fresh fruits and fewer dried fruits, more popcorn or toast and fewer sweet rolls or cookies, more sugar-free soft drinks and fewer drinks flavored with caloric sweeteners.[2]

Although these three areas—obesity, displacement of foods that contribute a variety of nutrients, and dental caries—may be related to excess sugar consumption, the questions outlined at the beginning of this Highlight

[2]*A Snacking Guide More or Less* (Chicago: American Dental Association, 1975).

remain. Let us examine each of these.

How Much Sugar Do We Consume? During the last 60 years, the pattern of carbohydrate consumption in the U.S. has shifted, with potato and cereal consumption dropping about 50 percent, vegetable (other than the potato) and fruit consumption remaining about the same, and sugar consumption rising about 20 percent. The effect is shown in Figure 1. The rise in sugar consumption does not include the sugar used in the manufacture of alcoholic beverages. Dr. John Yudkin, of the Department of Nu-

trition, London University, has estimated that if alcoholic beverages are included, the consumption of sugar per person averages about 126 lb.[3]

You may be able to say truthfully that you have not eaten 126 lb of sugar in a year, that you drink your coffee black, that you don't eat much cake or pie, and that you never drink cola or alcoholic beverages. However, if Dr. Yudkin's estimate is correct, this means that for every person like you there is

[3]U.S. Senate, Select Committee on Nutrition and Human Needs, *Nutrition and Diseases* (Washington, D.C.: Government Printing Office, 1973), p. 147.

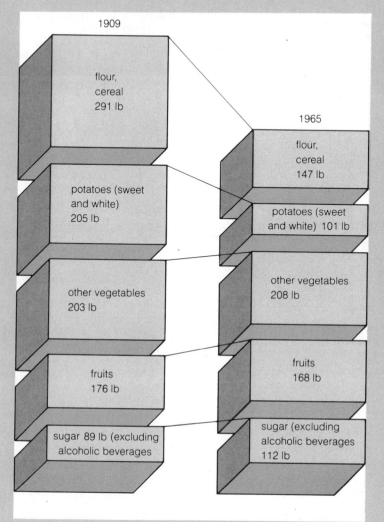

1909

flour,
cereal
291 lb

potatoes (sweet
and white)
205 lb

other vegetables
203 lb

fruits
176 lb

sugar 89 lb (excluding
alcoholic beverages

1965

flour,
cereal
147 lb

potatoes (sweet
and white) 101 lb

other vegetables
208 lb

fruits
168 lb

sugar (excluding
alcoholic beverages
112 lb

Figure 1 Trends in average yearly carbohydrate consumption per person.

Adapted from Berta Friend, Nutrients in U.S. food supply, *American Journal of Clinical Nutrition* 20(1967):8.

that sugar consumption rose markedly prior to 1925, but he believes that it has not increased appreciably since then.[5] Food consumption tables published by the U.S. Department of Agriculture really concern the disappearance of the food from the market, he points out, and do not accurately reflect the food actually consumed. Dr. Stare estimates that the average per capita intake of sugar is about 80 lb per year in the United States.

Dr. Louise Page and Dr. Berta Friend, nutrition analysts with the Consumer and Food Economics Institute of the U. S. Department of Agriculture, state that there has been a one-third increase in the amount of refined sugar used per capita in this century, even though the consumption of all carbohydrates has dropped by about one-fourth. At the present time, each person consumes approximately 102 lb of refined sugar per year, they say. Beverages account for the largest industrial use of sugar, about one-fifth; cereal and bakery goods account for

another who consumes enormous amounts of sugar, thereby bringing the average up to 126 lb. It has been estimated that some teenage boys consume about 400 lb of sugar a year, mostly in the form of carbonated beverages and snack foods.[4].

[4]J. Yudkin, in U.S. Senate, Select Committee on Nutrition and Human Needs, *Dietary Sugar and Disease (Hearings)* (Washington, D.C.: Government Printing Office, 1973), pp. 233-236.

Figure 2 shows the consumption of soft drinks by individuals of different ages in Canada and the United States. Note that adult males in Canada and adolescent males in the United States have the highest consumption.

Other scientists disagree with Yudkin's claim. Notable among them is Dr. Frederick J. Stare, Department of Nutrition, Harvard School of Public Health. Dr. Stare agrees

[5]F. J. Stare, Role of sugar in modern nutrition, in *World Review of Nutrition and Dietetics* 22, ed. G. F. Bourne (Basel: S. Karger, 1975), pp. 239-247.

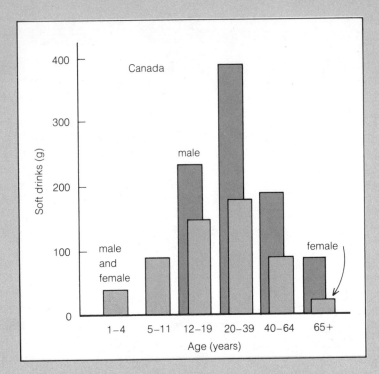

Adapted from *Food Consumption Patterns Report*, a report from Nutrition Canada by the Bureau of Nutritional Sciences, Health Protection Branch, Department of National Health and Welfare, 1970-1972.

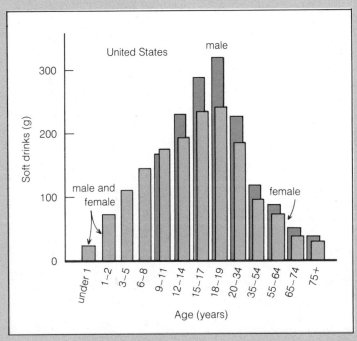

From L. Page and B. Friend, Level of use of sugars in the United States, in *Sugars in Nutrition*, ed. H. L. Sipple and K. W. McNutt (New York: Academic Press, 1974), chap. 7.

Figure 2   Average daily consumption of soft drinks per person in Canada and the United States.

about one-sixth of the total used.[6]

In neighboring Canada, a study of food consumption patterns was conducted using a method of gathering data that Dr. Stare would approve of. People in various regions were asked to name the exact quantities of the foods they had eaten on the previous day. From this diet recall study it was determined that adolescent males in Canada consume about 210 lb a year of foods that are primarily sugar (such as candy and cake icings), and sugar in soft drinks, on cereal, and in coffee. Adult males, ages 20 to 39 years, consume about 165 lb of such foods a year.[7] It is impossible to compare pounds of sugar disappearing from the market (the U.S. study) with pounds of sugary foods that have been eaten (the Canadian study), and it is equally difficult to compare the average amount of sugar consumed by all ages with the amount used by a single age group. Nevertheless, the

[6]Page and Friend, 1974, p. 96.
[7]Department of National Health and Welfare, *Food Consumption Patterns Report*, a report from *Nutrition Canada* by the Bureau of Nutritional Sciences Health Protection Branch, 1970-1972.

data show that the Canadian consumption of sugar was not dramatically lower than U.S. consumption. The one observation that can be made is that both these countries, with their similar lifestyles and exposure to the same sort of advertising, consume large quantities of caloric sweeteners.

Is Increased Consumption of Refined Sugar Causing a Rising Incidence of Diabetes and Cardiovascular Disease?

Diabetes and cardiovascular disease account for a much larger percentage of deaths than they did half a century ago. About half of all the people who die in the United States today die of heart disease. It is very likely that diabetes contributes to a number of these deaths but does not appear on the death certificate as the primary cause.

Concern over the rising incidence of these two diseases and consumption of sugar prompted the United States Senate in 1973 to form a select committee to conduct hearings on "Sugar in Diet, Diabetes, and Heart Disease." Scientists from various parts of the world who had been studying the relationship of sugar to these diseases were invited to appear before the committee. Among the many interesting testimonies presented was one by Dr. Aharon M. Cohen of the Hebrew University, Hadassah

---

Mini-Glossary

caloric: containing energy or kcalories.

calor = heat

(**noncaloric:** kcalorie-free)

cardiovascular disease: a disease affecting the heart or circulatory system. (See the description of atherosclerosis in Highlight 6.)

correlation: the simultaneous increase or decrease of two variables.

dental caries (CARE-eez): tooth decay, cavities.

diabetes (dye-uh-BEET-eez): a hereditary metabolic disease characterized by an inadequate supply of effective insulin, which renders an individual unable to regulate blood glucose level normally. Diabetes affects carbohydrate, fat, and protein metabolism and gives rise to pathological changes in nerves and blood vessels. Diabetes is properly called diabetes mellitus.

empty-kcalorie food: a popular term used to denote foods contributing kcalories relatively empty of the nutrients protein, vitamins, and minerals. The most notorious empty-kcalorie foods are sugar, fat, and alcohol.

epidemiology (ep-uh-deem-ee-OLL-uh-gee): the study of the incidence and distribution of disease in a population.

etiology (ee-tee-OLL-uh-gee): causation, the study of all of the causes. The term is used especially with respect to disease.

junk food: a popular term used to denote foods that are "bad" for you—for example, foods high in salt, sugar, or fat content.

variable: a factor that may vary (increase or decrease). One variable may depend on another; for example, the height of the average child depends on his age. One variable may be independent of another; for example, the intelligence of a child is independent of his height.

Medical College of Jerusalem, Israel.[8]

Dr. Cohen had had the opportunity to study in his homeland the changes in dis-

[8]A. M. Cohen, High sucrose intake as a factor in the development of diabetes and its vascular complications, in U.S. Senate, Select Committee on Nutrition and Human Needs, *Dietary Sugar and Disease (Hearings)* (Washington, D.C.: Government Printing Office, 1973), pp. 167-198.

eases that occur when a group of people emigrate to a new culture. He studied the immigrants flowing from Yemen and the West into Jerusalem. Over a period of ten years, he tested 16,000 immigrants for diabetes. None of the 5,000 newly arrived Yemenites he tested had diabetes, although there was a remarkably high number of cases among the settled

Yemenites. A dietary study revealed that the Yemeni immigrants had not consumed sucrose before coming to Israel but soon afterward adopted a more Western diet, particularly in the use of sugar. Many of them, he found, drank large quantities of coffee, stirring five or six spoonfuls of sugar into each cup; moreover, they ate little other food in the early part of the day.

This digression is intended to help you learn to evaluate what you read about nutrition from experimental results. In Cohen's long-term study two variables increased at the same time: sugar consumption and diabetes. But noting a correlation between two variables does not necessarily mean that there is a cause-and-effect relationship between them. For example, you may notice that the sun always rises shortly after the milkman has made his delivery to your doorstep. This does not mean that the milkman causes the sun to rise. Further investigation would show that the milkman's coming and the sun's rising are independent events; either can happen without the other, although both tend to correlate with a third variable, the time of day. In

the same manner, noting that a rise in sugar consumption correlates with a rise in the incidence of diabetes does not proove that the sugar has caused the diabetes.

CAUTION WHEN YOU READ!

If A increases as B increases, or if A decreases as B decreases, it does not follow that A causes B. When you note such an association, ask yourself: Are there other variables with which both A and B may correlate?

There are many factors in the etiology of diabetes. One of these is age; another is heredity. Diabetes is usually an adult-onset disease. It may be that the cause of the diabetes in those Yemenites who immigrated to Israel was simply that they had become older; perhaps if they had remained in Yemen they would have developed diabetes with the same incidence. This possibility was studied; it was found that diabetes developed uniquely in the immigrants and not in those of the same age who remained in Yemen.

The factor of heredity was also considered. Those who developed diabetes and

those who did not had a common racial background; but if they had come from different racial groups, the fact that one group (consuming sucrose) had become diabetic while the other group (consuming no sucrose) had not might reflect differences in their genetic makeup and be unrelated to the differences in their diets.

In epidemiological studies of human beings, many variables are present that are not identified. Dr. Cohen could not expect that the 5,000 Yemenites he tested had lived lives in every respect identical to those of their countrymen who had stayed in Yemen. It might be that some other unidentified factor in their new environment was responsible for their becoming diabetic after living some years in Jerusalem.

CAUTION WHEN YOU READ!

When epidemiological studies are made, many variables are present that are not identified. Ask yourself: Did the researcher consider the many possible variables that might have had an effect on the results?

One way to test theories resulting from an epidemiological study on human beings is to design an experiment using animals in which all variables other than the one in question (in this case, sugar in the diet) can be kept constant. Animals with physiological systems similar to the human system under study are excellent subjects for examining a human disease theory. Such animals can share a common heredity, their life span is short compared to that of human beings, and they can be maintained in laboratory conditions, where most variables can be controlled.

CAUTION WHEN YOU READ!

When animals are used as experimental subjects, most variables can be controlled. Ask yourself: Did the researcher design the experiment so that the variables critical to this study were controlled?

To test the theory that diabetes is more likely to result when sucrose replaces complex carbohydrates in a diet, Dr. Cohen designed an experiment using rats. He controlled the genetic factor by breeding a uniform strain of rats that were particularly sensitive to sucrose feeding. He divided this new strain into two groups: One group was fed a high-starch diet, and the other group was fed a diet in which sugar, providing the same number of kcalories, replaced the starch.

In the animals fed the starch diet, the tissues of the kidney and the retina of the eye remained normal. However, in the animals fed a high-sucrose diet, these tissues showed a type of damage similar to that seen in the diabetic human; that is, the blood vessels were constricted, and there were deformities in the tissues of the kidneys and the retina.

Cohen came to the conclusion that this experiment offered hope to potential diabetics: If from birth they consume a low-sucrose diet, they may never become diabetic.

Has it then been firmly established that the rising intake of sugar has precipitated the rise in the incidence of diabetes? No. Certainly Cohen's studies suggest a correlation and point toward the use of complex carbohydrates instead of refined sugar in the diet. However, it is not clear that sugar consumption in the United States has risen in parallel with the rise in diabetes. Even if it has, what has been observed in the United States and Israel is a correlation, not a cause-and-effect relationship. Perhaps both diabetes and cardiovascular disease are on the rise because they are more often correctly diagnosed than formerly or because the incidence of other diseases, such as tuberculosis and diphtheria, has fallen. Perhaps early diagnosis and treatment of diabetics is allowing them to live long enough to produce offspring who carry the genes for the disease, thus adding to the number of potential diabetics in the population.

Some competent authorities dispute the view that sugar intake causes diabetes. Dr. E. L. Bierman and Dr. R. Nelson, of the University of Washington School of Medicine and the Mayo Clinic, state that "the cause of primary diabetes mellitus in man remains unknown. There is no evidence that excessive consumption of sugar causes diabetes."[9]

Similarly, Dr. F. Grande, School of Public Health, University of Minnesota, does not attribute significance to the correlation between rising sugar consumption and rising deaths from coronary heart disease. He states that the true rate of individuals' consumption of sugar is unknown and that the rise in deaths from coronary heart disease may be due in

[9]E. L. Bierman and R. Nelson, Carbohydrates, diabetes, and blood lipids, in *World Review of Nutrition and Dietetics* 22, ed. G. F. Bourne (Basel: S. Karger, 1975), pp. 280-287.

changes in medical diagnosis of the causes of death.[10] The whole question of cardiovascular disease is so complex that further discussion of it has been reserved for Highlight 6. Meanwhile, the third question concerning the value of sugar in the diet needs to be discussed.

Is Sugar "Physiologically Worthless" and a Contributor of "Empty kCalories"?   Sugar, in the process of metabolism, eventually becomes the equivalent of two molecules of glucose. Glucose is used for energy to power the body. If glucose is needed, then the sucrose that provides it is not physiologically worthless.

The term *empty kcalories* (or a similarly pejorative term like *junk food*) is often used to denote foods that contribute no nutrients like amino acids, vitamins, and minerals. Some nutritionists object to the use of the term, since a large portion of the world's population is kcalorie-poor. They believe that sugar's relatively cheap kcalories could protect the small amount of locally available protein from use as an energy source. There is some merit to this point of

view, but it does not hold for the developed countries, where kcalories are abundant. Meanwhile, the original question remains.

Is Sugar "Bad" for You?
There is no reason to believe that the moderate consumption of sugar (5 to 10 percent of kcalories) is in any way dangerous to the normal, healthy human being.[11] Clearly, however, it may be associated with other factors that are harmful: obesity, the displacement of needed nutrients and fiber, and dental decay. If on these grounds you conclude that sugar is indeed to be avoided, it is important to recognize that other caloric sweeteners, such as honey, are no better.

You should also note that sugar is hidden in many supposedly healthful products. The advertising industry would have us believe that some products provide an excellent replacement for a balanced meal. One such product, advertised as a substitute for breakfast, contains more sugar than any other single ingredient. Labeling laws require that food ingredients be listed on the container in the order of their weight, with the ingredient

in the largest amount listed first. In the breakfast substitute just mentioned, the first three ingredients are refined sugar, vegetable shortening, and water. The recommended serving contains 370 kcal. For only 335 kcal, you could have 1/2 c orange juice (60), a poached egg on toast (150), a pat of margarine (35), and a cup of skim milk (90). This breakfast of real foods provides complex carbohydrate in contrast to the simple sugar in the substitute. The fat in the foods is less saturated (see Chapter 2) than in the substitute. The protein from eggs and milk is of high quality, and the bread contributes needed fiber. As for the vitamins and minerals, you can be sure that the foods contain many, whereas the substitute may contain only those listed on the label. In reality, then, although you can't tell from the label, the substitute is far inferior.

The dieter who is limiting his kcalories needs especially to choose nutritious foods because he has a smaller kcalorie allowance within which to get his nutrients. Weight Watchers, Inc. recommends refusing foods when the label puts sugar in the first or second place. Sugar is "bad" for the dieter, not because it is poisonous but because it displaces nutritious foods.

On the other hand, energy is the prime nutritional need of humans. People in many countries suffer severe

[10]F. Grande, Sugar and cardiovascular disease, in *World Review of Nutrition and Dietetics* 22, ed. G. F. Bourne (Basel: S. Karger, 1975), pp. 248-269.

[11]W. E. Connor and S. L. Connor, Sucrose and carbohydrate, in *Nutrition Reviews' Present Knowledge in Nutrition* (New York: The Nutrition Foundation, Inc., 1976), pp. 33-42.

malnutrition from an energy deficit. If sugar is available to make up this deficit, it may be considered a life-saving resource.

In answer to the question Is sugar "bad" for you? we have to say we don't know. But if you turn the question around to ask Is sugar "good" for you? we can answer a definite no. Except for energy, refined sugar contributes nothing. And the body can derive all the energy it needs from nutritious food.

Carbohydrate

If you have decided to study your own diet as you read this book, then you have already recorded your food intakes for three days and determined your average intakes for several nutrients, as instructed in the Self-Study following the introduction to Part One. Exercises 1 to 6 make use of the information you recorded there.

1. How many grams of carbohydrate do you consume in a day?

2. How many kcalories does this represent? (Remember, a gram of carbohydrate contributes 4 kcal.)

3. One estimate sets the amount of carbohydrate needed every day at no less than 500 kcal.[1] How does your intake compare with this minimum?

4. What percentage of your total kcalories is contributed by carbohydrate? (To figure this, divide your carbohydrate kcalories by your total kcalories, then multiply by 100.)

5. A dietary goal quoted in Chapter 1 was for carbohydrate to contribute about 60 percent of the total kcalories (58 percent, to be exact). How does your carbohydrate intake compare with this recommendation? (Note: If you are on a diet to lose weight, then this goal does not apply to you. See the

[1]N. Kretchmer, Lactose and lactase, *Scientific American* 227 (1972):71-78.

exercises in Self-Study: Diet Planning, which begins on p. 310.

6. Another dietary goal was for no more than 10 percent of total kcalories to come from refined and other processed sugars and foods high in such sugars. The other 48 percent or more was to come from complex carbohydrates and naturally occurring sugars, such as those in fresh fruits. To compare your carbohydrate intake with these goals, study the records you made on Form 1 (p. 14). List all the foods you consumed that provided carbohydrate (for simplicity's sake, you could omit those that provided fewer than, say, 5 g carbohydrate). Divide these foods into two categories: "sugary foods" and "complex carbohydrate-natural sugar foods." Compute how many grams of carbohydrate you consumed in each of these categories for the three-day period you studied and divide by three to find out how many grams of each type you consume in a day.

Now convert these gram figures to kcalories.

Finally, determine what percentages of your total

kcalorie intake these figures represent. How do these intakes compare with the dietary goals of 10 percent from "sugars" and 48 percent from "complex carbohydrate-natural sugars"? What implications do you find here for changing your diet, if any? If a change should be needed, what foods should be emphasized?

Optional Extras

● You can also estimate, if you wish, how many pounds of sugar you eat in a year (1 lb = 454 g). How does your yearly sugar intake compare with the estimated averages cited in Highlight 1? (If you need additional information on the sugar contents of foods you eat, try looking in Appendix F.)

● To reduce your sugar purchases, learn to read labels. If sugar is listed first or second on the list of ingredients, then it is the most or second-most abundant ingredient in the package. Next time you go shopping, compare brands to see if you can buy the items you want with less sugar. For example, frozen strawberries can be bought with or without sugar.

● Appendix F lists about 80 cereals and shows the percentage of sucrose in each. How many of these cereals are primarily a sugar product and not a grain product? Can you find others in the supermarket that have sugar listed third or below third in the ranking of ingredients? Are there any cereals that do not list sugar at all? (At last inspection we were able to find only three such cereals.) Remember to include sugar's sisters—honey, corn syrup, and the like—when you do this exercise.

● Notice your own serving sizes. Many people think that the spoon they use for sugar holds 1 tsp, but when it is heaped high with sugar it may hold more nearly 2 tsp. Using your sugar spoon as you usually do, spoon ten helpings of sugar into a bowl. Now measure this sugar with a measuring spoon, using level spoonfuls. How many teaspoons is a spoonful of sugar as you use it.

● Visualize your sugar intake. Having calculated (in Exercise 6) how many grams of sugar you consume in a day, you can now look at this amount of sugar and see how much it is. Measure into a glass or jar the amount of sugar you consume in a day (it may help you to know that 1 tsp is about 5 g). People often find this to be a surprising experience.

● We have emphasized the digestible carbohydrates in this Self-Study, but you may be interested in computing fiber intake as well. To get a rough idea of the amount of fiber you consume, turn to Appendix K. We can offer no guidelines for the appropriate amount of fiber for a day, but it might be interesting to compare your fiber intake with the estimated 6 g (crude fiber) provided by the typical U.S. diet in about 1900 and with the estimated 4 g provided today. Some authorities believe that 6 or more grams per day is a desirable intake.[2]

[2]We offered a more complete discussion of the fiber question in E. M. N. Hamilton and E. N. Whitney, Controversy 2: Fiber, *Nutrition: Concepts and Controversies* (St. Paul: West, 1979), pp. 78-80.

CHAPTER 2

CONTENTS

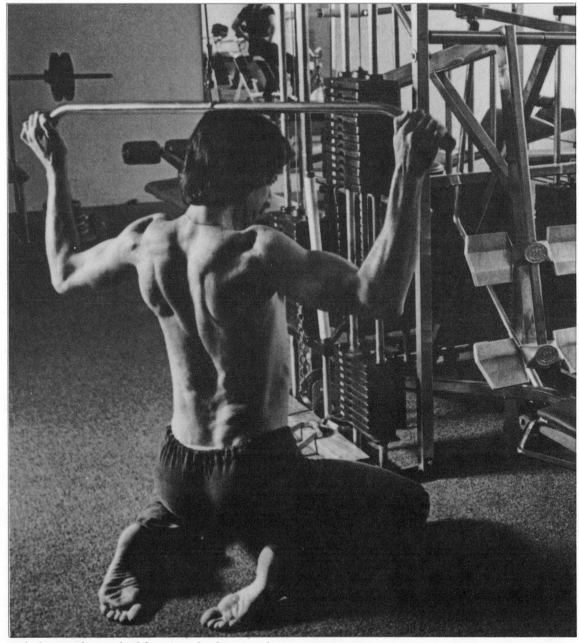

Body fat provides much of the energy for these muscles.

THE LIPIDS: Fats and Oils

The notion that matter is something inert and uninteresting is surely the veriest nonsense. If there is anything more wonderful than matter in the sheer versatility of its behavior, I have yet to hear tell of it.

FRED HOYLE

You have been conditioned to believe that slim is beautiful. The less fat you carry on your frame, the lovelier (sexier, healthier) you are thought to be. On the other hand, your body fat does things for you that you would be hard put to do without. If you carry neither too much nor too little body fat, you will enjoy the benefits nature intended in providing stores of this very important nutrient.

Although a third of the world's population is underfed, at least a third of our population is overfed. And indeed, overweight is a major health problem in the developed countries, contributing to the incidence of heart disease, diabetes, and many other ills.

Fat in the Body: Pros and Cons

The fats—more properly called the lipids—are actually a family of compounds that include both fats and oils. Both fats and oils occur in your body, and both help to keep it healthy. Natural oils in the skin provide a radiant complexion; in the scalp they help nourish the hair and make it glossy. The layer of fat beneath the skin, being a poor conductor of heat, insulates the body from extremes of temperature. A pad of hard fat beneath each kidney protects it from being jarred and damaged, even during a motorcycle ride on a bumpy road. The soft fat in the breasts of a woman protects her mammary glands from heat and cold and cushions them against shock. The fat that lies embedded in the muscle tissue shares with muscle glycogen the task of providing energy when the muscle cells are active.

An uninterrupted flow of energy is so vital to life that in a pinch any other function is sacrificed to maintain it. If a growing child is fed too little food, for example, the food she does consume will be used for energy to keep her heart and lungs going, but her growth will come to a standstill. To go totally without an energy supply, even for a few

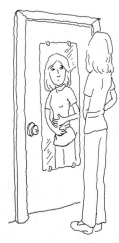

"I have *got* to go on a diet."

minutes, would be to die. The urgency of the need for energy has ensured, over the course of evolution, that all creatures have built-in reserves to protect themselves from ever being deprived of it. One provision against this sort of emergency has already been described in Chapter 1: the stores of glycogen—chains of sugar (glucose) units—in the liver that can be returned to circulation whenever the blood glucose supply runs short.

Fat cells are often called **adipose** (ADD-hi-poce) **cells.**

However, the liver cells can store only a limited amount of energy as glycogen; once this is depleted, the body must receive new food or turn to its backup reserve, the body fat. Unlike liver cells, fat cells have an unlimited storage capacity. During a prolonged period of food deprivation fat stores make an important contribution to energy needs.

1 lb "body fat" = 3,500 kcal (but see p. 238).

The average 20-year-old woman needs about 2,000 kcal a day to fuel her body's maintenance and activities. If she fasts (drinking only water to flush out her metabolic wastes), she will rapidly oxidize her own body fat. A pound of body fat provides 3,500 kcal. In conditions of enforced starvation, say, during a siege or famine, the fatter person has a better chance of surviving.

If you happen to be acquainted with a polar bear, you will be aware that the same thing is true for him. As he lumbers about on his iceberg, great masses of fat ripple beneath his thick fur coat. When he hibernates, he oxidizes that fat, extracting tens of thousands of kcalories from it to maintain his body temperature and to fuel other metabolic processes while he sleeps. Come spring, he is several hundred pounds thinner than when he went to sleep.

Since we do not yet anticipate facing a famine in this country, the thinner person actually has most of the advantages. To lose 50 pounds, you would have to deprive yourself of all food for at least three months—and for much longer if you didn't elect total starvation. No one acquainted with the risks of this course would undertake such a program except under close medical supervision.

ketones (KEE-tones): a condensation product of fat metabolism produced when carbohydrate is not available (see Chapter 7).

Living on body fat has other disadvantages. Fat can provide energy—but not as glucose, the form from which the brain and nerve cells can best extract energy. After a long period of glucose deprivation, these cells develop the ability to derive about half of their energy from a special form of fat known as ketones, but they still require glucose as

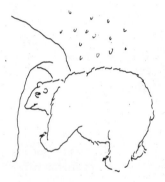
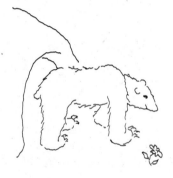

well. With the available glycogen long gone, they demand this glucose from the only alternative source—protein. And since no protein is coming in from food, the only supply is in the muscle and other lean tissues of the body. With the demand for body protein, these tissues atrophy, bringing on weakness, loss of function, and ultimately—when half the body protein has been used up—death. Death from loss of lean body mass will occur even in a fat person if a fast is too prolonged.

To sum up what's good about body fat: It helps maintain the health of the skin and hair, protects body organs from temperature extremes and mechanical shock, and provides a reserve fuel supply for use whenever body carbohydrate is depleted. As for what is bad about body fat: There can simply be too much of it. When fat is being oxidized for energy in the absence of glucose, ketones are formed to meet about half of the energy needs of the brain and nervous system. Protein released from wasting muscle and other lean tissue provides the other half.

atrophy (ATT-ro-fee): to waste away.

  a = without
  trophy = growth

For more about the dangers of fasting, see Highlight 8.

Fat in Foods: More Pros and Cons

Many of the compounds that give foods their flavor and aroma are found in fats and oils; they are fat-soluble. Four vitamins—A, D, E, and K—are also soluble in fat. Understanding this fact provides insight into many different areas in nutrition, so let us spend a moment here considering the phenomenon of fat solubility.

As you know, fats and oils tend to separate from water and watery substances. The oil floats to the top when salad dressing stands. As hot meat drippings cool, the fat separates and hardens on top of the other juices. You can probably think of many other examples of this phenomenon. Whenever a mixture of a fatty liquid and a watery liquid separates in this manner, the other compounds in the mixture must go with either the fat or the water. The nutritional significance of this is evident if you think what happens when the fat is removed from a food.

In general, foods from which the fat or oil has been removed lack much of their original flavor, aroma, and fat-soluble vitamin content. If you skin chicken meat before cooking it, the layer of fat is removed with the skin. The result is a tasteless, odorless meat. Chicken meat without its fat is almost indistinguishable from defatted veal or lamb or water-packed tuna; many of the compounds that give the meat its flavor are removed with the fat. The aromatic nature of many fat-soluble compounds becomes obvious when foods are cooking. Meat fat, especially from bacon, ham, pork, and fatty beef (hamburgers), and the fat added to vegetables—onions smothered in butter, french fries—all contribute to a "good food" smell. Milk when skimmed loses much of its buttery flavor too, and more importantly, it loses all of the vitamins A and D that the cow secreted into the milk. To make skim milk nutritionally equivalent to whole milk, these vitamins must be

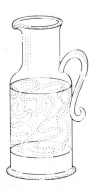

Fat solubility. Oil and water separate; fat-soluble compounds stay dissolved in the oil, water-soluble compounds in the water.

Fortification actually involves adding back more vitamin D than was in the whole milk originally (see Highlight 13).

Remember, fat is a more concentrated energy source than the other energy nutrients:

1 g carbohydrate = 4 kcal
1 g fat   = 9 kcal
1 g protein   = 4 kcal

mixed in; hence the "vitamin A & D fortified" label you see on skim milk.

An additional feature is lost when fat is removed: kcalories. A medium pork chop with the fat trimmed to within a half inch of the lean meat contains 260 kcal; with the fat trimmed off completely it contains 130 kcal. A baked potato with butter and sour cream (1 tbsp each) is 260 kcal; plain, it is 90 kcal. So it goes. The single most effective step you can take to reduce the energy (kcalorie) value of a food is to eat it without the fat.

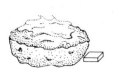

Pork chop with 1/2" fat (260 kcal)   Potato with 1 tbsp butter and 1 tbsp sour cream (260 kcal)   Whole milk, 1 c (170 kcal)

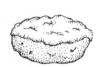

Pork chop with fat trimmed off (130 kcal)   Plain potato (90 kcal)   Skim milk, 1 c (80 kcal)

The Chemist's View of Fats

For a precise definition of triglycerides, the major class of dietary lipids, see p. 64.

"Your blood triglycerides are up." If a doctor says this, the patient may be alarmed, perhaps rightly. Most of us are aware nowadays that there is a close relationship between the fats in the blood and the health of the heart. A closer look at the fats will lay the foundation for an understanding of this relationship.

When we speak of fats, we are usually speaking of triglycerides. Almost all (95 percent) of the lipids in the diet are triglycerides. The other two classes of dietary lipids are the phospholipids—of which lecithin is one—and the sterols, including cholesterol. Phospholipids and sterols amount to only 5 percent of the dietary lipids. Because the triglycerides predominate in the diet, the following section focuses on them.

For a precise definition of phospholipids, a minor class of dietary lipids, and of sterols (including cholesterol), see p. 73-74.

Fats (lipids) in foods:

95 percent triglycerides (synonymous with fats and oils)

5 percent phospholipids (example: lecithin)
sterols (example: cholesterol)

The Triglycerides Triglycerides come in many sizes and several varieties, but they all share a common structure; they all have a "backbone" of glycerol to which three fatty acids are attached. All glycerol molecules are alike, but the fatty acids may vary in two ways: length and degree of saturation.

To understand the fats and the beneficial and harmful effects they have on your body, you must understand their molecular structure. It is not so complicated as it may seem at first. If you follow the few steps of reasoning presented here, you can reap an appreciation for the whole subject—and for its beauty—that you may never otherwise enjoy.

A fatty acid is a chain of carbon atoms with hydrogens attached and with an acid group (COOH) at one end. The fatty acid shown here is acetic acid, the compound that gives vinegar its sour taste:

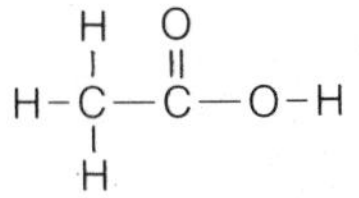

Acetic acid (a 2-carbon fatty acid)

This is the simplest of the fatty acids; the chain is only two carbon atoms long. A longer fatty acid may have four, six, eight (they mostly come in even numbers), or more carbon atoms. Among those common in dairy products are fatty acids that are six to ten carbons long. Butyric acid, which is present in butter, is a four-carbon fatty acid. Fatty acids that predominate in meat and fish are 14 or more carbon atoms long.

To illustrate the characteristics of these fatty acids, let us look at the 18-carbon series. Stearic acid is one of these:

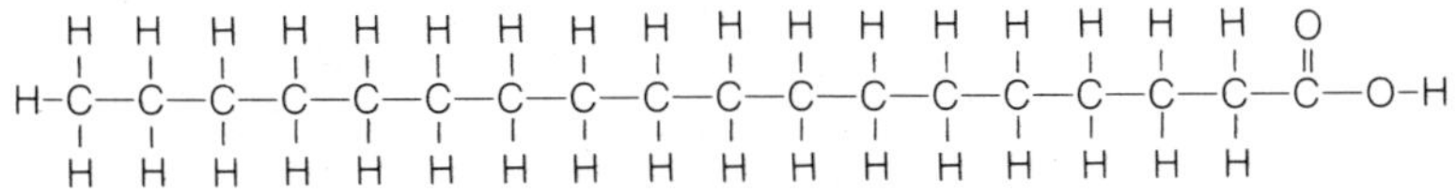

Stearic acid (an 18-carbon fatty acid)

A simpler way to depict this structure:

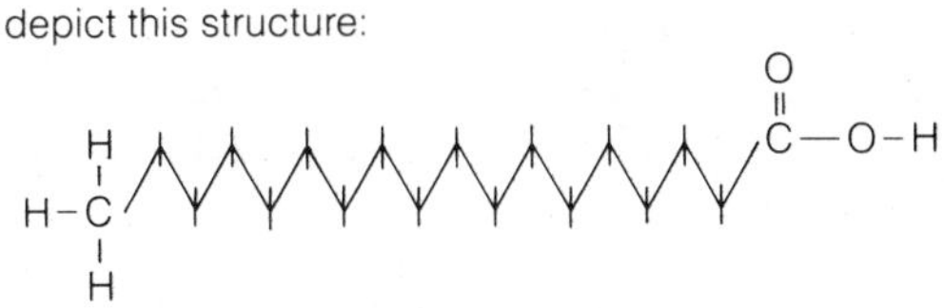

Each "corner" on the zigzag line represents a carbon atom with 2 attached Hs.
Still more simply, the lines representing bonds to the Hs can be left out:

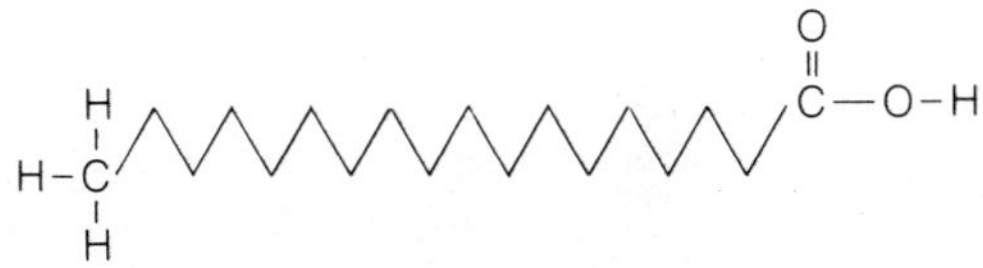

If you count the "corners," you will see that this still represents an 18-carbon fatty acid. This is the way fatty acids will be represented in many of the following diagrams.

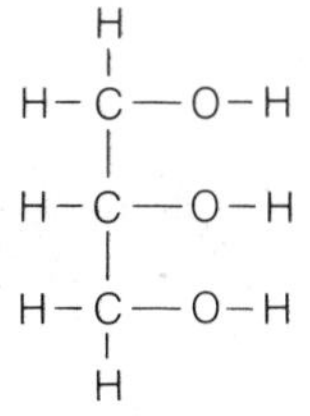

Glycerol

glycerol (GLIS-er-ol): a organic alcohol composed of a 3-carbon chain, each with an alcohol group attached. An alcohol is a compound containing a reactive OH group.

ol = alcohol

acid: a compound that tends to ionize in water solution, releasing H^+ ions. The more H^+ ions that are free in the water, the stronger the acid (see Appendix B).

acid group: the COOH group of an organic acid, which can also be represented

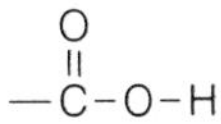

fatty acid: an organic compound composed of a carbon chain with hydrogens attached and an acid group at one end.

When a triglyceride forms, three fatty acids attach to a molecule of glycerol. A triglyceride composed of glycerol and three molecules of stearic acid is shown forming below. The resulting structure is called a fat (triglyceride).

triglyceride (try-GLIS-uh-ride): a compound composed of carbon, hydrogen, and oxygen arranged as a molecule of glycerol with three fatty acids attached to it.

tri = three (fatty acids)
glyceride = a compound of glycerol

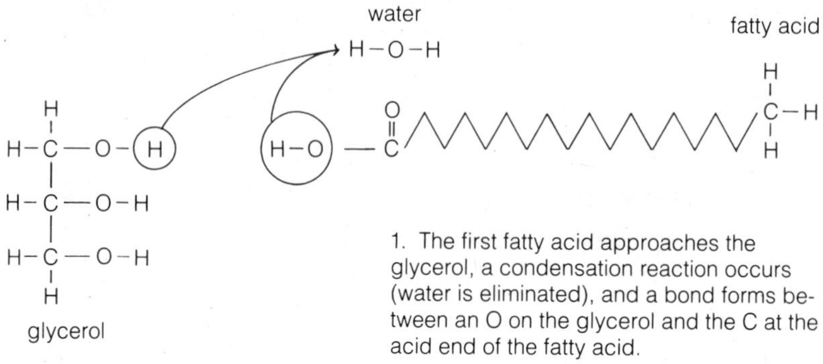

1. The first fatty acid approaches the glycerol, a condensation reaction occurs (water is eliminated), and a bond forms between an O on the glycerol and the C at the acid end of the fatty acid.

2. Later, 2 more fatty acids attach themselves to the glycerol by the same means; the resulting structure is a triglyceride.

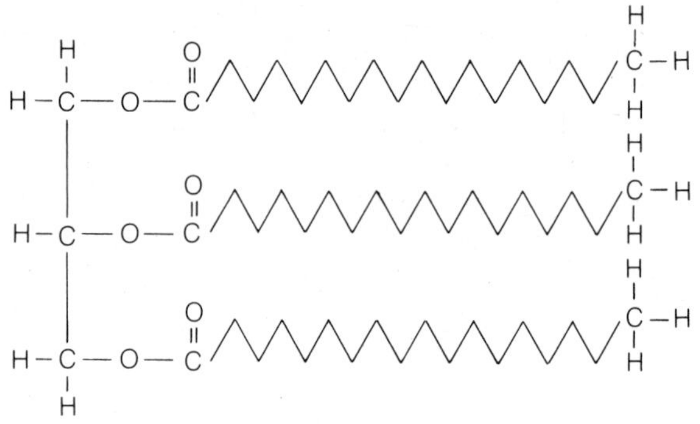

Formation of a fat (triglyceride).

A fat (triglyceride) that might be found in butter

saturated fatty acid: a fatty acid carrying the maximum possible number of hydrogen atoms—for example, stearic acid. Thus a **saturated fat** is composed of triglycerides in which a majority of the fatty acids are saturated.

fat: a mixture of mixed triglycerides.

impossible structure

People threatened with heart trouble may be told to reduce their intake of saturated fats and to increase their intake of polyunsaturated fats. Cutting out butter and using vegetable oil in its place is one way to do this. The triglyceride just shown is a saturated fat; it is loaded, or saturated, with all the hydrogen (H) atoms it can carry.

Some soft margarines are rich in polyunsaturated fats, triglycerides in which the fatty acids are carrying less than their full complement of hydrogens. To understand them, let us consider stearic acid once more. If we remove two Hs from the middle of the carbon chain, we are left with a compound that looks like this:

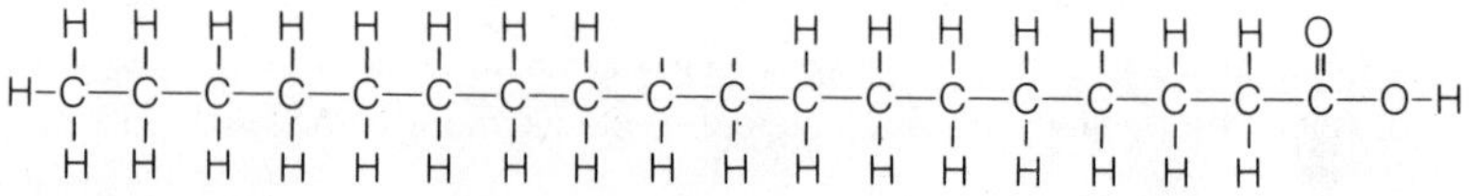

The two carbon atoms that formerly held the Hs are, in a sense, empty-handed. Each has a bond that is going unused. Such a compound cannot exist in nature. But an extra bond can be formed between the two carbons to satisfy nature's requirement that every carbon must have four bonds connecting it to other atoms. There is then a "double bond" between them:

Simplified diagram:

Oleic acid

(The same situation exists in the acid group at the end of the chain, where an O is double-bonded to the terminal C. That carbon has its full four bonds, and the oxygen meets its requirement of having two.) The resulting structure is an unsaturated (in this case *mono*unsaturated) fatty acid, oleic acid, which is found abundantly in the triglycerides in olive oil.

The heart patient is advised to eat *poly*unsaturated fats, because they seem to reduce the risk of artery disease. A polyunsaturated fat is a triglyceride in which the fatty acids have two or more points of unsaturation. An example is linoleic acid, which lacks four Hs and has two double bonds:

Simplified diagram:

Linoleic acid, the essential fatty acid

Linoleic acid is found in the triglycerides of most vegetable oils—corn oil, safflower oil, and the like. It is the most common of the polyunsaturated fatty acids in foods and the most important. In fact it is an *essential nutrient*. (We will discuss it further at the end of this section.)

Having looked at three of the most common fatty acids in foods, you can probably anticipate what the others look like. The fourth member of the family of 18-carbon fatty acids is linolenic acid, which has three

monounsaturated fatty acid: a fatty acid that lacks two hydrogen atoms and has one double bond between carbons—for example, oleic acid.

polyunsaturated fatty acid (PUFA): a fatty acid that lacks four or more hydrogen atoms and has two or more double bonds between carbons—for example, linoleic acid (2 double bonds) and linolenic acid (3 double bonds). Thus a **polyunsaturated fat** is composed of triglycerides containing a high percentage of PUFA.

Note: Linoleic acid (18 C, 2 double bonds) should not be confused with linolenic acid (18 C, 3 double bonds). The shorthand way of describing these two fatty acids is 18:2 and 18:3.

double bonds. A similar series of 20-carbon fatty acids exists, as well as a series of 22-carbon fatty acids. These are the long-chain fatty acids. In lesser amounts, medium-chain (14 to 16 Cs) and short-chain (8 to 12 Cs) fatty acids are also present in foods.

To repeat, the fats and oils in foods are mostly (95 percent) triglycerides: glycerol backbones with fatty acids attached. To complete the picture, it only remains to say that any combination of fatty acids is possible in a fat or oil. A mixed triglyceride, one that contains more than one type of fatty acid, is shown here:

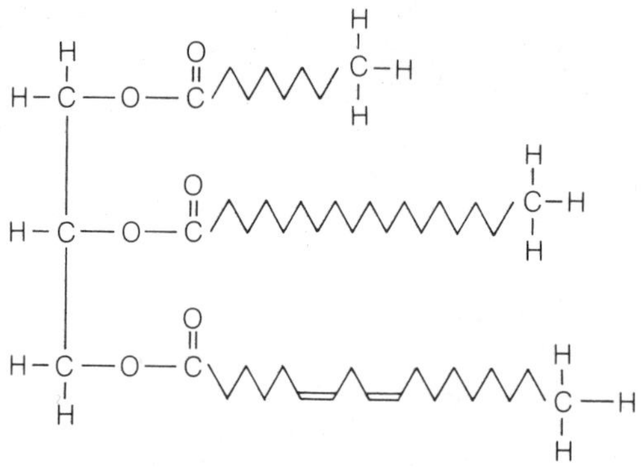

For these series, names, and structures, see Appendix C.

A mixed triglyceride typical of those found in foods.

essential nutrient: a compound that cannot be synthesized in the body in amounts sufficient to meet physiological needs. Many nutrients are needed by the body, but the word *essential* refers only to those that must be supplied by eating food.

dermatitis (derm-uh-TIGHT-us): infection or inflammation of the skin evidenced by itching, redness, and various skin lesions.

derma = skin
itis = infection or inflammation

Acetic acid, or acetyl CoA, is formed from glucose (see Chapter 7 and Highlight 7).

Linoleic Acid: The Essential Nutrient   Because the concept of essential nutrients pervades much of nutrition science, let us devote our attention to it for a moment. Why is this fatty acid essential for health, whereas a lack of any of the others would produce no ill effects?

When polyunsaturated fatty acids are missing from the diet, the skin reddens and becomes irritated and the liver develops abnormalities. Adding the fatty acids back to the diet clears up these symptoms. It turns out that what the body cells need is arachidonic acid (20 Cs, four double bonds); you can make this compound for yourself if linoleic acid is supplied in your diet.

The body's cells are equipped with many enzymes that can convert one compound to another. To make body fat or oil—triglycerides—all the enzymes need is a usable food source containing the atoms that triglycerides are composed of: carbon, hydrogen, and oxygen. Glucose does perfectly well. In fact, given an excess of blood glucose (and a filled glycogen storage space), this is precisely what the enzymes do: They cleave the glucose to make the two-carbon compound acetic acid and then combine many acetic acid molecules, with the appropriate alterations, to make long-chain fatty acids. (This is why most fatty acid carbon chains come in even numbers.) But the cells do not possess an enzyme that can arrange the double-bonding of linoleic acid.

Linoleic acid has thus come to be considered "the essential fatty acid,"[1] although arachidonic acid alleviates the dermatitis and, to a

[1]R. B. Alfin-Slater and L. Aftergood, Fats and other lipids, in *Modern Nutrition in Health and Disease*, 5th ed., eds. R. S. Goodhart and M. E. Shils (Philadelphia: Lea and Febiger, 1973), pp. 117-141.

limited extent, linolenic acid also helps. Nearly all diets supply enough linoleic acid to meet the requirement. Deficiencies are usually seen only in infants fed a formula that lacks this nutrient and in hospital patients who have been fed through a vein for prolonged periods using a formula that provides no essential fatty acids. Even in a totally fat-free diet, only 1 tsp (5 g) of corn oil would be sufficient to supply the needed amount of linoleic acid.

A (linoleic acid) →
B (arachidonic acid)

Compound A is the **precursor** of compound B.

The relief of dermatitis by linoleic acid might suggest to the unwary observer that all cases of dermatitis indicate a deficiency of this nutrient. Not so! Dermatitis is, by definition, a skin condition; the word does not imply a single cause. Actually there are more than a hundred body compounds — including other oils, vitamins, minerals, and hormones — that are needed in certain proportions to ensure the health of the skin. A deficiency or imbalance of any of these, caused either by a dietary lack or by failure of the body to produce necessary compounds in the normal way, may create a dermatitis condition. Bacterial and viral infections, allergens, physical agents such as radiation, and chemical irritants also cause dermatitis. There may also be a "psychosomatic" cause, as when excessive nervous activity in the brain (mind) generates a hormone imbalance that affects the skin (body). (See Highlight 5.) For these reasons, when you notice a symptom, never conclude that the cause is necessarily one that you are familiar with.

allergen (AL-er-gen): an agent that provokes an allergic reaction.

A distinction must be made between a symptom and a disease. A symptom can be alleviated (soothing oils can be applied to the skin to make it feel better, for example), but until you have identified the disease, you cannot achieve a cure. The rule is that if a certain nutrient clears up the symptom, then a deficiency of that nutrient may have been the cause.

symptom: the outward manifestation of a disease condition.

disease: the impairment or failure of a vital function, due to viral or bacterial infection, lack of an essential nutrient, genetic abnormality, or other causes.

A symptom is not a disease. Prescription of a cure depends on correct diagnosis of the disease.

diagnosis: identification.

You can also be fooled into thinking that a particular food — safflower oil, for example — is essential for healthy skin. Health food stores make millions of dollars a year promoting misconceptions like this. Actually, of course, safflower oil is not essential at all; you need never taste a drop of it all your life. All you need, to avoid a deficiency of linoleic acid, is to eat an ordinary mixed diet; it will inevitably include some polyunsaturated fat. The chance that you will then lack linoleic acid is virtually nil, since it is found in almost all oils (Appendix H).

The distinction between foods and nutrients has been emphasized once before (page 4). The implication that any specific food has magical, miraculous, or curative powers is false.

A FLAG SIGN OF A SPURIOUS CLAIM IS THE IMPLICATION THAT:

Any specific food is needed for any reason.

Processed Fat Ever since researchers first began to conclude that saturated fats were linked to heart disease and that polyunsaturated fats might be preventive, advertisers have been proclaiming the value of their margarines and oils as "high in polyunsaturates." Indeed, margarines made from vegetable oils and plant foods such as peanut butter do contain unsaturated fatty acids, and this is why they spread and melt more easily than foods that contain saturated fats. But virtually all margarines and all the leading peanut butters are at least partially hardened, and in the process they lose much of their polyunsaturated character.

Unfortunately, however, whatever you may gain in health from polyunsaturated fats, you lose in keeping quality. The more double bonds there are in a fatty acid, the more easily oxygen can destroy it.

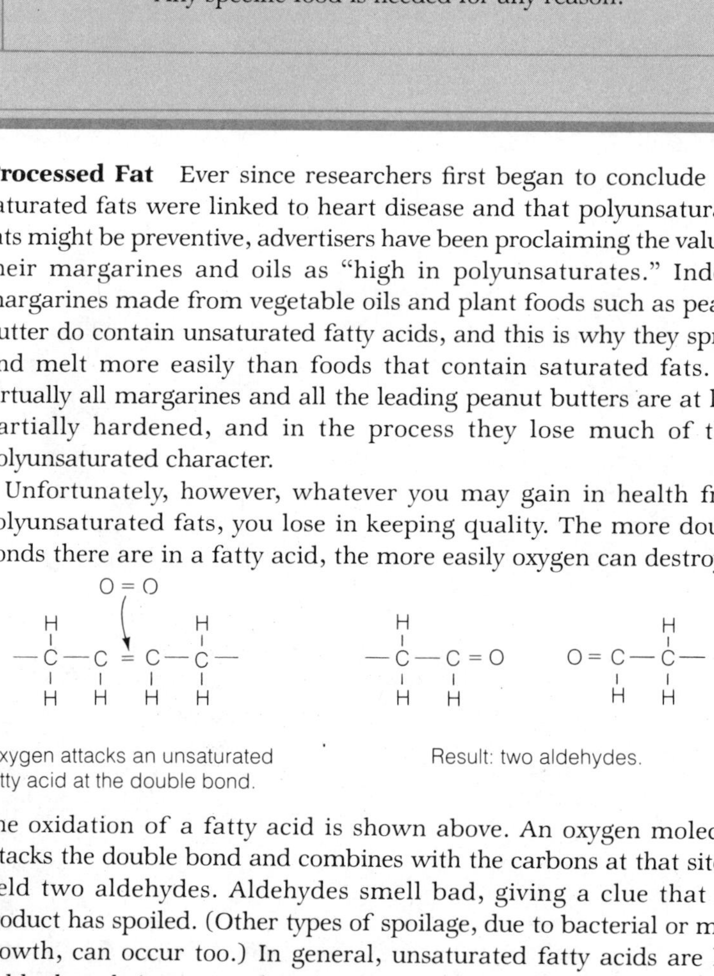

One way to determine the degree of unsaturation of a fat is to perform a chemical test using iodine to obtain the "iodine number." The higher the iodine number, the greater the degree of unsaturation:

safflower oil	= about 140
other vegetable oils (except coconut and palm)	= about 110-120
soft margarines	= about 90
olive oil	= about 75
hard margarines	= about 70
butter	= about 25-40
coconut and palm "oil"	= about 10-15

Oxidation of a fatty acid.

Oxygen attacks an unsaturated fatty acid at the double bond.

Result: two aldehydes.

The oxidation of a fatty acid is shown above. An oxygen molecule attacks the double bond and combines with the carbons at that site to yield two aldehydes. Aldehydes smell bad, giving a clue that the product has spoiled. (Other types of spoilage, due to bacterial or mold growth, can occur too.) In general, unsaturated fatty acids are less stable than their saturated counterparts.

aldehyde (AL-duh-hide): an organic compound containing a CHO group:

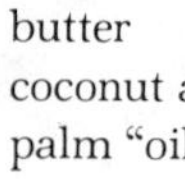

For the disadvantages of these additives, see Highlight 13.

Marketers of fat-containing products have three alternatives, none perfect. They may keep the product tightly sealed and under refrigeration—an expensive storage system. The consumer will have to do the same, and most people prefer not to buy a product that spoils readily. Marketers may also protect the fat by adding preservatives and antioxidants, but there are disadvantages to this course too. Finally, they may increase the product's stability by extracting the unsaturated fat and replacing it with a more saturated one, or by chemically hydrogenating it. Either method makes it more solid, which is often desirable. Margarine made from vegetable oils is solid at room temperature because the oils have been partially hydrogenated, and this improves its usefulness for some purposes. Hydrogenation, however, diminishes the margarine's polyunsaturated fat content and possibly, therefore, its health value. Moreover, new evidence suggests that there may be other concerns about hydrogenated oils.

hydrogenation (high-dro-gen-AY-shun): a chemical process by which hydrogens are added to unsaturated or polyunsaturated fats to make them more solid and more resistant to oxidation.

The new evidence on the processed fats began surfacing in the late 1970s, when reports began to appear of an unexpected effect of fat processing. When vegetable oils are partially hydrogenated, some of the fatty acids that remain unsaturated may undergo a change at their double bonds. The significance of this change is still poorly understood and its occurrence would be of no interest to anyone other than the theoretical chemist except for one thing: There is an association between the consumption of processed vegetable fats and the incidence of certain kinds of cancer, and it is possible that the changed fatty acids are responsible for the connection.

At the outset we promised that the chapters of this book would deal with known facts and that the Highlights would take up current controversies. Notice how carefully the statements above are worded: "There is an association" and "it is possible that the changed fatty acids are responsible." These statements are tentative, and the rest is speculation. To learn more about the status of fat/cancer research, turn to Highlight 2.

Meanwhile, it is hoped that your curiosity about the shift in fatty acids has been sufficiently aroused to motivate you to read a little more chemistry. It is actually quite a simple matter.

The change that occurs at a double bond during processing can be understood by way of an analogy. A single bond is like a dowel stick between two blocks. The blocks attached by such a stick can rotate. A double bond is like two dowel sticks between the blocks; the blocks can't rotate. (You may remember discovering these rules while playing with your Tinker Toy set.) The double bond between carbons in an unsaturated fatty acid holds the carbons and hydrogens in a fixed position and determines the shape of the molecule.

Almost all unsaturated fatty acids occur in nature in the *cis* form; that is, the hydrogens on the carbons adjacent to the double bond stick out on the same side of the molecule. During processing, one of the two double bonds may be broken and reformed. As this happens, the groups may rotate so that they become fixed in the *trans* position— across from each other. This changes the shape of the molecule.

cis (sis): same side.

trans: opposite sides.

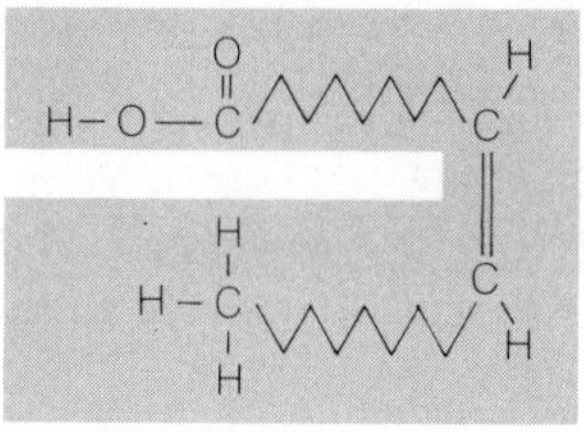

cis-fatty acid

The Hs are on the same side of the double bond, forcing the molecule to assume a horseshoe shape.

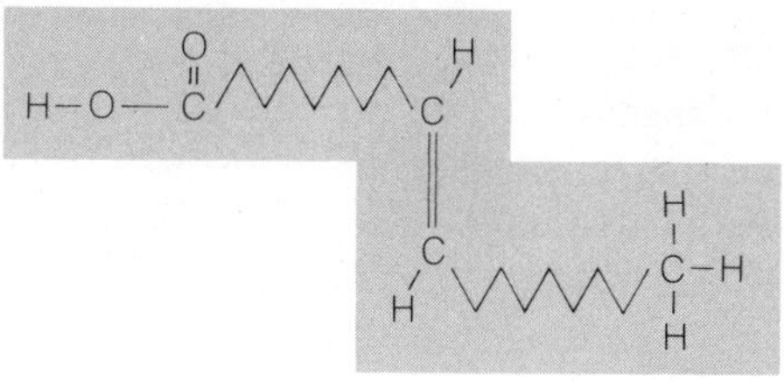

trans-fatty acid

The Hs are on opposite sides of the double bond, forcing the molecule into an extended position.

One effect of this change is to create a more solid product while still leaving double bonds in the fatty acids—so the manufacturer can still say his product is unsaturated or polyunsaturated. But *trans* fatty acids are not made by the body's cells, and they are rare in foods. It is not clear that our bodies are equipped to deal with large quantities of these *trans* fatty acids; the presence of these unusual molecules in our cells and tissues may create problems.[2] As yet this issue is poorly understood.

It is as frustrating for us to have to write the statement "we don't know" as it is for you to read it. This short discussion of a new finding in lipid research is intended to alert you to new developments that will occur after this book is in print and to help you understand what you read about them. You are urged to withhold judgment regarding the risks of using processed fats and not to jump to conclusions. If you are curious about the possible relationship of diet to cancer, read the Highlight at the end of this chapter. It won't give you the answers, but it will help to give you an overview of the whole area and to put these few facts in perspective.

In the meantime, a prudent and practical course is doubtless one of moderation. A principle of wise diet planning is the principle of dilution. Almost any substance—even water, even "natural," unadulterated, unprocessed foods—could be harmful in large quantities. To minimize the probability of accumulating any single substance, choose from a wide variety of foods. In the process, you will maximize the likelihood of obtaining all the nutrients you need for optimum nutrition.

[2] M. G. Enig, R. J. Munn, and M. Keeney, Dietary fat and cancer trends: A critique, *Federation Proceedings* 37 (1978): 2215-2220.

If you wish to avoid using processed fats, you can adopt some additional strategies. Rather than margarine, for example, you can mix warm butter with vegetable oil in equal amounts, producing a spread that is cheaper than butter, spreads well, has the same degree of polyunsaturation as margarine but more linoleic acid, and contains no *trans* fatty acids. The only disadvantage of this spread is that it contains cholesterol (and the question of whether this is a disadvantage is still being debated). As for peanut butter, it is possible to find unhydrogenated varieties on the shelf. The peanut mash and the oil separate readily in these products, but you can stir them back together before using them or pour off the oil for a product lower in kcalories.

Ultimately, if fat processors wish to produce margarines that are free of *trans* fatty acids, they will use an alternative process that hydrogenates double bonds without producing the *cis-trans* change. But because this process is a little more expensive and technically more difficult than the one presently in use, it has not been employed on a wide scale.

How the Body Handles Fat

The body has a problem in digesting and using fats—how to get at them. Substances that are soluble in fat are called water-fearing, and among these substances are, of course, the fats themselves. Fats in any compartment of the digestive tract tend to float to the top of that compartment, clumping together and separating themselves as far as possible from the watery digestive juices. On the other hand, the enzymes that digest fats are water-loving. Water molecules tend to ionize, to separate into positively charged H^+ and negatively charged OH^- ions, both of which attract their opposites. Enzymes also have positively and negatively charged groups on their surfaces, and so they mix comfortably with the ions in water. What the body needs to help mix them together is a substance that is friendly with both water-fearing and water-loving substances. The bile acids meet that need.

Manufactured by the liver and stored in the gallbladder until needed, the bile acids are released into the intestine whenever fat arrives there. Not surprisingly, they are made largely from lipids themselves. The system seems to have been designed for maximum efficiency and balance. The more fat you eat, the more is available to manufacture the bile acids needed to prepare the fat for digestion.

Each molecule of bile acid has at one end an ionized group that is attracted to water and at the other end a fatty acid chain that has an affinity for fat. Just as a skilled hostess will take your hand, draw you away from the company of your old friends, and leave you shaking hands with a new acquaintance, so a molecule of bile acid will attach itself to a lipid molecule in a droplet and draw it into the surrounding water solution where it can meet an enzyme. The process is known as emulsification (see Figure 1).

Water-fearing substances are known to chemists as **hydrophobic**.

hydro = water
phobia = fear

They may also be called **lipophilic**.

lipo = lipid
phile = friend

Water-loving substances are known as **hydrophilic.**

Ionize: see Appendix B.

enzyme: a large protein molecule that facilitates the making or breaking of chemical bonds (in this case the digestion, or breaking). Enzymes are fully defined and described in Chapter 3.

bile: the emulsifying compound manufactured by the liver, stored in the gallbladder, and released into the small intestine when fat is present there. Bile contains no enzymes. Bile appears sometimes in acid form, sometimes in salt form; for our purposes these are interchangeable.

Figure 1 Emulsification of fat by bile. Detergents work the same way (they are also emulsifiers), which is why they are so effective in removing grease from clothes and dishes. Molecule by molecule, the grease is dissolved out of the spot and suspended in the water, where it can be rinsed away. You can guess where the manufacturers of "detergents with enzymes" got their idea.

1. Fats and water separate; enzymes (E) are in water:

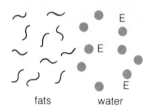

fats　　　water

2. Emulsifier has an affinity for both:

emulsifier with fat and water

3. Emulsifier helps distribute fats in water, where enzymes can work on them:

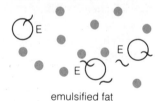

emulsified fat

emulsify (ee-MULL-suh-fye): to disperse and stabilize fat droplets in a watery solution.

Lipoproteins: see also pp. 75, 200.

Now, after all of this preparation, the enzymes can get at the triglycerides. The enzymes digest each triglyceride by removing two of its fatty acids, leaving a monoglyceride, or by removing all three of them, leaving a molecule of glycerol. As with the carbohydrates, the digestive process requires the participation of water, as shown in Figure 2. Finally the monoglycerides, glycerol, and fatty acids pass into the cells of the intestinal wall.

The products of lipid digestion are then released for transport through the body. Some of the larger ones are packaged in protein for this purpose. The protein-wrapped packages, called lipoproteins, are the subject of intensive research as laboratory sleuths seek to detect their structure and their relationships to heart and artery disease. The lipoproteins will appear again later in this chapter and are fully described in Chapter 6.

The Phospholipids and Sterols

The preceding pages have been devoted to one of the three classes of lipids, the triglycerides. The other two classes, the phospholipids and sterols, comprise only 5 percent of the lipids in the diet, but they are interesting and important and receive a lot of attention in the press.

lecithin (LESS-uh-thin): one of the phospholipids.

The Phospholipids　One of the "magical" nutrients that periodically receives much attention is lecithin. You are told that this nutrient is a major constituent of cell membranes (true), that the functioning of all cells depends on the integrity of their membranes (true, and on a great many other structures), and that you must therefore include large quantities of lecithin in your daily meals (false). You might as well believe that in order to grow healthy hair or to maintain the brain you must eat hair or brains! The enzyme lecithinase in the intestine takes lecithin apart before it passes into the body fluids anyway, so the lecithin you eat does not reach the body tissues intact. The lecithin you need for building cell membranes and for other functions is made from

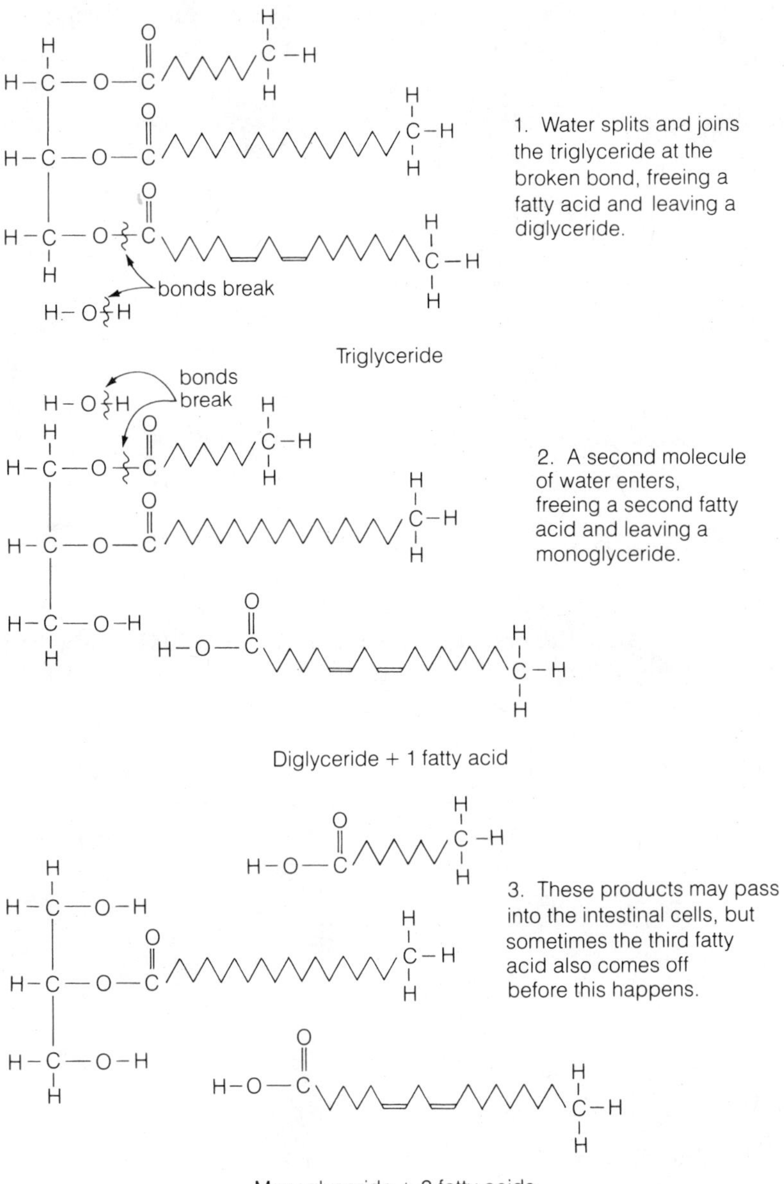

Figure 2 Digestion (hydrolysis) of a fat (triglyceride).

1. Water splits and joins the triglyceride at the broken bond, freeing a fatty acid and leaving a diglyceride.

Triglyceride

2. A second molecule of water enters, freeing a second fatty acid and leaving a monoglyceride.

Diglyceride + 1 fatty acid

3. These products may pass into the intestinal cells, but sometimes the third fatty acid also comes off before this happens.

Monoglyceride + 2 fatty acids

scratch by the liver. In other words, the lecithins are not essential nutrients.[3]

Like the triglycerides, the lecithins and the other phospholipids have a backbone of glycerol; they are different because they have only two fatty acids attached to them. In place of the third fatty acid is a molecule of choline or a similar compound containing phosphorus (P)

phospholipid: a compound similar to a triglyceride but having choline or another phosphorus-containing acid in place of one of the fatty acids.

Choline: see also p. 346.

[3]D. C. Fletcher, Lecithin for hyperlipemia: Harmless but useless (questions and answers), *Journal of the American Medical Association* 238 (1977): 64.

and nitrogen (N) atoms. A diagram of a lecithin molecule follows (others differ in the nature of the attached fatty acids):

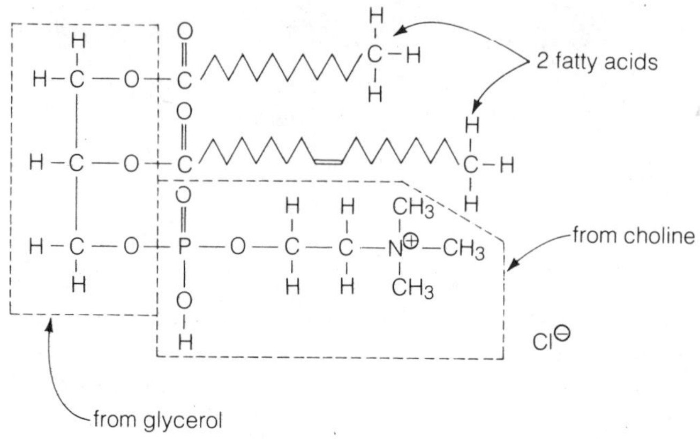

Lecithin.

(The plus charge on the N is balanced by a negative ion—usually chloride—that stays nearby.)

sterol: a compound composed of C, H, and O atoms arranged in rings like those of cholesterol, with any of a variety of side chains attached.

The Sterols: Cholesterol A student observing the chemical structure of cholesterol for the first time once remarked, "Would you believe dimethyl dihydroxy chicken wire?" He was not far wrong; chemists do remarkable "terminologizing." According to them, cholesterol is a member of the cyclopentanoperhydrophenanthrene family, whose particular designation is 3-hydroxy-5,6-cholestene. Never mind. It is not necessary to memorize a structure as complex as this one. But once having viewed it, you can say, "I have seen the structure of cholesterol."

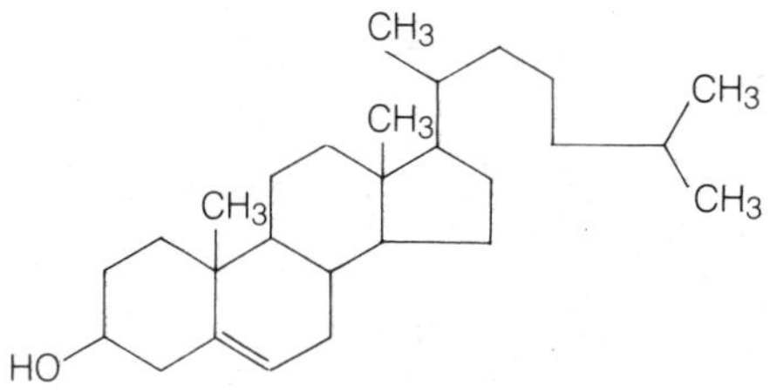

Cholesterol.

cholesterol: one of the sterols.

All of the carbons in cholesterol come from acetyl CoA (see Chapter 7), which in turn can be derived from several different compounds in the body besides glucose and fatty acids.

Cholesterol is not at all an unusual type of molecule. There are dozens of similar ones in the body; all are interesting and important. Among them are the bile acids, the sex hormones (such as testosterone), the adrenocortical hormones (such as cortisone), and vitamin D.

Like lecithins, cholesterol is needed metabolically but is not an essential nutrient. Your liver is manufacturing it now, as you read, at the rate of perhaps 50,000,000,000,000,000 molecules per second. The raw materials that the liver uses to make cholesterol can all be taken from glucose or saturated fatty acids.

After manufacture, cholesterol either is transformed into related compounds like the hormones just mentioned or leaves the liver. The cholesterol that leaves the liver has three possible destinations: (1) It may be excreted, (2) it may be deposited in body tissues, or (3) it may wind up accumulating in arteries and causing artery disease.

How Cholesterol Is Excreted   Most of the cholesterol that the liver makes becomes part of the bile salts, and these are released into the intestine to emulsify fat. After doing their job, some of the bile salts reenter the body with absorbed products of fat digestion. The cholesterol is thus recycled—back to the liver, once again into bile salts, back to the intestine, again into the body, and once more back to the liver.

The recycling of cholesterol and bile is diagramed on p. 203.

Once out in the intestine, however, some of the bile salts can be trapped by certain kinds of dietary fibers, which carry them out of the body with the feces. The excretion of bile salts reduces the total amount of cholesterol remaining in the body.

How Cholesterol Is Deposited in the Body   Some cholesterol leaves the liver packaged with other lipids for transport to the body tissues. These packages are the lipoproteins. The blood carries them through all the body's arteries, and any tissue can extract lipids from them.[4] To pass into the cells, lipids must first cross the artery walls, and it is here that they may be implicated in artery disease.

Both the intestine and the liver make lipoproteins to transport fat.

How Cholesterol Relates to Artery Disease   Artery disease often begins with a condition called atherosclerosis—hardening of the arteries. Atherosclerosis denotes the soft lipid accumulations called plaques on the inner wall of the arteries. As these plaques enlarge, the artery walls lose their elasticity, and the passage through them narrows.

Normally, blood surges through the arteries with each beat of the heart, and the arteries expand with each pulse to accommodate the flow. Arteries hardened and narrowed by plaques cannot expand, and so the blood pressure rises. The increased pressure can damage the artery walls further.

In addition to being elastic, the inner walls of the arteries must be glass-smooth so that the blood can move over the surface with as little friction as possible. Clotting of blood is an intricate series of events triggered when the blood moves past a rough surface, such as the edge of a cut. As long as the inner wall remains smooth, clotting will not occur inside the vessel, but if the plaques encroach on the bore of the vessel, the roughness of these plaques can cause the clotting reactions to begin.

atherosclerosis (ath-er-oh-scler-OH-sis): a type of artery disease characterized by patchy nodular thickenings of the inner walls of the arteries, especially at branch points.

athero = porridge
scleros = hard
osis = too much

plaques (PLACKS): mounds of lipid material mixed with smooth muscle cells and calcium, which are lodged in the artery walls. The same word is also used to describe an entirely different kind of accumulation of material on teeth, which causes dental caries.

[4]Some lipoproteins enter the body cells whole, as described in M. S. Brown and J. L. Goldstein, Receptor-mediated control of cholesterol metabolism, *Science* 191 (1976): 150-154.

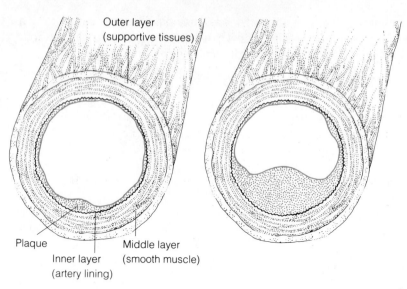

Outer layer
(supportive tissues)

Plaque

Inner layer
(artery lining)

Middle layer
(smooth muscle)

An artery (section) with plaque just beginning to form. Plaques could easily appear in a person as young as 15.

The same artery, years later, almost completely blocked by plaque.

Development of atherosclerosis.

A stationary clot is called an **embolus** (EM-boh-luss): When it has grown enough to close off a blood vessel, it is an **embolism**. An embolus that breaks loose is a **thrombus**; the kind of heart attack described here may be called a **coronary thrombosis**.

coronary = crowning (the heart)
thrombo = clot

A stroke is a **cerebral thrombosis**.

cerebrum = part of the brain

multifactorial: having many causes.

risk factors: factors known to be related to (or correlated with) a disease but not proven to be causal.

The clot thus formed may linger, attached to a plaque, and gradually grow until it shuts off the blood supply to that portion of the tissue supplied by the artery. That tissue may die slowly and be replaced by scar tissue. Or the clot may break loose and travel along the system until it reaches an artery too small to allow its passage. Then the tissues fed by this particular artery will be robbed of oxygen and nutrients and will die suddenly. Should such a clot lodge in an artery of the heart, we would say that the person had a heart attack. If the clot should lodge in an artery of the brain, we would call this event a stroke.

More than half of the people who die each year in the United States and Canada die of heart and blood vessel disease. The underlying condition that contributes to most of these deaths is atherosclerosis, which is now so widespread that it has been called an epidemic.[5] This disease, which takes its heaviest toll among men in the most productive period of their lives, has been called the number-one killer, and many health agencies have devoted millions of hours to the battle against it.

So far, all that can be said for sure about the causes of atherosclerosis is that it is multifactorial in origin. There are many risk factors—smoking, gender (being male), heredity (including diabetes), high blood pressure, lack of exercise, obesity, stress, high blood cholesterol and triglyceride concentrations, and some 30 others.[6] But it is not at all

[5]Alfin-Slater and Aftergood, 1973.

[6]E. M. N. Hamilton and E. N. Whitney, Atherosclerosis: What causes it, and can we prevent it? in *Nutrition: Concepts and Controversies* (St. Paul: West, 1979), pp. 105-108.

clear which of these is caused by what; they are only correlations. Highlight 6 delves into the many lines of inquiry. We do not know whether reducing any of the risk factors will actually reduce the risk of dying of heart disease.

An analogy may help you to understand this important point. Suppose that there is an outbreak of crime in a certain city—arson, for example. Someone is setting fires, and the police are after him. It is observed that a certain person, Mr. A, is always seen in the neighborhoods when the fires start, and he is deemed guilty of the crimes. However, it may be that a very sneaky individual, Ms. B, is the real culprit and that Mr. A is only following her around. Mr. A is associated with but not a causal agent in the setting of the fires. The evidence against him is only circumstantial (correlational) unless we can show that whenever he is locked up there are no fires and that whenever he is let out the fires start again. Better yet, we will know for sure if we catch him pouring the gasoline and lighting the match. You may recall that this point has been made before: Correlation is not cause.

In light of all the evidence relating to plaque formation, it seems more than likely that dietary fat (triglycerides) and possibly cholesterol are among the contributing factors in atherosclerosis. Plaques are composed largely of cholesterol, and this cholesterol is manufactured largely from fragments derived from saturated fat. Thus limiting your consumption of fat will do no harm, and it may do some good. And on the assumption that some of the body's cholesterol may come from the diet, it may make sense to limit your cholesterol intake as well. It is on this reasoning that three of the U.S. Dietary Goals are based.

Fat: Goals and Guidelines

The U.S. Dietary Goals make three recommendations relating to lipids in the diet. According to the Goals, you should

- Reduce consumption of fat, so that it contributes only 30 percent of the kcalories in your diet (at present, the U.S. average is 42 percent).
- Reduce saturated fat intake, so that it contributes only 10 percent of total kcalories, letting the remaining fat come from mono- and polyunsaturated fat sources.
- Reduce cholesterol consumption to about 300 mg a day (the present U.S. average is about 600 mg).

When these goals were translated into the more moderate guidelines of 1979 (pp. 34-35), the resulting practical recommendation was simply to avoid excess fat, saturated fat, and cholesterol.

The Fats in Foods

The exchange system presented in Chapter 1 provides a useful means of learning where the fats are in foods. Three of the six lists in the exchange system—the milk list, the meat list, and the fat list—include foods containing appreciable amounts of fat. The items on the milk list contain protein, carbohydrate, and fat; those on the meat list contain protein and fat; and those on the fat list contain only fat. Table 1 shows the fat content of each of these groups of foods in the context of their overall energy-nutrient composition.

Milk List   The foods on the milk list contain variable amounts of fat. A cup of skim milk has negligible fat, a cup of 2% fortified milk has 5 g, and a cup of whole milk has 10 g. Users of the exchange system think of this added fat as being equivalent to teaspoons of fat (fat "exchanges"). Thus, a cup of 2% milk is like skim milk plus 1 tsp fat, and a cup of whole milk is like skim milk plus 2 tsp fat.

Foods containing fat:

10 g in 1 c whole milk

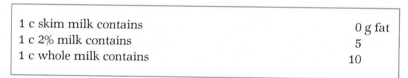

1 c skim milk contains	0 g fat
1 c 2% milk contains	5
1 c whole milk contains	10

Table 1.   Fat Content of the Six Exchange Groups

Exchange group	Serving size	Carbohydrate (g)	Protein (g)	Fat (g)	Energy (kcal)
(1) **Skim milk***	1 c	12	8	0	80
(2) Vegetables	1/2 c	5	2	0	25
(3) Fruit	varies	10	0	0	40
(4) **Bread†**	1 slice	15	2	0	70
(5) **Meat‡**	1 oz	0	7	3	55
(6) **Fat**	1 tsp	0	0	5	45

*Skim milk is the standard milk item in diet planning. Planners are encouraged to think of low-fat or whole milk as "milk with added fat." A cup of low-fat milk contains 5 g fat (1 fat exchange), and 1 c whole milk contains 10 g fat (2 fat exchanges).

†Ordinary bread items contain low or negligible fat, but some baked goods, such as baking powder biscuits, have enough added fat to count as an additional fat exchange (see the exchange lists in Appendix L).

‡An ounce of low-fat meat contains 3 g fat. An ounce of medium-fat meat contains 2 1/2 additional grams (1/2 fat exchange), or 5 1/2 g in all. An ounce of high-fat meat contains 5 g more than the lean, or 8 g in all. Peanut butter is included on the meat list because it is a protein-rich food, but it is higher in fat than any other item: 2 tbsp peanut butter are equivalent to 1 oz meat in protein but contain 13 g fat.

The fat in milk is mostly saturated fat; the cholesterol content is 25 mg per cup of whole milk or 7 mg per cup of skim milk. Thus choosing skim in place of whole milk reduces your intakes of both saturated fat and cholesterol.

Meat Lists   The meats have been sorted into three lists depending on their fat content. An ounce of lean meat has 3 g of fat, an ounce of medium-fat meat has about 2 1/2 g more or 5 1/2 g total, and an ounce of high-fat meat has 8 g of fat. Peanut butter, which is a protein-rich food grouped with meat, has 15 1/2 g of fat per 2-tbsp serving.

1 oz lean meat contains	3 g fat
1 oz medium-fat meat contains	5 1/2
1 oz high-fat meat contains	8
2 tbsp peanut butter contains	15 1/2

3 g in 1 oz lean meat

All of these items are equivalent in protein content, however. One can be exchanged or traded for another in a menu without changing the amount of protein that is delivered.

A person studying the meat list for the first time may be surprised to note how many fat kcalories are in meat. An ounce of lean meat supplies 28 kcal from its protein and 27 kcal from its fat. An ounce of high-fat meat supplies the same number—28 kcal—from protein but 72 kcal from fat. Two tablespoons of peanut butter, also with 28 kcal from protein, supply 117 kcal from fat! Thus meat, which is often thought of as a protein food, actually contains more fat energy than protein energy and is an unexpectedly fattening food, often accounting for the excess weight that meat eaters tend to gain.

1 oz = about 30 g (see Appendix D) An ounce (30 g) of lean meat contains 5 g protein and 3 g fat. The rest, of course, is largely water.

Note that the unit by which meat is measured in this system is only an ounce. To use this system you need to be aware of serving sizes. An egg is like one ounce of meat. A hamburger is usually three or four ounces. A dinner steak may be six or eight ounces or even larger.

The fats in meats and eggs are mostly saturated; those in poultry and fish have a better balance between saturated and polyunsaturated fats. (A rank listing of fats from most to least saturated is presented in Appendix G.) As for cholesterol, the foods that contain the highest amounts are such organ meats as liver and kidneys and such shellfish as lobster, oysters, and shrimp. Lower but still significant levels of cholesterol are contained in beef, ham, lamb, veal, and pork, followed by poultry and fish. (The cholesterol contents of foods are also presented in Appendix G.) As a general rule, however, a person wishing to reduce cholesterol and saturated fat intake could accomplish both objectives by eating less meat and more poultry and fish (except shellfish).

Fat List   In addition to the obvious items (butter, margarine, and oil), this list includes bacon, olives, and avocados. These foods are grouped together because the amount of lipid they contain makes them essentially pure fat contributors. An eighth of an avocado or one slice of bacon contains as much fat as a pat of butter, and like butter, they contain negligible protein and carbohydrate. Hence when you eat bacon you are not eating a protein food; you are eating a fat food.

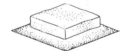

5 g in a pat of butter
or margarine

1 tsp butter or margarine (or any other serving of food listed on the fat list) contributes:	5 g fat

Saturated fats have a high melting point and are solid at room or body temperature.

Polyunsaturated fats have a low melting point and are liquid at room or body temperature.

A rule of thumb in determining the degree of saturation of a fat is to observe how hard it is at room temperature. Chicken fat is softer than pork fat, which is softer than beef tallow. Of the three, beef tallow is the most and chicken fat the least saturated. The double bonds in polyunsaturated fats make them melt more readily. Generally speaking, vegetable and fish oils are rich in polyunsaturates, whereas the harder fats—animal fats—are more saturated.

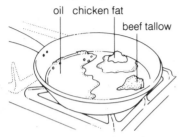

oil   chicken fat

beef tallow

The most polyunsaturated fat melts soonest.

If you wish to make choices consistent with the recent goals or guidelines, you should learn how to read food labels. But beware: Words like *vegetable fat* and *unsaturated fat* can be used to mislead you. Not all vegetable oils are polyunsaturated. Coconut oil, for example, is often used in nondairy creamers, and coconut oil is a saturated fat. Vegetable oils that are hydrogenated may have lost their polyunsaturated character. Another exception to the rule is olive oil, widely used in salad dressings and in Greek and Italian foods. The predominant fatty acid in olive oil is the *mono*unsaturated fatty acid oleic acid. Thus olive oil can claim to be *un*saturated but not to be *poly*unsaturated.

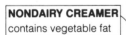

NONDAIRY CREAMER
contains vegetable fat

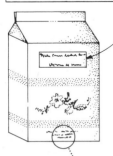

Ingredients:
corn syrup solids, hydrogenated vegetable oils (palm kernel, coconut)

Here's the truth. Notice, too, that sugar is listed first!

Estimating Fat with the Exchange System   The values presented above provide a way to estimate the amount of fat eaten at a meal or in a day. Two reminders are needed. First, fat is often hidden in cooked vegetables. As a rule of thumb, vegetables served with butter or margarine can be assumed to contain one fat exchange (1 tsp) per half-cup serving. Second, some baked goods also contain appreciable fat; these are listed on the bread list in Appendix L.

Using these values, let us see how much fat was provided by the day's meals described on page 43. Adding up the meat exchanges for the egg, peanut butter, and steak; taking into account the extra fat in these meats, the whole milk, and the shortcake biscuit; adding the fat used in frying the egg and flavoring the beans and potato; and finally adding a fat exchange for the heavy cream—we reach a total of 109 g fat for the day:

Breakfast	Exchanges	Grams fat
1 egg fried in 1 tsp fat	1 meat + 1/2 fat	5 1/2
1 piece toast with 1 tsp margarine	1 fat	5

Lunch		
2 slices bread		
2 tbsp peanut butter	1 meat + 2 1/2 fat	15 1/2
2 tsp jelly		
1 c milk	2 fat	10

Dinner		
6-oz steak	6 meat + 6 fat	48
1/2 c green beans served with		
1 tsp margarine	1 fat	5
1 c mashed potato served with		
1 tsp margarine	1 fat	5

Dessert		
2-inch diameter biscuit	1 fat	5
3/4 c strawberries		
1 tbsp heavy cream	1 fat	5
6 tsp sugar		
Total		104 g fat

The day's meals thus supplied about 936 kcal from fat (9 times 104). The day's total from all these foods was about 1,930 kcal, so this eater consumed about 50 percent of her kcalories from fat.

In addition to facilitating calculations of this kind, the exchange lists divide fats into two classes—saturated and polyunsaturated—to aid in meal planning for the diabetic. The importance of being aware of the quality of dietary fat as well as its quantity must be abundantly evident by now.

Each culture has its own favorite food sources of fats and oils. In Canada, rapeseed oil is popular and is enjoying increasing use. The peoples of the Mediterranean (Greeks, Italians, and Spaniards) rely heavily on olive oil, which is high in monounsaturates, and the Orientals use the polyunsaturated oil of soybeans. Jewish cookery traditionally employs chicken fat, whereas U.S. Southerners rely heavily on pork fat—lard and bacon. The saturated fat consumption of blacks is cause for concern among health authorities who note a high incidence of hypertensive heart disease among these people. This high rate of heart disease may be diet-related, genetically caused, or both.

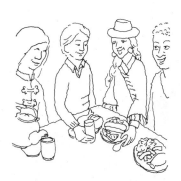

hypertension: high blood pressure. This problem may also be related to salt (sodium) intake;[7] thus the Dietary Goals and the Guidelines recommend limiting salt (see Chapter 14).

[7]Y. K. Seedat and J. Reddy, A study of 1000 South African nonwhite hypertensive patients, *South African Medical Journal* 48 (1974): 816-820.

Summing Up

Lipids in the body serve as a major energy reserve and also provide structural material for many tissues; in specific locations body fat protects organs from heat, cold, and mechanical shock. The oxidation of a pound of human body fat supplies 3,500 kcal to meet energy needs.

The lipids are known familiarly as the fats and oils. In foods they are not soluble in water but serve as a solvent themselves for the fat-soluble vitamins and for the aromatic compounds that give foods their flavor and aroma. About 95 percent of them are triglycerides, compounds composed of glycerol with three fatty acids attached. The fatty acids may be long-, medium-, or short-chain fatty acids, and they may be saturated or mono- or polyunsaturated. Triglycerides are classed by the nature of the fatty acids they contain. For example, a triglyceride containing polyunsaturated fatty acids is a polyunsaturated fat. The other 5 percent of dietary lipids are the phospholipids and sterols, cholesterol being a member of the latter group.

During digestion, the triglycerides must be emulsified (dispersed in water) by bile before they can be hydrolyzed by enzymes to diglycerides and then to monoglycerides and fatty acids, which are absorbed into the intestinal cells. Phospholipids also undergo hydrolysis, but cholesterol is absorbed virtually as is. All three classes of lipid are carried in lipoproteins that circulate in the body fluids.

Deficiencies of essential fatty acids manifest themselves in dermatitis and liver abnormality. The symptoms can be cleared up by administering linoleic acid, which has therefore come to be called "the" essential fatty acid.

Food fats containing unsaturated fatty acids spoil easily but may be processed (hydrogenated) to make them less vulnerable to oxidation. In the processing, *trans* fatty acids may be formed, whose effects on health are as yet unknown.

Cholesterol is normally made in the body by the liver and is transported to all tissues, where it is picked up and used for cell functions. Abnormal deposition of cholesterol in artery walls, together with smooth-muscle cells and other constituents, forms plaques characteristic of atherosclerosis, the major killer disease of the developed countries. Research shows atherosclerosis to be multifactorial in origin, with smoking and high blood pressure among the major risk factors; a diet high in saturated fat and cholesterol is also implicated. The U.S. Dietary Goals and the Guidelines that evolved from them suggest limiting intakes of total fat, saturated fat, and cholesterol as a preventive measure.

In the exchange system, the foods that contribute fat to the diet are found mainly on the milk list, the meat list, and the fat list. The size of a milk exchange is a cup; an exchange of 2% milk contains 5 g fat, and an exchange of whole milk contains 10 g fat. For meat, the size of an exchange is an ounce or the equivalent; an exchange of lean meat contains 3 g, of medium-fat meat 5 1/2 g, and of high-fat meat 8 g of fat. An exchange (2 tbsp) of peanut butter contains 15$1/2$ g fat. For fat itself, the exchange size is a teaspoon or the equivalent, and one fat exchange contains 5 g of fat. When fat is added to vegetables, the amount is usually 5 g per half-cup serving. Some baked goods also contain fat (see the bread list in Appendix L).

For the most part, meats and animal fats are the main contributors of saturated fat to the diet. Foods containing cholesterol include most notably the organ meats, shellfish, and eggs, with meats and other animal fats also containing significant amounts. Vegetable oils, with a few exceptions, contain more polyunsaturated fats, and no plant product contains cholesterol.

"Why is there a Highlight on cancer in a nutrition text?" you may say. "I want to learn about food—not disease." Or maybe you're thinking, "First you took away my cigarettes, then my cyclamates, and now you are asking me to face the possibility of cancer from the fat in my diet. I'm scared of cancer. I don't want to hear any more about it." These are normal human responses to the subject of cancer.

Before you close the book with a shudder, let us explain our placing this segment here. As always, we want you to be informed about the latest research in our field. We also want you to become familiar with the thinking behind the research so that you can respond intelligently to the stories that link ordinary elements of your life with frightening diseases. If you face your own fear, you may be able to take the positive step of planning changes in your lifestyle that will harmonize with the best evidence on cancer and diet that is currently available.

What Is Cancer?   Cancer is not a single disease. There are cancers—plural. The word *cancer* refers to any growths, tumors, or neoplasms that grow wild. It is correct to speak of cancers in the plural because there are different kinds of tumors, many of which are specific to certain parts of the body. When a neoplasm grows, it

HIGHLIGHT 2

Dietary Fat and Cancer

We ought to be developing a much better system for general education about human health, . . . even some celebration of the absolute marvel of good health that is the real lot of most of us, most of the time.

LEWIS THOMAS

interferes with the normal functioning of an organ or tissue. The growth seemingly has no built-in brakes, as normal growth does. Furthermore, cancerous cells are alive, and as they grow they take nutrients from the host's diet or body reserves.

Full-blown cancer develops from some initiating event. That event may be radiation, either the general radiation that is always present or medical or industrial radiation. Or the event may be the intrusion of a chemical—a carcinogen—into the cell.

Either radiation or a carcinogen may alter the protein-making machinery of the cell, so that the DNA produces a new, "foreign" protein. Since this is an unfamiliar protein, the cell has no way to tell the DNA to halt its production. Normally, when you cut your finger, the DNA in the cells alongside

the cut receives a signal to step up cell division in order to fill in the space. When that has been accomplished, the DNA receives another signal to resume ordinary, slow cell division. But if some random event disrupts the orderly operation of the cell, a new protein is produced that has no such feedback system to control it.

After the initiating event, conditions within the cell determine which of several different courses the cancer will follow. Healthy tissue has automatic immune responses to foreign substances, and these often destroy the early clone of a tumor cell so that it doesn't develop at all.[1] And sometimes conditions within the tissue may be such that the neoplasm grows very slowly, taking many years to make itself known. But at other times, a "favorable" environment stimulates rapid growth of the tumor, with resultant dysfunction and death.

Thus scientists may pursue several avenues in search of cancer causes. The task can be compared to the detective work needed to solve a murder mystery: Scientists must look for clues. They may try to identify substances or events that initiate cancer; or the cellular conditions that permit it to get started; they

[1] R. L. Phillips, Role of life-style and dietary habits in risk of cancer among Seventh Day Adventists, *Cancer Research* (1975):3513-3522.

may look for the protective factor that some people have which could keep cancer from starting; or they may examine the immunological system to see why this foreign material is not destroyed at the outset. All of these lines of investigation pursue clues to understand the initiating phase of cancer development. (Scientists also want to know what conditions aid or suppress the growth once it has begun so that it can be treated successfully—but this is an entirely distinct research question.)

Nutrition and Cancer.

How can nutrition play a role in cancer initiation? There seem to be three possibilities.[2] First, food may be the vehicle for bringing carcinogens into the body. These carcinogens may be nutrients themselves, additives that are used to preserve or enhance processed foods, or accidental contaminants of food. Until they are tested, we cannot be sure of their guilt or innocence. (Some suspects are discussed in Highlight 13.)

Second, nutrient deficiencies may favor cancer development. For example, if a nutrient is necessary for the synthesis of an anticancer compound, then a deficiency of that nutrient may enable

[2]Symposium: Nutrition in the causation of cancer, *Cancer Research* 35 (2) (1975), entire issue.

Mini-Glossary

carcinogen (car-SIN-uh-jen): a cancer-causing substance.

carcin = cancer
gen = gives rise to

case-controlled study: an epidemiological study that matches groups with respect to all variables except the one of interest.

clone: a group of identical cells descended asexually from a single ancestor.

initiating event: an event caused by radiation or chemical reaction that can give rise to cancer.

metabolite (meh-TAB-oh-light): a substance produced by the physical and chemical processes involved in the maintenance of life. In the sequence of chemical conversions from A to B to C to D, B, C, and D are metabolites of A.

neoplasm (NEE-oh-PLAZ-um): a tumor in an animal or plant.

neo = new
plasm = tissue

promoter: a substance that does not initiate cancer, but that favors its development once the initiating event has taken place.

radiation the emission of energetic particles that can penetrate living tissue.

selective permeability: the property of a living cell membrane that enables it to "choose" which substances to allow or move in or out.

---

the cancer to get started or to grow. For another example, a nutrient deficiency may cause the buildup of an intermediate metabolite that is itself a carcinogen or a promoter.

Imagine that a substance in a food, compound A, enters a healthy, well-nourished body. Somewhere along the digestive tract an enzyme working with a vitamin or a mineral attacks one of A's bonds, breaking it into two molecules of compound B. (How enzymes work is described on p. 101. Later on, other enzymes acting in collaboration with a different vitamin or mineral attack bonds in the two molecules of compound B, converting them into compound C. In a similar experience involving different enzymes, minerals, and vitamins, compound C becomes compound D. Although the body is unable to make use of the predecessors (precursors) of compound D, it is able to absorb D out of the intestinal tract and put it to good work in the cells.

Now suppose there is a nutrient deficiency: A mineral or vitamin that was meant to help the enzyme break the bonds in compound C is not present. The result is an accumulation of compound C and a deficiency of compound D. Suppose that compound C is a weak carcinogen. As long as everything proceeds normally from A to B to C to D, there is no buildup of C and the carcinogen is not absorbed; or if it is, the immune system destroys it at an early stage. But when the cells are overloaded with C, then it has time to initiate a neoplasm. The "guy in the black hat" is not compound A, which came in food, or even compound C, which the body can handle under ordinary circumstances, but a deficiency of a mineral or vitamin.

The third possibility is that excesses of some of the nutrients may induce abnormalities that favor cancer development. Human evolutionary design has been toward the economical use of nutrients; excesses are so new that we have no history with which to evaluate their significance. It may be, for example, that the present overuse of animal protein in some way changes the immune surveillance system, so that it does not recognize and destroy foreign (protein) tumor cells. Or perhaps excess vitamin and mineral supplements somehow alter the absorptive system, so that it allows carcinogens or cancer promoters to enter the body.

Epidemiological Studies
The scientist/detective's task is mind-boggling, but there are several data-gathering techniques available for tracking down the possible connections between nutrition and cancer. These range from asking broad, general questions to discover the background of cancers to searching for specific, tiny clues to piece together small parts of the puzzle. These methods all have their limitations, but they form necessary links in the chain of studies that may finally solve a scientific mystery.

A newspaper or magazine article giving the exciting news of a breakthrough in the search for cancer causes is often reporting on just one study. You should be aware that what is being reported is a clue, not a solution. How often do you jump to the conclusion that a murder mystery has been solved when you hear that the murder weapon has been found? This point is developed further in Highlight 10. In reading, meanwhile, keep an open mind.

Major efforts to discover the conditions that favor cancer have been made by epidemiologists. They try to identify groups of people who have a high incidence of cancer and those who have a low incidence and then try to identify all the differences between these groups' lifestyles, including their eating habits. Then they try to match high-risk and low-risk groups as closely as possible in terms of sex, age, socioeconomic background, and other variables so that only the groups' food habits will be different. (A study of matched groups like this is called a case-controlled study.) The final step is a series of questionnaires and interviews, designed to pinpoint the differences in diet that may account for the different cancer risks.

Early epidemiological studies showed that the incidence of certain cancers varied by geographic area[3] and by racial group. Japanese immigration to the United States after World War I provided a fertile field for such study. The Japanese have a high incidence of stomach cancer and a low incidence of colon cancer when compared with people in the United States and other Western countries. If this were the only clue from these studies, it might be reasonable to conclude that the Japanese carry special genes for certain cancers or for protection against some of them. However, it has been found that the incidence of stomach and colon cancers among second-generation Japanese-Americans more nearly approaches the rate of these cancers in the Western World. What changed the susceptibility of Japanese immigrants? It was not their heredity. Nor was it pollution, because Japan and the United States are both in-

[3]D. Burkitt, Epidemiology of cancer of the colon and rectum, *Cancer* 28 (1971):3-13.

dustrial countries. However, something in the environment had changed, and an obvious candidate was their diets.

(Some interesting questions arose from this study that are still not answered. Curiously, even though the incidence of colon cancer rose in the immigrants, Japanese women of the second generation retained a rate of breast cancer more nearly like that of their homeland.[4] This was in contrast to the fact that, worldwide, breast and colon cancer correlate, rising and falling together in the same population. Does this show that breast cancer is more genetically based than other cancers? Is there some cultural factor that Japanese women retain after immigrating to the United States? Do they, for example, continue to breastfeed instead of adopting the Western practice of bottle-feeding? Answering one question only raises more questions.)

What factors in the Japanese diet favored stomach cancer and protected against colon cancer? Was it their high salt intake? Their low intake of animal protein? Their high vegetable intake?

Other population studies

provided additional clues for the cancer detectives. Some of these studies showed that Seventh-Day Adventists have a remarkably lower death rate from cancers of all kinds than the general population of the United States. This religious sect has, as a part of its church doctrine, rules against smoking, using alcohol, and using hot condiments and spices. It especially forbids pork, which is spoken of in the Bible as "unclean meat." It encourages a lacto-ovo-vegetarian diet. Even Seventh-Day Adventists who do not strictly adhere to church tenets eat meat very sparingly. When the cancers linked to smoking and alcohol are discounted, Seventh-Day Adventists still have a mortality rate due to cancer about one-half to two-thirds that of the rest of the population.

In this case, as with all epidemiological studies, many questions were raised. Is the group's low cancer mortality rate due to its low consumption of meat and high consumption of vegetables and cereal grains? Or is there some factor other than diet that makes this group unique? The Seventh-Day Adventists are of a higher-than-average socioeconomic level, and more are college-educated; what influence might these factors have on their incidence of cancer?[5]

In order to track down the factors that are associated

with cancers in some populations, Draser and Irving studied the diets of people in 37 countries.[6] They documented the food available per person per day, as well as other indicators of lifestyle, such as possession of radio receivers and motor vehicles. They found a high positive correlation between colon cancer and breast cancer, which would suggest a common environmental factor. They also found that these two have a high positive correlation with atherosclerosis but a negative correlation with stomach cancer.

The most interesting correlation they found showed both breast and colon cancer to be strongly associated "with indicators of affluence, such as a high-fat diet rich in animal protein and the availability of motor vehicles. However, the correlation with fat and animal protein was higher than for the other factors."[7] Other investigators have reported similar findings.[8]

However, any attempt to link dietary components with disease should be ap-

[4]W. M. Haenszel and M. Kurihara, Studies of Japanese migrants: 1. Mortality from cancer and other diseases among Japanese in the U.S., *Journal of the National Cancer Institute* 40 (1968):43-67.

[5]Phillips, 1975.

[6]B. S. Drasar and D. Irving, Environmental factors and cancer of the colon and breast, *British Journal of Cancer* 27 (1973):167-172.

[7]Drasar and Irving, 1973.

[8]K. K. Carroll, Experimental evidence of dietary factors and hormone-dependent cancers, *Cancer Research* 35 (2) (1975):3374-3383.

proached with caution. An increase in one component of the diet causes increases or decreases in others.[9] If a high correlation is shown between a disease and, say, the consumption of animal protein, how can you be sure that the critical factor is the animal protein? It may be the increased fat consumption; fat goes with animal protein in foods. Or the disease may be correlated with what is crowded out: the vitamins, minerals, or fiber contained in the missing fruits, vegetables, and cereals.

Drasar and Irving were not able to find a negative correlation between fiber in the diet and these two cancers (of the breast and the colon), although they had expected it. They felt that their failure might be due, in part, to the lack of definition as to the nature of fiber[10] (see p. 40). Their failure somewhat weakens the claim of the fiber enthusiasts that fiber protects against cancer and shows how important it is to withhold judgment about claims like this until more is known.

If a certain diet appears causally linked to a disease, you can't be sure immediately whether the

cause is the presence of something or the absence of something else. You have to separate the two possibilities by further testing.

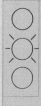

CAUTION WHEN YOU READ!

Remember that a diet high in some nutrients or foods must be low in others.

Another problem inherent in epidemiological studies is that they depend on dietary recall. People tend to have trouble remembering how much of each food they ate.[11] And in the case of cancer studies, the need is not so much to know what the diet is like now but what it was like at an earlier time, say, 30 years ago, when the initiating event may have occurred.[12] In this connection, study of the Seventh-Day Adventists offers hope of clarifying the relationship between animal protein and cancer. Most of

them can tell you exactly when they quit eating meat—they quit when they joined the church. Another difficulty with epidemiological studies is the finding of a control group that matches the experimental group in enough ways to make the comparison valid.

Animal Studies   After an epidemiological study has tentatively identified a dietary factor, researchers often turn to experiments with laboratory animals. Animal researchers can control many variables while manipulating only the dietary factor.

When the Western diet was first implicated in breast and colon cancer, many scientists looked at the studies and said, "Ah yes, of course, fat must be the culprit. Look at the low-meat diet of the low-risk groups. And look at the Western world's increasing use of meat, which correlates with the rising incidence of cancer. It must be the high-meat diet that puts the Western world at high risk." So they were off and running to try to link meat, especially animal fat, with cancer. (Nobody suspected vegetable fat.)

Laboratory studies using animals confirmed suspicions that fat, of all the dietary components, is uniquely correlated with cancer. For example, Carroll found that he could increase the number of mammary tumors induced in rats by a single dose of a carcinogen if he raised their

[9]Carroll, 1975; and B. Modan, Role of diet in cancer etiology, *Cancer* 40 (1977):1887-1891.

[10]Drasar and Irving, 1973.

[11]Modan, 1977.

[12]A. B. Miller, Role of nutrition in the etiology of breast cancer, *Cancer* 39 (1977):2704-2708; and B. Armstrong and R. Doll, Environmental factors and cancer incidence and mortality in different countries, with special reference to dietary practises, *International Journal of Cancer* 15 (1975):617-631.

dietary fat.[13] Both animal protein and high kcalories had previously been shown to be correlated with breast and colon cancer. In foods these are both associated with fat, so the relationship between fat itself and cancer was not surprising.

Retrospective Studies   An unexpected variable found by Carroll and other investigators was polyunsaturated fats (PUFAs).[14] They found that PUFAs had a greater effect on tumor yield than saturated fats did. In light of findings that the Japanese and Seventh-Day Adventists have both the lowest risk of colon cancer and diets low in saturated fats (a lot of vegetables and little animal protein), this finding was baffling.

This new piece of evidence also struck fear. Many people had been put on high-PUFA diets for the reduction of serum cholesterol following heart attacks. The response was quick. Immediately, several retrospective studies were made. Pearce and Day-

ton in Los Angeles looked at the eight-year records of 846 heart patients who had been put randomly on two different diets.[15] The only difference in the diets was that vegetable oil had been substituted for saturated fats. They found that patients who had been using vegetable oil had a higher incidence of death from cancer than the patients who had been using saturated fats.

Retrospective studies are those in which data previously gathered for one purpose are reexamined with a new purpose in mind. Retrospective studies can be valuable, because long-term data have already been gathered. However, such data are sometimes of questionable validity when they are used for another purpose.

The eight-year Los Angeles study just mentioned was originally undertaken in a veteran's hospital to determine whether a change from saturated fat to polyunsaturated fat would affect the longevity of heart patients. The intent was to study heart problems—not cancer.

Pearce and Dayton

pointed out in their report that their use of elderly men was not a good design for a cancer study.[16] Cancer is the second leading cause of death in the United States,[17] and it would be expected that a large number of the men in both diet groups would die of cancer, with about the same frequency as in the total population. Other writers, citing Pearce and Dayton, spoke of the results—31 out of 174 deaths due to cancer in the experimental group and 17 out of 178 deaths in the control group—as being "significant." But Pearce and Dayton thought these results were of "borderline significance," because the data were not originally collected to study cancer.[18]

CAUTION WHEN YOU READ!

Data collected for one purpose may not be valid when used for another purpose.

[13]Carroll, 1975.

[14]K. K. Carroll and H. T. Khor, Effects of level and type of dietary fat on incidence of mammary tumors induced in female Sprague-Dawley rats by 7,12-dimethylbenz-α-anthracene, *Lipids* 6 (6) (1971):415-420; and E. B. Gammal, K. K. Carroll, and E. R. Plunkett, Effects of dietary fat on mammary carcinogenesis by 7,12-dimethylbenz-α-anthracene in rats, *Cancer Research* 27 (1967):1737-1742.

[15]M. Pearce and S. Dayton, Incidence of cancer in men on a diet high in polyunsaturated fat, *Lancet* 1 (1971):464-467.

[16]Pearce and Dayton, 1971.

[17]E. N. Alcantara and E. W. Speckmann, Diet, nutrition and cancer, *American Journal of Clinical Nutrition* 29 (1976):1035-1047.

[18]Pearce and Dayton, 1971.

Results from three other retrospective studies analyzed by Ederer contradicted the results of the Los Angeles study.[19] Ederer came to the comforting conclusion that "the evidence does not support the hypothesis that cholesterol-lowering diets are carcinogenic." This finding allayed fears that we were in a double bind—that we would either have to eat saturated fats and get heart disease or have to eat polyunsaturated fats and get cancer. But nutritionists still wondered how a diet high in polyunsaturated fatty acids could initiate or promote breast and colon cancer.

The Role of Processed Fats Writing in Federation Proceedings in 1979, Enig and his co-workers reminded us that polyunsaturates are not always so unsaturated as advertised and pointed up some fallacies that had been widely accepted about the consumption of fats in the United States.[20] Raw vegetable oils, they said, contain about 10 percent saturated fatty acids and may contain up to 25 percent saturated fatty acids after refining, depending on the form in

which the oil is to be marketed (margarines, oils, or shorteneings). It may be that research animals' diets reported to be "high in polyunsaturates" were, in fact, mixtures of saturated and unsaturated fats. Enig and his co-workers also thought that there had been a misconception about the increasing use of animal fat in Western countries. They showed that the major change in fat consumption in the United States during the twentieth century has been an increase in the use of partially hydrogenated vegetable fats and that the use of animal fat has decreased.[21]

Perhaps it is processed vegetable oils that are the villains in our cancer mystery! In processing and refining vegetable oils, some of the double bonds are changed from *cis* to *trans*. (See pp. 69-70 for a discussion of *cis* and *trans* bonds.) It may be the *trans* configuration that sets the stage for cancer. The *cis* configuration is generally considered the natural bond (even though the *trans* is present in some natural products); it is changed to *trans* during processing or prolonged heating. Enig and his co-workers calculated that the consumption of *trans* fatty acids in the United States has risen from 4.14 g per person per day in 1910 to 12.1 g in 1972.[22]

```
H–C —COOH      C—COOH
   ‖              ‖
H–C —COOH      C—COOH
```

cis configuration
(maleic acid)

```
H–C —COOH
   ‖
HOOC— C–H
```

```
          C—COOH
          ‖
HOOC— C
```

trans configuration
(fumaric acid)

This new idea may account for results reported as many as forty years ago. In 1942, Tannenbaum had reported that total dietary fat correlated with cancer.[23] Few people took much notice of the article at the time; fewer still, including Tannenbaum himself, noticed that he had used hydrogenated cottonseed oil for the total fat. (However, being a meticulous researcher, he recorded this information in a footnote.) So his "total fat" was vegetable, not animal, and processed, not raw. Perhaps what he had found was a correlation between *trans* fatty acids and cancer!

What possible difference could rearrangement of the fatty acid chain around a double bond make in the incidence or growth of tumors?

---

[19]F. Ederer, Cancer among men on cholesterol-lowering diets, *Lancet* 2 (1971):203-206.

[20]M. G. Enig, R. J. Munn, and M. Keeney, Dietary fat and cancer trends: A critique, *Federation Proceedings* 37 (9) (1978):2215-2220.

[21]Enig, Munn, and Keeney, 1978.

[22]Enig, Munn, and Keeney, 1978.

[23]A. Tannenbaum, The genesis and growth of tumors: III. Effects of a high-fat diet, *Cancer Research* 2 (1942):468-475.

How can a cell know whether the hydrogen atoms are on the same side or on opposite sides of a bond? Several suggestions have been made.[24]

One way that the type of fat may influence cancer proneness is by altering cell membranes. Farmers have known for decades that certain kinds of feed produce animals for market that have a particular quality of fat. "Corn-fed beef," for example, is considered especially desirable because of the texture bestowed on the meat by the

PUFA of corn. The cell's membrane is its gatekeeper; it allows some substances to pass through freely, it ushers some in like VIPs, and it excludes some. (This role of the membrane in the life of the cell is called selective permeability.) If the structure of this membrane is altered, then the selection of substances is altered. Thus a high-PUFA diet might make cells more permeable to carcinogens. Or the changes in fatty acids in the interior of the cell might be more conducive to tumor growth. Another suggestion is that increased PUFA content in the blood may suppress the immune system, allowing a tumor to grow more freely.

The effects ascribed to a high-PUFA diet may apply only to processed PUFA and may be due to their *trans* bonds. The *cis* to *trans* alter-

ation occurs when vegetable oils are hydrogenated for a particular use or when they are heated for a long time, as in a fast-food restaurant. It may be that these altered fatty acids, incorporated into cell membranes, alter enzymes and the protein carriers mounted in cell membranes; the shape of the membranes depends on their *cis* and *trans* content.[25] It may be that the altered membrane structure affects the activity of these proteins. Hsu and Kummerow have shown that animals fed hydrogenated vegetable fats have at least one altered enzyme function, and they believe that an altered membrane structure may be the cause.[26]

Fats in Your Diet   Through some 40 years of trying to unravel the cancer mystery, researchers have moved from studying human populations to studying animals and cells. In the process they have altered their idea of the villain in this particular piece of the cancer story from animal protein, to animal fat, to high total fat, to polyunsaturated (vegetable) fat, and now to processed vegetable fat. This is as far as the story

[24]The more fat is eaten, the more bile is manufactured to emulsify it, and bile is returned to the body from the GI tract mostly in the lower colon. One theory has it that bile is carcinogenic and that the relationship of dietary fat to colon cancer is explained this way (Burkitt, 1971). Another possibility is that the kind of fat in the diet influences the kind of bacteria present in the lower colon and that the bacteria in turn alter the colon chemistry (Gammal, Carroll, and Plunkett, 1967). Colon bacteria act on the fecal matter, producing substances that may be carcinogenic (Burkitt, 1971), but some indications are that they are anticarcinogenic (Alcantara and Speckmann, 1976). Still another possibility is that fat acts by displacing fiber, and that it is the lack of fiber, not the presence of fat, that facilitates cancer initiation. Fiber is thought to speed up the transit time of all materials through the colon, thus reducing the period of exposure of the colon walls to cancer-causing substances (see Chapter 1).

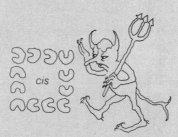

Curses! Foiled again!

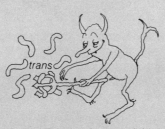

Aha! This time I can get in!

[25]H. A. Harper, *Review of Physiological Chemistry* (Los Altos, Calif.: Lange Medical Publications, 1971), p. 505.

[26]C. M. L. Hsu and F. A. Kummerow, Influence of elaidate and erucate on heart mitochondria, *Lipids* 12 (6) (1977):486-494.

has progressed; if you want to know more, you will have to stay tuned to new research in the years to come.

This Highlight has covered a lot of ground, perhaps telling you more than you wanted to know about cancer research. But we believe that only when you understand research can you appreciate the tentativeness of the result from a single experiment. "Tentativeness," you may say, "is a fine intellectual game to play. But when you are discussing the possibility of my diet causing me to develop cancer, I don't want you to be tentative. I want answers. I want to be told what changes I should make in my life in order to avoid cancer."

We wish we had answers. So do all the scientists around the world who are laboring to discover the cause of cancer. However, we promised at the beginning that we would help you to look at the evidence and make some decisions in light of that evidence.

We have seen that epidemiological studies do not speak to an individual about his probability of developing a disease. Such studies speak only about large groups of people and serve principally as pointers for the next research. Animal research cannot be translated literally into human terms until the research is repeated with humans. Human research involving the initiating

phase of cancer is obviously unthinkable. So what do you do with your diet?

There are two questions you should ask before making a decision to change your diet. First, of the material presented in this Highlight, which facts can be said to be generally accepted as true and what change in diet do these imply as advisable? Second, what are the risks connected with the change you propose to make, and do the benefits outweigh the risks?

As a preface to answering the first question, you should know that you have not been exposed here to all the viewpoints and research on the controversy over fat and cancer. We selected what we considered representative views. Another reviewer might have made a different and equally valid selection.

With this limitation in mind, let us look at the evidence. First it has not been shown that dietary fat causes cancer. A high-fat diet is linked in some way to a higher risk of breast and colon cancers—but not to all cancers. The type of fat implicated—polyunsaturated or saturated, vegetable or animal—is still being questioned. Whether or not the *trans* configuration in double bonds is the culprit (if we accept the theory that polyunsaturated fatty acids are more dangerous than saturated) is a question for much more research. It was

included here as an exciting new possibility. Conclusion: The general consensus gathered from this search of the literature is that a high-fat diet, even when it is made up mostly of polyunsaturated fats, puts you at risk for breast and colon cancer.

If you decide that your diet is high in total fat, you may want to (1) lower (not eliminate) your consumption of meat, (2) eliminate fried foods, especially from fast-food restaurants, and (3) increase your consumption of fresh fruits, vegetables, and cereals. Then you would be eating foods more nearly like the ones that the human digestive system was using as it evolved, and you would be ingesting fewer of the chemicals that have been introduced into the food supply so recently that we have no adequate information about their effect. There is no risk that we know of connected with such a change. The benefits would be lowered weight (probably), increased dietary fiber, and increased vitamins and minerals, all of which have been recommended by health professionals for years. In times of rising food prices, your new diet may even cost you less money.

It may seem that we are fudging on our promise by giving you such a simple recommendation for helping to reduce the risk of cancer. Actually we are being true to our promise. If we were economists, we would say that we are teaching you to diversify your investments, or if we were gamblers, to hedge your bets. Nutritionists call this principle dilution. We are recommending that you increase your intake of fresh fruits, vegetables, and cereals so as to crowd out—dilute—the meat and fat in your diet. There is a wide variety of fruits and vegetables on the market, so they can be varied from season to season; you would be diluting them by eating as many different ones as possible. If you were to eat a wider variety of meats and not just beef, you would be diluting the beef in your diet. This is insurance. If one of the nutrients in these foods, or a chemical that has been added to one, is found to be carcinogenic at some future date, you would not have accumulated a large amount of that chemical or nutrient in your body.

It is easy for the contemporary, well-read individual to develop paranoia from the bombardment of news about possible carcinogens. From your reading of this Highlight, we hope that you have gained an understanding of the complexity of cancer research and can now recognize the inconclusiveness of the results from a single study. We also hope that you are now a better judge of your own diet and can make intelligent, sensible alterations in it if that is necessary.

To Explore Further

The proceedings of the Conference on Nutrition in the Causation of Cancer, sponsored by the American Cancer Society and the National Cancer Institute in 1975, are published in *Cancer Research* 35 (November 1975).

Dunn, J. E., Jr., Cancer epidemiology in populations of the United States—with emphasis on Hawaii and California—and Japan, *Cancer Research* 35 (2) (November 1975):3240-3245, gives a complete discussion of population studies.

These articles report research that show roles for specific foods in the genesis of tumors:

Alcantara, E. N., and Speckman, E. W., Diet, nutrition, and cancer, *American Journal of Clinical Nutrition* 29 (1976):1035-1047.

Graham, S., Dayal, H., Mittelman, A., Swanson, M., and Wilkinson, G., Diet in the epidemiology of cancer of the colon and rectum, *Journal of the National Cancer Institute* 61 (1978):709-714.

Lowenfels, A. B., and Anderson, M. E., Diet and cancer, *Cancer* 39 (1977):1809-1814.

Carroll, K. K., Experimental evidence of dietary factors and hormone-dependent cancers, *Cancer Research* 35 (2) (November 1975):3374-3383, discusses the genesis of tumors more fully.

Many writers on nutrition and cancer relationships have recommended the use of a "prudent" diet. Some of these, notably Wynder writing in *Cancer Research* (November 1975), are referring to the following:

Bennett, I., *The Prudent Diet* (New York: David White, 1973).

Exercises 1 to 6 make use of the information you recorded on Forms 1 to 3 in the Self-Study at the end of the introduction to Part One.

1. How many grams of fat do you consume in a day?

2. How many kcalories does this represent? (Remember, 1 g fat contributes 9 kcal.)

3. What percentage of your total kcalories is contributed by fat? (To figure this, divide your fat kcalories by your total kcalories, then multiply by 100.)

4. A dietary goal quoted in Chapter 2 was for fat to contribute not more than 30 percent of total kcalories. How does your fat intake compare with this recommendation? If it is higher, look over your food records and answer the following questions: What specific foods should you cut down on or eliminate, and what foods should you increase or add to your diet in order to bring your total fat intake into line?

5. Within total fat, a 1:1:1 ratio of polyunsaturated, monounsaturated, and saturated fat is sometimes recommended. Using the averages you computed on Form 2 at the end of the introduction to Part One (p. 16), you can compare your intakes of linoleic acid (polyunsaturated), oleic acid (monounsaturated), and saturated fat to see what ratio is characteristic of your diet. The lowest of these three numbers should appear as 1 in expressing the ratio. To express the ratio, therefore, divide all three numbers by the lowest of the three. (For example, if the three numbers were 10, 20, and 30, you would divide all three by 10, arriving at a ratio of 1:2:3.)

6. Does the ratio agree reasonably well with the 1:1:1 ratio recommended? Or is your polyunsaturated fat intake higher than 1 in comparison with your saturated fat intake? If so, okay. But if not—if your saturated fat intake is relatively high—then answer the following questions: What specific foods should you cut down on or eliminate, and what foods should you increase or add to your diet in order to bring your fat intake into better balance? (Look over your food records to see which foods are the greatest contributors of the various kinds of fat.)

Optional Extras

● You can also estimate, if you wish, how much cholesterol you consume daily, using Appendix G. How does your cholesterol intake compare with a dietary goal of not more than 300 mg a day?

● It is usually recommended that 2 percent of your kcalories come from the essential fatty acid, linoleic acid. Is your diet in accord with this recommendation?

● You may not be aware of how large your meat portions are. Weigh them for a day or so to see. Then calculate how much fat you derive from meat in a day. To visualize this amount of fat, measure it from your butter or margarine dish onto a plate.

CHAPTER 3

CONTENTS

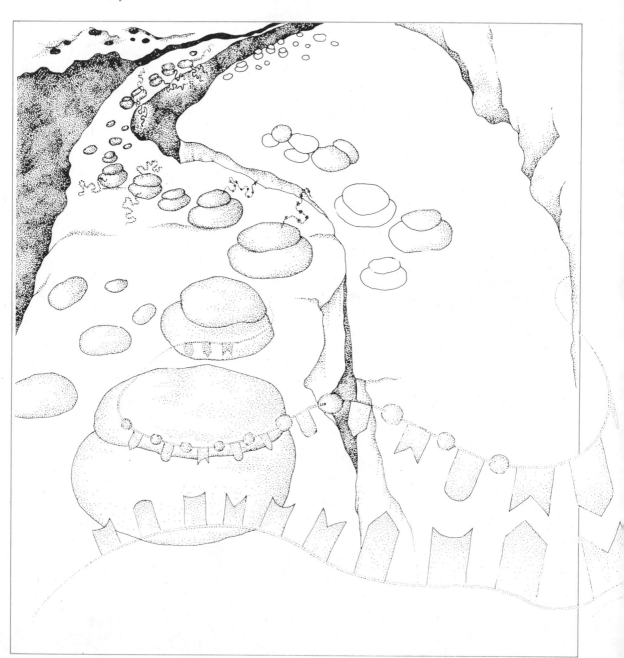

PROTEIN: Amino Acids

To make an organism demands the right substances in the right proportions and in the right arrangement. We do not think that anything more is needed — but that is problem enough.

GEORGE WALD

Everybody knows that protein is important. It is advertised on every cereal box; it is said to "build strong bodies" and to provide "super go power." In fact, as you will see, protein has been so overemphasized that many people eat more than enough, sometimes at the expense of other nutrients that are equally important. An understanding of the quantity and quality of protein will help put it in its proper place — as only one of the many essential nutrients needed in correct proportions to achieve a balanced diet.

The preceding two chapters, on carbohydrates and lipids, began with sections describing the roles of these nutrients in the body, then moved on to a consideration of their structure. This chapter, on the contrary, describes the structure of protein first, because protein's structure enables it to play many more roles than carbohydrate or lipid. All three nutrients are important, and all three share the common function of providing energy, but protein is far more versatile.

Protein structure is also far more interesting than that of carbohydrate or lipid. The regularity and simplicity of protein structure have yielded only recently to human investigation. Those who have worked on elucidating the structure of protein have been rewarded with a rare insight into the elegance of nature's designs.

The Chemist's View of Protein

A protein is a chemical compound composed of the same atoms as carbohydrate and lipid—carbon, hydrogen, and oxygen—but protein also contains nitrogen atoms. These C, H, O, and N atoms are arranged into amino acids, which are linked into chains to form proteins. It is easy to construct a protein once we know what an amino acid looks

protein: a compound composed of C, H, O, and N, arranged into amino acids linked in a chain. Proteins also contain some S (sulfur).

like, and the unit structure of an amino acid is simpler than that of either carbohydrates (monosaccharides) or lipids (glycerol and fatty acids).

Amino Acid Structure   An amino acid has a backbone of one nitrogen and two carbon atoms linked together. Recall that carbons must form four bonds with other atoms, oxygens two, and hydrogens one. In amino acids, nitrogens form three bonds with other atoms. The structure that all amino acids have in common fulfills these requirements:

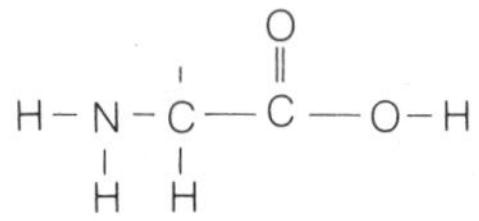

amino (a-MEEN-oh) **acid:** a building block of protein; a compound containing an amino group and an acid group attached to a central carbon, which also carries a distinctive side chain.

amino = containing nitrogen

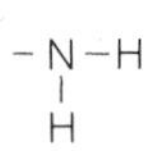

At one end is an amino group (NH_2); at the other is an acid group (COOH). Both are attached to a central carbon that also carries a hydrogen (H). As you can see, on this drawing one position is left unfilled: The central carbon atom must have another atom or group of atoms attached to it to make a complete structure.

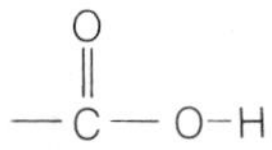

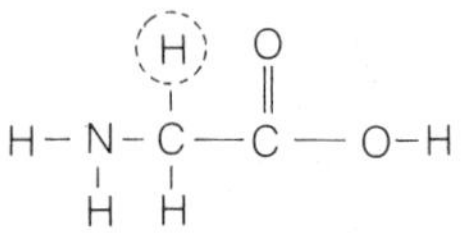

This central carbon atom and the attached structures are what make proteins so different from either carbohydrates or lipids. A polysaccharide (starch, for example) is composed of glucose units one after the other. It may be 100 or 200 units long, but every unit in the chain is a glucose molecule just like all the others. In a protein, on the other hand, 22 different amino acids may appear. Each differs from the others in the nature of the side group that it carries on the central carbon. The simplest amino acid, glycine, has a hydrogen atom in that position. A slightly more complex amino acid, alanine, has an extra carbon with three attached hydrogen atoms. Other amino acids have still more complex side groups. For example, one amino acid may have an acid group, another may have an amino group. Still others may have aromatic ring structures. Thus although the basic structure of an amino acid is simple, the side groups may be quite elaborate.

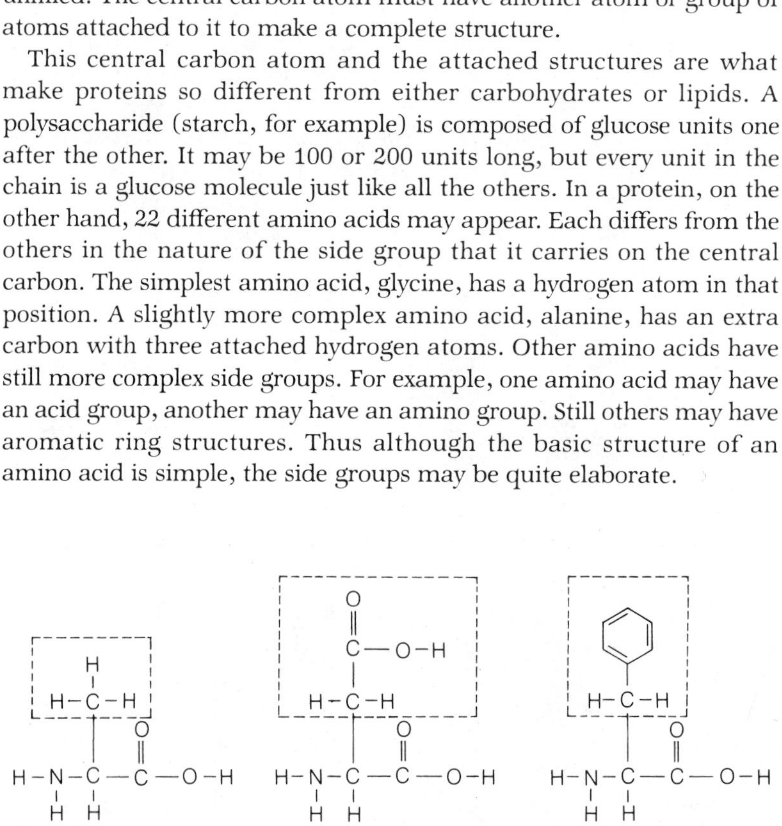

Amino group   Acid group

Glycine

Examples of amino acids.

Alanine   Aspartic acid   Phenylalanine

Amino Acid Sequence   The 22 different common amino acids may be linked together in a great variety of ways to form proteins. They connect by means of a condensation reaction similar to those you have seen before. An OH is removed from the acid end of one and an H from the amino group of another amino acid. A bond forms between the two amino acids, and the H and OH join to form a molecule of water. The resulting structure is called a dipeptide:

Condensation reactions: see pp. 27, 64.

dipeptide: two amino acids bonded together. The bond between two amino acids is a **peptide bond**.

di = two
peptide = amino acid

Formation of a dipeptide by condensation of two amino acids.

By the same reaction, the OH can be removed from the acid end of the second amino acid and an H from the amino group of a third to form a tripeptide. As additional amino acids are added to the chain, a polypeptide is formed. Most proteins are polypeptides, 100 to 300 amino acids long.

It would be misleading, however, to end the description here, because in showing the structures on paper we have drawn a straight, flat chain. Actually, polypeptide chains fold and tangle so that they look not like rods but like crazy jungle gyms or tangled balls of yarn. The sequence of amino acids in a protein determines which specific way the chain will fold.

tripeptide: three amino acids bonded together by peptide bonds.

tri = three

polypeptide: many amino acids bonded together by peptide bonds. *Many* refers to 10 or more. An intermediate string of between 4 and 10 amino acids is an **oligopeptide**.

poly = many
oligo = few

Folding of the Chain   The chain structure can best be visualized by keeping in mind that each side group on the amino acids has special characteristics that attract it to other groups. Some side groups are negatively charged, others are positively charged, and the aromatic rings are attracted to other aromatic rings. As amino acids are added to a polypeptide chain and the chain lengthens, the acids that are negatively charged move as close as possible to those that are positively charged. Since the molecule is in a watery solution, these charged groups, being hydrophilic (see p. 71), tend to expose themselves on the outer surface of the completed protein; the aromatic groups, being hydrophobic (see p. 71), tend to tuck themselves inside. The shape the polypeptide finally assumes is usually globular, giving it the maximum stability possible in water solution. Finally, two or more of these giant molecules may associate to form a still larger working aggregate. Thus

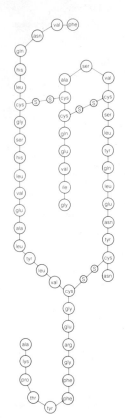

(Figure at left)
The complete amino acid sequence of insulin, a small protein. S-S represents the cross-links between cystine molecules, known as disulfide bridges. (For structures and abbreviations of the individual amino acids, see Appendix C.)

the completed protein is one or more very complex tangled chains of amino acids, bristling on the surface with positive and negative charges.

When a protein molecule is subjected to heat, acid, or other conditions that disturb its stability, it uncoils or changes its shape, thus losing its function to some extent. That is what happens to an egg when it is cooked; alterations of the egg proteins during cooking largely account for the observable changes in the egg white and yolk.

The Completed Protein If you could step onto a carbohydrate molecule like starch and walk along it, the first stepping stone would be a glucose. Your next stepping stone would be glucose again, and then glucose, and then glucose, and then glucose. But if you were to step onto one end of a polypeptide chain, your first stepping stone might be a glycine. Your second might be an alanine. The third might be a glycine again, and the fourth a tryptophan, then a serine, and so on. In other words, the variety of units in a protein, in both their nature and their sequence, is far greater than it is in a carbohydrate molecule.

By way of another analogy, if you were to try to make a sentence using only the letter G, you could only speak gibberish: G-G-G-G-G-G. But with 26 different letters available, you can say, "To be or not to be, that is the question"—or on a different plane, "The way to a man's heart is through his stomach." The Greek alphabet contains only 24 letters, and all of Homer was written with it.

The variety of sequences in which the 22 amino acids can be linked together is even greater than that possible for letters in a sentence, because proteins do not have to be pronounced. This gives them a tremendous range of possible surface structures, which in turn enable them to perform very distinct, individual, and specialized functions.

The change in a protein's shape brought about by heat, acid, or other conditions is known as **denaturation**. Past a certain point, denaturation is irreversible.

tryptophan (TRIP-toe-fane) and **serine** (SEAR-een): amino acids. A complete list of the amino acids, with their structures, appears in Appendix C.

maltase: the enzyme that hydrolyzes maltose to two glucose units.

maltose: the disaccharide composed of 2 glucose units (see p. 32).

ase: a suffix denoting an enzyme, usually identifying the compound that the enzyme works on. Thus maltase is the enzyme that works on maltose.

Enzymes: A Function of Protein

In Chapter 1 we mentioned enzymes for the first time, and we promised that we would look at these magnificent molecules more closely when protein structure had been explained. Let's start by looking at the enzyme maltase.

A typical protein, maltase is a tangled ball-shaped polypeptide chain, 100 or so amino acids long. The little molecule maltose, on the other hand, is a disaccharide perhaps 100 times smaller. If you were one of the glucoses in maltose, you would be joined to the other glucose like a Siamese twin, incomplete and unable to stand alone for lack of an H or an OH. Suppose you were swallowed by a person: You would travel down her esophagus, and after spending some time in her stomach, you would find yourself floating around in the watery medium of her small intestine. Looking about, you would see many giant enzymes working on, breaking down, and putting together a variety of other compounds like yourself. Sooner or later you would find yourself snapping into position on the surface of a maltase, an enzyme custom-designed to fit your contours. On this surface you would encounter a molecule of water, and as you split away from your glucose twin, the water would also split apart, its H being added to one of you and its OH to the other. Released as a free glucose, you might turn around to see other pairs being attracted into that same position and being hydrolyzed just as you had been.

Enzymes and what they do are so fundamental to all life processes that it may be worthwhile to introduce a somewhat fanciful analogy in order to clarify two important characteristics they all share. Enzymes could be compared to the ministers and judges who respectively make and dissolve human matrimonial bonds. When two individuals come to a minister to be married, the couple leaves with a new bond between them. They are joined together. But the minister is only momentarily involved in this process and remains unchanged and available to perform other ceremonies between other pairs of people. One minister can perform thousands of marriage ceremonies. In a divorce court, the judge plays a similar but opposite role. A couple enters the court, the judge performs the dissolution, and the couple leaves as two separate individuals. Like the minister, the judge may decree many divorces before he dies or retires.

The minister represents enzymes that synthesize larger compounds from smaller ones—the synthetases, which build body structures. The judge represents enzymes that hydrolyze larger compounds to smaller ones—the proteases, lipases, carbohydrases, disaccharidases, and others. Maltase is a disaccharidase.

The first point to be learned is that some enzymes put compounds together and others take them apart. Since you yourself are a very "put-together" kind of organism, superbly organized out of billions of molecules that have been bonded together to make muscle, bone, skin, eyes, and blood cells, you can imagine how numerous and very active in your body are the enzymes that put things together.

The second point to be learned is that the enzymes are not themselves affected in the process of facilitating chemical reactions: They are catalysts. The technical definition of an enzyme, which biologists and chemists use, is a protein catalyst.

What makes you unique and distinct from any other human being is minute differences in your body proteins (enzymes, antibodies, and others). These differences are determined by the amino acid sequences of your proteins, which are written into the genetic code of the DNA you inherited from your parents and ancestors. Each person receives at conception a unique combination of DNA codes for these sequences. The DNA code directs the making of all the body's proteins, as shown in Figure 1.

An apology for the use of fanciful descriptions appears in the Note to the Student.

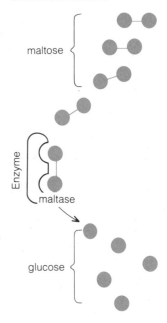

Model of enzyme action.

synthetase (SIN-the-tase): an enzyme that synthesizes compounds.

protease (PRO-tee-ase): an enzyme that hydrolyzes proteins.

lipase (LYE-pase): an enzyme that hydrolyzes lipids.

The definitions of **carbohydrase, disaccharidase, sucrase, lactase,** and **phospholipase** are self-evident.

catalyst (CAT-uh-list): a compound that facilitates chemical reactions without itself being destroyed in the process.

enzyme: a protein catalyst.

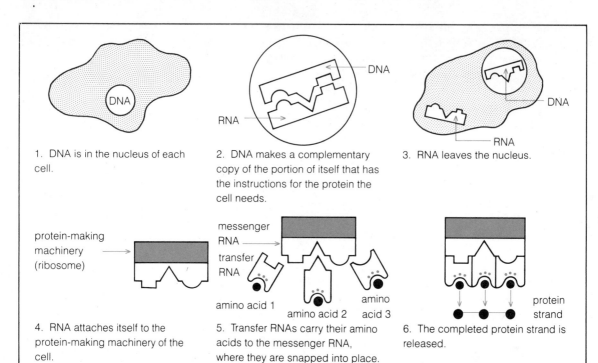

1. DNA is in the nucleus of each cell.

2. DNA makes a complementary copy of the portion of itself that has the instructions for the protein the cell needs.

3. RNA leaves the nucleus.

4. RNA attaches itself to the protein-making machinery of the cell.

5. Transfer RNAs carry their amino acids to the messenger RNA, where they are snapped into place.

6. The completed protein strand is released.

Figure 1 Protein synthesis. The instructions for making every protein in a person's body are transmitted in the genetic information he or she receives at conception. This body of knowledge is filed away in the nucleus of every cell. The master file is the DNA (deoxyribonucleic acid), which never leaves the nucleus. The DNA is identical in every cell and is specific for each individual. Each specialized cell has access to the total inherited information but calls on only the instructions needed for its own functions.

In order to inform the cell of the proper sequence of amino acids for a needed protein, a "photocopy" of the appropriate portion of DNA is made. This copy is messenger RNA (ribonucleic acid), which is able to escape through the nuclear membrane. In the cell fluid it seeks out and attaches itself to one of the ribosomes (a protein-making machine, itself composed of RNA and protein). Thus situated, the messenger RNA presents the specifications for the amino acids to be linked into a protein strand.

Meanwhile, another form of RNA, called transfer RNA, collects amino acids from the cell fluid and brings them to the messenger. For each of the 22 amino acids there is a specific kind of transfer RNA. Thousands of these transfer RNAs, with their loads of amino acids, cluster around the ribosomes, like vegetable-laden trucks around a farmer's market awaiting their turn to unload. When an amino acid is called for by the messenger, the transfer RNA carrying it snaps into position. Then the next and the next and the next loaded transfer RNAs move into place. Thus the amino acids are lined up in the right sequence. Then an enzyme bonds them together.

Finally, the completed protein strand is released, the messenger is degraded, and the transfer RNAs are freed to return for another load. It takes many words to describe these events, but in the cell, 40 to 100 amino acids can be added to a growing protein strand in only a second.

Perhaps you have realized by now that the protein story moves in a circle. All enzymes are proteins. All proteins are made of amino acids. Amino acids have to be put together to make proteins. Enzymes put together the amino acids. Only living systems work with such self-renewal. A broken toaster cannot be fixed by another toaster. A car cannot make another car. Only living creatures and those parts that they are composed of—the cells—can duplicate themselves and make the parts of which they are made. To follow the circle in nutrition, start with a person eating proteins. The proteins are broken down by proteins (enzymes) into amino acids. The amino acids enter the cells of the body, where proteins (enzymes) put them together in long chains with sequences specified by DNA. The chains fold and become enzymes themselves. These enzymes may then be used to break apart other compounds or to put other compounds together. Day by day, billion reactions by billion reactions, these processes repeat themselves and life goes on.

A Closer Look at Enzyme Action

If you look closely at the details of the reaction sequences governed by enzymes, some additional important facts emerge. The following description is an example of the way enzymes work to alter the structure of a compound. It is the only example in this book of biochemistry at the level biochemists actually think about it. The object is to give you an insight into the kinds of processes that account for human nutritional needs.

Let's look at a biochemical pathway partway along its length and see how each enzyme alters the structure of a compound until one thing has been converted into another quite different thing. Beginning with glucose, a six-carbon compound, enzymes add a phosphate group, altering and breaking this structure until a three-carbon compound results—which looks like compound A.

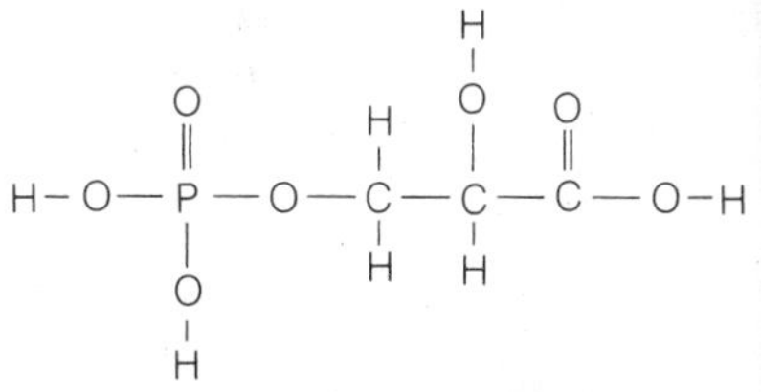

An intermediate in glucose metabolism (compound A).

Compound A floats around until it encounters an enzyme with the specialized function of removing hydrogen atoms (from these compounds). The encounter results in the altered compound, compound B.

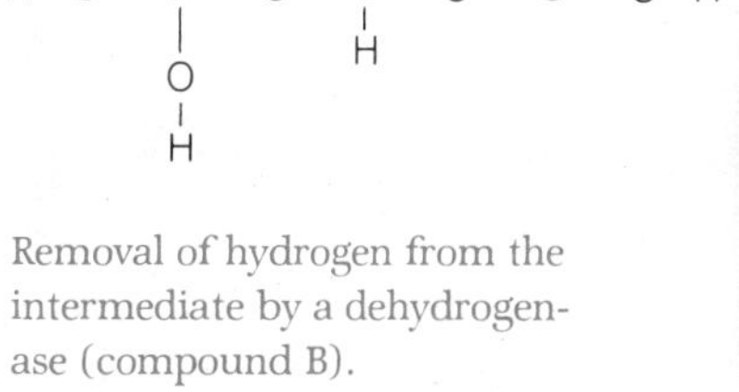

Removal of hydrogen from the intermediate by a dehydrogenase (compound B).

Compound B is released from the enzyme and later encounters another enzyme, which removes oxygens and substitutes amino groups. What results is compound C.

The structure for compound C (phosphate-amino acid intermediate) is shown.

Removal of oxygen and substitution of H and NH_2 by a transaminase (compound C).

The structure for compound D is shown.

Removal of phosphate by a phosphatase (compound D).

The structure for compound E is shown.

What is it (compound E)?

essential amino acid: an amino acid that the body cannot synthesize in amounts sufficient to meet physiological need. The eight amino acids known to be essential for human adults:

methionine (meh-THIGH-o-neen)
threonine (THREE-o-neen)
tryptophan (TRIP-toe-fane)
isoleucine (eye-so-LOO-seen)
leucine (LOO-seen)
lysine (LYE-seen)
valine (VAY-leen)
phenylalanine (fee-nul-AL-uh-neen)

Infants also require **histidine** (HISS-tuh-deen).[1]

Students attempting to learn these by heart often use the device "TV TILL PM" to recall their first letters.

The next enzyme removes the phosphate group from the end carbon and replaces it with a hydrogen, leaving compound D.

If you look closely at the picture of compound D, you may recognize its characteristics and not be surprised by the statements that follow. But first let us take the process one more step. Another enzyme, whose function is to remove CH_2OH groups from these molecules, forms compound E. Look at this product closely. It is one that you may recognize because you have seen it before. It has an amino group at one end, an acid group at the other, and a central carbon carrying two Hs. It is the amino acid glycine (p. 98).

Well, how about that! We started with a molecule of glucose, a derivative of dietary carbohydrate, and by making one minute change after another, we transformed it into an amino acid, a member of the protein family.

The lesson to be learned from this sequence of events is that the body can make, from glucose and nitrogen-containing compounds, many of the amino acids needed to build body proteins. Glycine is one of those. Compound D, which precedes glycine, is the amino acid serine (which has a CH_2OH on its central carbon). This too is an amino acid the body can make.

The Essential Amino Acids

It should now be clear that the role of protein in food is not to provide body proteins directly but to supply the amino acids from which the body can make its own proteins. Since the body can make glycine and serine for itself, the proteins in the diet need not contain these two amino acids. But there are some amino acids that the body cannot make at all, and some that it cannot make fast enough to meet its need. (This is because the body does not possess the genetic code for making the enzymes necessary to synthesize these amino acids, or because the enzymes it does make work too slowly.) These amino acids are referred to as essential amino acids; it is essential that they be included in the diet.

[1]R. E. Olson, Clinical nutrition: An interface between human ecology and internal medicine, *Nutrition Reviews* 36 (June 1978): 161-178.

In Chapter 2, one fatty acid was singled out as a dietary essential for the same reason: because it cannot be synthesized in the body. All compounds in your body are needed for your health, but those that you cannot make for yourself are needed in your diet, and these are called essential nutrients. With the addition of the eight essential amino acids, your list of essential nutrients has now expanded to nine.

To make body protein, a cell must have all 22 amino acids available simultaneously. The first important characteristic of dietary protein is therefore that it should supply at least the eight essential amino acids plus enough additional nitrogen for the synthesis of the others.

Protein Quality

A complete protein is a protein that contains all of the essential amino acids; it may or may not contain all of the others. A high-quality protein is one that is not only complete but also contains the essential amino acids in amounts proportional to the body's need for them.

Ideally, dietary protein would supply each amino acid in the amount needed for protein synthesis in the body. If one amino acid is supplied in an amount smaller than is needed, the total amount of protein that can be synthesized from the others will be limited. By analogy, suppose that a signmaker plans to make 100 identical signs, each saying LEFT TURN ONLY. He needs 200 Ls, 200 Ns, 200 Ts, and 100 of each of the other letters. If he has only 20 Ls, he can make only 10 signs, even if all the other letters are available in unlimited quantities. The Ls limit the number of signs that can be made. If he doesn't get some more Ls, he will have to throw away all his other letters.

When the body uses a protein of poor quality, it wastes many of the amino acids. What happens is that enzymes strip off the nitrogen-containing amino groups and fix them into the compound urea, and the urea is excreted in the urine. The carbon skeletons that remain can be used to make glucose or fat, but the nitrogen from amino acids cannot be stored in the body. The amount of urea excreted is thus a measure of the number of wasted amino acids.

The quality of dietary protein thus depends partly on whether the protein supplies all the essential amino acids and, more important, on the extent to which it supplies them in the needed proportions. An excellent protein by these standards is egg protein, whose nitrogen tends to be retained in the body. Egg protein has been designated the reference protein and has been assigned a biological value of 100 by the Food and Agriculture Organization of the United Nations, which sets world standards.

The amino acid composition of a test protein can be compared with the composition of egg protein, and a chemical score can be derived to express the theoretical value of the test protein. A test protein with a chemical score of 70, for example, contains a limiting amino acid, and

complete protein: a protein containing all of the amino acids essential for humans.

high-quality protein: a complete protein whose amino acids fit the pattern needed by humans. (A true high-quality protein is also easily digestible.)

EFT TURN ON Y

limiting amino acid: the amino acid found in the shortest supply relative to the amounts needed for protein synthesis in the body.

How urea is made: see Chapter 7.

reference protein: egg protein; used by FAO/WHO as a standard against which to measure the quality of other proteins.

chemical score: a rating of the quality of a test protein arrived at by comparing its amino acid pattern with that of a reference protein.

that amino acid is present in only 70 percent of the amount found in the ideal amino acid pattern. If you fed that test protein to a human being, you could expect 30 percent of its amino acids to be wasted (30 percent of its nitrogen to be excreted in the urine).

In a world where food is scarce and where many people's diets contain marginal or inadequate amounts of protein, it is important to know which foods contain the highest-quality protein. It is now possible to determine the amino acid composition of any protein relatively inexpensively, but unfortunately chemical scoring does not always give an accurate reflection of the way a protein will be used by the body. One reason is that proteins also differ in digestibility. If a protein can't be digested to small fragments—amino acids, dipeptides, and tripeptides—then its amino acids will not pass across the intestinal wall into the blood but will be lost in the feces.

digestibility: the amount of protein absorbed from a given intake. To learn why liquid protein is less digestible than whole protein, even though it is delivered in small fragments, turn to p. 163.

To determine the actual value of a protein as it is used by the body, it is therefore necessary to measure not only urinary but also fecal losses of nitrogen when that protein is actually fed to human beings under test conditions. (Even then, small additional losses from sweat, shed skin, and the like will be missed.) This kind of experiment provides the determinations of biological value (BV) of protein that are used internationally. (The mathematics of chemical scoring and biological value determinations are presented in Appendix E for those who are interested.) The biological values of the protein in some sample foods are shown below. Generally, a biological value of 70 or above indicates acceptable quality.

biological value (BV): the amount of protein retained from a given amount absorbed. BV is more fully explained in Appendix E.

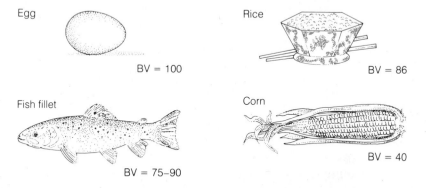

Egg   Rice

BV = 100   BV = 86

Fish fillet   Corn

BV = 75–90   BV = 40

As you may well imagine, determining the biological value of a protein is a cumbersome and expensive procedure. A different laboratory test involves feeding a test protein to young animals (usually rats) and measuring their growth rate. This measure, the protein efficiency ratio (PER), is used to qualify statements about daily protein requirements in the United States. You are assumed to eat protein with a PER of 70 or above; if the PER is lower, you need more protein.

protein efficiency ratio (PER): a measure of protein quality derived by feeding a test protein to growing animals and determining their weight gain.

For those who choose not to tangle with the formulas for BV and PER, a convenient way to distinguish among proteins is to think of animal proteins as being generally of higher quality than plant proteins. However, the educated vegetarian can design a perfectly acceptable diet around plant foods alone.

Diet planning for the vegetarian: see Highlight 3.

This statement, like all generalizations, will not quite stand up to close inspection. One animal protein that is not complete is gelatin (it lacks tryptophan). Ironically, this is the protein often recommended for correcting cracked nails and dull or brittle hair. The logic is that, because these tissues are made of protein, a drink of protein will improve their texture. Even if this were the case, however—and a symptom, you remember, is not a deficiency disease—gelatin supplements would help only if protein containing tryptophan had already been supplied. And if that protein were complete, then the gelatin would not be needed!

There is a place for low-quality proteins in the diet, however. An excellent way to support the efficient use of high-quality animal protein is to eat plenty of plant protein along with it. Research has shown that expensive meat protein is far more efficiently used when ample bread, cereal, and vegetable protein accompanies it. An adult needs only 20 percent of his total protein as essential amino acids.[2]

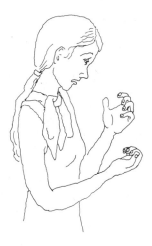

There is one circumstance in which dietary protein—no matter how high the quality—will not be used efficiently by the body and will not support growth: when energy from other energy nutrients is lacking. The body assigns top priority to meeting its energy needs, and when kcalories from other sources are not available, it will break down protein to meet this need. Stripping off and excreting the nitrogen from the amino acids, it will use their carbon skeletons in much the same way it uses those from glucose or from fat.

Other conditions may also affect the body's use of protein. The presence of other nutrients—vitamins, minerals, and water—is needed to process the protein, and the body itself must be in a healthy state in order to absorb and assimilate it. Cooking methods affect digestibility: Moist heat enhances it, and dry heat may reduce it.

In summary, to be used with maximum efficiency a protein must contain an amino acid pattern tailored to meet the body's needs; it must be digestible; it must be consumed with sufficient kcalories from other sources so that it will not be used for energy; it must be accompanied by the needed vitamins, minerals, and water; and it must be received by a body that is healthy and equipped to use it.

Carbohydrate and fat allow amino acids to be used to build body proteins. This is known as the **protein-sparing action** of carbohydrate and fat.

Energy value of protein: 1 g provides 4 kcal.

[2]M. C. Crim and H. N. Munro, Protein, in *Nutrition Reviews' Present Knowledge in Nutrition*, 4th ed. (Washington, D. C.: Nutrition Foundation, 1976), pp. 43-54.

Recommended Protein Intakes

nitrogen balance: the amount of nitrogen consumed (N-in) as compared with the amount of nitrogen excreted (N-out) in a given period of time. To learn about nitrogen balance and the athlete, turn to Chapter 16.

The average amino acid weighs about 6.25 times as much as the nitrogen it contains, so the laboratory scientist can estimate the protein in food by multiplying the weight of the food nitrogen by 6.25.

nitrogen equilibrium (zero nitrogen balance): N-in = N-out.

positive nitrogen balance: N-in > N-out.

negative nitrogen balance: N-in < N-out.

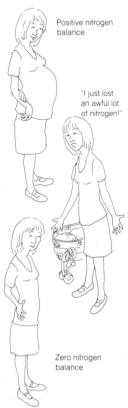

Positive nitrogen balance

"I just lost an awful lot of nitrogen!"

Zero nitrogen balance

Quality and total kcalories are not the only important factors in selecting protein for your diet. The quantity of protein that you need depends on the amount of lean tissue in your body. Fat tissue requires relatively little protein to maintain itself, but the muscles and blood and other metabolically active tissues must be maintained by a continuous supply of essential amino acids. To determine how much protein a person needs, the laboratory scientist can perform a nitrogen balance study.

Protein is the only one of the three energy nutrients that contains nitrogen, so it is possible to follow its path through the body simply by following the nitrogen. Furthermore, the amount of nitrogen in a mixture of substances can easily be measured. When we measure the amount of nitrogen in a meal, we are also measuring indirectly the amount of protein in the meal. When we measure the nitrogen excreted by a person in feces and urine (and to a lesser extent in hair, fingernails, and perspiration), we are indirectly measuring the amount of protein that is being lost from the body.

Under normal circumstances healthy adults are in nitrogen equilibrium or zero nitrogen balance—they have at all times the same amount of total protein in their bodies. When nitrogen-in exceeds nitrogen-out, they are said to be in positive nitrogen balance; this means that somewhere in their bodies more proteins are being built than are being broken down and lost. When nitrogen-in is less than nitrogen-out, they are said to be in negative nitrogen balance. Let's consider some of the circumstances in which these non-zero balances occur.

Growing children add to their bodies every day new blood, bone, and muscle cells. Since these cells contain protein, children must have in their bodies more protein (and therefore more nitrogen) at the end of each day than they had at the beginning. A growing child is therefore in positive nitrogen balance. Similarly, when a woman is pregnant she is in essence growing a new organism; she too must be in positive nitrogen balance (although on the day she gives birth she loses at one fell swoop a tremendous amount of the protein she has accumulated). When she is lactating, she may be in equilibrium again, but it is a sort of enhanced equilibrium. She is eating more protein than before to make her milk and is excreting it whenever the baby nurses.

Negative nitrogen balance occurs when muscle or other protein tissue is broken down and lost. When people have to rest in bed for a period of time, their muscles atrophy, and they suffer a net loss of protein. One of several problems faced by nutritionists responsible for the welfare of the astronauts was that of the negative nitrogen balance that occurred when they were confined for days in the space capsule; their muscles failed to receive enough exercise to maintain themselves.

On the basis of nitrogen balance studies and other experiments, governments attempt to set recommendations for people's protein intakes. Some of these recommendations are described in the following sections.

U.S. Recommendations One recommendation for protein intake has already been mentioned in the preceding chapters. The Senate committee that published the Dietary Goals for the United States observed that protein intake has been relatively constant in U.S. diets for many decades, representing about 12 percent of the total kcalories consumed. In setting the Dietary Goals for protein, fat, and carbohydrate, the committee recommended that you continue to consume about 12 percent of your kcalories from protein. They reasoned that your intakes need not be higher in protein than they already are and that a reduction in protein intake, which might require drastic alterations in your lifestyle, would not pay off in any predictable benefits. The Dietary Goals for the three energy nutrients, then, were:

- *Protein.* 12 percent of kcalories (more loosely, 10 to 15 percent is fine).
- *Carbohydrate.* 58 percent of kcalories (or more).
- *Fat.* 30 percent of kcalories (or less).

A much more formal recommendation for protein intake is the Recommended Dietary Allowance (RDA). (Don't confuse the RDA with the U.S. RDA used on labels: see pp. 440-441.) Protein is the first nutrient discussed in this book for which there is an RDA, so some discussion of the RDA is in order here. The agency that has responsibility for setting formal recommendations for nutrient intake for U.S. citizens is the Committee on RDA of the Food and Nutrition Board. Its most recent recommendations for protein intakes were published in 1979-1980. The Committee on RDA stated that a generous protein allowance for a healthy adult would be 0.8 g of high-quality protein per kilogram of ideal body weight per day. Suppose that your ideal weight is 50 kilograms; your protein RDA would then be 0.8 times 50, or 40 g of protein each day.

The Committee uses the ideal, not the actual, weight for this calculation because that weight is proportional to the lean body mass of the average person. If you gain weight, your fat tissue increases in mass; but fat tissue is composed largely of fat—C, H, and O—and does not require much protein for maintenance.

The RDAs have been much misunderstood. One young woman, on first learning of their existence, was outraged: "You mean Uncle Sam tells me that I must eat exactly 40 g of protein every day?" This is not the government's intention, and the RDAs are not commandments. The following facts will help put the RDAs in perspective:

- They are published by the government, but the study group that recommends them is composed of nutritionists and other scientists, not politicians.

Recommended Dietary Allowances (RDA): published by the Food and Nutrition Board (FNB) of the National Academy of Sciences/National Research Council (NAS/NRC).

To figure your protein RDA, follow the directions in Exercise 5 in the Self-Study at the end of Highlight 3.

● They are based on available scientific evidence to the greatest extent possible and are revised about every five years for this reason.

● They are recommendations, not requirements, and certainly not minimum requirements. They are thought by the Food and Nutrition Board to include a margin of safety for most people, being perhaps about 30 percent higher than the average requirement.

● They are based on the understanding that people's nutrient needs are not identical but fall within a range. They recommend an intake thought to be near the upper end of that range.

● They are for healthy persons only; medical problems alter nutrient needs.

RDA tables: see the inside front cover.

RDAs are published for protein and several vitamins and minerals as well as for kcalories. Separate recommendations are made for different groupings of people. Children 4 to 6 years old are distinguished from men 19 to 22, for example. Each individual can look up the recommendations for his or her own age-sex group. No RDA is set for carbohydrate or fat. The assumption is that you will use a certain number of kcalories meeting your protein needs and then will distribute the remaining kcalories among carbohydrate and fat and possibly alcohol, according to your personal preference, to meet your energy RDA.

The RDA for Protein

The most important thing to understand about the RDA at first is the way the numbers were chosen, and a theoretical discussion will illustrate this.

Suppose we were the Committee on RDA and we had the task of setting an RDA for nutrient X. Ideally, our first step would be to try to find out how much of that nutrient individual people need. We might review and select the most valid balance studies. We would note the subjects' losses of the nutrient and determine exactly what intake they needed to stay in balance. For each individual subject, we could determine a *requirement* for nutrient X. Below the requirement, that person would slip into negative balance and begin to develop a deficiency.

requirement: the amount of a nutrient that will just prevent the development of specific deficiency signs.

We would find that different individuals have different requirements. Mr. A might need 40 units of the nutrient each day to maintain balance, Ms. B might need 35, and Mr. C, 65. If we looked at enough individuals, we might find that their requirements fell into a normal distribution, that most were somewhere close to the mean and only a few were at the extremes. Figure 2 depicts this situation.

normal distribution: a distribution in which the majority of points cluster near the mean. The graph of this distribution is symmetrical and bell-shaped.

Then we would have to decide what intake to recommend for everybody: We would have to set the RDA. Should we set it at the mean (shown in Figure 2 at 45 units)? This is the average requirement for

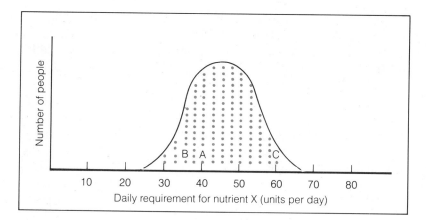

nutrient X; it is the closest to everyone's need. But if people took us literally and consumed exactly this amount of nutrient X each day, half of the population would develop deficiencies, Mr. C among them.

Perhaps we should set the RDA for nutrient X at or above the extreme—say, at 70 units a day—so that everyone would be covered. (Actually, we didn't study everyone, so we would have to worry that some individual we didn't happen to test would have a still-higher requirement.) This might be a good idea in theory, but what if nutrient X is expensive or scarce? A person like Ms. B, who needs only 35 units a day, would then try to consume twice that, an unnecessary strain on her resources. Or she might overeat as a consequence or overemphasize foods containing nutrient X to the exclusion of foods containing other valuable nutrients.

The choice we would finally make, with some reservations, would be to set the RDA at a reasonably high point so that the bulk of the population would be covered. In this example, a reasonable choice might be to set it at 63 units a day. By moving the RDA further toward the extreme, we would pick up very few additional people but inflate the recommendation as it applies to most people (like Mr. A and Ms. B).

It was this kind of choice that the Committee made with respect to protein. They set the RDA two standard deviations above the mean requirement, as best they could determine it from the available data. (Actually, they didn't even have enough data to be sure that the population's requirements fit the normal distribution.) Assuming a normal distribution of requirements, this choice would theoretically meet the needs of 97.5 percent of the population.[3]

The RDA for protein, then, is 0.8 g per kilogram of ideal body weight, but this number cannot be taken literally by any individual. Remember, no individual knows exactly what his or her personal requirement may be. Remember, too, that the Committee on RDA made several assumptions that would not apply to all real situations: They assumed,

[3]A. E. Harper, Those pesky RDAs, *Nutrition Today*, March/April 1974, pp. 15-16, 19-22, 27-28.

standard deviation: describes the spread of a distribution. If the standard deviation is small, the curve is narrow; if large, the curve is broad. One standard deviation each side of the mean includes 68 percent of the sample; two include 95 percent. To determine the standard deviation of a particular distribution, the statistician adds up the squares of all the deviations from the mean, divides that total by the number of cases minus one, and finds the square root of the resulting number. The square root figure equals the standard deviation.

among other things, that the protein would be of high quality (a PER of 70 or above), that it would be consumed with adequate kcalories from carbohydrate and fat, and that other nutrients in the diet would be adequate.

The RDAs have many uses. One use is to provide a yardstick against which the nutrient intakes of segments of the population can be measured. If, for example, all the children in a community are healthy and all are consuming over 100 percent of the RDA for protein, we can assume that we have no need to worry about their diets with respect to this nutrient. But if half the children are consuming less than 75 percent of the RDA for protein, we have cause for alarm because as many as half of these children may not be meeting their needs fully.

Another use of the RDAs is to set a standard for diet planning. In feeding large groups of people, a planner is well advised to aim at providing 100 percent of the recommended intakes for each nutrient to each person each day.

Before applying these numbers to individuals, however, it is important to understand that any application of statistical norms to individuals has inherent limitations. The RDAs have been so widely misinterpreted, misunderstood, and misused that the American Dietetic Association has published a paper titled "The RDAs Are Not for Amateurs."[4]

Note: The RDA is not the same as the U.S. RDA. To use the U.S. RDA for interpreting labels, see Highlight 12.

There are two important cautions to apply when the RDAs are used as a yardstick to measure individual intakes:

● The RDAs are not minimum daily requirements. Most people do not have to consume 100 percent of their RDAs for all nutrients in order to be adequately nourished.

CAUTION WHEN YOU READ!

A margin of safety is built into the RDAs. R stands for Recommended—not for Required.

● The RDAs apply only to healthy persons. Illness, malnutrition, or other stress may greatly increase an individual's needs for certain nutrients.

The Minimum Daily Requirements (MDR), formerly used for purposes similar to the RDA, have been discontinued.

[4]R. M. Leverton, The RDAs are not for amateurs, *Journal of the American Dietetic Association* 66 (1975): 9-11.

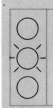

CAUTION WHEN YOU READ!

The RDAs apply to healthy persons only.

Additional cautions regarding interpretation of the RDAs are offered in later chapters.

Canadian Recommendations The Canadian equivalent to the RDAs is the Dietary Standard for Canada, a table of Recommended Daily Nutrient Intakes (shown in Appendix O). The Canadian recommendations differ from the RDAs in several important respects, because conditions in Canada differ somewhat from those in the United States. The protein recommendation, however, is similar to the RDA.

FAO/WHO Recommendations The protein recommendation of the Food and Agriculture Organization and the World Health Organization is considerably lower than the RDA for protein: 0.57 g per kilogram for the adult male and 0.52 for the adult female. These figures are much closer to the average *requirement* for protein and are not a generous *allowance* like the RDA. FAO/WHO has a somewhat different task from that of the Committee on RDA, however. It must find acceptable levels of nutrient intakes for a world in which poverty makes generous intakes a luxury. FAO/WHO carefully defines its protein recommendation in terms of egg or milk protein and also publishes a set of graded recommendations for proteins of lower quality. There is some concern that the FAO/WHO recommendation is too low to support health, and this matter is still under study.[5]

The FAO/WHO tables are shown in Appendix O. What may interest you the most about them is the way they differ from the U.S. and Canadian standards, a difference that reflects realities in the societies they are designed for.

Protein in Foods

In the exchange system, the foods that supply protein in abundance are those in the milk and meat lists. One milk exchange provides 8 g of protein; one meat exchange provides 7 g, as shown in Table 1.

[5] N. S. Scrimshaw, Strengths and weaknesses of the committee approach: An analysis of past and present Recommended Dietary Allowances for protein in health and disease, *New England Journal of Medicine* 294 (1976): 136-142.

Table 1. Protein Content of the Six Exchange Groups

Exchange group	Serving size	Carbohydrate (g)	Protein (g)	Fat (g)	Energy (kcal)
(1) **Skim milk**	1 c	12	8	0	80
(2) Vegetables	1/2 c	5	2	0	25
(3) Fruit	varies	10	0	0	40
(4) Bread	1 slice	15	2	0	70
(5) **Lean meat**	1 oz	0	7	3	55
(6) Fat	1 tsp	0	0	5	45

Foods containing protein:

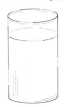

8 g in 1c milk

7 g in 1 oz meat

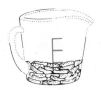

2 g in 1/2 c vegetables

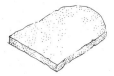

2 g in a slice of bread

As the table also shows, the foods in the vegetable and bread lists contribute small but significant amounts of protein to the diet.

The exchange system provides an easy way to estimate the amount of protein a person consumes in a day. For example, the day's meals described on p. 43 supplied the following amounts.

Breakfast	*Exchanges*	*Grams Protein*
1 egg	1 meat	7
1 slice toast	1 bread	2
Lunch		
2 slices bread	2 bread	4
2 tbsp peanut butter	1 meat	7
1 c milk	1 milk	8
Dinner		
6-oz steak	6 meat	42
1/2 c beans	1 vegetable	2
1 c mashed potato	2 bread	4
Dessert		
shortcake	1 bread	2
	Total	78 g protein

This menu provides more than enough protein for the day.

Recall from the discussion of the RDAs that the protein recommendation is a generous intake for most people. If your recommended intake is 40 g, then you will need only about 14 g of protein at each meal—provided, of course, that the protein is of high quality. From the exchange lists it is clear that 1 c milk or 1 oz meat along with the incidental additional protein provided by a few servings of vegetables, bread, or cereal will provide this amount. This means that 2 c milk and a very small serving of meat would suffice for a day. Needless to say, most people in the developed countries consume a great deal more high-quality protein than they need. Further considerations relating to the consumption of protein and to the special needs and problems of vegetarians are offered in the Highlight at the end of this chapter.

Too Much Protein?

As the essential nutrients were discovered early in the history of nutrition, great emphasis was placed on the concept of minimum intakes. It was important to get enough. More recently the notion has arisen that it is possible to get too much, even of a valuable nutrient such as protein. One authority puts it this way:

> As the amount of any nutrient in the diet is increased from zero, a level is approached that prevents clinical symptoms and is considered the minimal requirement. With further additions of the nutrient, when body stores are saturated, the optimal requirement is reached. Still further nutrient additions may result in toxic or adverse effects.[6]

Is it possible to consume too much protein? Research designed to answer this question is now under way, and several facts are already known. Infants and children do not adjust well to diets containing large amounts of protein.[7] Animals fed high-protein diets experience a "protein overload effect," seen in the hypertrophy of their livers and kidneys. There are evidently no benefits to be gained by consuming a diet that derives more than 15 percent of its kcalories from protein, and there are possible risks.[8] The higher a person's intake of such protein-rich foods as meat and milk, the more likely it is that fruits, vegetables, and grains will be crowded out of the diet, making it inadequate in other nutrients. And diets high in protein necessitate higher intakes of calcium as well because such diets promote calcium excretion.

This discussion illustrates a point to remember about nutrient needs. It is naive to think only in terms of minimum intakes. A more accurate view is to see one's nutrient needs as falling within a range, with danger zones below and above it. The figure in the margin illustrates this point.

At the end of Chapter 2 we recommended that the diet be designed around the principles of dilution and variety. To these should now be added two more watchwords for diet planning: moderation and balance.

hypertrophy (high-PURR-tro-fee): growing too large.

hyper = too much
trophy = growth

Nutrient needs:

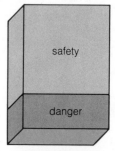

Naive view

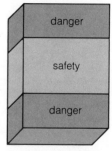

Accurate view[7]

[6]M. E. Swendseid, Nutritional implications of renal disease: 3. Nutritional needs of patients with renal disease, *Journal of the American Dietetic Association* 70 (1977): 488-492.

[7]A. A. Albanese and L. A. Orto, The proteins and amino acids, in *Modern Nutrition in Health and Disease*, 5th ed., eds. R. S. Goodhart and M. E. Shils (Philadelphia: Lea and Febiger, 1973), pp. 28-88; and L. E. Holt, Jr., Protein economy in the growing child, *Postgraduate Medicine* 27 (1960): 783-798.

[8]J. G. Chopra, A. L. Forbes, and J. P. Habicht, Protein in the U.S. diet, *Journal of the American Dietetic Association* 72 (1978):253-258.

[9]Holt, 1960.

Summing Up

Proteins are composed of carbon, hydrogen, oxygen, and nitrogen atoms arranged as amino acids, which are linked in chains some 100 to 300 amino acids long. The sequence of a protein's amino acids determines how it folds. The final configuration establishes the surface characteristics that enable the protein to act in specific ways—for example, as an enzyme that catalyzes a particular chemical reaction. (Other roles of protein are described in Chapter 4.)

Many amino acids can be synthesized in the body from other energy nutrients and a nitrogen source. Eight (listed on p. 104) cannot; these are the essential amino acids. An additional amino acid, histidine, is required by infants. The major role of dietary protein in human nutrition is therefore to supply amino acids for the synthesis of proteins needed in the body, although dietary protein can also serve as an energy source, providing 4 kcal per gram.

A complete protein is defined as one that supplies all of the essential amino acids; a high-quality protein is one that not only supplies them but also provides them in the appropriate amounts relative to human physiological need. When one essential amino acid is in short supply relative to the others in a protein source, it is said to be a limiting amino acid; that is, it limits the total amount of protein that can be synthesized from that source. Egg protein is the World Health Organization's reference protein; it is a high-quality protein used as a standard for measuring the quality of other proteins.

Ways of measuring protein quality include chemical scoring; measuring the extent to which protein supports growth in a young animal (protein efficiency ratio, or PER); or measuring nitrogen intake and losses under test conditions (biological value, or BV). Animal protein sources are generally of higher quality than vegetable protein sources, but a vegetarian can design a diet that is adequate in protein by exercising some care.

The amount of protein needed by humans can be determined by nitrogen balance studies. The RDA for protein for the healthy adult is 0.8 g of protein per kilogram of ideal body weight (determined by the Committee on RDA of the Food and Nutrition Board). This is a generous allowance, set high enough to cover even people whose individual needs for protein (as determined by nitrogen balance and other studies) reach as high as two standard deviations above the mean. The Canadian recommendation for protein is similar; the FAO/WHO recommendation is lower and is heavily qualified to ensure consumption of proteins of acceptable quality.

In the exchange system, the exchange groups that supply protein in abundance are the milk list (8 g per exchange, or per cup) and the meat list (7 g per ounce and therefore 28 g per 4-oz serving). Vegetable and bread exchanges contribute 2 g protein per exchange. Most people's average consumption of protein is considerably higher than the RDA and is largely from high-quality sources. Diets that are especially high in protein might actually be hazardous. The Highlight that follows this chapter deals with some aspects of protein overnutrition and the special needs of vegetarians.

To Explore Further

A paperback that offers a clear picture of our new and profound understanding of how genes code for enzymes, which in turn determine the structure and function of cells, tissues, and whole organisms:

Watson, J. D., *Molecular Biology of the Gene*, 3rd ed. (Menlo Park, Calif.: W. A. Benjamin, 1976).

An amusing autobiographical account (paperback) of Watson and Crick's discovery of the structure of DNA:

Watson, J. D., *The Double Helix* (New York: Atheneum, 1968).

The 1980 RDA book provides readable and interesting accounts of the reasoning behind the latest recommendations:

Recommended Dietary Allowances, 9th ed. (Washington, D.C.: National Academy of Sciences, 1980).

Meat Eaters versus Vegetarians

"Boy!" said the cave lady, as we stood with them before the solemn, clergyman-like head of an enormous moose. "Would he be good with onions!"

ALDOUS HUXLEY

The middle-aged man who says with braggadocio that he is a "meat and potatoes man" and the college-aged person who almost defiantly disdains any restaurant that will not serve a meal of vegetables, fruit, and nuts have a lot more in common than either would like to believe. Both are extremists in their use of a valuable class of food—protein—and both could be suffering from malnutrition due to the rigidity of their ideas about what constitutes a "good" food plan.

In today's world, where overconsumption in affluent nations contrasts with famines in poorer nations, there is a need for better understanding of protein nutrition by everyone, from policymakers to consumers.

In earlier times, recommendations on proper diet were made on the basis of observation only. A doctor might have noted, for instance, that people who ate meat and eggs and drank milk were healthier, stronger, taller, or more resistant to infections. Therefore, he might have recommended to all his patients that they needed more protein and should include animal and dairy products in their diets. Later, when more sophisticated laboratory tests had been developed, it became clear that it was necessary to include certain amino acids in the diet and that animal and dairy products contained all of these essential amino acids. Vegetables, it was found, were lacking in one or more of these. Another observation was that populations existing on cereal diets, for reasons either of meat taboos or of economic necessity, were malnourished. The

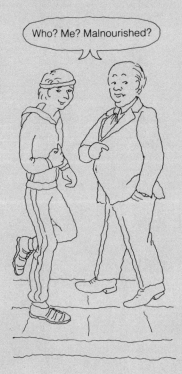

Who? Me? Malnourished?

evidence was their shorter stature, lower resistance to diseases, shorter life span, and higher infant mortality. All these observations and supporting laboratory work underscored a common belief that animal and dairy products were "good" protein foods and that plants were "poor" protein foods. Present-day clinical tests have shown that this notion was not entirely justified.

It is true that animal and dairy foods contain complete proteins; it does seem to be true that populations that eat milk and meat are generally healthier than grain-eating populations. But it has been shown by clinical tests that if the vegetables, legumes, fruits, and grains are wisely chosen, children grow as well on a diet devoid of animal protein as on one that includes milk and other animal proteins.[1]

In the United States and Canada, a love affair with meat has been flourishing for a century or more. No doubt the wide expanses of grazing land and the easy availability of wild animals to be had for the hunting (especially in earlier times) contributed to the acquisition of a taste for meat three times a day. In this century in the United States, the amount of protein coming from animal sources has increased from 52 percent to 69 percent; protein

[1]U. D. Register and L. M. Sonnenberg, The vegetarian diet, *Journal of the American Dietetic Association* 62 (1973):253-261.

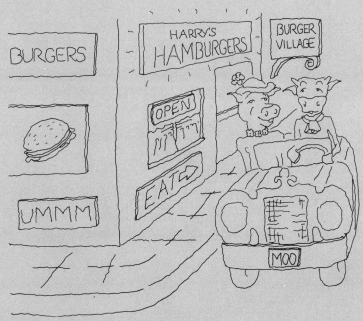

"This neighborhood always makes me nervous."

from plant sources has decreased from 48 percent to 31 percent.[2]

However, a countertrend has been developing among young people, who are turning from the meals made up of eggs and bacon, hamburger and french fries, and steak and potatoes toward vegetarian diets. There is a wide variation in the reasons for this change given by the "new" vegetarians:[3] Some have been influenced by Eastern religions; some eschew meat on humanitarian grounds; some are expressing

antiestablishment feelings; and some are merely caught up in a new fad. There is also a wide variation in the extent to which meat and dairy products are excluded from these diets, ranging from the highest "Zen" macrobiotic diet, made up exclusively of cereals, to those that eliminate animal meat but include animal products such as eggs, milk, and cheese.

In order to help us gain an understanding of the nutritional problems of these two groups, let's examine the kcalorie, protein, and fat content of a "meat-and-potatoes" diet and a "vegetables, fruits, and nuts" diet to see why anyone who relies on either may be malnourished.

To make a valid comparison, we must use people of the same age and sex. If both are men under 35 and their ideal weight is 70 kilograms (154 pounds), their daily kcalorie allowance would be 2,700 kcal (see Appendix O). The RDA for protein is 0.8 g for each kilogram of ideal body weight, or 56 g protein for our subjects. If we assume that each eats a third of his kcalorie and protein allowance at each meal, then dinner should provide 900 kcal, and 19 g of protein.

[2]B. Friend and R. Marston, *Nutritional Review 1975*, bulletin of the Consumer and Food Economics Institute, U.S. Department of Agriculture, 1976.

[3]J. T. Dwyer, R. F. Kandel, L. D. V. H. Mayer, and J. Mayer, The new vegetarians, *Journal of the American Dietetic Association* 64 (1974):376-381.

Table 1. The Meat-and-Potato Dinner

Food	Exchanges*	Energy (kcal)	Protein (g)	Fat (g)
6 oz boneless	6 lean meat	330	42	18
beefsteak	6 fat	270	—	30
1 large baked potato	2 bread	140	4	—
2 tsp margarine	2 fat	90	—	10
1 lettuce salad	vegetable (free)	—	—	—
2 tbsp French dressing	2 fat	90	—	10
1 slice (1/7) apple pie†		350	3	15
TOTAL		1,270	49	83

*Food composition values are from the exchange lists in Appendix L.
†Calculated by using the Table of Food Composition (Appendix H).

By examining the meat-and-potatoes man's consumption of one meal, what implications can we see for his future health? The first observation must concern his excess *kcalories*. It is relatively easy to exceed the energy allowance when a large portion of the kcalories comes from animal meat, particularly beef and pork. Some fat can be trimmed from the meat, but much of it is in the marbling. Marbling deceives the eater who doesn't realize that he is consuming considerable invisible fat. The fat also contributes to palatability, which encourages larger servings.

The *protein* needs for the entire day have almost been met in this one meal alone—49 g when only 56 g were needed for the entire day. You will recall that protein is important in the diet because of its contribution of essential amino acids and nitrogen. The ease with which a person can derive the essential amino acids from animal products is one of the advantages of including such products in the diet. But if more amino acids are present than are needed by the body for several hours after ingestion, these amino acids will be degraded to carbon fragments that will be used for energy. If the carbon fragments are not needed for energy, they will be used to build body fat. Thus, overconsumption of essential amino acids, even

though they are valuable, can lead to obesity.

Beef used for *kcalories* is costly. If a cut of beef costs $2.75 a pound, its cost is 23 cents for 100 kcal; if an 18-oz box of rolled oats costs $0.75, its cost is 3 cents for 100 kcal. If it is energy rather than amino acids you are buying, it is obvious which of these is the better buy.

Plant kcalories also cost less land. A million kcalories in wheat can be produced on less than an acre of land; a million kcalories in beef require 17 acres.[4] (These figures have some harsh implications for groups interested in solving the nutrition problems in developing countries; introducing meat into a vegetarian economy may worsen the food balance. [See Highlight 4.] Even in the United States we may soon find that we cannot afford the luxury of using 17 times as much land to produce the same amount of energy food.)

As for *fat*, 83 g were consumed in this meal. Each gram of fat produces 9 kcal, so about 750 out of 1,270 kcal in this meal came from fat—more than 55 percent. It is recommended that fat contribute no more than 30 percent of the total kcalories and, furthermore, that satu-

rated fat consumption be reduced. This meal is not only high in total fat but also contains virtually all saturated fat. This has serious implications for the development of atherosclerosis (see Highlight 6). Fat also has a high satiety value, but this is not desirable when the appetite is satisfied before enough vegetables, fruits, and grains have been consumed to ensure that all the needed vitamins and minerals have been included.

Finally, this is a low-*fiber* meal. Only the lettuce has appreciable fiber content. Fiber aids in digestion and may be important for the prevention of diverticulosis and cancer of the colon,[5] as well as atherosclerosis.[6] People who are interested in prevention of these diseases would be wise to increase their consumption of vegetables, fruits, and grains.

In summary, this meal contains more than enough protein. There is no need to be concerned that all essential amino acids are present, because the protein is predominantly of animal origin. There is, however, an excess of kcalories, largely from

[4]F. J. Stare, Sugar in the diet of man, in *World Review of Nutrition and Dietetics* 22, ed. G. F. Bourne (Basel: S. Karger, 1975), pp. 239-247.

[5]D. P. Burkitt, Relationships between diseases and their etiological significance, *American Journal of Clinical Nutrition* 30 (1977):262-267.

[6]D. Kritchevsky and J. A. Story, Binding of bile salts in vitro by nonnutritive fiber, *Journal of Nutrition* 104 (1974):458-462.

saturated fat, which leads to a concern about obesity and atherosclerosis. There may not be enough vegetables and fruits in the diet as a whole to ensure that all essential nutrients and adequate fiber are present, but you cannot make this judgment without knowing the intake for the other meals of the day.

In the introduction to Part One we stated that the only unequivocal statement about the nutritive quality of a food is a statement of the specific nutrients it contains and the amount of each. In this Highlight the nutritive quality of two diets is being examined, and the above statement can be amplified. In assessing these diets it is useful (1) to note the specific nutrients they contain and (2) to state the amount of each. We also undertake two additional means of evaluation: (3) to examine the quality of the nutrients (complete or incomplete protein, saturated or polyunsaturated fat) and (4) to compare the amounts of the nutrients with the recommended intakes. Each of these two additional judgments deserves a comment.

Notice that in assessing the quality of the nutrients we are not concerned

Mini-Glossary

diverticulosis (DYE-ver-tick-yoo-LO-sis): a condition in which the walls of the intestines are weakened in spots and form "blowouts," or outpocketings. These may become inflamed or infected, a condition known as **diverticulitis** (DYE-ver-ti-cu-LIE-tis), which is dangerous because the intestinal walls may rupture.

extrapolation (ex-trap-oh-LAY-shun): an educated guess, from a known series of numbers, as to what others may be. For example, knowing that the world population was 2 billion in 1930, 3 billion in 1960, and 4 billion in 1977, we can extrapolate that it will be 6 billion in 2000.

lacto-ovo-vegetarian: a vegetarian who excludes animal flesh but eats such animal products as milk and eggs.

lacto = milk
ovo = eggs

lacto-vegetarian: a vegetarian who excludes animal flesh and all animal products except milk.

marbling: a lacy network of fat embedded in meat, sometimes so fine as to be invisible. Sometimes called **invisible fat**, in contrast to the visible fats—butter, margarine, oil, and the fats removable from meat.

mutual supplementation: the strategy, used by vegetarians, of combining two incomplete protein foods in a meal so that each food provides the essential amino acid(s) lacking in the other.

ovo-vegetarian: a vegetarian who excludes animal flesh and all animal products except eggs.

satiety (suh-TIE-uh-tee): the feeling of fullness or satisfaction after a meal. Fat provides satiety more than carbohydrate or protein because it slows gastric motility.

vegan (VAY-gun, VEJ-an): a strict vegetarian; one who excludes all animal flesh and animal products, eating only plant foods.

about their source but about their molecular characteristics. The food sources of amino acids need not be "organically grown," but they do need to contribute a complete and balanced spectrum of essential amino acids. The

fat need not be "natural," but it does need to have a high percentage of polyunsaturated fatty acids. These observations reinforce the points made in the Digression on pp. 67-68.

In comparing the

amounts of the nutrients with the RDAs, we can make a meaningful statement about their contribution to a person's needs. Failing to use such a yardstick can cause serious misunderstanding on the part of a careless reader/consumer. For example, when you read that a diet pill contains "570 mg of solid natural protein," you may believe that you are taking a pill that will protect your tissues while you are reducing. Only when you measure this amount against the RDA for protein (56,000 mg for each of our subjects) do you realize that you would have to take nearly a hundred diet pills a day to meet the protein recommendation.

CAUTION WHEN YOU READ!

Make a habit of using a yardstick to measure quantities.

Many food companies make statements about their products that can be critically analyzed this way. A "high-protein cereal" may sound like a cereal that provides a lot of protein for human

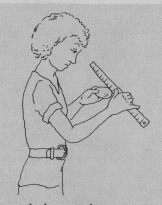

needs, but on closer examination it turns out to be high in protein only when compared with other cereals. In small lettering on the side panel, the label of such a cereal may reveal that one serving, even including the milk added to it, supplies only 10 percent of the RDA for protein!

If there is no statement of quantity on the label or in the advertisement, beware. The statement that a food contains a nutrient, without specifying how much, may be intended to mislead.

A FLAG SIGN OF A SUSPECT CLAIM IS THE STATEMENT THAT:

This product contains X (with no amount specified).

Now let's look at the "vegetables, fruits, and nuts" diet.

Table 2. The Vegetables, Fruits, and Nuts Dinner

Food	Exchanges*	Energy (kcal)	Protein (g)	Fat (g)
1 c cooked cabbage	2 vegetable	50	4	—
1 tsp safflower oil	1 fat	45	—	5
1/2 c cooked carrots	1 vegetable	25	2	—
1 large baked potato	2 bread	140	4	—
1 tbsp margarine	3 fat	135	—	15
fruit salad:				
1 small banana	2 fruit	80	—	—
1 small apple	1 fruit	40	—	—
1/2 c pineapple	1 fruit	40	—	—
2 tbsp raisins	1 fruit	40	—	—
6 nuts	1 fat	45	—	5
TOTAL		640	10	25

*See the exchange lists in Appendix L.

This one meal is not typical of a knowledgeable vegetarian's meal, but it illustrates several of the difficulties an amateur vegan may encounter. There is a very large quantity of food in this meal, yet the energy is deficient by about 250 kcal. This deficiency, amounting to about 750 kcal per day, could result in a loss of about a pound every four to five days—unless, of course, it is corrected at the other meals. This is, as a matter of fact, a common observation about vegans: They are usually underweight and must eat huge amounts of food if they are to maintain their weight.

Another obstacle the vegetarian faces in planning meals is obtaining sufficient protein. This vegetarian dinner provides about half the recommended amount of protein. Furthermore, the protein that is present has a poor combination of essential amino acids. Vegetables must be chosen carefully if they are to be the only source of protein. Potatoes and carrots provide many important nutrients as well as adding to the fiber content of the diet, but a child would not grow properly on a diet in which the only sources of protein were potatoes and carrots.

If you examine the vegetable list in Appendix L, you will note that a few vegetables provide such an insignificant amount of protein and kcalories that they are treated as having no protein

or kcalories. Quite a few vegetables provide only 2 g of protein and 25 kcal per half cup. The bread list contains still other vegetables (legumes, tubers, and other starchy vegetables) that provide 2 g of protein and 70 kcal per exchange.

In selecting protein sources for the diet, you must not only know the amount of protein in the source but also be certain that the essential amino acids are present. Most of the vegetables and grains are low in such essen-

tial amino acids as lysine, methionine, threonine, or tryptophan; however, by eating specific combinations at the same meal, you can obtain the equivalent of a complete protein. Use of two protein sources that each lack a different amino acid, so that each provides the amino acid missing from the other, is called mutual supplementation. A rule of thumb: Mixtures of grains and legumes eaten at the same meal provide a fairly good proportion of the essential amino acids.

Mutual supplementation.

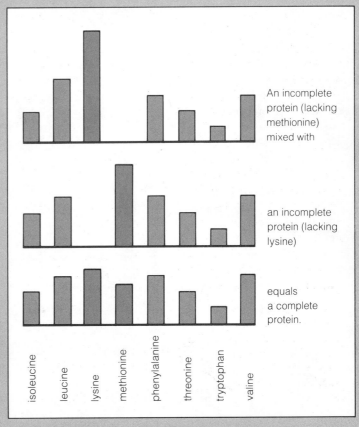

An incomplete protein (lacking methionine) mixed with

an incomplete protein (lacking lysine)

equals a complete protein.

isoleucine   leucine   lysine   methionine   phenylalanine   threonine   tryptophan   valine

Also most of are degraded
to meet energy demands.
no v.t B₁₂

Some sincere vegetarians, when they first learn how important it is to eat complementary proteins at the same meal, are eager to know how much of each essential amino acid is required daily. They also want to know exactly how much of each is contained in their favorite plant foods.

This information is available. The laboratory work has been done, and the results are contained in advanced nutrition references.[7] However, much time can be squandered calculating the amino acid content of a meal. The calculations won't be useful because they tell you only how much amino acid is present, not how much your body will receive. The way the digestive system handles proteins is highly complex. For example, on some plant proteins the exposed bonds may resist early digestive steps, so that the entire protein remains intact. In this instance, even if the amino acids were present in the diet, they would not be available to

[7]A. A. Albanese and L. A. Orto, The proteins and amino acids, in *Modern Nutrition in Health and Disease*, 5th ed., eds. R. S. Goodhart and M. E. Shils (Philadelphia: Lea and Febiger, 1973), pp. 28-88.

the body; they would simply be excreted in the feces.

Rather than going through the hassle of computing specific amino acid quantities from tables, the vegetarian should adopt the strategy of eating a wide variety of protein sources in generous servings. It is also practical to ask the question, What mixtures of plant foods contain a complete spectrum of essential amino acids? Armed with these strategies, the vegetarian can plan a menu that provides for his body's protein needs. Here is an answer to that question:[8]

Peanut protein	+ Wheat, oats, corn, rice, or coconut
Soy protein	+ Corn, wheat, rye, or sesame
Legumes	+ Cereals
Leafy vegetables	+ Cereals

Another point to consider in planning the protein for a meal is that there must be sufficient kcalories so that the amino acids will not be degraded for energy. With a

[8]Register and Sonnenberg, 1973.

250-kcal deficit, the 10 g protein in this vegetarian's meal will most likely be used for energy rather than for building and maintaining his body tissues.

When we examine the fat content of the vegetarian's meal, we find only 25 g; this amount supplies 225 kcal, or about 35 percent of the total kcalories for the meal. This approaches the optimum fat consumption. In addition, about a third of the fat is the essential fatty acid, linoleic acid, whereas only a sixth of the fat in the meat-and-potatoes diet is linoleic acid. Also, there is no cholesterol in this meal. These are among the advantages of the vegetarian diet as compared to the meat-and-potatoes diet: Plant sources contain no cholesterol and, except for coconuts, very little saturated fat.

You have seen that this one meal of vegetables, fruits, and nuts contains a large quantity of food but a deficit of kcalories. This deficit could lead not only to loss of weight but also to poor utilization of the protein that is present. The minimal amount of protein has a poor amino acid spectrum, since the two protein sources are not mutually supplemental. The meal does, however, contain a wide variety of fruits and vegetables, which would ensure an ample supply of vitamins and minerals and a good fiber content.

Four Food Group Plan for the Vegetarian[9]

2 servings milk or milk products (or soy milk fortified with vitamin B_{12})

2 servings protein-rich foods (include 2 c legumes daily to help meet women's iron requirements; count 4 tbsp peanut butter as a serving)

4 servings whole-grain foods

4 servings fruits and vegetables (include 1 c dark greens to help meet women's iron requirements)

The vegan faces some problems with other nutrients; these will be discussed later but should be recognized here. With the absence of milk and milk products, calcium, riboflavin, and vitamin B_{12} must be obtained in other ways. Occasional use of dark-green leafy vegetables, legumes, and nuts will not supply enough calcium and riboflavin, but the daily use of 2 c soybean milk will protect against deficiencies of these two nutrients.[10] Soybean milk has been on the market for many years as a milk substitute for infants who are allergic to cow's milk. Soybean milk contains no vitamin B_{12}, however, so all vegans should supplement their diets with this vitamin or make a point of getting specially fortified soy milk.[11]

The vegan should take one other precaution in menu planning: Avoid the use of empty-kcalorie foods. Vegans must eat large quantities of food to meet their protein needs. They are dependent on the accumulation of small amounts of amino acids from each of many items. Empty-kcalorie foods would make no contribution of any nutrient except glucose or fat.

The ideal diet lies somewhere between the two examples we've just studied. The person on a diet of meat and potatoes should select smaller servings of meat and include a variety of vegetables, fruits, and cereals. Substituting meats that are lower in saturated fats (such as fish, chicken, and veal) for beef and pork would lower the fat and cholesterol content of this diet as well as the total kcalorie content. If vegans would decide to become lacto-ovo-vegetarians, they could easily correct most of the deficiencies noted in the vegetarian menu. One egg and 2 c milk (2% fat) would provide 23 g of complete protein and 305 kcal as well as other valuable nutrients.

If vegetarians insist on omitting all animal and dairy products, they should be especially careful to meet their protein needs, should use a vitamin B_{12} supplement, and should meet their energy needs without resorting to empty-kcalorie foods. They must also be willing to become very well informed on nutrition and strict about including, at every meal, plant proteins that supplement one another.

The lesson from these two examples seems to be that people can get into trouble nutritionally when they emphasize foods from just one or two categories, even if these are high-quality, important foods. By the same token, if they avoid one entire group of foods, as some vegetarians do, they are likely to develop deficiencies. The old maxim among nutritionists appears to be true: Good nutrition depends mostly on including a wide variety of foods in the diet.

To Explore Further

An easy book for the vegetarian, with an especially good discussion of complementarity of amino acids, is the paperback:

Lappé, F. M., *Diet for a Small Planet* (New York: Ballantine Books, 1971).

[9]Register and Sonnenberg, 1973.

[10]Shands Teaching Hospital and Clinics, Food and Nutrition Service, *Vegetarian Food Choices* (Gainesville: University of Florida, 1976).

[11]Register and Sonnenberg, 1973.

Lappé's ideas are translated into attractive recipes in the paperback:

Ewald, E. B., *Recipes for a Small Planet* (New York: Ballantine Books, 1973).

Two other cookbooks that we like are:

Robertson, L., Flinders, C., and Godfrey, B., *Laurel's Kitchen: A Handbook for Vegetarian Cookery and Nutrition* (Berkeley, Calif.: Nilgiri Press, 1976).

Thomas, A., *The Vegetarian Epicure* (New York: Knopf, 1972) (paperback).

An excellent alternative to the two extreme diets described in this Highlight is presented by Chinese cookery, which uses small amounts of meat in dishes with great varieties of vegetables. The advantages of Chinese cookery are well described in the article:

Newman, J. M., Chinese-American food: The diet of the future? *Journal of Home Economics* 68 (November 1976):39-43.

Exercises 1 to 6 make use of the information you recorded on Forms 1 to 3 in the Self-Study at the end of the introduction to Part One.

1. How many grams of protein do you consume in a day?

2. How many kcalories does this represent? (Remember, 1 g protein contributes 4 kcal.)

3. What percentage of your total kcalories is contributed by protein? (To figure this, divide your protein kcalories by your total kcalories, then multiply by 100.)

4. A dietary goal quoted in Chapter 3 was for protein to contribute about 10 to 15 percent of total kcalories. How does your protein intake compare with this recommendation? (Note: If you are on a kcalorie-restricted diet, then this goal does not apply to you. See the Self-Study at the end of Chapter 8.) If your protein intake is out of line, what foods should you consume more of—or less of—to bring it into line?

5. Calculate your protein RDA as follows: Look up your ideal weight on the inside back cover, and convert pounds to kilograms (remember, 2.2 lb = 1 kg). The RDA for protein for a healthy adult is 0.8 g per kilogram of ideal body weight. Your RDA, in grams, then, is 0.8 g × your ideal body weight in kilograms.

6. Compare your average daily protein intake with your RDA. On the average, about what percentage of your RDA for protein are you consuming each day? If you are "average" and healthy, the RDA is probably a generous recommendation for you. And if you are "typical," your intake of protein is higher than the recommendation. This means that you may be spending protein prices for an energy nutrient. What substitutions could you make in your day's food choices so that you would derive from carbohydrate, rather than from protein, the kcalories you need for energy?

Optional Extras

● How many of your protein grams are from animal and how many from plant sources? Should the proportion be changed? (Not more than half of an adequate protein intake need come from animal sources.) If you decreased your intake of animal protein and increased your plant protein, what effect would this have on the ratio of polyunsaturated to saturated *fat* in your diet?

● How is your protein intake distributed throughout the day? (Study the record you made of your food intake.) Do you have amino acids at breakfast time to help maintain your blood glucose supply from carbohydrate? at lunchtime, to replenish dwindling pools? at dinnertime, to sustain you through the evening?

● A "high-protein supplement" advertises that it supplies "an unbelievable 690 mg of purified high-quality protein in every tablet!" Using the RDA as a yardstick, what percentage of a person's daily need for protein does a tablet supply? (Check the inside back cover to compare milligrams with grams.)

● Protein food is one of the most costly items in the food budget. To cut down on food costs, calculate the cost per gram of the protein delivered by various foods. Form 1 will help in making these comparisons. You might wish to enter your own food choices in the spaces at the top.

Form 1. Calculating the Relative Costs of Protein

	Regular hamburger	Low-fat milk	Plain cornflakes	Peanut butter	Eggs	Canned pork and beans
Grams protein per measure	$\dfrac{23\ g}{3\ oz}$			$\dfrac{4\ g}{1\ tbsp}$		
Amount of food to provide 40 g protein						
Cost of unit amount of food						
Cost of amount of food to provide 40 g protein						
Cost of 1 g protein						

CHAPTER 4

CONTENTS

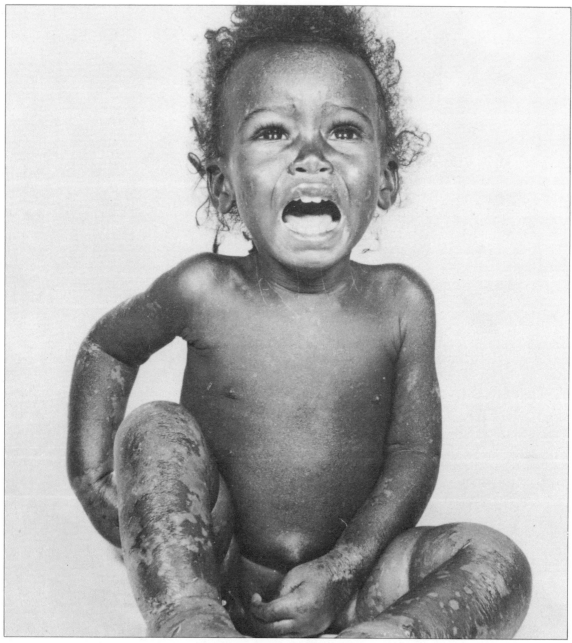

Protein deficiency.

PROTEIN IN THE BODY

There is present in plants and in animals a substance which . . . is without doubt the most important of all the known substances in living matter, and, without it, life would be impossible on our planet. This material has been named Protein.

GERARD JOHANNES MULDER, 1838

The elaborately coiled configuration of the body's gigantic protein molecules enables them to do the thousands of tasks that maintain life. This chapter describes a few of those tasks so that you may understand the tremendous importance of obtaining the amino acids you need. The following discussion focuses on the tasks performed by protein in which other nutrients (vitamins and minerals) cooperate. The minerals sodium and potassium, for example, help proteins maintain the water balance; vitamin C helps make the protein collagen which is involved in scar formation. For the present, we suggest that you read the following with the thought in mind that "proteins do all these things." Then you will have the background to appreciate the roles of the helper nutrients, details of which are given in Chapters 9 through 14. When you read those chapters, you can recall that "these other nutrients help the proteins do all these things." Margin references in this chapter show where each of the helper nutrients is described.

Some proteins act as enzymes. Our earlier description of enzyme molecules depicted them as giant tangled chains of amino acids, bristling with positive and negative charges, and bouncing about in the fluids of the body. Because of their differing surface characteristics, each enzyme is able to perform a different role. Each can work on a different compound—to break it apart into smaller compounds, to add something to it and make it larger, or to change some part of it in order to change its chemical identity.

There are many other proteins besides enzymes in the body. The roles of some of these are understandable at the molecular level if you keep this "bristling ball" picture in mind.

Enzyme: see pp. 100-104.

Helper nutrients: coenzymes (like the B vitamins) and cofactors (minerals). See Chapters 9, 12, and 13.

Fluid Balances

Proteins help maintain the water balance. To understand how this extremely important function is managed, you must know that there are three principal compartments for fluids in the body: the intravascular space, the intracellular space, and the interstitial space. In normal, healthy people, each of these compartments contains the

water balance: distribution of body water among the body compartments.

intravascular space: the continuous space inside the circulatory system (heart, arteries, capillaries, and veins).

intra = inside (within)
vascular = vein

intracellular space: the spaces inside the cells.

131

interstitial (in-ter-STISH-ul) **space:** the spaces between the cells and outside the vascular system.

interstice = space between

Minerals are helper nutrients (see pp. 494-508).

The flow of water across a membrane in the direction of a solute, such as protein or minerals, is due to osmotic pressure (see Chapter 14).

edema (uh-DEE-muh): accumulation of fluid in the interstitial spaces. In the special case where edema occurs in the abdomen, it is known as **ascites** (uh-SITE-eez).

diuretic (dye-yoo-RET-ic): a drug that stimulates increased renal water excretion.

renal = kidney

Kidneys: see the illustration on p. 197.

proper amount of fluid. Fluid can flow back and forth across the boundaries between them, but whenever the volume of fluid deviates, it is rapidly brought back to normal. Protein (with certain minerals) helps to maintain the amount of water at the proper volume in each compartment.

The way this works is neat and simple. Proteins are so large that they cannot pass freely across the walls or membranes that separate the compartments. They are trapped where they are. They are also hydrophilic, or attractive to water molecules, so the water molecules stay with or near the proteins. By regulating the amount of protein (and minerals) in each compartment, the body indirectly regulates the amount of water.

When something goes wrong with this system—when a person is suffering from a condition in which the blood protein concentration falls, for example—fluid may leak out of the vascular system and accumulate in the interstitial tissues. The result is a symptom known as edema, a visible swelling or puffiness in the tissues. It is not uncommon for pregnant women to suffer a swelling of the ankles, which reflects fluid leakage from the leg veins. In other people fluid may leak out of the veins into the abdominal cavity, resulting in a swollen "pot belly." In others the hands may swell or the face may become puffy.

The uninformed person may believe that the way to prevent this swelling is to drink less water or to increase excretion by taking a diuretic. If edema has become extreme, these measures, as well as salt restriction, may indeed be a necessary part of treatment. Yet you can never cause edema by drinking too much water. The more you drink, the more you carry in your vascular system, and (because the vascular fluid is circulated through your kidneys) the more you automatically excrete.

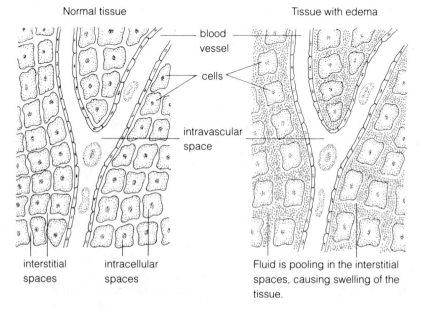

Normal tissue — blood vessel — Tissue with edema

cells

intravascular space

interstitial spaces   intracellular spaces

Fluid is pooling in the interstitial spaces, causing swelling of the tissue.

This discussion illustrates a principle that pervades the study of health. Provided that you are healthy, your body will maintain its own health. No known drug renders the healthy body more capable of regulating its own functions than it is already. Drugs are needed only to remedy situations in which body functions have become impaired. Diuretics may be needed only when excess fluid has already accumulated. They are not useful as preventive medicine.

Since the taking of a diuretic increases water excretion, it causes a sudden weight loss. A healthy person who fails to distinguish between loss of body fat and loss of water may see this as a desirable effect and start using diuretics for this purpose. But because the only loss induced is water loss, the only achievement gained is dehydration.

So what does cause edema? One thing is a protein-deficient diet. When protein intake falls below a certain limit, blood proteins become depleted and the body's hormonal balance becomes upset. The water that should be held within the bloodstream then leaks into the interstitial space causing swelling. This water is not available to the kidneys to excrete; the kidneys do not "know" it is there. (Remember, the kidneys can only "see" what is in the bloodstream that travels through them.) Hence the remedy may not be less water but more protein.

Another fluid balance that proteins help maintain is that between acids and bases. An acid solution is one in which there are hydrogen ions floating around. The more hydrogen ions, the more concentrated the acid. Proteins (and minerals), which have negative charges on their surfaces, attract hydrogen ions, and hydrogen ions in turn attract proteins. As long as the concentration of hydrogen ions—that is, the strength of the acid—stays within certain limits, the proteins maintain their integrity. If the acid becomes too strong, however, the extra positive charges surrounding the protein molecules deform them and, so to speak, pull them out of shape. When this happens the proteins can no longer function.

Of all the consequences that stem from exceeding the normal limits of acid-base balance in the body, the most direct and serious is a disturbance of the shapes of the proteins that carry out so many of the vital body functions. Acidosis and alkalosis both are lethal if unchecked. The proteins in the plasma, such as albumin, help to prevent these conditions from arising. In a sense the proteins protect one another by binding or sequestering extra hydrogen ions when there are too many in the surrounding medium and by releasing them when there are too few. This ability to regulate the acidity of the medium is known as the buffering action of proteins.

acid-base balance: the balance maintained in the body between too much and too little acid. Blood pH, for example, is regulated normally between 7.38 and 7.42 (pH: see below).

Minerals are helper nutrients (see pp. 494-508).

Ion: see p. 71, Appendix B.

pH: the concentration of H^+ ions (see Appendix B). The lower the pH, the stronger the acid. Thus pH 2 is a strong acid, pH 6 a weak acid (pH 7 is neutral). A pH above 7 is alkaline, or basic (a solution in which acid-accepting ions such as OH^- predominate).

acidosis: too much acid in the blood and body fluids.

alkalosis: too much base in the blood and body fluids.

lethal: causing death.

sequester (see-KWES-ter): to hide away or take out of circulation.

buffer: a compound that can reversibly combine with H^+ ions to help maintain a constant pH. Figure 1 in Chapter 14 shows how a buffer works.

1. Body is challenged with foreign invaders.

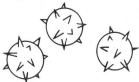

2. Body makes code for manufacturing antibody.

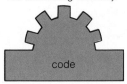

3. Code makes antibody.

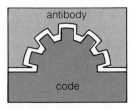

4. Antibody inactivates foreign invader.

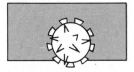

Crunch!

5. Code remains to make antibodies faster the next time this foreign invader attacks.

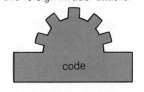

Development of immunity.

Antibodies and Hormones

Other major proteins found in the blood—the antibodies—act against disease agents. When a body is invaded by a virus—whether it is a flu virus, smallpox virus, measles virus, or virus that causes the common cold—the virus enters the cells and multiplies there. One virus may produce a hundred replicas of itself within an hour or so. These burst out and invade a hundred different cells, soon yielding ten thousand virus particles, which invade ten thousand cells. After several hours there may be a million viruses and then a hundred million and so on. If they were left free to do their worst, they would soon overwhelm the body with the disease they cause.

The antibodies, giant protein molecules circulating in the blood, are a defense against viruses, bacteria, and other "foreign agents." The surface of each antibody molecule has characteristics that enable it to combine with and inactivate a specific foreign protein, like that in a virus coat or bacterial cell membrane. The antibodies work so efficiently that in a normal healthy individual the many disease agents that attempt to attack never have a chance to get started. If a million bacterial cells are injected into the skin of a healthy person, fewer than ten are likely to survive for five hours.[1]

Once the body has manufactured antibodies against a particular disease agent (such as the measles virus), the cells never forget how to produce them. The next time the antibodies will respond even more quickly. The immunological response of the antibody-producing cells and the way they achieve their molecular memory of the body's enemies is beyond the scope of this book, but references at the end of this chapter will lead you further, if you like.

Hormones are also carried by the blood, and some are pure protein. Among them are the familiar thyroid hormone and insulin. The thyroid hormone regulates the body's metabolic rate—the rate of the chemical reactions that yield energy. Insulin regulates the concentration of the blood glucose and its transportation into cells, upon which the functioning of the brain and the nervous system depend. Hormones have many other profound effects on the body, which will become evident as you read further.

Transport Proteins

Some proteins move nutrients into and out of cells. There are proteins in the membrane of every cell of the body, each one specific for a certain compound (or group of related compounds). Each of these proteins is confined to the membrane but can rotate or shuttle from one side to the other. These protein "pumps" can pick up a compound on one side of the membrane and release it on the other, thus enabling the cells to

[1] R. Y. Stanier, M. Doudoroff, and E. A. Adelberg, *The Microbial World*, 3rd ed. (Englewood Cliffs, N.J.: Prentice-Hall, 1970), p. 784.

choose what substances to take up and what to release. For example, the glucose pump and the potassium pump transport glucose and potassium into cells faster than they can leak out, and the sodium pump transports sodium out of cells. Thanks to these pumps, a higher concentration of glucose and potassium is maintained inside than outside the cells, and the reverse is true of sodium. It may not be obvious why the cells go to so much trouble to maintain these concentration gradients, but many reasons will become apparent in later chapters. To anticipate one of them very simplistically: The sodium-potassium distribution across the membranes of nerve cells is what makes it possible for nerve impulses to travel—and so for you to think.

The mineral calcium enters the body with the help of a protein too, the calcium-binding protein in the intestinal tract. In fact, almost every water-soluble nutrient seems to have its own pump in cell membranes. (By contrast, lipids can cross membranes without the help of pumps if they are small and simple enough. Cells seem to regulate lipid transport by taking them apart so they can move across the membranes, then putting them back together again to keep them from escaping.)

Many of the cell membrane pumps can be switched on or off according to the body's needs. Often hormones do the switching, with a marvelous precision. Suppose, for example, there is too much glucose in the blood. High blood glucose causes the pancreas to step up its output of the hormone insulin; the insulin stimulates glucose uptake in the membranes of the liver and fat cells (and is destroyed in the process); these cells pick up the excess glucose; then when the blood glucose concentration is normal, the pancreas reduces its insulin output. The absorption of calcium is regulated by the hormones calcitonin and parathormone in a similar manner. These examples illustrate how hundreds of different body proteins maintain the distribution of substances into the various body spaces.

Another type of transport protein is the carriers in the body fluids. Many nutrients travel freely in the vascular system, but others have to be carried. The lipids are an example. You have already read about the problem these cumbersome molecules pose for the digestive system: They have to be emulsified in order to be made accessible to the enzymes that hydrolyze them. Even after absorption they require special handling. Each major lipid has to be wrapped in protein before it can be transported in the blood. These complexes are called lipoproteins. They are giant aggregates, much larger than lipids by themselves, but they travel easily in water because their protein coats are hydrophilic. (Only the smaller lipids—monoglycerides, glycerol, and fatty acids—can travel freely without carriers.) The fat-soluble vitamins are also carried by special proteins.

The mineral iron is a nutrient whose handling in the body illustrates especially well how precisely proteins operate. On leaving the intestine, iron is picked up by an iron-carrying protein in the bloodstream known as transferrin. Transferrin may transfer the iron to a storage protein in

antibody: a large protein of the blood, produced in response to invasion of the body by foreign protein; inactivates the foreign protein.

immunology (im-yoo-NOLL-uh-gee): the study of immunity and the way in which it is achieved by antibodies and other agents of disease resistance.

Hormone: see p. 165.

Iodine (part of the thyroid hormone) and zinc (part of insulin) are helper nutrients (see pp. 465-470).

These membrane-associated proteins are variously called **permeases, vectorial enzymes,** and **transferases.**

concentration gradient: a difference in concentration of a **solute** (SOLL-yoot), a dissolved substance, on two sides of a semipermeable membrane.

Regulation of calcium absorption: see p. 425.

Emulsification: see pp. 71-72.

Lipoprotein: see p. 200.

hydrophilic (high-dro-FILL-ic): water-loving (see also pp. 71-72).

the bone marrow known as ferritin. This protein finally releases the iron to become part of the protein hemoglobin, which is synthesized in new red blood cells as they are formed.

The protein hemoglobin is a giant molecule that contains four atoms of iron. The iron can combine with oxygen and then release it. As the red cells flow through the lungs, the hemoglobin iron picks up oxygen. Then as the red cells flow through the tissues, the iron releases the oxygen into the body cells, where it can oxidize other nutrients to provide energy. (As a carbon-hydrogen-oxygen compound such as carbohydrate or fat is oxidized, the H combines with O to form water—H_2O—and the C combines with O to form carbon dioxide—CO_2.) The blood plasma then dissolves the carbon dioxide released by the cells. When the blood returns to the lungs, this carbon dioxide is released into the air spaces in the lungs and exhaled. The oxygen carrier of muscle, myoglobin, is also a protein.

Other Proteins

Proteins perform many other roles in the body. Only a few more examples will serve to illustrate their diversity.

thrombin: a protein carried in the blood, involved in blood clotting.

thrombo = clot

The other protein circulating in the blood, ready to react with thrombin is **fibrinogen** (fye-BRIN-o-gen). The reaction between these two and other protein factors produces **fibrin** (FYE-brin), the protein material of the clot.

fibr = fibers
ogen = gives rise to

Vitamin K (involved in the production of thrombin) and calcium (needed for blood to clot) are helper nutrients (see p. 409).

Collagen: see also p. 363.

Vitamin C (needed to form collagen) and minerals (to calcify bones and teeth) are helper nutrients (see pp. 363-403).

Blood Clotting   Blood is unique and wonderful in its ability to remain a liquid tissue even though it carries so many large molecules and cells through the circulatory system. But blood can also turn solid within seconds when the integrity of that system is disturbed. If it did not clot, a single pinprick could drain your entire body of all its blood, just as a tiny hole in a bucket makes the bucket forever useless for holding water. When you cut yourself, the injured blood cells react immediately by releasing a protein called thrombin. The thrombin encounters another protein already circulating in the fluid part of the blood and converts it to fibrin, a stringy, insoluble mass of fibers that plugs the cut and stops the leak. Later, more slowly, a scar forms to replace the clot and permanently heal the cut.

Connective Tissue   Proteins help make scar tissue, bones, and teeth. When the construction of a bone or a tooth begins, the shape is first roughed out by laying down a protein matrix known as collagen, which forms a cartilage. Later, crystals of calcium, phosphorus, fluoride, and other minerals are laid down on this matrix, and the hardened bone begins to form. When a bone breaks, again the protein collagen precedes the bony material in the mending process. Collagen is also the mending material in torn tissue, forming scars to hold the separated parts together. It forms the material of ligaments and tendons and is a strengthening constituent between the cells of the artery walls, which must be able to withstand the pressure of surging heartbeats.

Visual Pigments   The light-sensitive pigments in the cells of the retina are molecules of the protein opsin. Opsin responds to light by changing its shape, thus initiating the nerve impulses that convey the sense of sight to the higher centers of the brain.

Opsin: see p. 391.

Vitamin A is a helper nutrient (see pp. 389-392).

Growth and Maintenance

Proteins are needed for growth and maintenance of all body tissues. Whenever you take a bath, you wash off whole cells from the surface layers of your skin, losing protein. Your hair and fingernails are growing constantly; since you ultimately cut them off (or break or chew them), these processes also result in a net loss of body protein. Similar processes occur inside your body. When you swallow food, it passes down your intestinal tract. Ultimately the undigested materials—fiber, water, and waste—leave your body, carrying with them cells that have been shed from the intestinal lining. Both inside and outside you must constantly build new cells to replace those lost from the exposed surfaces. In fact, it is said that a person's skin is replaced totally every seven years.

Given either fat or carbohydrate (composed of C, H, and O) as an energy source, the body can construct many of the materials (also composed of C, H, and O) needed to replace these lost cells. But to replace the protein, it must have protein from food, because food protein is virtually its only available source of nitrogen.

If the body is growing, it must manufacture more cells than are lost. Children end each day with more blood cells, more muscle cells, more skin cells than they had at the beginning of the day. So protein is needed both for routine maintenance (replacement) and growth (addition) of body tissue.

The above list of protein functions is by no means exhaustive, but it does give some sense of the immense variety and importance of proteins in the body. With this information as background, you are in a position to appreciate the significance of the world's most serious malnutrition problem: protein-kcalorie deficiency.

Protein-kCalorie Deficiency

The most ominous specter haunting the populations of the world's underdeveloped countries is protein-kcalorie malnutrition. Protein and kcalories (energy) are all-pervasive in human nutrition; they are involved in every body function. When children are deprived of food and suffer a kcalorie deficit, they degrade their own body protein for

protein-kcalorie malnutrition: a deficiency of protein or kcalories or both.

energy and thus indirectly suffer a protein deficiency as well as a kcalorie deficiency.

Protein and kcalorie deprivation go hand in hand so often that public health officials have adopted an abbreviation for the overlapping deficiency: PCM (protein-calorie malnutrition). Cases are observed at both ends of the spectrum, however. The classic kcalorie deficiency disease is marasmus, and the protein deficiency disease is kwashiorkor.

Classical marasmus is discussed in the chapter on energy balance (Chapter 7), because it can more easily be understood after some facts about energy metabolism have been presented. Kwashiorkor, however, is understandable on the basis of what we have already said about protein. These two diseases have a tremendous impact on the world's people and serious implications for the future of humankind. The problem is so complex that it requires separate emphasis; it is the subject of Highlight 4.

Kwashiorkor   The word *kwashiorkor* originally meant "the evil spirit which infects the first child when the second child is born." It is easy to see how this superstitious belief arose among the Ghanaians who named the disease. When a mother who has been nursing her first child bears a second child, she weans the first and puts the second on the breast. The first child soon begins to sicken and die, just as if an evil spirit had accompanied the new baby into the world and set out to destroy the older child. What actually happens, of course, is that protein deficiency follows soon after weaning. Breast milk provides a child with sufficient protein, but these children are generally weaned to a starchy, protein-poor gruel. The gruel does not supply enough amino acids even to maintain a child's body, much less enough to enable it to grow.

Kwashiorkor occurs not only in Africa but also in Central America, South America, the Near East, the Far East—and in some wealthier countries as well. In all these regions, mother's milk is the only reliable and readily available source of protein for infants. Thus kwashiorkor typically sets in around the age of two. By the time the child is four, his growth is stunted; he is no taller than he was at two. His hair has lost its color; his skin is patchy and scaly, sometimes with ulcers or open sores that fail to heal. His belly, limbs, and face become swollen with edema; he sickens easily and is weak, fretful, and apathetic. Figure 1 is a picture of such a child.

The body follows a priority system when there is not enough protein to meet all its needs. It abandons its less vital systems first. When it cannot obtain enough amino acids from dietary sources, the body switches to a "metabolism of wasting": It begins to digest its own protein tissues in order to supply the amino acids needed to build the most vital internal proteins and thus to keep itself alive. Hair and skin pigments (which are made from amino acids) are dispensable and are not manufactured. The skin needs less integrity in a life-or-death situation than the heart does, so its maintenance ceases and skin sores

PCM: protein-calorie malnutrition.

Marasmus: see also p. 235.

kwashiorkor (kwash-ee-OR-core, kwash-ee-or-CORE): the protein-deficiency disease.

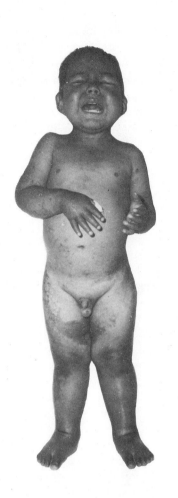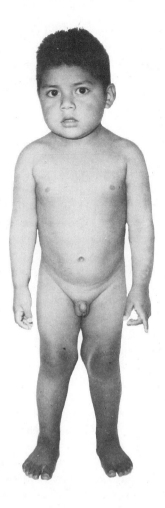

Figure 1 Kwashiorkor. The child at left has the characteristic "moon face" (edema) and the edematous swelling, which stretches the skin of his hands, belly, legs, and feet. His skin shows the typical patchy dermatitis of kwashiorkor. Without the swelling of edema, he would appear emaciated. At right, the same child after nutritional therapy.

Courtesy of Dr. Robert S. Goodhart, M.D.

fail to heal. Many of the antibodies are also degraded so that their amino acids may be used as building blocks for heart and lung and brain tissue. A child with a lowered supply of antibodies cannot resist infection and readily contracts dysentery, a disease of the digestive tract. Dysentery causes diarrhea, leading to rapid loss of nutrients— including amino acids—that the child may be receiving in food. Thus dysentery worsens the protein deficiency, and the protein deficiency in turn increases the likelihood of a second or third or tenth attack of dysentery.

The water loss in diarrhea increases losses of the water-soluble B vitamins and vitamin C. The child's inability to manufacture protein carriers for the fat-soluble vitamins creates a deficiency in vitamins A and D as well. The child's inability to manufacture protein carriers for fat often leaves him with fat accumulated in the liver tissue, from which it would normally be carried away. As the liver clogs with fat, its cells lose their ability to carry out their other normal functions, and gradually they atrophy and die.

dysentery (DIS-en-terry): an infection of the gastrointestinal tract caused by an amoeba or bacterium and giving rise to severe diarrhea.

When two variables interact so that each increases the other, they are said to be acting synergistically. Malnutrition and infection are a deadly combination because they work this way.

synergism (SIN-er-jism): the effect of two factors operating together in such a way that the sum of their actions is greater than the actions of the two considered separately.

A malnourished child who contracts measles cannot fight it off. In our country, where protein deficiency is not a problem, the child with measles may expect to recover within five to seven days; the kwashiorkor child dies within the first two days. Other diseases also take their toll.

Edema: see pp. 132-133.

The swollen belly of the kwashiorkor child is due to edema; blood protein is low and hormonal balance is disturbed so that fluid leaks out of the blood vessels into the body tissues and spaces. The child is too weak to stand much of the time, so the fluid settles in the belly—the lowest available space. Thus a child with this problem often has skinny arms and legs and a greatly swollen belly. On first glance you might think the child is fat, but if the fluid could be drawn off, his true condition would be revealed: He is actually a wasted skeleton, just skin and bones.

Adult Protein Deficiencies   Kwashiorkor is only one of several diseases associated with protein deficiency. Another that is closer to home for most of us is the nutritional liver disease associated with alcoholism. The alcoholic person, like the kwashiorkor child, consumes abundant kcalories, but up to three-fourths of his kcalories may come from alcohol, a nonprotein substance. Like the kwashiorkor child, the malnourished alcoholic may have a swollen belly; puffy hands, feet, and face; skin sores; and a reduced ability to withstand infection. Also like the kwashiorkor child, the chronic alcoholic develops a fatty liver. If the situation goes unremedied for too long, the liver cells ultimately die and are replaced by inert scar tissue. This is the progression to cirrhosis, which is so often caused by alcoholism.

The "beer belly" of the alcoholic sometimes reflects ascites (edema in the abdomen), although it is usually rightly attributed to an excess of kcalories.

cirrhosis (seer-OH-sis): irreversible liver damage involving death of liver cells and their replacement by scar tissue (see also p. 355).

For the effects of alcohol on the liver, see Highlight 9.

Adult kwashiorkor and marasmus also occur in hospital patients whose diets have been inadequate. A person undergoing surgery or fighting an infection has a greatly increased need of protein and kcalories. At the same time, she may feel too sick to eat or may be fed only liquids or intravenous fluids, which are not nearly nutritious enough even to maintain a healthy body. Hospital malnutrition occurs in up to 50 percent of the patients in some hospitals and increases the risks associated with surgery and infection. Physicians, whose medical school training has until recently almost totally neglected nutrition, are now becoming increasingly aware of its importance in the treatment of the sick. Some hospitals now maintain staffs to assess the nutritional status of their patients and to provide nutritional support.[2]

It must now be abundantly clear that protein is more than just an energy source. The profound consequences of protein deficiency are suffered by millions of people in the world. They are the subject of the Highlight that follows.

[2]G. L. Blackburn and B. R. Bistrian, Nutritional support resources in hospital practice, in *Nutritional Support of Medical Practice*, eds. H. A. Schneider, C. E. Anderson, and D. B. Coursin (Hagerstown, Md.: Harper & Row, 1977), chap. 10.

Summing Up

In addition to acting as enzymes, as described in Chapter 3, proteins perform many other functions in the body. They provide osmotic pressure, which regulates the distribution of water in the various body compartments (the water balance). They provide a buffering action in the body fluids, which helps to maintain the acid-base balance. Antibodies, which convey immunity, and some hormones, such as thyroid hormone and insulin, are made of protein. In the cell membrane, protein "pumps" confer on the cell the ability to select and take up specific compounds while excluding others, thus establishing concentration gradients. The absorption of many nutrients from the gastrointestinal tract depends on this function. Protein carriers are necessary to transport fats and fat-soluble vitamins in the circulatory system. Proteins are hydrophilic and so can carry these compounds in the watery fluid of the blood. The body's oxygen carriers, the hemoglobin of red blood cells and the myoglobin of muscles, are also proteins. Other important body proteins include collagen—the building material of scar tissue, cartilage, ligaments, bones, and teeth—and the light-sensitive pigments of the retina.

Since all body cells contain protein, routine maintenance and repair of body tissues requires a continual supply of amino acids to synthesize proteins. Growth of new tissue requires additional protein.

Kwashiorkor is the name for the disease in which protein is lacking but kcalories are adequate. (kCalorie deficiency, known as marasmus, is treated in Chapter 7.) Kwashiorkor typically occurs in children after weaning, with severest symptoms being observed after the age of two. Symptoms include stunted growth, loss of pigment in the hair and skin, ulceration of the skin, edema, weakness, and apathy. The kwashiorkor victim often develops a fatty liver caused by a lack of the protein carriers that transport fat out of the liver. Reduced antibody formation makes the child extremely vulnerable to such diseases as dysentery and measles. These diseases work synergistically with the malnutrition, leaching nutrients from the body. Similar symptoms are seen in the alcoholic with nutritional liver disease and in the undernourished hospital patient.

Protein deficiency occurs whenever protein itself is lacking in the diet or when kcalories are inadequate. In the latter case, amino acids are degraded for energy, causing protein deficiency indirectly. The two deficiencies of protein and kcalories, which often go hand in hand, are together called PCM (protein-calorie malnutrition); this is the world's most serious malnutrition problem. PCM afflicts millions of people, especially children.

To Explore Further

The chapter on immunology in Stanier, R. Y., Doudoroff, M., and Adelberg, E. A., *The Microbial World*, 3rd ed. (Englewood Cliffs, N.J.: Prentice-Hall, 1970) provides a clear and understandable explanation of the way antibodies are constructed and how they work.

A detailed treatment of antibodies written for the general reader is Nossal, G. J. V., *Antibodies and Immunity* (New York: Basic Books, 1969).

A dramatic article exposing the prevalence of hospital malnutrition in the United States for the first time was Butterworth, C. E., The skeleton in the hospital closet, *Nutrition Today*, March/April 1974, pp. 4-8.

The next two issues of *Nutrition Today* included confirmations of Dr. Butterworth's findings, and the next year he and his colleague Dr. Blackburn published a set of guidelines for identifying undernourished patients:

Butterworth, C. E., and Blackburn, G. L., Hospital malnutrition, *Nutrition Today*, March/April 1975, pp. 8-18.

An excellent film on the subject, *An Illusion of Nutritional Health*, is available from Ross Laboratories (address in Appendix J).

For an overview of the problem of educating doctors about nutrition, see Hamilton, E. M. N., and Whitney, E. N., Controversy 18: Doctors, in *Nutrition: Concepts and Controversies* (St. Paul: West, 1979).

The story is told of a woman, well educated and beautifully dressed, who parked her car in front of a doctor's office. Late for her appointment, she rushed out of the car and bumped her knee on the door handle. She dabbed at the bleeding knee with a tissue and hurried into the office. The cut continued to ooze blood; a nurse bandaged it. When an hour had gone by and the knee was still bleeding, the doctor admitted her to a hospital for further tests. The diagnosis? Vitamin C deficiency. Prescription? Drink plenty of orange juice. Time to effect recovery? A few days.

Although we ordinarily do not expect to find nutritional deficiencies like this in well-to-do persons, we have come to expect that nutritional deficiencies will present easily identifiable symptoms that can be cured dramatically by adding the missing nutrient to the diet. The history of nutrition science is filled with such simple and direct stories: the addition of butter to the diet curing infections of the eye, the addition of a lime a day to British sailors' diets preventing scurvy on long voyages, or the addition of the polishings of rice to the diet curing beriberi.

However, the story of protein-kcalorie malnutrition (PCM) does not present a few observable symptoms that would lead to laboratory tests for confirmation. As you

HIGHLIGHT 4

World Protein-kCalorie Malnutrition

[Man] alone by his own efforts can enlarge the bounds of empire, to the effecting of all things possible, to remolding this sorry scheme of things nearer to the heart's desire. He alone can see himself and his world in width and depth. He alone can choose, out of his vision of the present and the past, his future course.
HOMER SMITH

have seen in Chapter 4, a lack of protein food affects every nook and cranny of the body, causing a vast array of symptoms.

A story about PCM might go like this: A happy little one-year-old-girl lives in a shack with several brothers and sisters and her parents in Biafra (or Cambodia or the United States). A new baby has just arrived and is now nestled close to the mother, being fed from the breast where once the little girl was held and fed. She has been banished. She must somehow learn to use a hard utensil to spoon a thin, tasteless cereal into her mouth. She pouts and cries with hunger, but no one listens. Finally she quits trying to acquire the new skill of eating from a bowl or spoon. She doesn't follow her brothers and sisters outside to play but wanders off into a

corner and plays alone. The mother is disgusted with her churlishness and doesn't try anymore to entice her to eat. "She will eat when she is hungry," thinks the mother. Sometimes the mother forgets about her altogether, the little girl is so quiet.

The little girl's body defends itself from destruction by adapting to the lower energy input with a lower energy output: She keeps still. She ingests few amino acids with which to build body tissue (hormones, enzymes, new cells). The amino acids she does receive and her entire body's resources are directed toward supplying energy to her brain, heart, and lungs. There is no energy left for the muscular activity of playing with her brothers and sisters or for smiling at her mother or even for crying for food. Apathy is the body's way of conserving energy. Its danger, in the case of an infant who depends on the mother to give it food, is that apathy can damage the mother-child relationship to the point where the mother rejects the child. The downward spiral that is PCM has thus begun. If the little girl would eat the gruel, she might receive enough kcalories, but without a protein source she would probably develop kwashiorkor.

Textbooks usually describe marasmus and kwashiorkor as the two endpoints on a spectrum—lack of kcalories

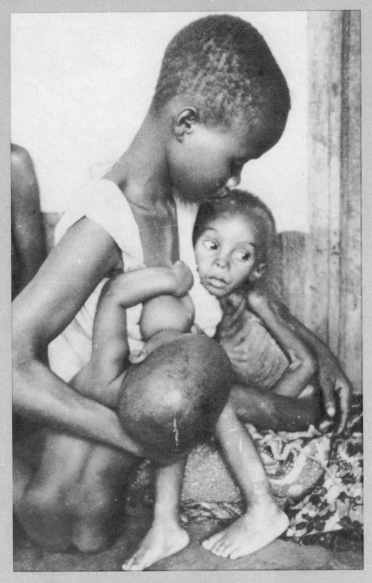

The sickness that invades the first child when the second child is born. (Wide World Photos.)

on correcting the underlying social, political, and economic causes.[1]

Protein-kcalorie malnutrition particularly affects vulnerable groups in the community, such as pregnant and lactating women, nursing infants, just-weaned children, and children in periods of rapid growth. These groups have a greater need for protein than the rest of the population because of the new tissues being formed in their bodies. They need ample kcalories to protect that protein from degradation, yet in many cultures they are the very ones who are denied protein.

The Effects of PCM

Apathy like that of the little girl in our story is just one symptom of PCM. Other symptoms result from the disturbance of the water balance (edema), reduced synthesis of key hormones (lowered body temperature), lack of proteins to transport nutrients into and out of the circulatory system (anemia), lack of protein to carry oxygen to the cells (muscular weakness) or to carry away carbon dioxide (sleepiness), and lack of protein to build collagen for scar formation (poor healing of cuts) and for growth of bones and teeth (stunted growth).

However, one of the most insidious and far-reaching effects of PCM lies in the

at one end and lack of protein at the other—with PCM occupying the central region. In clinical practice these distinctions are not so easily made. At all points between marasmus and kwashiorkor, protein deficiency produces symptoms, whether the underlying cause is lack of dietary protein or lack of kcalories to protect the dietary protein. It seems to us that Cicely Williams had the right idea in urging that we quit worrying about the descriptions and the pathology of the diseases and spend our energies instead on delivering the care that is needed and

[1] C. D. Williams, On that fiasco, *Lancet* I (1975):793-794.

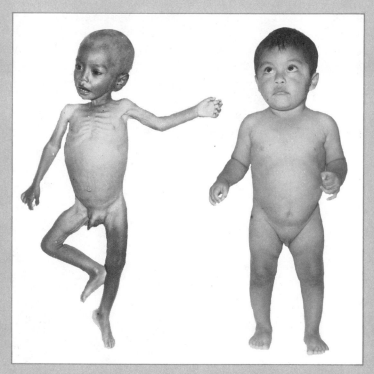

A child suffering from the extreme emaciation of marasmus.

Courtesy of Dr. Robert S. Goodhart, M.D.

The same child after nutritional therapy.

growth, Winick and his associates analyzed the brain tissue of young children who had died of severe marasmus as well as brain tissue from otherwise healthy accident victims (children of comparable ages).[3] They found that the number of brain cells of the marasmic children was significantly lower than the number in the well-fed children (See Figure 1). Since the number of brain cells does not increase significantly after about one year of age,

[3]M. Winick, P. Rosso, and J. Waterlow, Cellular growth of cerebrum, cerebellum, and brain stem in normal and marasmic children, *Experimental Neurology* 26 (1970):393-400.

possibility of its causing intellectual dysfunction. If the time of the insult occurs at a critical period of brain growth, children may never attain their intellectual potential—even if they are well nourished later. It is difficult to determine whether mental deficiencies observed in children are due to PCM or to other disadvantages, since social deprivation often goes hand in hand with malnutrition.[2]

In order to study the effects of PCM on brain

[2]J. Tizard, Early malnutrition, growth and mental development in man, *British Medical Bulletin* 30 (2) (1974):169-174.

Figure 1   DNA content of cerebellum in brain, which indicates the number of brain cells.

From M. Winick, P. Rosso, and J. Waterlow, Cellular growth of cerebrum, cerebellum, and brain stem in normal and marasmic children, *Experimental Neurology* 26 (1970):393-400.

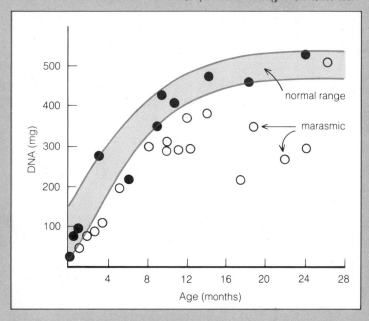

this finding has serious implications for the intellectual development of the child who is deprived of protein and/or kcalories during gestation and the first year of life.

PCM in the Modern World PCM did not gain much attention until after World War II. At that time increasing numbers of health teams sponsored by the United Nations and religious groups carried a message of better sanitation and improved medical care around the world. The postwar development of pesticides and antibiotics also helped raise the standards of health in many countries. Infant mortality was lowered, and recovery from infectious diseases became common.

These lowered mortality rates, combined with already-high birth rates, posed a new threat: severe food shortages. There probably had always been a shortage of food, especially of high-quality protein, but the problem had been masked by the more obvious one of infectious diseases. Figure 2 shows the prevalence of PCM in 59 countries in the decade 1963 to 1973.

The factors that contribute to the development of PCM are as varied and complex as the physical symptoms observed in people suffering from it. No one factor can be singled out as the only cause. Geography, education, traditions, economics, and birth rates are involved, all of which are interdependent.

Figure 2 Prevalence of severe and moderate protein/kcalorie malnutrition, compiled from the results from 101 surveys in 59 countries, 1963-1973.

Adapted from J. M. Bengoa and G. Donoso, Prevalence of protein-calorie malnutrition 1963-1973, *PAG Bulletin* 4 (1) (1974):25-35.

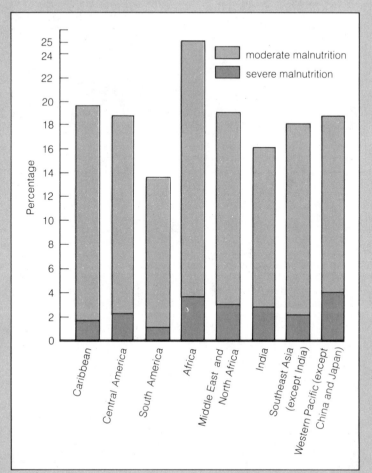

Geography If the land is rocky or barren, it may require enormous effort to produce the minimum amount of food needed to support human life. Many of the developing countries are in the subtropical or tropical regions. With their high temperatures and rainfall, they may produce an abundant harvest. However, crop pests and bacteria also thrive in a warm humid climate, and they may substantially reduce the harvest. If the region is near the sea, fish may be plentiful, but again, in a warm climate spoilage will take its toll.

Education Certainly the lack of education is part of

the evil cycle contributing to PCM. Poorly nourished people are too sick to use the educational opportunities open to them and so become more poorly nourished. They may lack knowledge of birth control methods or may fail to understand that delaying the birth of the next child until the mother has replenished her body's supply of nutrients will be an advantage to the health of subsequent children. In any case, ignorant people continue to produce children destined to die or to live out their lives under great hardships.

People in the regions of the world where PCM is rampant have no knowledge of efficient ways to plant, fertilize, and harvest crops and no capital with which to buy technology. Once the crops are harvested, the people do not know how to store them where insects and rodents will not destroy them or how to preserve them by drying or canning. These people suffer alternating periods of plenty and starvation, because one year's harvest, even if it is bountiful, cannot be made to stretch until the next harvest. With no knowledge of nutrition, they greatly reduce by improper handling the nutrient levels of the food they do have.

Traditions Probably the saddest causes of PCM are human traditions. In many communities meat is for males; females are not allowed to eat meat during their reproductive years, which is the very time when they and their future offspring most need the complete spectrum of amino acids offered by meat.

Traditions within a group also produce food prejudices or beliefs that limit the use of valuable food. For example, some peoples of Southeast Asia view milk as belonging to the animal's offspring and thus as not rightfully theirs to take. If urged to drink it, they will admit that they think of it as an unclean body secretion.[4] Other groups have such a reverence for all life that they refuse to use pesticides. Thus a farmer's crop may support the lives of the crop insects while his own children die for lack of food.

Economic Systems Countries need to have a marketable export item, even if the item is a food badly needed by their own people, in order to produce a balance of payments with which to import other needed items. Some of these import-export exchanges are difficult to understand. For instance, Africa imports high-carbohydrate foods, which its own land could produce, and exports pulses (peas or lentils), meat, and groundnuts, which its own people need. It has been estimated that a handful of groundnuts per person per day would solve India's protein problem,[5] yet India exports its groundnuts.

An effort by the government of Java to increase its total food supply produced a situation in which a large part of its malnourished population lost a major source of protein—soybeans. About 75 percent of Java's soybeans were grown in East Java during the dry season. Rice was a second crop grown during the rainy season. Then a high-yield variety (HYV) of rice seed was developed, and it was hailed as an answer to Java's need for more food. The government offered farmers fertilizer, seeds, and technical advisers to persuade them to irrigate their lands so that the HYV rice could be grown even during the dry season. Once the land was irrigated, however, farmers could no longer grow soybeans; soybean production decreased. Furthermore, the farmworkers then had no dry land to live on and were forced to live in the cities, paying cash for food they had formerly produced themselves.[6] Thus government intervention, although it increased the amount of food, decreased the protein supply and increased PCM.

[4]F. J. Simoons, The geographic approach to food prejudices, *Food Technology* 20 (1966):42-44.

[5]I. Palmer, UNRISD studies on the "green revolution," *Food and the New Agricultural Technology* No. 5, Report No. 72.9 (Geneva: United Nations Research Institute for Social Development, 1972).

[6]Palmer, 1972.

Birth Rates As mortality from infectious diseases has decreased, more people have lived more years. But they have had to be fed from the same amount of land. The late Dr. Grace Goldsmith, Dean of the School of Public Health and Tropical Medicine of Tulane University, stated, "Population growth must be slowed, or all efforts to augment agricultural production will merely postpone mass starvation."[7] Numerous other specialists agree.

When it became evident in the early 1950s that the world's population was going to "explode," many people were not concerned. "Science will find a solution," they thought, just as it had found the solution to so many other plagues. It was thought that through better fertilizers and higher-yield seeds, the "Green Revolution" would produce enough food to take care of the population increase.[8] However, the picture is even more gloomy today than it was in the 1950s. The world's grain stores are depleted, and since 1971 only three countries—the United States, Canada, and Australia— have had net exports of grain.[9] It is estimated that half the world's people live in perpetual hunger.[10]

In spite of the introduction in the 1950s of improved contraceptive methods, which have received worldwide dissemination through the efforts of such organizations as the Planned Parenthood Association, populations have continued to increase faster than food production. The population of the United States is still increasing too. It has been predicted that our population, which in 1973 was 209 million, will be 321 million by the year 2000.[11] This prediction is based on an average of three children per family, all other variables remaining the same. If, however, the birth rate declines to two children per family, which it appears to be doing, our population size will be 266 million in the year 2000.

Figure 3 compares the size of the U.S. population in 2070 assuming a birth rate of three children per family to its size assuming a birth rate of two children per family. This difference can be likened to placing the population of seven more New York Cities into the United States between 1973 and 1998.

Visualize the problems connected with feeding seven new cities the size of New York. Land will be taken out of food production and covered with concrete; land will be taken away from forests and put into food production; the water needed for growing the food will run

[7]F. H. Quimby and C. B. Chapman, in U.S. Senate, Select Committee on Nutrition and Human Needs, *National Nutrition Policy: Nutrition and the International Situation* (Washington, D.C.: Government Printing Office, 1974).

[8]Palmer, 1972.

[9]F. H. Sanderson, The great food fumble, *Science* 188 (1975):503-509.

[10]Quimby and Chapman, 1974.

[11]Quimby and Chapman, 1974.

Figure 3 Comparison of U.S. population in 2070 with birth rate of three children per family and two children per family.

From F. H. Quimby and C. B. Chapman, *National Nutrition Policy: Nutrition and the International Situation*, Select Committee on Nutrition and Human Needs (Washington, D.C.: Government Printing Office, 1974).

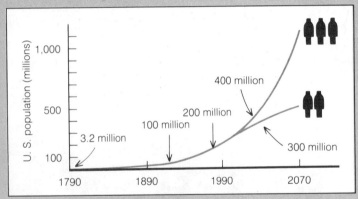

off into the ocean because of the loss of forests; more highways and trucks will be needed for transporting the food into the cities and the garbage out; additional energy will be required for this transportation network, as well as for cooking the food and for fertilizers. The problems seem insurmountable even for a rich country. How can we hope to feed the burgeoning populations of the rest of the world? As King wrote in 1960, "This is an historical era . . . to be witnessed in the biological realm . . . in the explosive increase of the world's population, and the concomitant spectre of slow and corrosive famine."[12]

Translating numbers of people into numbers of kcalories needed to feed those people illustrates the contribution of high birth rates to the prevalence of PCM. India's concern over its population growth may be translated into a limit on the number of children a family may have. Figure 4 shows that even if India lowers its birth rate by 30 percent from its 1965 level, it will still need 88 percent more kcalories in 1985 than it used in 1965. If its birth rate remains the same, it will need more than double its 1965 kcalories.

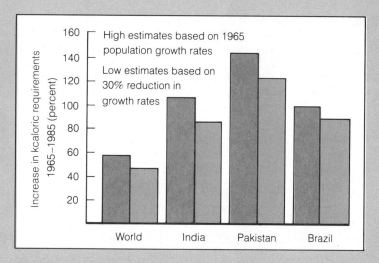

Figure 4   Projection of kcaloric requirements for the world, India, Pakistan, and Brazil.

Adapted from J. M. Bengoa and G. Donoso, Prevalence of protein-calorie malnutrition 1963-1973, *PAG Bulletin* 4 (1) (1974):25-35.

Transportation   Then there is the problem of distribution. Food must go from where it is plentiful to where it is in short supply. The solution to this problem involves other areas: economics (Who is to bear the cost? Are the recipients able to pay?), modern technology (food must remain edible in transit, vehicles for transport must be affordable), and, of course, energy (petroleum for fertilizers, insecticides, farm machinery, and transport).

Advertising   One bizarre cause of protein-kcalorie malnutrition is the advertising of food products. Mothers in low-income groups around the world are buying infant formula instead of breast-feeding their babies, because of intensive advertising campaigns. This advertising

shows pictures of fat rosy-cheeked babies and white-coated milk "nurses" who entice a mother into using the product and letting her own milk dry up. Her decision is irrevocable. She has decided to give up a perfect combination of high-quality protein and a kcalorie source suited to the baby's early digestive system for a costly product that requires safe water, sanitary care of expensive bottles, and ability to follow mixing directions. Not only that, she has given up a natural contraceptive; ovulation starts soon after the breasts have ceased lactation.[13] The fight against this particular cause of PCM has engendered a controversy

[12]C. G. King, in *Human Nutrition Historic and Scientific*, ed. I. Goldston (New York: International Universities Press, 1960):Introduction.

[13]D. B. Jelliffe and E. F. P. Jelliffe, "Breast is best": Modern meanings, *New England Journal of Medicine* 297 (1977):912-915.

over advertising ethics. Does a corporation have the right to direct its advertising to a population that is unable to make informed decisions? (This question is being directed also to the makers of sugary snacks who advertise on children's television programs.) Many are beginning to believe that it is immoral to persuade children and illiterate people to buy products that are detrimental to their health.

How Can We Fight PCM?

Such is the maze of modern life that what started out as a discussion of protein and kcalorie deprivation has become a debate on questions of economics, politics, human rights, and finally, corporate responsibility. If it seems to you that we have gone too far afield, our excuse is that we wanted you to realize that there are no simple solutions. Our country's sending wheat to a starving population is analogous to giving a beggar at your door a sandwich. Neither act helps to solve the underlying condition, even though both are acts of kindness that cannot be withheld by caring persons or nations. What is needed is for policymakers to attack the problems of malnutrition on many fronts.

Hundreds of experts from different walks of life have become involved in and concerned about world hunger. Dozens of international conferences have been held, and policies have emerged from them that promise to benefit nations that are enlightened enough to adopt them. At one conference, it was concluded that "there are now so many possible ways to go . . . that the setting of priorities has become a major problem," but hope was derived from the fact that "the questions are at last here."[14]

There is no consensus regarding "the" solution to the crisis or even about whether it can be solved. Many feel that it is too late and that it is only a matter of limited time before the human race enters a new Dark Age, beset by disease and starvation such as have never before been seen.[15] Others find cause for hope. The U.S. National Research Council has conducted a comprehensive study of the problem and has reached a conclusion of guarded optimism. The Council recommends "a massive research and development effort to expand world food supply, reduce poverty, and curb soaring population growth."[16] In other words, we should go beyond feeding the hungry beggar at the door and help him solve his problems so that he can feed himself.

The National Research Council recommends that research based in this country should emphasize four concerns: (1) nutrition, (2) food production (especially genetic manipulation, pest control, and soil improvement in the tropics), (3) food marketing and waste reduction, and (4) mechanisms to improve distribution. Given a commitment by the U.S. government and parallel commitments from other government agencies, the Council states that "it should be possible to overcome the worst aspects of widespread hunger and malnutrition within one generation."[17] This seems to be an optimistic view. But what is most required now is the political will to take the initiative. So we must move from the scientific into the political arena.

On the personal level, if you are concerned about

---

[14]Interdisciplinary Cluster on Nutrition, President's Biomedical Research Panel, Assessment of the state of nutrition science, part 1, *Nutrition Today*, January/February 1976, pp. 18-19, 25-27.

[15]W. Paddock and P. Paddock, *Time of Famines* (Boston: Little, Brown, 1976).

[16]Steering Committee, National Research Council Study on Food and Nutrition, National Academy of Sciences, World food and nutrition study: The potential contributions of research. Cited in *The Wilson Quarterly*, Autumn 1977, p. 55.

[17]National Research Council, 1977.

malnutrition, you can investigate the various movements that are attacking world hunger and can align yourself with the organization that best reflects your own philosophy. You can make your concerns known to political leaders, perhaps by joining a political action group. You can also implement ecologically sound conservation and nutritional programs in your own life. Don't be afraid to show your concern. The words of Benjamin Franklin, spoken in another context, apply to the world's PCM problem as well: "We must all hang together, or, assuredly, we will all hang separately."

CHAPTER 5

CONTENTS

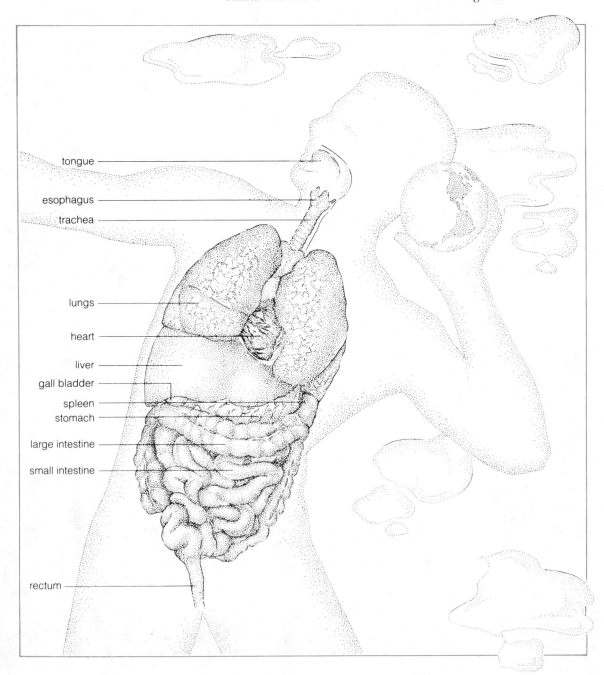

tongue

esophagus

trachea

lungs

heart

liver

gall bladder

spleen

stomach

large intestine

small intestine

rectum

DIGESTION

Food does not become nutrition until it passes the lips.

RONALD M. DEUTSCH

Lynn, age one, is playing with her mother's necklace. As one-year-olds do, she puts it in her mouth and chews on it. The necklace breaks. Lynn puts the beads into her mouth one by one and swallows them. An hour later her mother finds her with only a few of the hundred beads left on the table. In a panic, her mother calls the doctor. "Doctor," she says, "my daughter has just swallowed a necklace!" "Don't panic," says the doctor. "What was the necklace made of?" "Glass beads," says the mother. "And how big were the beads?" "About the size of a pea," says the mother. "That's all right then," says the doctor. "You'll get them back. Just watch her diapers for a day or so."

One of the beauties of the digestive tract is that it is selective. Materials that are nutritive for the body are broken down into particles that can be assimilated into the bloodstream. Those that are not are left undigested and pass out the other end of the digestive tract. In a sense, the human body is doughnut-shaped, and the digestive tract is the hole through the doughnut. You can drop beads through the hole indefinitely, and none of them will ever enter the doughnut proper. Two days after Lynn has swallowed them, her mother has recovered and restrung all the beads—and is again wearing the necklace!

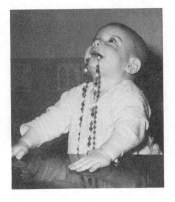

The problems associated with the nonnutritive dietary contaminants that can be absorbed are treated in Highlight 13.

The Problems of Digestion

Should you ever accidently swallow a necklace, you would be protected from any serious consequences by the design of your digestive tract. The system solves many other problems for you without your having to make any conscious effort. In fact, the digestive tract is the body's ingenious way of getting the nutrients ready for absorption. Let's consider the problems that are involved:

1. Human beings breathe as well as eat and drink through their mouths. Air taken in through the mouth must go to the lungs; food and liquid must go to the stomach. The throat must be arranged so that food and liquid do not travel to the lungs.

Diaphragm: see p. 170.

2. Below the lungs lies the diaphragm, a dome of muscle that separates the upper half of the major body cavity from the lower half. Food must be conducted through this wall to reach the abdomen.

3. To pass smoothly through the system, the food must be ground to a paste and must be lubricated with water. Too much water would cause the paste to flow too rapidly; too little would compact it too much, which could cause it to stop moving. The amount of water should be regulated to keep the intestinal contents at the right consistency.

4. When digestive enzymes are working on food, it should be very finely divided and suspended in a watery solution so that every particle will be accessible. Once digestion is complete and all the needed nutrients have been absorbed out of the tract into the body, only a residue remains, which is excreted. It would be both wasteful and messy to excrete large quantities of water with this residue, so some water should be withdrawn, leaving a paste just solid enough to be smooth and easy to pass.

5. The materials within the tract should be kept moving, slowly but steadily, at a pace that permits all reactions to reach completion. The materials should not be allowed to back up, except when a poison or like substance has been swallowed. At such a time the flow should reverse, to get rid of the poison by the shortest possible route (upward). If infection sets in farther down the tract, the flow should be accelerated, to speed its passage out of the body (downward).

6. The enzymes of the digestive tract are designed to digest carbohydrate, fat, and protein. The walls of the tract, being composed of living cells, are made of the same materials. These cells need protection against the action of the powerful juices that they secrete.

7. Once waste matter has reached the end of the tract, it must be excreted, but it would be inconvenient and embarrassing if this function occurred continuously. Provision must be made for periodic evacuation.

The following sections show how the body solves these problems, with elegance and efficiency.

GI tract: the gastrointestinal tract or alimentary canal; the principal organs are the stomach and intestines.

gastro = stomach
aliment = food

Anatomy of the Digestive Tract

The gastrointestinal (GI) tract is a flexible muscular tube measuring about 26 feet in length from the mouth to the anus. The voyage of the blue glass beads traces the path followed by food from one end to the other (see Figure 1).

When Lynn swallowed the beads, they first slid across her epiglottis, bypassing the entrance to her lungs. This is the body's solution to problem 1: Whenever you swallow, the epiglottis closes off your air passages so you do not choke. (You may wonder, however, what happens when a person does choke; that question is answered later in this chapter.)

Next the beads slid down the esophagus, which conducted them through the diaphragm (problem 2) to the stomach. There they were retained for a while. The cardiac sphincter at the entrance to the stomach closed behind them so that they could not slip back (problem 5). Then one by one they popped through the pylorus into the small intestine, and the pylorus too closed behind them. At the top of the small intestine they bypassed an opening (entrance only, no exit) from a duct (the common bile duct), which was dripping fluids (problem 3) into the small intestine from two organs outside the GI tract—the gallbladder and the pancreas. They traveled on down the small intestine through its three segments—the duodenum, the jejunum, and the ileum—a total of 20 feet of tubing coiled within the abdomen.

Having traveled through these segments of the small intestine, the beads arrived at another sphincter (problem 5 again)—the ileocecal valve—at the beginning of the large intestine (colon) in the lower right-hand side of the abdomen. As the beads entered the colon they passed another opening. Had they slipped into this opening they would have ended up in the appendix, a blind sac about the size of your little finger. They bypassed this opening, however, and traveled along the large intestine up the right-hand side of the abdomen, across the front to the left-hand side, down to the lower left-hand side, and finally below the other folds of the intestines to the back side of the body, above the rectum.

During passage through the colon, water was withdrawn, leaving semisolid waste (problem 4). The beads were held back by the strong muscles of the rectum. When the child chose to defecate, this muscle relaxed (problem 7), and the last sphincter in the system, the anus, opened to allow their passage.

To sum up, the path followed by the beads was

Esophagus

Epiglottis

Cardiac sphincter
Stomach
Pylorus

Common bile duct

Gallbladder
Pancreas   see
Duodenum   Figure 1.
Jejunum
Ileum
Ileocecal valve
Colon

Appendix

Rectum

Anus

> Mouth (epiglottis) → esophagus (cardiac sphincter) → stomach (pylorus) → small intestine (duodenum, with entrance from gallbladder and pancreas → jejunum → ileum) → large intestine (appendix) → rectum (anus)

This is not a very complex route, considering all that happens on the way. If you understand the anatomy of the system and the way the parts are connected, you can understand a number of common experiences: what happens when you choke on food (and what to do about it), when you vomit, when you get constipated, or when you have an ulcer. These experiences are explained in the last section of this chapter.

epiglottis (epp-ee-GLOT-is): cartilage in the throat that guards the entrance to the trachea and prevents fluid or food from entering it when a person swallows.

epi = upon (over)
glottis = back of tongue

trachea (TRAKE-ee-uh): windpipe.

esophagus (e-SOFF-uh-gus): food pipe.

cardiac sphincter (CARD-ee-ack SFINK-ter): sphincter muscle separating the esophagus from the stomach.

cardiac = near the heart

sphincter: circular muscle surrounding and able to close a body opening.

sphincter = band (a binder)

pylorus (pie-LORE-us): sphincter muscle separating the stomach from the small intestine.

pylorus = gatekeeper

Gallbladder and pancreas: see pp. 161-162.

duodenum (doo-oh-DEEN-um, doo-ODD-num): the top portion of the small intestine (about "12 fingers' breadth" long).

duodecim = twelve

jejunum (je-JOON-um): the first two-fifths of the small intestine beyond the duodenum.

ileum (ILL-ee-um): the last segment of the small intestine.

ileocecal (ill-ee-oh-SEEK-ul) **valve:** sphincter muscle separating the small and large intestines.

colon (COAL-un): the large intestine. Its segments are the ascending colon, the transverse colon, the descending colon, and the sigmoid colon.

sigmoid = shaped like the letter S (sigma)

appendix: a narrow blind sac extending from the beginning of the colon; a vestigial organ with no function.

rectum: the muscular terminal part of the intestine, from the sigmoid colon to the anus.

anus (AY-nus): terminal sphincter muscle of the GI tract.

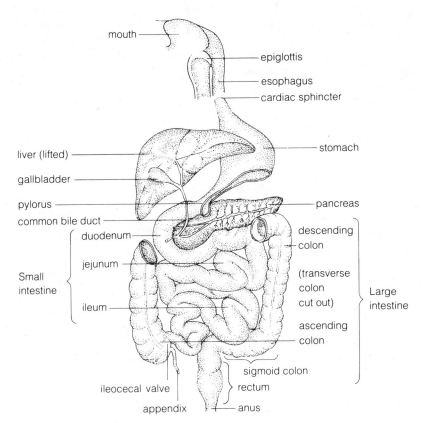

Figure 1   The flexible muscular tube called the alimentary canal, with associated structures.

The Involuntary Muscles and the Glands

You are usually unaware of all the activity that goes on between the time you swallow and the time you defecate. Like so much else that goes on in the body, the muscles and glands of the digestive tract meet internal needs without your having to exert any conscious effort to get the work done.

Chewing and swallowing are under conscious control, but even in the mouth there are some automatic processes that you have no control over. The salivary glands squirt just enough saliva into each mouthful of food so that it can pass easily down your esophagus (problem 3). (Occasionally, as you have noticed, they will squirt when you definitely do not want them to—when your mouth is open.) After a mouthful of food has been swallowed, it is called a bolus.

At the top of the esophagus peristalsis begins. The entire GI tract is ringed with muscles that can squeeze it tightly. Within these rings of muscle lie longitudinal muscles. When the rings tighten and the long muscles relax, the tube is constricted. When the rings relax and the long muscles tighten, the tube bulges. These actions follow each other so

gland: a cell or group of cells that secretes materials for special uses in the body. The salivary glands are **exocrine** (EX-o-crin) glands, secreting saliva "out" (not into the blood) into the mouth.

exo = outside

endocrine: secreting into the blood.

endo = within

bolus (BOH-lus): the portion of food swallowed at one time.

peristalsis (peri-STALL-sis): successive waves of involuntary contraction passing along the walls of the intestine.

peri = around
stellein = to wrap

that the intestinal contents are continuously pushed along (problem 5). (If you have ever watched a lump of food pass along the body of a snake, you have a good picture of how these muscles work.) The waves of contraction ripple through the GI tract all the time, at the rate of about three a minute, whether or not you have just eaten a meal. Peristalsis—along with the sphincter muscles that surround the tract at key places—prevents anything from backing up.

Peristalsis.

Tube with longitudinal (L) and circular (C) muscles

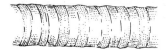

bolus

C muscles contract, L muscles relax.

L muscles contract, C muscles relax.

bolus

Wave moves along, pushing bolus ahead of it.

segmentation: a periodic squeezing or partitioning of the intestine by its circular muscles.

During the pushing motion, the intestines also periodically squeeze in short bands—as if you had put a string around them and pulled it tight. This motion, called segmentation, forces their contents backward a few inches at intervals, mixing them and allowing the digestive juices and the absorbing cells of the walls to make better contact with them.

Four major sphincter muscles work along the tract. The cardiac sphincter prevents reflux of the stomach contents into the esophagus. The pyloric sphincter, which stays closed most of the time, also prevents backup of the intestinal contents into the stomach and holds the bolus in the stomach long enough so that it can be thoroughly mixed with gastric juice and liquefied. At the end of the small intestine, the ileocecal valve performs a similar function. Finally, the tightness of the rectal muscle is a kind of safety device; together with the anus, it prevents elimination until you choose to perform it voluntarily (problem 7).

Smaller and Smaller

Besides forcing the bolus along, the muscles of the GI tract help to liquefy it so that the digestive enzymes will have access to all the nutrients. The first step in this process takes place in the mouth, where chewing, the addition of saliva, and the action of the tongue reduce the food to a coarse mash suitable for swallowing. A further mixing and kneading action then takes place in the stomach.

Of all parts of the GI tract, the stomach has the thickest walls and strongest muscles; in addition to the circular and longitudinal muscles, it has a third layer of transverse muscles that also alternately contract and relax.

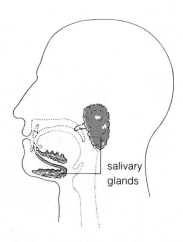

salivary glands

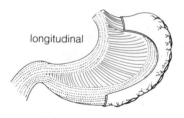
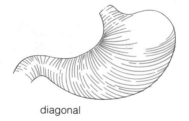
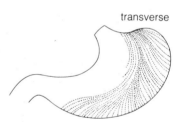

longitudinal

diagonal

transverse

Stomach muscles.

While these three sets of muscles are all at work forcing the bolus downward, the pyloric sphincter usually remains tightly closed, preventing the bolus from passing into the duodenum. Meanwhile, the gastric glands release juices that mix with the bolus. As a result, the bolus is churned and forced down, hits the pylorus, and bounces back. When the bolus is thoroughly liquefied, the pylorus opens briefly, about three times a minute, to allow small portions through. From this point on the intestinal contents are called chyme. They no longer resemble food in the least.

How Food Becomes You

One person may be a vegetarian, eating only fruits, vegetables, legumes, and nuts; another may have a meat-and-potatoes diet, eating very few fruits and vegetables. Whatever the diet—as long as it provides the needed nutrients in one form or another—people's body composition remains very much the same. It is impossible to tell from looking at a person whether he has just eaten a bowl of spaghetti and meatballs or a mixed green salad; in either case he has converted the materials in his food into the flesh, skin, and bones he is made of. How does he do it? It all comes down to the fact, of course, that the body renders food—whatever it was to start with—into the basic units that carbohydrate, fat, and protein are composed of. The body absorbs these units and builds its tissues from them. The final problem of the GI tract is to digest the food.

For this purpose there are five body components that contribute digestive juices: the salivary glands, the gastric glands, the intestinal glands, the liver, and the pancreas.

In addition to water and salts, saliva contains amylase, an enzyme that hydrolyzes starch to maltose. The digestion of starch thus begins in your mouth. In fact, you can taste the change if you choose. Starch has very little taste, but maltose has a subtly sweet flavor that you may associate with malted milk. If you hold a piece of starchy food like white bread in your mouth without swallowing it, you can taste it getting sweeter as the enzyme acts on it.

gastric glands: exocrine glands in the stomach wall that secrete gastric juice into the stomach.

gastro = stomach

chyme (KIME): the semiliquid mass of partly digested food expelled by the stomach into the duodenum.

chymos = juice

(1. Salivary glands already shown)

2. Gastric glands (stomach)

4. Liver

3. Pancreas

5. Intestinal glands

Organs that secrete digestive juices.

saliva: the secretion of the salivary glands; the principal enzyme is salivary amylase.

amylase (AM-uh-lase): an enzyme that hydrolyzes amylose (a form of starch). An older name for salivary amylase is **ptyalin** (TY-uh-lin).

hydrolyze (HIGH-dro-lies): to split by hydrolysis (see p. 27).

Mouth:	
Carbohydrate	Starch $\xrightarrow{\text{amylase}}$ maltose
Fat	No chemical action
Protein	No chemical action
Vitamins	No chemical action
Minerals	No chemical action
Water	Added
Fiber	Remains

gastric juice: the secretion of the gastric glands. The principal enzymes are rennin (curdles milk protein, casein, and prepares it for pepsin action), pepsin (acts on proteins), and lipase (acts on emulsified fats).

pH: see p. 133.

mucus (MYOO-cuss): a mucopolysaccharide secreted by cells of the stomach wall. The cellular lining of the stomach with its coat of mucus is known as the mucous membrane.

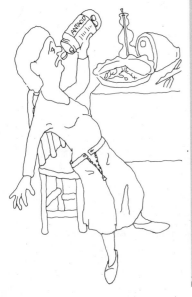

Gastric juice is composed of water, enzymes, and hydrochloric acid. The acid is so strong (at or below pH 2) that if it chances to reflux into the mouth, it burns the throat. To protect themselves from gastric juice, the cells of the stomach wall secrete mucus, a thick, slimy, white polysaccharide that coats the cells, protecting them from the acid and enzymes that would otherwise digest them (problem 6).

It should be noted here that the strong acidity of the stomach is a desirable condition—television commercials for antacids notwithstanding. A person who overeats or who bolts her food is likely to suffer from indigestion. The muscular reaction of the stomach to unchewed lumps or to being overfilled may be so violent as to cause regurgitation (reverse peristalsis, another solution to problem 5). When this happens, the overeater may taste the stomach acid in her mouth and think she is suffering from "acid indigestion." Responding to TV commercials, she may take antacids to neutralize the stomach acid. The consequence of this action is a demand on the stomach to secrete more acid to counteract the neutralizer and enable the digestive enzymes to do their work. So the consumer ends up with the same amount of acid in her stomach but has had to work against the antacid to produce it.

Antacids are not designed to relieve the digestive discomfort of the hasty eater. Their proper use is to correct an abnormal condition, such as that of the ulcer patient whose stomach or duodenal lining has been attacked by acid. Antacid misuse is similar to the misuse of diuretics already described.

> A FLAG SIGN OF A SPURIOUS CLAIM IS THE IMPLICATION THAT:
>
> Medication designed to correct an abnormal condition is needed for the normal, healthy person.

What our misguided consumer actually needs to do is to chew her food more thoroughly, eat it more slowly, and possibly eat less at a sitting.

All proteins are responsive to acidity; the stomach enzymes work most efficiently in a fluid of pH 2 or lower. However, salivary amylase—which is swallowed with the food—does not work in acid this strong, so the digestion of starch gradually ceases as the acid penetrates the bolus. In fact, salivary amylase becomes just another protein to be digested; its amino acids end up being recycled into other body proteins.

The major digestive event in the stomach is the hydrolysis of proteins. Both the enzyme pepsin and the stomach acid itself act as catalysts for this reaction. Minor events are the hydrolysis of some fat by a gastric lipase, the hydrolysis of sucrose (to a very small extent) by the stomach acid, and the attachment of a protein carrier to vitamin B_{12}.

Stomach:	
Carbohydrate	Minor action
Fat	Minor action
Protein	$Protein \xrightarrow[\text{HCl}]{\text{pepsin}}$ smaller polypeptides
Vitamins	Minor action
Minerals	No chemical action
Water	Added
Fiber	Remains

By the time food has left the stomach, digestion of all three energy nutrients has begun. But the action really gets going in the small intestine, where three more digestive juices are contributed. Glands situated in the intestinal wall secrete a watery juice containing all three kinds of enzymes—carbohydrases, lipases, and proteases—and others as well. In addition, both the pancreas and the liver make contributions by way of ducts leading into the duodenum. The pancreatic juice also contains enzymes of all three kinds, plus others.

Food evidently needs to be digested completely. The presence of two sets of enzymes for this purpose at this point underscores the body's determination to get the job done. If the pancreas fails, the intestine can largely carry on; if the intestine fails, the pancreas can substitute at least in part. Such duplication of effort is never seen in nature unless the job is absolutely vital, as it is in this case.

In addition to enzymes, the pancreas secretes sodium bicarbonate, which neutralizes the acidic chyme leaving the stomach. From this point on the contents of the digestive tract are at a neutral or slightly alkaline pH. The enzymes of both the intestine and the pancreas work best at this pH.

Bile, a secretion from the liver, also flows into the duodenum. The liver secretes this material continually, but it is needed only when fat is present in the intestine. The bile is concentrated and stored nearby, in the gallbladder, which squirts it into the duodenum on request. As explained in Chapter 2, bile is not an enzyme but an emulsifier; it brings fats into suspension in water so the enzymes can work on them.

pepsin: a gastric protease. It circulates as a precursor, pepsinogen, and is converted to pepsin by the action of stomach acid.

Vitamin B_{12} and the intrinsic factor: see Chapter 9.

intestinal juice: the secretion of the intestinal glands; contains enzymes for the digestion of carbohydrate and protein and a minor enzyme for fat digestion.

pancreatic (pank-ree-AT-ic) **juice:** the exocrine secretion of the pancreas, containing enzymes for the digestion of carbohydrate, fat, and protein. (The pancreas also has an endocrine function, the secretion of insulin and other hormones; see p. 21). Juice flows from the pancreas into the small intestine through the pancreatic duct. When the pancreas fails, fat digestion is seriously impaired, since the intestine has no major lipase.

bicarbonate: an alkaline secretion of the pancreas, part of the pancreatic juice. Bicarbonate also occurs widely in all cell fluids.

bile: an exocrine secretion of the liver (the liver also performs a multitude of metabolic functions). Bile flows from the liver into the gallbladder, where it is stored.

gallbladder: an organ that stores and concentrates bile. The gallbladder has no secretory function. Bile flows from the gallbladder into the small intestine through the bile duct.

The pancreatic and bile ducts conduct pancreas and liver secretions into the duodenum.

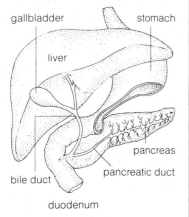

Details of pancreas, liver, gallbladder, and ducts.

Thanks to all these secretions, all the energy nutrients are digested in the small intestine.

Small intestine:		
Carbohydrate	All carbohydrates ⟶ monosaccharides	
Fat	All fats ⟶ (bile) emulsified fats	
	Emulsified fats ⟶ monoglycerides or glycerol and fatty acids	
Protein	All proteins ⟶ di- and tripeptides and amino acids	
Vitamins	No chemical action	
Minerals	No chemical action	
Water	Added	
Fiber	Remains	

Denaturation: see p. 100.

Most proteins are broken down to di- and tripeptides and amino acids before they are absorbed. With this in mind, you will be in a position to refute certain untrue claims made about foods. For instance:

"Don't eat store-bought beef. They injected a tenderizer into the blood of the steer before they killed it. When it gets into your blood, this enzyme will digest and destroy your tissues."

Just before slaughtering, pancreatic enzymes are sometimes injected into the steer's circulatory system; they do digest tough connective tissue in the vessel walls and make the meat easier to chew. But when you eat the meat, these enzymes have been denatured by cooking and cannot function as enzymes. They are but a few among thousands of different proteins in your digestive tract; they are broken down to amino acids identical to those from the other proteins you eat. Your body cannot tell the source of a particular amino acid any more than it can tell where its vitamin C comes from (Introduction).

"Eat brains. The materials they are made of will nourish your brain."

Like any other nutrients, the proteins, fats, and carbohydrates in brain tissue will be digested and absorbed and will nourish the body. But they are no better than hamburger, in the sense that both are digested to basic units before absorption. Each body builds its own brain tissue from basic units that can be obtained as well from hamburger as from brains.

"Eat predigested protein as amino acid mixtures so your digestive tract won't have to work so hard to digest protein."

It used to be believed that protein was digested all the way to amino acids before it was absorbed. Now we know that protein digestion in the fluid of the intestinal tract proceeds only as far as small peptides in many cases. These then enter the cells of the intestinal lining, and there they are digested further to amino acids. As a matter of fact, whole proteins are better absorbed and utilized, even by the body of a very sick, malnourished person, than are hydrolyzed amino acid mixtures.[1] This surprising finding has come to light through actual experiments, not through the exercise of reasoning from what was known before. It has given the lie to advertisers who try to sell protein supplements to athletes, sick people, dieters, and others. The "best" protein is food protein. The reasons why will be made clearer in Chapter 6, where a closer look at the intestinal cells shows how they handle protein.

This discussion stresses a point that is important for the informed consumer to remember. The argument that a food (tenderized beef) is harmful or that a food (brains) is beneficial can be identified as spurious by the flag sign mentioned before (p. 68). In addition, although these arguments are logical, they are not based on evidence. They sound convincing, as logical statements do, but if you know the facts of nutrition you can see through them.

A FLAG SIGN OF A SPURIOUS CLAIM IS:

The use of logic rather than evidence.

Such mistaken notions are as old as humankind. Will eating beets build good red blood? Will eating polished rice rather than brown rice give you a clear white complexion? Will you get pregnant from drinking cow's milk? You know these statements are preposterous, but all of them are still believed by thousands of people less well informed than yourself. The level of misleading statements now being circulated to our better-educated public has also been raised.

On the other hand, once logical statements are tested, they often prove true. In a susceptible or upset system, especially in that of a young infant, whole proteins from an uncooked food such as milk may be absorbed. They may be beneficial, as when antibodies from the mother's milk confer immunity on the infant. But they may cause allergy; in fact, the most common cause of food allergy is milk

Milk allergy: see p. 429.

[1]E. M. N. Hamilton and E. N. Whitney, Controversy 6: Liquid protein, in *Nutrition: Concepts and Controversies* (St. Paul: West, 1979), pp. 144-145.

protein "leaking" into the system through a defect in the wall. When a question like this is raised, experimental research must be undertaken to ascertain what really happens.

This Digression is not intended to review the evidence on protein absorption but to remind you that questions regarding whether or not a constituent of food is harmful can be answered only by experimentation.

The story of how food is broken down into nutrients that can be absorbed is now nearly complete. All that remains is to recall what is left in the GI tract. The three energy nutrients—carbohydrate, fat, and protein—are the only ones that must be disassembled to basic building blocks before they are absorbed. The other nutrients—vitamins, minerals, and water—are mostly absorbable as is. The function of the indigestible residues, such as fiber, is not to be absorbed but rather to remain in the digestive tract—mainly to provide a semisolid residue that can stimulate the muscles of the tract so that they will stay in tone and perform peristalsis. Fiber also retains water, keeping the stools soft. Furthermore, it carries bile acids, sterols, and fat with it out of the body.[2]

However there are some alterations made in the form of some minerals and vitamins. For oxidative changes of iron, see p. 454; for the binding of iron, p. 456. For the B_{12} carrier, or intrinsic factor, see p. 344.

Small Intestine:	
Carbohydrate	Almost completely absorbed (as basic units)
Fat	Almost completely absorbed (as basic units)
Protein	Almost completely absorbed (as basic units)
Vitamins	Almost completely absorbed
Minerals	Mostly absorbed
Water	Remains
Fiber	Remains

The process of absorbing the nutrients presents its own problems, which are taken up in Chapter 6. For the moment, let us assume that the digested nutrients simply disappear from the GI tract as soon as they are ready. Virtually all are gone by the time the contents of the GI tract reach the end of the small intestine. Little remains but water, a few dissolved salts and body secretions, indigestible materials such as fiber, and an occasional blue glass bead. These enter the colon, where intestinal bacteria degrade some of the fiber to simpler compounds.

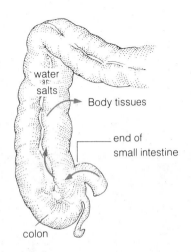

Detail of the large intestine.

[2]J. Scala, Fiber, the forgotten nutrient, *Food Technology* 28 (1974): 34-36.

The colon retrieves from its contents the materials that the conservative body is designed to recycle—much of the water and the dissolved salts (problem 4).

Large Intestine (Colon):
Minerals	Reabsorbed
Water	Some reabsorbed
Fiber	Some digested by bacteria; some remains

At the end of the colon what is left is a semisolid waste of a consistency suitable for excretion.

The Regulation of GI Function

This is the first chapter of the book that takes you inside the body. While you are there, watching the motions of the muscles and the secretion of the digestive juices responding to the presence of food, it is only fair to give you a glimpse of the puppeteers who pull the strings. The story of digestion told above, although complete in outline and fair in emphasis, fails to give credit to the two marvelous systems that coordinate all the digestive processes and ensure that nothing goes wrong: the hormonal (or endocrine) system and the nervous system. This is not the place for a detailed description of advanced physiology; accordingly, the five examples given below are intended only as vignettes to illustrate the principles of the body's regulation of its internal environment.

The stomach normally remains at pH 1.5 to 1.7. How does it stay that way? One of the regulators of the stomach pH is a hormone, gastrin, produced by cells in the stomach wall. The entrance of food into the stomach stimulates these glands to release the hormone. The hormone in turn stimulates other stomach glands to secrete the components of hydrochloric acid. When pH 1.5 is reached, the gastrin-producing cells cannot release the hormone, so they stop. (The acid itself turns them off.) The acid-producing glands, lacking the hormonal stimulus, then stop secreting hydrochloric acid. Thus the system adjusts itself automatically.

Another regulator consists of nerve receptors in the stomach wall. These receptors respond to the presence of food and stimulate activity by both the gastric glands and muscles. As the stomach empties, the receptors are no longer stimulated, the flow of juices slows, and the stomach quiets down.

hormone: a chemical messenger. Hormones are secreted by a variety of endocrine glands in the body. Each affects a specific target tissue or organ and elicits a specific response.

gastrin: a hormone produced by cells in the stomach wall. Target organ: the stomach. Response: secretion of gastric juice.

Gastrin regulation of stomach pH.

1. Food enters stomach.

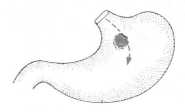

2. Stomach wall secretes gastrin into blood.

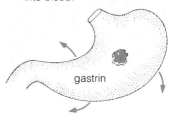

gastrin

3. Stomach glands respond by secreting acid.

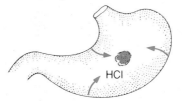

HCl

4. Acid stops gastrin secretion. Digestion proceeds at pH 1.5.

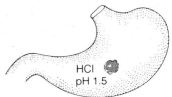

HCl
pH 1.5

The pylorus opens to let out a little chyme. How does it know when to close? When the pylorus relaxes, acidic chyme slips through. The acid itself touching that muscle on the far side causes the pylorus to close tightly. Only after the chyme has been neutralized by pancreatic bicarbonate and the medium surrounding the pylorus has become alkaline can the muscle relax again. This process ensures that the chyme will be released slowly enough to be neutralized as it flows through the small intestine. This is important because the small intestine has less of a mucous coating than the stomach does and therefore is not so well protected from acid.

Acid regulation of pylorus opening.

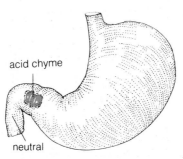

acid chyme

neutral

1. Pylorus opens.

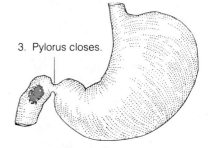

3. Pylorus closes.

2. Acid chyme passes through, touches far side of pyloric muscle.

secretin (see-CREET-in): a hormone produced by cells in the duodenum wall. Target organ: the pancreas. Response: secretion of pancreatic juice.

As the chyme enters the intestine, the pancreas adds bicarbonate to it, so that the intestinal contents always remain at a slightly alkaline pH. How does the pancreas know how much to add? The duodenal contents stimulate cells of the duodenum wall to release the hormone secretin into the blood. As this hormone circulates through the pancreas, it stimulates the pancreas to release its juices. Thus whenever there is an acid in the duodenum, the pancreas responds by sending bicarbonate to neutralize it. When the need has been met, the secretin cells of the duodenal wall are no longer stimulated to release the hormone, the hormone no longer flows through the blood, the pancreas no longer receives the message, and it stops sending pancreatic juice. Nerves also regulate pancreatic secretions.

acid chyme in duodenum

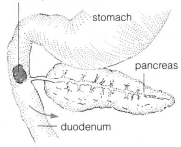

stomach

pancreas

duodenum

1. Duodenal wall releases secretin into blood.

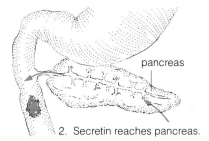

pancreas

2. Secretin reaches pancreas.

3. Pancreas secretes juice into duodenum.

4. Acid chyme is neutralized. Secretin release (1) stops.

Secretin regulation of pancreatic secretion.

When fat is present in the intestine, the gallbladder contracts to squirt bile into the intestine, to emulsify the fat. How does the gallbladder get the message that fat is present? Fat in the intestine stimulates cells of the intestinal wall to release the hormone cholecystokinin. This hormone, reaching the gallbladder by way of the blood, stimulates it to contract, releasing bile into the small intestine. Once the fat in the intestine is emulsified and enzymes have begun to work on it, it no longer provokes release of the hormone, and the message to contract is canceled.

cholecystokinin (coal-ee-sis-toe-KINE-in): a hormone produced by cells of the intestinal wall. Target organ: the gallbladder. Response: release of bile.

Cholecystokinin regulation of bile secretion.

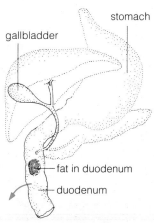

stomach

gallbladder

fat in duodenum

duodenum

1. Duodenal wall releases cholecystokinin into blood.

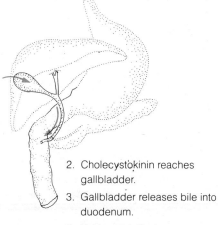

2. Cholecystokinin reaches gallbladder.

3. Gallbladder releases bile into duodenum.

4. Fat is emulsified. Cholecystokinin release (1) stops.

enterogastrone (enter-oh-GAS-trone): a hormone believed to be produced by the intestine in response to the presence of fat. Target organ: the stomach. Response: slowing of peristalsis.

The digestion of fat takes longer than that of carbohydrate. When fat is present, intestinal motility slows to allow time for its digestion. How does the intestine know when to slow down? Fat stimulates the release of the hormone enterogastrone, which suppresses the nerves that stimulate gastrointestinal motility, thus keeping food in the stomach longer. You may recall that a mixed breakfast of carbohydrate, fat, and protein was recommended in Chapter 1, partly because fat slows the digestion of carbohydrate, helping to keep the blood glucose level steady. Hormonal and nervous mechanisms like these account for much of the body's ability to adapt to changing conditions.

Once you have begun asking questions like these, you may not want to stop until you have become a full-fledged physiologist. For now, however, these few will be enough to make the point. Throughout the digestive system and all other body systems, all processes are precisely and automatically regulated, without your conscious efforts. This leaves you free to compose a symphony or to gaze at the stars instead of tying up your energy in worrying about how much acid to secrete or when to close your pylorus. This remarkable arrangement once prompted the physiologist Claude Bernard to remark, "Stability of the internal environment is the condition of free life." Walter Cannon, another physiologist, wrote a whole book about these processes, aptly titled *The Wisdom of the Body*.

The kinds of regulation described are all examples of **feedback** mechanisms: a certain condition demands a response to change that condition. The change produced becomes itself the signal to cut off the response thus the system is self-corrective.

Common Digestive Problems

The facts of anatomy and physiology presented in this chapter are so easy to apply to some common situations that a few practical applications will be presented here. Knowing how the air and food passages cross in the throat, for example, you can see how it is that food may sometimes slip into the air passage and cut off breathing.

larynx: the voice box (see Figure 2).

Choking on Food Food can lodge so securely in the trachea that all air is cut off. No sound can be made because the larynx is in the trachea and makes sounds only when air is pushed across it. This has happened often enough so that the event has been given a name—cafe coronary. The scenario reads like this: A person is dining in a restaurant with friends. A chunk of food, usually meat, becomes lodged in his trachea so firmly that he cannot make a sound. Often he chooses to suffer alone rather than "make a scene in public." If he tries to communicate distress to friends, he must depend on pantomime. The friends are bewildered by his antics and become terribly worried when the victim "faints" after a few minutes without air. They call a doctor or an ambulance. However, by the time he arrives at the hospital the victim is usually dead—from suffocation. In the past many of these cases were diagnosed as "death by coronary thrombosis"—thus the name cafe coronary.

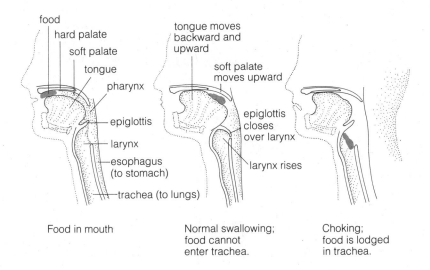

food
hard palate
soft palate
tongue
pharynx
epiglottis
larynx
esophagus
(to stomach)
trachea (to lungs)

tongue moves
backward and
upward
soft palate
moves upward
epiglottis
closes
over larynx
larynx rises

Food in mouth

Normal swallowing;
food cannot
enter trachea.

Choking;
food is lodged
in trachea.

To help a person who is choking, first ask this critical question: "Can you make any sound at all?" If the victim makes a sound, relax. You have time to continue with your questioning to see what you can do to help; you are not going to have to make a quick decision. But whatever you do, don't hit him on the back. If you do, the particle may become lodged more firmly in his air passage.

If the choking person is a child, pick her up by the ankles if you can do so without hurting her, so that gravity can aid the coughing reflex to expel the particle. If the choking person is an adult, lay him on his stomach across a table or bed with his head and neck off the support and almost vertical to the floor. Again, gravity will help. Now—and not before—you can thump him sharply between the shoulder blades to help dislodge the particle.

If the victim is unable to make a sound, you must act fast. The strategy most likely to succeed is the Heimlich maneuver. Get behind the victim and put your arms around the lower part of his rib cage. Make a fist with one hand and place the fist over the spot shown in Figure 2. Grasp the wrist of your balled-up hand with your other hand and give a sudden strong hug. What you are hoping to accomplish with this quick bear hug is to push the diaphragm upward, because this will expel air from the lungs. The hope is that this air will be effective in dislodging the stuck food particle in the same way that built-up gas pressure in a bottle of wine can push the cork out of the bottle. One word of caution: Be certain that your fist is in the correct position and is snugly against the person's body and that you proceed with the hug from that position. Do not slam your fist against the rib cage; this might cause the food to become more securely lodged in the trachea. It would be well to practice this technique at home, for there is no time to hesitate once you are called on to perform this death-defying act.

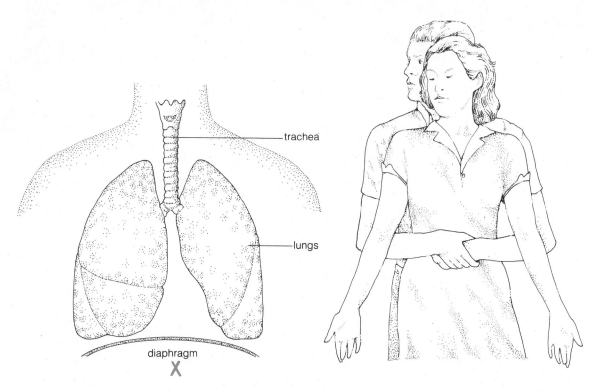

trachea

lungs

diaphragm

X

Figure 2 The Heimlich maneuver. Press fist on spot marked X, grasp wrist with other hand, and hug. Diaphragm should arch upward, forcing air out of the lungs through the trachea and dislodging the food.

If all else fails and time is running out, reach into the person's throat to try to pull out the lodged particle. You may scratch the tissues of the throat, but in a life-or-death situation this should not deter you. The scratches will heal if you can only save the person's life.

Vomiting Vomiting can be a symptom of many different diseases or may come from any situation that upsets the body's equilibrium, such as air or sea travel. For whatever reason, the waves of peristalsis reverse direction, and the contents of the stomach are propelled up through the esophagus to the mouth and expelled. If vomiting continues long enough or is severe enough, the reverse peristalsis will carry the contents of the duodenum, with its green bile salts, into the stomach and then up the esophagus. Simple vomiting is certainly unpleasant and wearying for the nauseated person, but it is no cause for alarm. Vomiting is one of the body's adaptive mechanisms to rid itself of something irritating.

Interstitial space: see p. 132.

But vomiting can be serious, and a doctor's care may be needed in some cases. When large quantities of fluid are lost from the gastrointestinal tract, fluid leaves the interstitial spaces to replace it. This interstitial water must be replaced from somewhere. The nearest supply is in the capillaries of the circulatory system. To resupply the circulatory system, fluid is drawn from the cells. The danger in prolonged vomiting is that eventually fluid is taken from every cell of the body. Leaving the cells with the fluid are electrolytes, particularly

Electrolyte: see p. 500.

sodium, potassium, chloride, and bicarbonate, which are absolutely essential to the life of the cells. These electrolytes and fluid must be replaced, which is difficult while the vomiting continues. Intravenous feedings of saline and glucose with electrolytes added are frequently necessary while the doctor is diagnosing the cause of the vomiting and instituting corrective therapy.

intravenous (in-tra-VEEN-us): into a vein.

saline (SAY-leen): a salt solution.

In an infant, vomiting is especially serious; a doctor should be contacted soon after onset. Babies have a higher proportion of fluid in the interstitial space, so it is much easier to deplete their body water and upset their electrolyte balance than it is with adults.

Projectile vomiting is another kind of vomiting that is not the simple type associated with nausea. In this type, the contents of the stomach are expelled with such force that they leave the mouth in a wide arc, arching far out from the body like a bullet leaving a gun. There are a number of causes for this type of vomiting, and all of them require immediate medical care.

Diarrhea   Diarrhea is the name given to the condition characterized by frequent, loose, watery stools. This sort of stool indicates that the intestinal contents have moved too quickly through the intestines for fluid absorption to have taken place or that water has been drawn from the cells lining the intestinal tract and added to the food residue. Diarrhea will be discussed in more detail in Chapter 14, but for the moment you should be aware that it can become serious if it continues. Diarrhea causes a depletion of the fluid and electrolyte content of the body cells in much the same way that vomiting does, and this condition is always serious. Diarrhea in an infant may quickly lead to dehydration so severe as to require emergency medical treatment.

Constipation   You may joke about or be irritated by the laxative commercials on television that frequently seem to appear on the screen at the dinner hour, but most persons believe the message the advertisements are sending—that Mrs. X must have a daily bowel movement or else she will be headachy and irritable and lose all her marvelous personality. The screen then shows Mrs. X the next day feeling her old jovial self because her pharmacist has persuaded her to take a laxative.

Each person's gastrointestinal tract responds to food in its own way, with its own rhythm, the fecal matter arriving at the rectal area in a fairly constant number of hours. Each GI tract thus has its own cycle, which depends on its "owner's" physical makeup and such environmental considerations as the type of food eaten, when it was eaten, and when the person's schedule allows time to defecate. If several days pass between movements but these movements take place without discomfort, then the person is not constipated, nor did she absorb any "toxins" that would cause irritable behavior. Nor does anyone need to worry about an inability to have daily movements—TV commercials notwithstanding.

constipation: the condition of having painful or difficult bowel movements (elapsed time between movements is not relevant).

defecate (DEF-uh-cate): to move the bowels, eliminate waste.

defaecare = to remove dregs

What then is constipation? When a person receives the signal that says to defecate and ignores it, the signal may not return for quite a few hours. In the meantime, water will continue to be withdrawn from the fecal matter, so that when the person does decide to defecate the movement will be drier and harder. If the bowel movement is hard and is passed with difficulty, discomfort, or pain, then it can be said that the person is constipated. (Note that in this definition of constipation no mention has been made of the amount of time that has elapsed since the previous bowel movement; that is irrelevant.)

What can be done about constipation? If discomfort is associated with passing fecal matter, a doctor's help should be sought in order to rule out the presence of organic disease. Once this has been done, dietary or other measures for correction can be considered.

Careful review of daily habits may reveal the causes of the constipation. Being too busy to respond to the defecation signal is a common complaint. One's daily regimen may need to be reexamined with the idea of instituting regular eating and sleeping times that will allow time in the day's schedule, at the dictate of the person's body, to have a bowel movement. This may mean going to bed earlier in order to rise earlier so that ample time is allowed for a leisurely breakfast and a movement.

There is a scarcity of laboratory research into the laxative quality of foods. It has been determined, however, that prunes contain a substance shown to be laxative.[3] If a morning defecation is desired, prune juice should be drunk at bedtime; if the evening is preferred, prune juice could be taken at breakfast.

Another cause of constipation that requires some rearrangment of lifestyle is the lack of physical activity. In modern society many people drive cars or ride buses to work, stand at assembly lines or sit behind desks, then sit in front of a television set in the evening. People who do not have the time or money to work out in a spa are finding that they can park their cars a distance from the office and walk the extra blocks, or they can walk up several flights of stairs rather than take an elevator. With such planning, much exercise can be incorporated into the day. The muscles that are responsible for peristalsis are improved by any activity that increases the muscle tone of the entire body.

Another helpful measure may be to increase the fiber content of the diet. During this century, two changes have occurred together (a correlation): a shift in food consumption away from vegetables, fruits, and grains and toward meats, fats, and sugar and a parallel increase in constipation.[4] You should be well aware by now that a correlation does not prove a causal relationship, but in the case of this relationship authorities at least agree that high-fiber diets do help to relieve constipation.[5] Fiber absorbs a lot of water and so softens the stools. A

[3]This substance is dihydroxyphenyl isatin.

[4]A. Tunaley, Constipation: The secret national problem, *Nutrition* 28 (1974): 91-96.

[5]L. Bass, More fiber—less constipation, *American Journal of Nursing* 77 (1977): 254-255.

gram of crude fiber increases stool weight by 15 g of water on the average, with cereal fiber being much more effective than that from fruits and vegetables.[6] It is proposed that an increase in the consumption of fruits, vegetables, and whole-grain cereals would overcome most constipation problems. Some African villagers who consume an unrefined diet pass soft stools over four times the volume of those of Westerners,[7] and the dietary fiber content of their diets is six times that of Westerners. It is also interesting to note that these villagers never have diverticular disease.[8]

Diverticulitis: see p. 121.

Some constipation may be relieved by the addition of fat to the diet. It was previously thought that the success of this regimen was due to its lubricating effect, but it now appears to be due instead to its stimulation of cholecystokinin, which causes bile to be secreted into the duodenum. The bile acts in the same way that a saline laxative does; that is, its high salt content draws from the intestinal wall an abundance of water, which stimulates peristalsis and softens the fecal matter.

Cholecystokinin: see p. 167.

Saline (SAY-leen): a salt solution. (See p. 171.)

Another recommendation for helping to ovecome constipation is to increase fluid intake. Since the fluid is reabsorbed in the lower colon, it has been difficult to understand how a greater intake of fluid would soften the fecal matter. However, it has now been suggested that the beneficial effect comes from the physical stimulation of the increased bulk on the upper gastrointestinal tract which promotes peristalsis throughout.

These suggested changes in diet or lifestyle should correct chronic constipation without the use of laxatives. One of the fallacies often perpetrated by television commercials is that one person's successful use of a laxative product is a good recommendation for another person to use that product. As a matter of fact, even diet changes that are successful in relieving constipation for one person may increase the constipation of another (see Figure 3). For instance, if a person has a spastic type of constipation, in which peristalsis promotes strong contractions that close off a segment of the colon and prevent passage, then increasing the fiber in the diet would be exactly the wrong thing to do. A good rule is that if laxatives seem to be indicated, a doctor's advice should be sought.

Ulcers   An ulcer can occur in many places outside and inside the body, but the term most often refers to an ulcer in the stomach (a gastric ulcer) or in the duodenum (a duodenal ulcer). The term *peptic ulcer* includes both of these. An ulcer is an erosion of the top layer of cells from an area, such as the wall of the stomach or duodenum, leaving the second and succeeding underlying layers of cells exposed, without protection. These exposed cells exude fluid, and anything that touches the eroded area causes pain. The erosion may proceed until the

peptic ulcer: an eroded mucosal lesion in the stomach or duodenum.

mucosal (myoo-COH-sul): of the mucous membrane.

lesion: an abnormal change in structure.

[6]Scala, 1974.

[7]Bass, 1977.

[8]Scala, 1974.

Figure 3 Different kinds of constipation require different treatments. Caution: Don't self-diagnose!

Adapted from M. V. Krause, *Food, Nutrition, and Diet Therapy*, 4th ed. (Philadelphia: Saunders, 1966), pp. 248-250. Courtesy of the author and publisher.

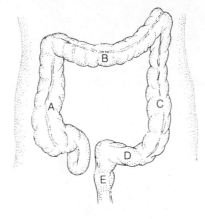

Normal colon: A, ascending colon; B, transverse colon; C, descending colon; D, sigmoid colon; and E, rectum.

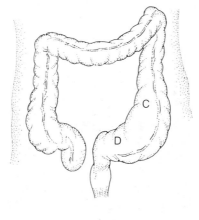

In the most common type of constipation, the muscles of the descending and sigmoid colon are loose and fail to push the contents along. This is **atonic constipation,** and it is helped by increasing the fiber content of the diet.

> *a* = without
> *tonic* = (muscle) tone

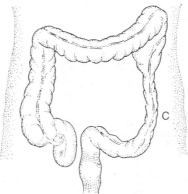

In a rarer kind of constipation, the descending colon is pinched closed by overreactive muscles. This is **spastic constipation,** and added fiber makes it worse.

capillaries that feed the area are exposed and bleeding or until there is a perforation (a hole) in the wall.

Some people naively believe that an ulcer is caused by the secretion of stomach acid, but this is not the case—at least not at first. The stomach lining of a healthy person is well protected by its mucous coat, as you learned earlier in this chapter. Why then do ulcers sometimes form? Two factors are required: first, a weakness in the stomach or duodenal wall; then the secretion of gastric acid to erode the weak spot. We are in the dark with respect to the cause of the initial weakness; it may be poor nutrition, lack of rest, or any other condition (including a genetic flaw) that hinders the maintenance of healthy tissue. But once an ulcer has started to form, the secretion of stomach acid can rapidly make it worse.

What is of interest about ulcers—and the reason why they are included here—is that their origin and development seem to be related more closely to stress than to diet. You may remember that the secretion of digestive juices is regulated by the master coordinators, the hormones and the nerves. Both hormonal secretions and nerve activity are profoundly influenced by a person's mental state. The brain, after all, is composed of nerves, including many that impinge on the endocrine glands. Excessive anxiety and worry may be the cause of the initial lesion of an ulcer; they are clearly related to the excessive acid secretion that makes an ulcer worse.

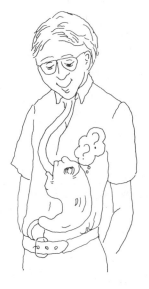

Dr. Sue Rodwell Williams, the author of a widely used textbook in diet therapy, puts it this way: "The individual's particular emotional make-up and his manner of dealing with life's day-to-day problems and challenges, will often be reflected in the functions of his digestive tract. . . . It is not what he eats, it's what is eating him that is important." Williams also reminds her readers to remember that "surrounding every stomach there is a person."[9]

Some interesting observations by two doctors, named Wolf and Wolff, set in motion the line of inquiry that was to culminate in today's agreement that stress is the primary factor that aggravates an ulcer. Wolf and Wolff were doctors at a hospital that admitted a most unusual patient one day in 1939. This patient, remembered in scientific circles only as "Tom," had had since childhood an opening from the outside of his body through the abdominal wall into his stomach. Through this opening, called a fistula, he had learned to feed himself and, keeping his condition secret, had grown to manhood and had lived a near-normal life.

At the age of 53, while performing hard manual labor, he tore the edge of the opening of the fistula and was taken to the hospital where Wolf and Wolff were on the staff. The two doctors managed to gain Tom's confidence. He cooperated with them by allowing them to make observations of his stomach lining through the fistula. As a result, they learned that emotions called forth unique responses from the stomach. Aggressive emotions, such as anger and hostility, made the capillaries in the stomach lining flush with blood and caused the gastric juices to pour forth as if food had been

[9]S. R. Williams, *Nutrition and Diet Therapy*, 3rd ed. (St. Louis: Mosby, 1977), p. 530.

introduced. However, when Tom was sad and depressed, there was no secretion of gastric juices, and the capillaries were pale pink instead of red. These emotional states and the stomach's responses to them were entirely independent of Tom's feelings of hunger.

This discovery was exceedingly important and was duly reported in the journals. Probably the most important result of these observations was the stimulus to experiment they gave to other doctors who had patients with fistulas. Thus researchers began to learn exactly which foods were irritating to the lining of the stomach and which foods neutralized the acidity, instead of relying on tradition and logical thinking for this knowledge. For instance, they found that the majority of the foods that had been classified as irritating to the stomach actually had more effect when applied to the skin of the arm! This story should remind you that caution must be applied when decisions are made on the basis of logic (see p. 163).

CAUTION WHEN YOU READ!

A logical conclusion cannot be accepted as true until it is supported by experimentation.

bland diet: the diet traditionally prescribed for peptic ulcer. Bland foods are literally dull and insipid, without strong flavor or odor. An even more restrictive diet is the Sippy diet, consisting of milk or milk and cream given in small amounts every one or two hours.

At the beginning of this century, ulcer patients were prescribed a rigid, restrictive bland diet consisting of foods believed to be nonirritating to the stomach. Experiments have shown, however, that such a diet does not hasten healing and have led to the conclusion that the ulcer patient needs instead to make some fundamental changes in lifestyle. Learning how to handle stress without overreacting and getting upset, learning to relax, to get enough sleep, to enjoy life—these are the therapeutic agents now advocated to aid recovery from ulcer disease. As far as diet is concerned, the only true irritants seem to be alcohol, caffeine-containing beverages, and meat extract such as bouillon. The only positive measure now recommended by the American Dietetic Association is to eat frequently—since food in the stomach gives the gastric acid something to work on other than the stomach lining itself.[10]

This discussion should help to reinforce a happy thought: that in at least some instances the diet that is best for your health may be the one you like. To promote the health of your digestive tract, you should indulge in eating as a pleasant experience that contributes to a tranquil

[10]American Dietetic Association, Position paper on bland diet in the treatment of chronic duodenal ulcer disease, reprint from the *Journal of the American Dietetic Association* 58 (1971).

state of mind. (The next chapter will provide reasons why you should also consume a wide and interesting variety of foods.) It is best to select mixed meals in which a multitude of colors, flavors, and aromas spark the appetite, stimulate the digestive juices to flow, relax the body into a state of enjoyment, and promote the healthful reception of valuable nutrients offered in a delicious form.

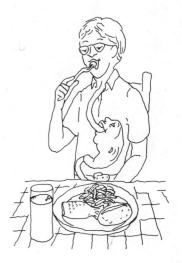

Summing Up

Let's follow some food through the digestive tract to the point where all needed nutrients have been absorbed. Whether it be a hamburger or a piece of chocolate cake, the same processes occur. The food is lubricated by saliva and broken up into particles by chewing. Starch digestion proceeds no farther than maltose in the mouth.

The food is swallowed and carried down the esophagus and through the cardiac sphincter by peristalsis, a muscular squeezing action that continues throughout the length of the tract. In the stomach further liquefication occurs, and the digestion of proteins begins through the action of pepsin and hydrochloric acid. The pylorus releases small portions of the liquefied acidic contents into the duodenum.

In the duodenum the emulsification of fats occurs—thanks to bile, a secretion of the liver that is concentrated and stored in the gallbladder until needed. Pancreatic bicarbonate neutralizes the intestinal contents to allow the enzymes of the intestinal and pancreatic juices to work, and fat, protein, and carbohydrate digestion all proceed further.

As the liquefied mixture of nutrients passes along the small intestine, the three energy nutrients continue being digested. By the time the mixture reaches the ileocecal valve, these nutrients have been almost completely rendered into the simpler compounds—the carbohydrates to monosaccharides; the lipids to monoglycerides, glycerol, and fatty acids; the proteins to di- and tripeptides and amino acids—and have been absorbed. The vitamins and minerals have also largely been absorbed by this time. For the most part, only water, fiber, and some dissolved salts remain.

In the large intestine, water and salts are reabsorbed, leaving a semisolid waste that is excreted from the rectum when the anus opens.

The regulation of GI functions is accomplished by various hormonal and nerve-mediated messages that coordinate the supply of digestive juices and the action of the tract's muscles with demand. Problems may arise, however. It is important to know when a problem must be handled immediately (as in using the Heimlich maneuver to dislodge a food particle stuck in the trachea); when it is of minor concern (as when temporary nausea arises as a consequence of motion sickness); and when a doctor should be consulted (with prolonged vomiting or diarrhea or when laxatives seem to be needed to alleviate constipation).

It is also important to distinguish between stress-induced illnesses and illness caused by malnutrition or poor eating habits. Peptic ulcers seem more related to stress than to diet, and a change in lifestyle, not just in diet, is often indicated.

To Explore Further

The early classic in physiology is Cannon, W. B., *The Wisdom of the Body* (New York: Norton, 1932), in which Cannon reveals and marvels at the ways the body maintains homeostasis.

One of many excellent recent physiology textbooks is Eckert, R., *Animal Physiology* (San Francisco: Freeman, 1978).

A teaching aid, *GI Function and Dysfunction*, includes four different slide presentations, each with an annotated syllabus. These can be purchased from the Nutrition Today Society (address in Appendix J).

A film, *The Heimlich Maneuver* (16 mins., 16 mm, color), is now being shown by local chapters of the American Red Cross. It can be obtained from Paramount-Oxford Films, 5451 Marathon Street, Hollywood, CA 90038.

An excellent reference for the way laxatives work is Corman, M. L., Veidenheimer, M. C., and Coller, J. A., Cathartics, *American Journal of Nursing* 75 (1975):273-279. It lists about 90 over-the-counter laxatives by brand name with classification and site of action.

Stress and Nutrition

This part of the soul which is the mind . . . being plunged within and mixed with the body and always having need of its help and its presence, . . . shall not reason nor understand nor do any other thing without its organ, the body.

JEAN FERNEL, 1656

Throughout recorded history, humans have expressed the intuitive knowledge that a person's state of mind affects the health of his body. Plato noted that "this is the great error of our day in the treatment of the human body that physicians separate the soul from the body." Religious sects have been founded on the belief that a person's state of mind (interpreted as a person's relationship to his God) can be used to cure illness without medical intervention. These ideas fell into disrepute with the coming of the scientific era, which considered only those factors that could be confined in a petri dish or reduced to a mathematical formula as "real" and worthy of scientific investigation.

In recent times, we have acquired a new awareness of the connection between mental stress and illness, especially as it pertains to hypertension, gastrointestinal illnesses, atherosclerosis, and cancer. However, as Greenberg wrote in *Science News*, "Although significant gains have been made in stress research, the field remains littered with contradictory, confusing studies that frequently inspire headscratching among the experts."[1] As bits and pieces of the stress-illness puzzle have been fitted together, nutritionists

[1]J. Greenberg, The stress-illness link: Not "if" but "how," *Science News* 112 (1977):394-398.

have attempted to discover how stress might alter nutritional requirements. These findings, too, are inconsistent.

What Is Stress? The word *stress* has many meanings. A building contractor considers stress to be the weight put on steel girders that tends to push them out of shape; a psychologist considers it the burdens carried by people who are experiencing major life-altering events. To a musician it is the accent on a note; to an orator the special emphasis put on a word. The struggle to win at tennis or to gain a promotion at work can also be considered stressful, and in this sense stress makes life interesting and invigorating. However, when stress pushes a person to the point where body processes are interrupted, it then becomes a cause of illness.

A patient may feel affronted if the doctor suggests that his illness is caused by stress, thinking that the doctor is saying his illness is imaginary. Another person may think that if there is stress in her life great enough to cause illness, it is because she is unable to cope with life's problems—she is inept. These views are widespread but are not based on current understanding of the body's physiological reaction to crisis.

Stress is always with us. The only way to avoid it is to be dead. To every influence pushing the body out of balance the body responds to restore itself to wholeness, just as the steel girder pushes back against the weight of the roof to maintain equilibrium. The maintenance of this equilibrium is called homeostasis. If you eat carbohydrate and your blood glucose is driven up, the pancreas secretes insulin to bring the blood glucose back to normal. If you walk into the winter cold without a coat, your body shivers to produce heat and sends the blood from the surface capillaries deep into your body so that its heat will not be lost to the air. Eating sugar and walking in the cold are stresses. They demand action to restore the status quo—normal blood glucose level and body temperature. Major physical stresses include pain, an illness of any kind, surgery, wounds, burns, infections, a very hot or humid climate, toxic compounds, radiation, and pollution.

The Stress Reactions   As our understanding of stress has expanded, we have come to realize that the body responds to every stress with the same set of reactions. It does not judge whether the event is happy or sad, whether it is physical or mental, or whether it will result in an advantage or a disadvantage. The body does respond differently, however, to different intensities of stress, so it is sensitive to the person's interpretation of the event.

The physiologist Cannon first described the set of stress reactions in the early twentieth century. He dubbed them the fight-or-flight reactions, because they help people mobilize their defenses to meet danger, either by staying to fight or by running away. Thus the danger

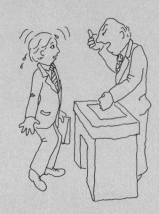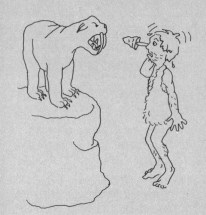

presented today by a boss who is vindictive or unfair calls forth the same physiological response as did the danger of a large aggressive animal to our cave-dwelling ancestors.

When a danger is present, the brain relays a message to the adrenal glands, which sit atop the kidneys. The adrenal medulla, the interior of the gland, then secretes the catecholamines, epinephrine and norepinephrine, into the bloodstream, which carries them to target areas all over the body. The results are (1) greater energy through the release of glucose from the liver; (2) greater protection

from blood loss by a faster clotting time, a conservation of fluid in the kidneys, and a retreat of blood from the periphery of the body to the vital organs and the legs; (3) increased ability to see through the widening of the pupils of the eyes; (4) increased catabolism of body fat for energy during a sustained crisis; (5) faster respiration to bring in more oxygen and to get rid of carbon dioxide; and (6) more powerful heartbeats to send nutrient- and oxygen-rich blood to the muscles faster. All these events (and more) enable a threatened person to escape danger or else to stand and fight the aggressor.

Modern urban societies do not present many situations that require actual fight-or-flight but the same reactions occur nevertheless. For the most part, you face stresses that demand calm, intelligent, rational behavior. When you are thwarted by the slowness of rush-hour traffic, you have no need for emergency action, for ele-

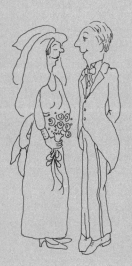

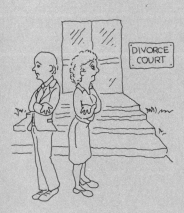

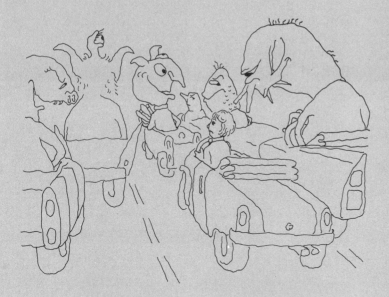

vated blood glucose, blood that clots faster, or additional fatty acids in the bloodstream. You must sit quietly behind the wheel and maneuver the car through traffic, even though your body is geared for heavy physical exercise.

The effect of *not* being active when under stress may be harmful. The fat depots are not receiving fat into storage while the stress reaction is active, so the fat must circulate in the bloodstream thus giving it more opportunity to enter the artery walls. The body generally treats the raised fat and glucose in the blood the same as if these had come from a recent high kcalorie meal. The health of the body depends on these excess energy nutrients being "worked off" by muscular activity. A recommendation, then, for mitigating the harmful effects of stress is to engage in heavy exercise such as jogging, dancing, skipping rope, or even punching a pillow until thoroughly fatigued, and to avoid the use of drugs such as alcohol and tranquilizers that would discourage exercise.

What are the life events that bring on the stress reactions? These differ for each individual. One person's past experience might make her perceive a particular event as one she can cope with successfully, but another person may view the same event as presenting danger. One criterion for judging an event as stressful is the amount of change in daily activities it entails and thus how much adaptive or coping behavior is necessary to deal with it. Holmes and Rahe developed "The Social Readjustment Rating Scale" and have used it with more than 5,000 patients to study the quality and quantity of life events that cluster at the onset of disease.[2] They noted a high degree of agreement about the significance of these life events, that cut across subgroups based on age, sex, religion, or race.

The 43 life events of the Social Readjustment Rating Scale are shown here arranged in order from the most stressful to the least stressful.[3]

1. Death of spouse
2. Divorce
3. Marital separation
4. Jail term
5. Death of close family member
6. Personal injury or illness
7. Marriage
8. Fired at work
9. Marital reconciliation
10. Retirement
11. Change in health of family member
12. Pregnancy
13. Sex difficulties
14. Gain of new family member
15. Business readjustment
16. Change in financial state
17. Death of close friend
18. Change to different line of work
19. Change in number of arguments with spouse

[2]T. H. Holmes and R. H. Rahe, The social readjustment rating scale, *Journal of Psychosomatic Research* 11 (1967):213-218.

[3]Holmes and Rahe, 1967.

20. Mortgage over $10,000
21. Foreclosure of mortgage or loan
22. Change in responsibilities at work
23. Son or daughter leaving home
24. Trouble with in-laws
25. Outstanding personal achievement
26. Wife begins or stops work
27. Begin or end school
28. Change in living conditions
29. Revision of personal habits
30. Trouble with boss
31. Change in work hours or conditions
32. Change in residence
33. Change in schools
34. Change in recreation
35. Change in church activities
36. Change in social activities
37. Mortgage or loan less than $10,000
38. Change in sleeping habits
39. Change in number of family get-togethers
40. Change in eating habits
41. Vacation
42. Christmas
43. Minor violations of the law

Stress and Illness

Research into psychosomatic illness has produced a flood of contradictory evidence. This is certainly to be expected in a field where the variables cannot be quantified. Some of these studies have purported to show that certain personality types develop certain diseases. Hard-driving, aggressive people have heart attacks;[4] emotionally immature, obsessive ones get ulcerative colitis;[5] and nervous, easily agitated people develop stomach ulcers.[6] Lately there have been reports that people who repress their emotions, especially anger, develop cancer.[7]

A major problem with these studies is that the psychological characteristics that are detected may be a direct result of having the disease rather than the cause of the disease.[8] In addition, these diseases develop over long periods of time, so there is a need to know the personality at the time of onset, which may have been many years prior to the outward manifestation of the disease. Before we can make sweeping generalizations about the kind of person who develops a disease, we need much more research using prospective studies.

One such study was undertaken at The Johns Hopkins University School of Medicine in 1946.[9] The purpose was to record genetic, physiological, metabolic, and psychological characteristics of healthy young medical students and then, by following them throughout their lives, to identify factors significantly associated with the early onset of disease. Originally the study was designed to find new approaches to the prevention of hypertension and coronary heart disease, but Thomas and Greenstreet reported in 1973 that the study had been extended to include three more disease states—suicide, mental illness, and tumor.[10] They concluded that many important psychobiological variables do characterize certain disease states and are not merely chance deviations. Among the predictive factors they found were total habits of nervous tension, blood pressure, closeness to parents, father's age at subject's birth, number of cigarettes smoked daily, relative body weight, depression, and insomnia.

[4]D. C. Glass, Review of *Behavior Patterns, Stress and Coronary Disease* (Hillsdale, N.J.: Lawrence Erlbaum Associates, 1977), in *Lancet* II (1978):924.

[5]M. V. Krause and M. A. Hunscher, *Food, Nutrition and Diet Therapy* (Philadelphia: Saunders, 1972), p. 357.

[6]Krause and Hunscher, 1972, p. 336.

[7]P. J. Rosch, Mind and cancer, *Lancet* I (1979):1302.

[8]Editorial: Mind and cancer, *Lancet* I (1979):706-707.

[9]C. B. Thomas and R. L. Greenstreet, Psychobiological characteristics in youth as predictors of five disease states: Suicide, mental illness, hypertension, coronary heart disease and tumor, *Johns Hopkins Medical Journal* 132 (1973):16-43.

[10]Thomas and Greenstreet, 1973.

This description of the prospective study carried out on medical students at The Johns Hopkins University is brief of necessity. It omits many important facts about the study, especially about its conclusions. It has been included here only as an example of a well-designed prospective study in the field of psychosomatic medicine. We urge you to refer to the original report as it appeared in *The Johns Hopkins Medical Journal* for a more complete account of the study's conclusions.

Two ideas about the relationship between stress and illness have been presented here: First, the body is sensitive to the individual's interpretation of an event; second, personal characteristics may potentiate a particular disease. If we accept these as true, then it seems that a person could prevent or cure certain diseases by changing his behavior. This idea has wide appeal and has led to a superabundance of popular manuals on how to cope with various diseases. People who have successfully waged war against cancer or other diseases are excited about their victories (and rightfully so) and enjoy recounting the details around the modern

version of the campfire—books and television talk shows. (They also enjoy the improvement in their bank balance.)

One of the best of these stories, in our opinion, is "Anatomy of an Illness" by Norman Cousins, editor of *Saturday Review*, which appeared in the *New England Journal of Medicine* in 1976.[11] Mr. Cousins was told he had an incurable collagen disease but chose not to surrender to it. He insisted on being active, not passive, in his own treatment. He is both an accomplished observer and an articulate writer, so that he was able to detail exactly what he had experienced without embellishing the truth, as most of us in our euphoria would have done. Among his strategies was that he took large doses of vitamin C—but the key to his success was not in what he did but rather in the fact that he acted vigorously in his own behalf. An editorial in *Lancet* expressed this opinion on the value of fighting for your life:

It is uncertain whether the benefit claimed for "fighting back" results mainly from a placebo effect, or from activation of the patients' homeostatic mechanisms by hope, expectation, and belief. Whether or not dynamic hope

or "fighting back" will prolong life in the cancer patient beyond its expected duration, it is almost certain that absence of hope can shorten life, apart from vitiating its quality.[12]

One negative aspect of these mind-over-matter stories is that some people may feel a distressing burden of guilt when they are not able to halt the progress of disease by their own mental efforts as the story teller has done. The listener should guard against having unrealistic expectations. There is no law that says what happens to one person must happen to another. But it will certainly do no harm to try using the power of positive thinking especially if it is used as an adjunct to the best modern medical care. As Mr. Cousins points up, we "need to encourage to the fullest the patient's will to live and mobilize all natural resources of body and mind to combat disease."[13] The effect of the state of mind on the body is a powerful natural resource. We need more scientific investigation into how to use it.

Stress and Energy Nutrients Stress, as you have seen, can cause multiple physiological changes in the body. Each of these changes involves hundreds of bio-

[11]N. Cousins, Anatomy of an illness as perceived by the patient, *New England Journal of Medicine* 295 (1976):1458-1463.

[12]Editorial, *Lancet*, 1979.

[13]Cousins, 1976.

Mini-Glossary

adrenal glands: a pair of endocrine glands situated on the kidneys.

ad = on (to)
renal = kidney

The adrenal cortex produces steroid hormones like the sex hormones; the adrenal medulla produces the catecholamines.

cortex = outer layer
medulla = inner layer

antidiuretic (an-tih-DYE-you-RET-ik) **hormone (ADH):** a hormone that promotes the conservation of water by the kidney.

anti = against
diu = to pass through
ouron = urine

catecholamines (cat-uh-COAL-uh-meens): **epinephrine** (ep-in-EFF-rin), and **norepinephrine** (NOR-ep-in-eff-rin). These hormones are neurotransmitters.

glycogenolysis: the breakdown of glycogen.

leukocyte (LOO-koh-SITE): a blood cell that fights infection.

leuko = white
cyte = cell

neurotransmitters: chemicals involved in sending messages along the nerves.

pituitary (pih-TOO-ih-TARE-ih) **gland:** a small endocrine gland attached to the base of the brain; influences growth, metabolism, and maturation.

prospective (prah-SPECK-tiv) **study:** a study designed and begun prior to an event, looking forward to unknown results.

proteolysis (pro-tee-OLL-uh-sis): the breakdown of protein.

psychosomatic (sigh-co-so-MAT-ic): relating to the interaction between mental and body phenomena, popular (and incorrect) meaning: imaginary.

psyche = mind, soul
soma = body

chemical reactions that rely on the availability of nutrients. If these nutrients are not replenished as they are used up, deficiencies will develop. These deficiencies may be the cause of some of the illness and tissue damage that have been noted in cases involving stress.

The answers to questions about nutrition and stress are just emerging from the laboratories; most of the studies use hospitalized patients for subjects. There is an abun-

dance of clues, some of them very promising, but there is no consensus among nutritionists that one or another nutrient is especially protective. Let's take a look at just one well known feature of stress—the raised blood glucose level. An examination of the nutritional implications of this change may help you understand why nutritionists have few absolute answers.

The raised blood glucose results when stress hormones and neurotransmitters

promote three actions in the body. First, liver glycogen breaks down to glucose. Second, while most cells drink up this glucose to speed up their work during the crisis, the storage cells—liver glycogen and fat cells—are prevented from taking up glucose. Third, body protein is broken down to amino acids. The amino acids are used for the synthesis of new proteins; for production of the TCA cycle (carbohydrate) intermediates, which must be continually replaced if ATP is to remain available; and of course for energy. If the stress continues or if the person was not in good nutritional status before the event, the ready supply of these two nutrients—glucose and amino acids—will be exhausted. In addition, the vitamins and minerals needed as catalysts will also be depleted.

Because glucose is the brain's preferred energy nutrient, stress-induced deficiencies may result in confusion or depression. As the body uses up its small pool of amino acids, muscles may waste and wounds may resist healing.

A logical nutritional therapy for the person under stress would be to eat carbohydrate and protein foods. However, this is not always recommended, because stress interferes with the digestive processes. (Digestion of food is not a top priority when you are being chased by a saber-toothed tiger.) Furthermore, the trauma may leave the person unable to eat.

If the patient cannot eat and cannot digest food, you might conclude that he could receive intravenous feedings of glucose to spare the body amino acids from being dismantled for energy. True, intravenous feeding of glucose has been the traditional procedure. However, doctors have noted that even with this help muscles continue to waste during the height of a crisis, such as during the first days following surgery.[14] So the glucose does not spare the muscle protein. Why is valuable lean body tissue sacrificed for kcalories when the kcalories are presented in glucose? And if the body needs kcalories so badly, why doesn't it burn its fat?

Some researchers have suggested that there is something special about infection. Normally, the peripheral tissues, especially the muscles, do use fat and carbohydrate very well—for example, during fasting or exercise.[15] (Most of our knowledge of

the protein-sparing action of carbohydrate and fat have come from studies of fasting and exercise.) But during the faster metabolism of infection, muscle tissue uses its own abundant amino acids in preference to fat.

It has been postulated that intravenous glucose raises the insulin level, which in turn interferes with fat mobilization. To test this hypothesis, Greenberg and coworkers used intravenous feedings of amino acids alone, amino acids with glucose, amino acids with lipid, and glucose alone.[16] They found that protein-sparing action was due to the presence of the amino acids and was not related to the mobilization of fat from the fat depots.

The only energy nutrient affected by the change in blood glucose level during stress seems to be protein. As Kaminski and his coworkers point out, "The patient's protein status, not his fat or glycogen stores, directly affects his ability to respond to stress."[17] As far as replenishing these proteins is concerned, we can talk only about people in hospitals under the extreme stress of surgery or infection as the only evidence we have comes from the study of such

people. Amino acid infusions seem to be indicated for these people, at least during the first several days.

What recommendation about protein can be made for people who are not hospitalized but are undergoing life-altering events? There is a strong temptation to jump directly from the evidence of a few studies to a recommendation for overusing a nutrient. As we see it, the truth that can be gleaned from the evidence presented here is that good protein status is protective in case stress occurs. Therefore, the consumption of adequate protein should be a daily objective. When stress does occur, listen to your body. If it says don't eat, then refrain. Perhaps your digestive processes are too upset right then to tolerate food. If you want food, include some high-quality protein food in small amounts. When the height of the crisis has passed, return to your normal eating pattern, which should include high-quality protein.

[14]G. R. Greenberg, E. B. Marliss, G. H. Anderson, B. Langer, W. Spence, E. B. Tovee, and K. N. Jeejeebhoy, Protein-sparing therapy in postoperative patients: Effects of added hypocaloric glucose or lipid, *New England Journal of Medicine* 294 (1976):1411-1416.

[15]T. F. O'Donnell, G. H. A. Clowes, G. L. Blackburn, N. T. Ryan, P. N. Benotti, and J. D. B. Miller, Proteolysis associated with a deficit of peripheral energy fuel substrates in septic man, *Surgery* 80 (1976):192-199.

[16]Greenberg et al., 1976.

[17]M. V. Kaminski, Jr., R. P. Ruggiero, and C. B. Mills, Nutritional assessment: A guide to diagnosis and treatment of the hypermetabolic patient, *Journal of the Florida Medical Association* 66 (1979):390-395.

Vitamins, Minerals, and Stress   Studies have been conducted with almost all the minerals and vitamins to uncover their roles during stress. Only one mineral, potassium, will be mentioned here, because its loss could be critical; and only one vitamin, vitamin C, is mentioned because today's rumor mills are connecting it to stress.

One of the physiological changes that occurs with stress is the retention of water, which protects the body against the consequences of blood loss (a good possibility if you are attacked by that saber-toothed tiger). When danger is perceived, the pituitary gland secretes the antidiuretic hormone (ADH). By its action on the kidneys, sodium is retained (and thus water), and in the ion exchange potassium is lost.[18] Therefore, if edema is seen during stress it may indicate that potassium is being lost. This sort of edema has been reported by people withdrawing from cigarettes, for example. Potassium-containing foods can be eaten for protection against this loss, but a doctor should also be consulted, since edema is a presenting symptom in some serious medical problems.

When you study the research on vitamin C it is easy to suspect that supplements should be given during stress. The adrenal glands, which produce the neurotransmitters epinephrine and norepinephrine, have the highest concentration of vitamin C in the body; the brain, which perceives danger and signals the adrenals, has the second highest concentration.

Vitamin C is a cofactor in a key step in the synthesis of norepinephrine and is important in the metabolism of all the neurotransmitters. According to Subramanian, the storage of epinephrine is known to be influenced by the presence of sodium, potassium, and calcium ions, and it may be that vitamin C plays a role in the active transport of these ions across the membranes in the brain. Subramanian believes that mental function and behavior are sensitive to the cerebral concentration of vitamin C, as shown in scurvy.[19] We also know that vitamin C can detoxify histamine, which is secreted under stress and accounts for many of the uncomfortable symptoms of allergy.[20]

Many clinical reports have claimed that large doses of vitamin C are beneficial in the stress conditions produced by burns, injuries, surgery, and infections. The theory is that vitamin C increases the bactericidal action of the leukocytes. However, when Shilotri and Bhat studied the effect of megadoses of vitamin C on leukocytes in humans, they did not find an increase in bactericidal action.[21] As a matter of fact, they found that bactericidal action was impaired when 2 g of vitamin C were given each day for two weeks and found no effect at all when 200 mg a day were given.

We conclude vitamin C is intimately involved in all levels of stress, but we believe there is no strong evidence for supplementation. However, there is no solid evidence that supplementation in the range up to 1,000 mg is harmful. Therefore we recommend the daily use of fruits and vegetables, with extra servings during times of stress, and if it makes you feel better, vitamin C supplements of about 100 mg per day.

Stress and Your Diet

Here, then, are our dietary recommendations for reasonably healthy people who are undergoing major life events:

● Trust in the wisdom of your own body. It may know more than you think it does.

● If you feel like eating, eat only small amounts, since

[18]S. R. Williams, *Nutrition and Diet Therapy* (St. Louis: Mosby, 1977), p. 187.

[19]N. Subramanian, On the brain ascorbic acid and its importance in metabolism of biogenic amines, *Life Sciences* 20 (1977):1479-1484.

[20]R. L. Pike and M. L. Brown, *Nutrition: An Integrated Approach* (New York: Wiley, 1975), p. 138.

[21]P. G. Shilotri and K. S. Bhat, Effect of mega doses of vitamin C bactericidal activity of leucocytes, *American Journal of Clinical Nutrition* 30 (1977):1077-1081.

stress slows down the production of digestive enzymes.

● Choose a variety of nutrient-dense foods as protection against what we don't yet know about nutrients and stress. Don't latch onto one item (for example, citrus) and eat it exclusively.

● Choose high-quality protein foods for protection against the breakdown of your own muscle protein.

● Drink plenty of fluids, especially water, to help prevent sodium retention, and fruit juices, for their vitamin C and potassium.

In conclusion we suggest that you watch these trends in stress and nutrition research in the 1980s. Researchers seem to be finding different reactions in the body to different levels of stress. The placebo effect is gaining respectability as it is shown that body systems return to normal when the patient is active in his own defense—even if that defense is sugar pills, vitamin supplements, meditation, or faith healing. Hospital diets are undergoing a revolution as patients are encouraged to actively participate in their own nutritional support. This is happening first with cancer patients who are hav-

ing radiation therapy or chemotherapy and are experiencing loss of appetite. Nutrition is increasingly being taught to patients in the hospitals and in doctors' offices. Finally, we hope that the day is coming when surgery will be delayed whenever possible until the patient is in good nutritional status and his will to live has been activated.

To Explore Further

Frieden, E., and Lippner, J., *Biochemical Endocrinology of the Vertebrates*, Foundations of Modern Biochemistry Series (Englewood Cliffs, N.J.: Prentice-Hall, 1971) is an excellent, readable text intended for college undergraduate chemistry students.

This article reports on one vitamin whose metabolism is affected by stress:

Hodges, R. E., Effect of stress on ascorbic acid metabolism in men, *Nutrition Today* 5 (1970):11.

This is the first study in which severe psychological stress has been shown to produce a measurable abnormality in immune function:

Bartrop, R. W., Lazarus, L., Luckhurst, E., Kiloh, L. G., and Penny, R., Depressed lymphocyte function after bereavement, *Lancet* 1 (1977):834-836.

This book is written for doctors by a doctor:

Altschule, M. D., *Nutritional Factors in General Medicine: Effects of Stress and Distorted Diets* (Springfield, Ill.: Charles C Thomas, 1978).

The following two articles tell the story of a prospective study of the stress created by the loss of a job:

Kasl, S. V., The experience of losing a job: Reported changes in health, symptoms and illness behavior, *Psychosomatic Medicine* 37 (1975):106-122.

Cobb, S., Physiologic changes in men whose jobs were abolished, *Journal of Psychosomatic Research* 18 (1974):245-258.

Written for the general reader, Selye, H., *Stress without Distress* (New York: Lippincott, 1974) tells how to use stress to achieve a rewarding life style (also in paperback).

A teaching aid, *Stress: On Just Being Sick*, by H. Selye, is a set of 13 slides designed to depict the consequences of stress. The set can be ordered from the Nutrition Today Society (address in Appendix J).

CHAPTER 6

CONTENTS

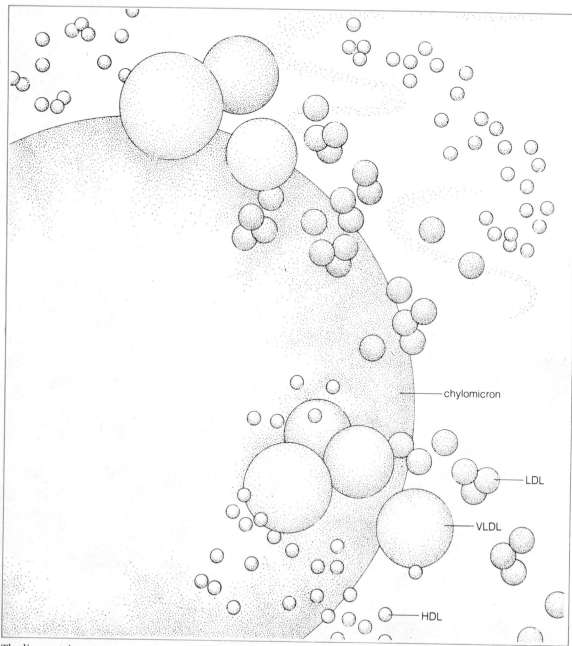

The lipoproteins.

ABSORPTION AND TRANSPORT

I know there have been certain philosophers, and they learned men, who have held that all bodies are endowed with sense; nor do I see, if the nature of sense be set alongside reaction solely, how they can be refuted.

THOMAS HOBBES

Problem: Given an elaborate production in which 1,000 actors are on stage at once, provide a means by which all can exit simultaneously! This is the problem of absorption. Within three or four hours after you have eaten a steak dinner with potato, vegetable, salad, and dessert, your body must find a way to absorb some two hundred thousand million, million, million amino acid molecules one by one, to say nothing of the other nutrient molecules. For the stage production, the manager might design multiple wings that all of the actors could crowd into, 20 at a time. If the manager were a mechanical genius, he might somehow design moving wings that would actively engulf the actors as they approached. The absorptive system is no such fantasy; in 20 feet of small intestine it provides over a quarter-acre of surfaces where the nutrient molecules can make contact and be absorbed. To remove them rapidly and provide room for more to be absorbed, a rush of circulation continuously bathes the underside of these surfaces, washing away the absorbed nutrients and carrying them to the liver and other parts of the body.

Anatomy of the Absorptive System

The inner surface of the small intestine looks smooth to the naked eye, but through a microscope it appears to be wrinkled into hundreds of folds. Each of these folds is covered with thousands of nipplelike projections, as numerous as the nap hairs on velvet fabric. Each of these small intestinal projections is a villus. If you could look still closer, you would see that each villus is covered with minute hairs, the microvilli.

villi (VILL-ee), singular **villus:** fingerlike projections from the folds of the small intestine.

microvilli (MY-cro-VILL-ee), singular **microvillus:** projections from the membranes of the cells of the villi.

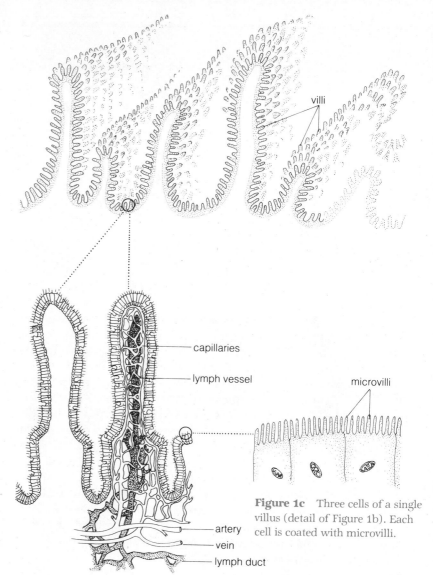

villi

capillaries

lymph vessel

microvilli

Figure 1c Three cells of a single villus (detail of Figure 1b). Each cell is coated with microvilli.

artery

vein

lymph duct

Figure 1b Two villi (detail of Figure 1a). Each villus is composed of several hundred cells.

A nutrient molecule, such as an amino acid, that encounters any part of this surface, is drawn into the cells that compose it.

The villi are in constant motion, waving, squirming, and wriggling like the tentacles of a sea anemone. They actively reach for and engulf nutrient molecules, aided by a thin sheet of muscle that lines each of them.

Once a molecule has entered a cell in a villus, the next problem is to transport it to its destination elsewhere in the body. Everyone knows that the bloodstream performs this function, but you may be surprised to learn that there is a second transport system—the lymphatic system. Both of these systems supply vessels to each villus, as shown in Figure

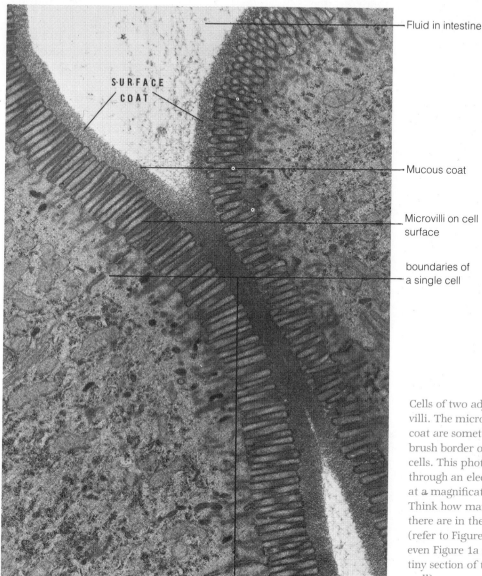

Fluid in intestine

Mucous coat

Microvilli on cell surface

boundaries of a single cell

Cells of two adjacent intestinal villi. The microvilli and mucous coat are sometimes called the brush border of the intestinal cells. This photograph was taken through an electron microscope at a magnification of 51,000X. Think how many of these cells there are in the small intestine (refer to Figure 1 and notice that even Figure 1a represents but a tiny section of the intestinal wall).

1b. When a nutrient molecule has crossed the cell of a villus, it may enter either the lymph or the blood. In either case the nutrients end up in the blood, at least for a while.

A Closer Look at the Intestinal Cells

The cells of the villi are among the most amazing in the body, for they recognize, select, and regulate the absorption of the nutrients the body needs. It is thanks to these cells that blue glass beads (see Chapter 5)

lymph (LIMF): the body's interstitial fluid, between the cells and outside the vascular system. Lymph consists of all the constituents of blood that can escape from the vascular system; it circulates in a loosely organized system of vessels and ducts known as the **lymphatic system.**

never enter the body proper to lodge in inconvenient places. But they are far more sophisticated in the distinctions they can make, and they not only absorb but also process many of the nutrients you consume in food. A closer look at them is worthwhile, because it will help to explode a number of common misconceptions about nutrition.

Some people believe, for example, that eating predigested protein—amino acid preparations such as the "liquid protein" products sold to dieters—saves the body the work of having to digest protein, so that the digestive system won't "wear out" so easily. Nothing could be further from the truth. Others believe that people shouldn't eat certain food combinations (for example, fruit and meat) at the same meal, because the digestive system can't handle more than one task at a time. The art of "food combining" is based on this gross underestimation of the body's capabilities.

Each cell of a villus is coated with thousands of microvilli (Figure 1c), which project from its membrane. In these microvilli and in the membrane lie hundreds of different kinds of enzymes and "pumps," which recognize and act on different nutrients. For example, one of the enzymes is lactase, which breaks apart the disaccharide lactose, or milk sugar. The presence of lactase at the cell surface ensures the efficient absorption of this sugar, because as soon as it is broken into its component parts (glucose and galactose), those parts are easily contacted by the nearby pumps, which move them into the interior of the cell.[1] This arrangement makes it easy for a newborn infant to absorb and use milk sugar, even though his gastrointestinal tract may in some ways still be immature.

Enzymes for cleaving di- and tripeptides also lie in the surface structures of the intestinal cells. Whole proteins—long polypeptides—are digested to shorter chains out in the fluid of the intestine, but once they have been rendered into short fragments, these fragments are contacted and trapped by the microvilli, where the final stages of digestion occur.[2] The cells' enzymes then can deliver the final products—amino acids—directly to the pumps, which carry them into the cells.

There is nothing random about this process. The anatomical arrangement guarantees not only digestion but also delivery of its products into the body. Digestion and absorption are coordinated.

When hydrolyzed proteins (that is, mixtures of amino acids) are consumed, there can be no such coordination. They arrive en masse in the intestine, presenting it with the problem of trying to absorb them all at once. At first, floating free in the fluid, they exert an

[1] R. Levine and D. E. Haft, Carbohydrate homeostasis (first of two parts), *New England Journal of Medicine* 283 (1970): 175-183.

[2] D. M. Matthews and S. A. Adibi, Peptide absorption, *Gastroenterology* 71 (1976): 151-161.

attractive force (remember that charged molecules attract water). As a result, excess water is drawn into the GI tract, causing at the least discomfort and at the worst cramping, nausea, and diarrhea.

This attractive force is osmotic pressure (see p. 500).

Chapter 3 showed that most people (in the developed countries) eat more protein than they need. Chapter 4, in describing the remarkable roles of protein, explained perhaps why they do: Protein is an impressively important nutrient, and the more we learn about it the more its importance staggers the imagination. Still, excess protein in any form does no good and may do harm; and protein in the form of artificially digested supplements is dangerous. Even in the hospital, in the treatment of very sick, starving people, it is now recognized that the well-meaning attempt to supply predigested proteins is outmoded. It was based on "a misconception concerning the digestive capacities of the human gastrointestinal tract in emaciation, disease, and after surgery. Actual feeding experiments have proven . . . that even in extreme starvation proteins can still be digested as long as food can be swallowed."[3]

It is unwise to try to second-guess the body. It has evolved over millions of years to derive its nutrients efficiently from foods. How could we presume, after five minutes of listening to a health food salesman or fad diet promoter, to improve on this natural capacity by feeding the body "liquid protein" or any other such nostrum?

An additional refinement of the system for digesting and absorbing protein gives a further reason for not tampering with it. The amino acid pumps are not specific for individual amino acids but for groups of them. For example, there is one pump for the basic amino acids and another for the neutral ones. Each group of amino acids with similar structures shares a carrier. This means that competition can occur: The amino acids within a group can interfere with each other's absorption.

For structures of these groups of amino acids, see Appendix C.

Normally, no problems arise with this arrangement. Food proteins deliver balanced assortments of amino acids to the GI tract, digestion occurs slowly, fragments are delivered in leisurely fashion to the microvilli, and the final steps of digestion-absorption occur without much mutual interference.

If, however, a person takes pure amino acids rather than protein, the competition for carriers is more severe and some amino acids are lost. If the person still more foolishly presumes to decide that she needs certain specific amino acids and takes an overdose of one, she may well precipitate a deficiency of the others that share its carrier. If the lost amino acids are essential ones, the net effect will be to reduce her total supply of usable protein.

Essential amino acids: see p. 104.

[3]A. A. Albanese and L. A. Orto, The proteins and amino acids, in *Modern Nutrition in Health and Disease*, 5th ed., eds. R. S. Goodhart and M. E. Shils (Philadelphia: Lea and Febiger, 1973), p. 37.

This is not to say that some food proteins can't be improved by amino acid supplementation. A plant protein of very poor quality may be better utilized by the body if the limiting amino acid(s) are added to it. In this instance, adding amino acids provides a balance closer to what the body needs. This theory has been scientifically tested and confirmed—for example, in growth experiments on children.[4]

"Very well, then, it is best to eat food proteins rather than artificial amino acid mixtures. But surely, if you ask the GI tract to perform all the fancy maneuvers of digesting and absorbing protein, it would be best not to ask it to handle other nutrients at the same time. Surely there is a limit to how much those little cells can do at once." (This is logic speaking.)

On the contrary, there seems to be no interference—other than the specific kind of competition just mentioned—between the absorption and utilization of one kind of nutrient and that of another. In fact they often seem to enhance each other. For example, sugars taken at the same time as protein (within four hours) seem to promote better retention of the protein.[5] The sugars may slow the digestive process so that it is more complete, or they may provide precursors for some nonessential amino acids so that whole proteins can be produced more readily and retained in the body. Whatever the mechanism, the facts support the practice of taking mixed meals composed of a wide variety of foods to supply nutrients together so that they can act cooperatively wherever possible. There is no basis in any known facts about the digestive system for thinking that combining foods (for example, fruit and meat) in a meal taxes the ability of the GI tract to handle them. More likely, the combination enhances its most efficient functioning.

Not only is there a beneficial interaction between the energy nutrients in these two foods (protein in meat and carbohydrate in fruit); there are others that have to do with the vitamins and minerals. For example, the vitamin C in one food enhances the absorption of the iron in another food. This phenomenon and many others like it are described in Part Two.

A FLAG SIGN OF A SPURIOUS CLAIM
IS THE IMPLICATION THAT:

We can second-guess the body and make its work easier.

[4]Albanese and Orto, 1973, p. 51.
[5]Albanese and Orto, 1973, p. 57.

The preceding discussion has illuminated some aspects of the absorption of carbohydrate and protein but has said nothing about lipids. The absorption of lipids differs in that pumps are not involved. Cell membranes dissolve lipids easily because they are made largely of lipid themselves. After the digestion of triglycerides to monoglycerides or to glycerol and fatty acids, for example, they simply diffuse across the cell membrane. The cell retains them by reassembling them.

As you can see, the cells of the intestinal tract wall are beautifully designed to perform their functions. A further refinement of the system is that the cells of successive portions of the tract are specialized for different absorptive functions. The nutrients that are ready for absorption early are absorbed near the top of the tract; those that take longer to be digested are absorbed farther down. Thus the top portion of the duodenum is specialized for the absorption of calcium and several B vitamins, such as thiamin and riboflavin; the jejunum accomplishes most of the absorption of triglycerides; and vitamin B_{12}, which requires extensive preparation, is absorbed at the end of the ileum. The rate at which these nutrients travel is finely adjusted to maximize their availability to the appropriate absorptive segment of the tract when they are ready. The lowly "gut" turns out to be one of the most elegantly designed organ systems in your body.

Vitamin B_{12} is first attached to a special carrier in the stomach. For further details about the absorption of vitamins and minerals, see Part Two.

Release of Absorbed Nutrients

Once inside the intestinal cells, the products of digestion must be released for transport to the rest of the body. The water-soluble nutrients—monosaccharides (from carbohydrate), amino acids (from protein), and small lipid components such as short-chain fatty acids and glycerol—are released directly into the bloodstream. The water-soluble vitamins and minerals also follow this route.

```
WATER-SOLUBLE NUTRIENTS

Carbohydrates
    monosaccharides ───────────────────────────►blood

Lipids
    glycerol
    medium- and short-chain fatty acids ───────►blood

Proteins
    amino acids────────────────────────────────►blood
Vitamins
    B vitamins ┐
               ├───────────────────────────────►blood
    vitamin C ┘
Minerals ──────────────────────────────────────►blood
```

Things get into cells in several ways:

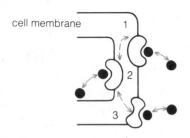

cell membrane

water ← water

water →

small lipids

Diffusion. Some substances cross membranes freely. Water is an example. The concentration of water tends to equalize on the two sides of a membrane: as long as it is higher outside the cell, it flows in; if it is higher inside the cell, it flows out. The cell cannot regulate the entrance and exit of water directly but can control it indirectly by concentrating some other substance to which water is attracted, such as protein or sodium. Thus the cell can pump in sodium, and water will follow passively. This is the way the cells of the wall of the large intestine act to retrieve water for the body. Since nearly all the sodium is taken into these cells before waste is excreted, nearly all the water is absorbed too. Small lipids also cross cell membranes by diffusion.

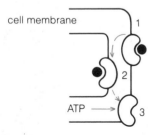

cell membrane   1

2

3

Facilitated diffusion. Other compounds cannot cross the membranes of the intestinal wall cells unless there is a specific carrier or facilitator in the membrane. The carrier may shuttle back and forth from one side of the membrane to the other, carrying its passengers either way, or it may affect the permeability of the membrane in such a way that the compound is admitted. Insulin probably works the latter way to facilitate the entrance of glucose into liver and other cells. The end result is the same as for diffusion: Equal concentrations are reached on both sides. By providing carriers only for the desired compounds, the cell effectively bars all others (except those to which it is freely permeable). Facilitated diffusion is also termed carrier-mediated diffusion or passive transport.

1. Carrier loads particle on outside of cell. 2. Carrier releases particle on inside of cell.   3. Or the reverse.

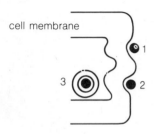

cell membrane   1

2

ATP →   3

Active transport. For compounds that must be absorbed actively, the two types of diffusion systems mentioned above will not suffice. The best a cell can do using only diffusion is to take up a compound until the concentration inside the cell is equal to that outside. An effective means of concentrating a substance inside the cell is to pump it in, consuming energy in the process. The monosaccharides, amino acids, and other nutrients are absorbed by intestinal wall cells in this manner.

1. Carrier loads particle on outside of cell. 2. Carrier releases particle on inside of cell. 3. Carrier returns to outside to pick up another, powered by the energy carrier, ATP (see p. 252).

cell membrane

3   1

2

Pinocytosis. This process involves a large area of the cell membrane, which actively engulfs whole particles and "swallows" them into the cell. Although it is not of great importance in the GI tract, this process is one way that the white blood cells are able to engulf invading viruses and bacteria in order to dispose of them.

1. Particle touches cell membrane. 2. Membrane wraps around particle. 3. Portion of membrane surrounding particle separates into cell.

The selective cell membranes.

As for the larger lipids and the fat-soluble vitamins, access directly into the bloodstream is impossible. They are apparently too insoluble and cumbersome to cross the walls of the blood vessels. Monoglycerides and long-chain fatty acids are assembled into larger molecules— triglycerides—the form in which the cells can best handle them. These and the other large lipids, cholesterol and the phospholipids, are wrapped in protein by a special arrangement (to be described beginning on p. 200) and are released into the lymphatic system. They can then "squish" through the lymph spaces until they move to a point of entry into the bloodstream near the heart.

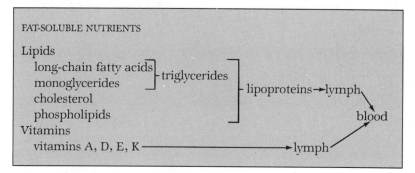

FAT-SOLUBLE NUTRIENTS

Lipids
    long-chain fatty acids
    monoglycerides ⎤ triglycerides
    cholesterol ⎦ → lipoproteins → lymph
    phospholipids → blood
Vitamins
    vitamins A, D, E, K —————————→ lymph

Anatomy of the Circulatory Systems

Once a nutrient has entered the bloodstream or the lymph circulatory system, it may be transported to any part of the body and thus become available to all the body cells, from the tips of the toes to the roots of the hair. To understand the way nutrients arrive at the toes or the hair roots, you must understand the anatomy of the circulatory systems.

The Vascular System The vascular or blood circulatory system is a closed system of vessels through which blood flows continuously in a figure eight, with the heart serving as a pump at the crossover point. The system is diagramed in Figure 2. As the blood circulates through this system it picks up and delivers materials as needed.

All the body tissues derive oxygen and nutrients from the blood and deposit carbon dioxide and other wastes into it. The lungs are the place for exchange of carbon dioxide (which leaves the blood to be breathed out) and oxygen (which enters the blood to be delivered to all cells). The digestive system is the place for nutrients to be picked up. The kidneys are the place where wastes other than carbon dioxide are filtered out of the blood to be excreted in the urine. There is something special about the routing of the blood past the digestive system that requires a little explanation.

Blood leaving the right side of the heart circulates by way of arteries into the lung capillaries and then back through veins to the left side of

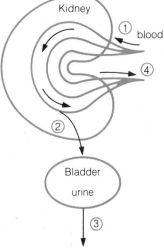

1. Blood enters the kidney by way of the arteries.
2. Waste is removed and sent as urine to the bladder.
3. Urine is periodically eliminated.
4. Cleansed blood is returned to the general circulation.

artery: a vessel carrying blood away from the heart.

capillary (CAP-ill-ary): a small vessel that branches from an artery. Capillaries connect arteries to veins. Exchange of blood and tissue components takes place across capillary walls.

vein: a vessel carrying blood back to the heart.

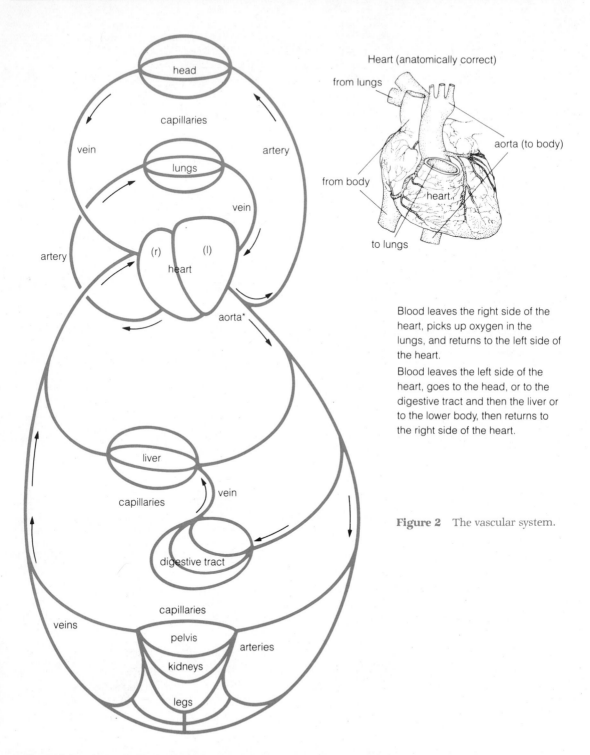

Heart (anatomically correct)

from lungs

aorta (to body)

from body

heart

to lungs

Blood leaves the right side of the heart, picks up oxygen in the lungs, and returns to the left side of the heart.

Blood leaves the left side of the heart, goes to the head, or to the digestive tract and then the liver or to the lower body, then returns to the right side of the heart.

Figure 2   The vascular system.

*The aorta is the main artery that launches blood on its course through the body. The picture is not anatomically correct but is drawn this way for clarity. The aorta arises behind the left side of the heart and arcs upward, then divides.

the heart. The left side of the heart then pumps the blood out through arteries to all systems of the body. The blood circulates in the capillaries and then collects into veins, which return the blood again to the right side of the heart (see Figure 2). In all cases but one, blood leaving the heart travels this simple route:

Heart → arteries → capillaries → veins → heart

Only in the case of the digestive system does the blood flow twice through a capillary bed before returning to the heart. Surrounding and supporting the stomach and intestines is the strong, flexible mesenteric membrane. A major artery from the heart leads into this membrane and branches into smaller arteries and then into tiny capillaries, which penetrate every villus of the intestine. These capillaries rejoin to form veins, which return to the mesenteric membrane and merge into a single large vein, the portal vein. This vein connects directly to the liver, where it again branches into capillaries. Thus all the blood leaving the digestive system must go through a second capillary bed in the liver:

Heart → arteries → capillaries (in intestines) → vein → capillaries (in liver) → veins → heart

An anatomist studying this system knows there must be a reason for it. He concludes that the liver is placed in the circulation at this point in order to have the first chance at the materials absorbed from the GI tract. In fact the liver has many jobs to do preparing the absorbed nutrients for use by the body. It is the body's major metabolic organ.

You might guess that in addition the liver may stand as a gatekeeper to waylay intruders that might otherwise harm the heart. Perhaps this is why, when people ingest poisons that succeed in passing the first barrier (the intestinal cells) and enter the blood, it is the liver that suffers the damage—from hepatitis virus, from drugs such as barbiturates, from alcohol, from poisons such as DDT, from toxic metals such as mercury. Perhaps, in fact, you have been undervaluing your liver, not knowing what quiet and heroic tasks it performs for you. (Highlight 9 focuses on the liver, in case you are interested in more information about this noble organ.)

The Lymphatic System   The lymphatic system is an open system that can be pictured simply as being similar to the spaces in a sponge. If you wet a sponge, its spaces fill with water. If you squeeze it, you can force the water from one end of the sponge to the other. Between the cells of the body there are spaces similar to those in the sponge; the fluid circulating in them is the lymph. This fluid is almost identical to the fluid of the blood except that it contains no red blood cells, because they cannot escape through the blood vessel walls. The spaces between the cells are somewhat imprecisely called lymphatic "vessels."

The lymphatic system has no pump; like the water in a sponge, lymph "squishes" from one portion of the body to another as muscles contract and create pressure here and there. Ultimately much of the

mesenteric (mez-en-TERR-ic) **membrane,** or **mesentery** (MEZ-en-terr-ee): the strong, flexible membrane that surrounds and supports the abdominal organs.

The vein that collects blood from the mesentery and conducts it to capillaries in the liver is the **portal vein.**

portal = gateway

The vein that collects blood from the liver capillaries and returns it to the heart is the **hepatic vein.**

hepat = liver

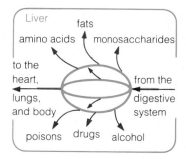

The liver removes many materials from the blood.

thoracic (thor-ASS-ic) **duct:** a duct of the lymphatic system that collects lymph that has circulated to the upper portion of the body. The **subclavian vein** connects this duct with the right upper chamber of the heart, providing a passageway by which lymph can be returned to the vascular system.

lipoprotein (lip-oh-PRO-tee-in): a complex of lipids with proteins. The lipids apparently orient with their hydrophobic ends in; the proteins associate with the outside of the cluster, rendering the entire complex water-soluble.

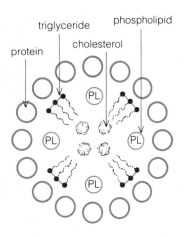

A lipoprotein.

chylomicron (kye-lo-MY-cron): the lipoprotein formed in intestinal wall cells following digestion and absorption of fat. Released from these cells, chylomicrons transport ingested fats to liver cells. The liver cells dismantle the chylomicrons and construct other lipoproteins for further transport.

lymph collects in a large duct behind the heart called the thoracic duct. This duct terminates in a vein that conducts the lymph into the heart. Thus materials from the GI tract that enter lymphatic vessels in the villi ultimately enter the blood circulatory system and then circulate through arteries, capillaries, and veins like the other nutrients. In other words, nutrients that are first absorbed into lymph soon get into the blood.

Transport of Lipids: A Special Arrangement

Once inside the body, the nutrients can travel freely to any destination and can be taken into cells and used as needed. What becomes of them is the subject of Chapter 7. Before leaving the transport system, however, you might be interested in looking more closely at the forms in which lipids travel.

Within the circulatory systems, lipids always travel from place to place wrapped in protein coats—that is, as lipoproteins. Lipoproteins are very much in the news these days. In fact, when the doctor measures a person's blood lipid profile, she is interested not only in the types of fat she finds (triglycerides and cholesterol) but also in the types of protein coats they are wrapped in. Newly absorbed lipids leaving the intestinal cells are mostly packaged in the lipoproteins known as chylomicrons. Lipids that have been processed or made in the liver are released in lipoproteins known as VLDL and LDL. Lipids returning to the liver from other parts of the body are packaged in lipoproteins known as HDL. The distinction of interest, because it has implications for the health of the heart and blood vessels, is the distinction between HDL and the other lipoproteins. Raised HDL concentrations are associated with a low risk of heart attack.[6]

A brief look at each of these types of particles will help you to interpret the news about them as new findings continue to emerge—and to understand the significance of tests the doctor may run to determine your own lipid profile. (An artist's conception of what they look like appears at the start of this chapter.)

Chylomicrons: From the Intestinal Cells The lipids you eat are in the form of water-insoluble triglycerides, cholesterol, and phospholipids, with the triglycerides predominating (composing about 95 percent of dietary fat). Both of the body's transport systems—lymph and blood—are watery fluids. Clearly, if the lipids were dumped "as is" into the bloodstream, they would clump together to form globs of fat that would clog the arteries. You are familiar with this effect if you have ever carelessly dumped greasy foods down the kitchen sink: The drain became clogged and the grease had to be removed, at great expense to you. The body is smarter with lipids than you may be with your kitchen

[6]High blood lipid levels can be good or bad—depending on the lipid, *Journal of the American Medical Association* 237 (1977):1066-1070.

grease. Although arteries sometimes clog (see this chapter's Highlight), it is not because pure, unadulterated grease ever travels through them.

An intestinal cell allows a cluster of triglycerides to form, then wraps the cluster with a protein coat to form a chylomicron. The fat-loving tails of the fatty acids position themselves as far away from the water as they can get, some phospholipids and cholesterol arrange themselves nearby, and the small skin of protein forms around the entire aggregate. In this ingenious configuration, the fat can be released from the intestinal cell and can travel through the lymph to the blood.

The protein of the chylomicrons is recognized by the liver cells, which make it their business to remove these lipoproteins from the blood, to dismantle them, and to custom-design new lipids for use by other body cells. Chylomicrons are large, fluffy particles that float at the top of a blood sample in a test tube. This floating layer of fat does not appear if blood is drawn 14 hours after a meal, for in this period of time the liver has completely disposed of all of it.

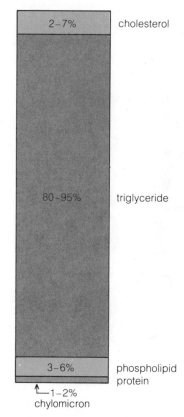

From the intestine:

The density of these particles is very, very low because they contain so little protein and so much triglyceride. You can see how the laboratory report that a person has "high blood triglycerides" might easily reflect a high concentration of chylomicrons in his blood.

VLDL: very low density lipoprotein. This type of lipoprotein is made by liver cells (and to some extent by intestinal cells[7]). An alternative name is "pre-beta" lipoprotein.

LDL: low-density lipoprotein. This type of lipoprotein may be made by liver cells or derived from VLDL as cells remove triglycerides from them.[8] An alternative name is "beta" lipoprotein.

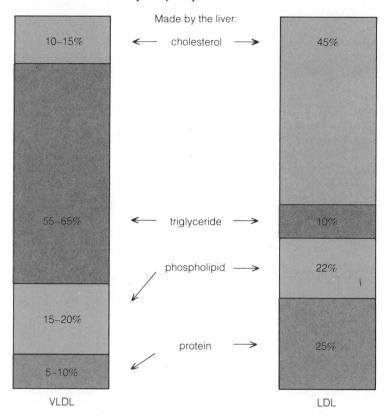

Compare these particles with the chylomicrons and HDL. Note that "high blood cholesterol" might easily reflect a high LDL concentration.

[7]H. B. Brown and M. Farrand, What a dietitian should know about hyperlipidemia, *Journal of the American Dietetic Association* 63 (1973): 169-170.

[8]An intermediate form, IDL, is now recognized by some authorities. A. K. Khachadurian, guest editor, Hyperlipoproteinemia, *Dietetic Currents, Ross Timesaver* 4 (July/August 1977).

Returned to the liver:

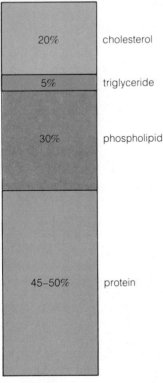

HDL

These particles are denser than the others because they contain such a high percentage of protein.

HDL: high-density lipoprotein. These lipoproteins seem to transport lipids back to the liver from peripheral cells. An alternative name is "alpha" lipoprotein.

VLDL and LDL: From the Liver The liver cells rearrange most of the triglycerides from the chylomicrons. They break the fatty acids down to fragments and use them to make other fatty acids, cholesterol, and other compounds. (At the same time, if they are metabolizing carbohydrates, they may be making lipids from some of these.) Ultimately, some of the lipids they manufacture will need to be used or stored in other parts of the body. To send them there, the liver once again wraps them in proteins, this time as VLDL and LDL.

The VLDL and LDL made by the liver contain relatively more cholesterol and phospholipid than the chylomicrons do. Released from the liver into the blood, they circulate throughout the body, making their fat available to all the body cells—muscle, including the heart muscle, adipose tissue, the mammary glands, and others. The body cells can select fat from these particles to build new membranes, to make hormones or other compounds, or to store for later use. Both VLDL and LDL are much smaller and denser than the chylomicrons, but the VLDL are still large enough to give the blood a milky appearance if there are enough of them.

HDL: From the Body Cells When energy is in short supply, the cells may have only their own stored fat to rely on. At such a time they mobilize fat; that is, they take it out of storage. Most of the triglycerides are used for energy, and the cells return the unused fat—mostly cholesterol and phospholipid—to the blood. The packages in which unused fats are returned are the HDL, and it is believed that these are returned to the liver for recycling or disposal.

Atherosclerosis and the Lipoproteins The lipoproteins have become headline news in recent years, as researchers have discovered that they may be an important clue to the risks of heart and artery disease. In the early years, scientists spoke of "hyperlipidemia"—too much lipid in the blood. Now they refer to "hyperlipoproteinemia," recognizing the carrier in which the lipid appears.

The formation of plaques in the artery walls is described in Chapter 2. The cholesterol deposited in these plaques is available to them from the lipoproteins that carry it in the bloodstream. Those that carry the most cholesterol are the LDL, and the LDL correlate most closely with atherosclerosis.[9] LDL have an affinity for the artery walls, perhaps because of the character of their protein.[10] Generally speaking, *high serum cholesterol* reflects a high LDL concentration.

But the HDL also carry cholesterol, and raised HDL concentrations represent lower total body cholesterol, a lower risk of developing atherosclerosis, and a lower risk of heart attack. It is clearly not useful

[9]Interdisciplinary Cluster on Nutrition, President's Biomedical Research Panel, Assessment of the state of nutrition science, part 2, *Nutrition Today*, January/February 1977, pp. 24-27.

[10]D. M. Small, Cellular mechanisms for lipid deposition in atherosclerosis (first of two parts), *New England Journal of Medicine* 297 (1977):873-877.

simply to measure the amount of cholesterol in the blood; it is necessary to know whether it is LDL or HDL cholesterol.

Some people have abnormal lipid profiles (high in chylomicrons, VLDL, or LDL) for genetic reasons, but apparently some may have them due to such poor health habits as overeating, overconsumption of fat, or underactivity. To normalize their blood lipid profiles, such people may need to eat less fat and lose weight. Activities that raise HDL concentrations—such as frequent, intensive, and sustained exercise—may help to reverse degenerative disease processes such as atherosclerosis. (For more about HDL and atherosclerosis, see Highlight 6.)

Excretion of Cholesterol with Fiber   Knowing how the digestive and circulatory systems are arranged, you can better appreciate the relationship of dietary fiber to the body's cholesterol content. Cholesterol is used by the liver largely to manufacture bile. The bile collects in the gallbladder and stays there until fat arrives in the intestine; then the bile is squirted into the intestine to emulsify the fat.

When emulsified fat is absorbed, some of the bile accompanies it into the intestinal cells. The cells can't use this bile, and they excrete some of it back into the GI tract and return the rest to the bloodstream, where it travels by way of the portal vein back to the liver. There it may either be degraded or returned once again to the gallbladder for further recycling to the intestine.

The bile that is left in the intestine travels down the GI tract with the waste materials and is excreted from the body with them. Certain kinds of fiber have an affinity for bile, and when the diet is rich in those fibers, more bile is excreted. This effectively reduces the total body cholesterol content and is one reason for interest in dietary fiber as a possible means of retarding the development of atherosclerosis.

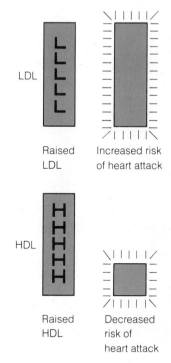

LDL

Raised
LDL

Increased risk
of heart attack

HDL

Raised
HDL

Decreased
risk of
heart attack

The circulation of bile from the liver to the gallbladder to the intestine and back to the liver is known as the **enterohepatic circulation** of bile.

enteron = intestines

People who have learned that "fiber lowers blood cholesterol" have not learned quite enough to take advantage of this knowledge. If you accept oversimplified statements like this one, you may find yourself on a bandwagon like the fiber fad. Faddists have for some years been buying purified fiber to sprinkle into their foods, in the hope of improving their health. But it happens that the purified fiber they buy is most often wheat bran, the only type known to have no such effect.[11] (Bran is, however, an excellent stimulator of peristalsis and promotes the maintenance of healthy muscle tone in the GI tract.) Fibers that do lower blood cholesterol levels include pectin (the fiber of apples and other fruits) and hemicellulose (a fiber found in cereal

[11]A. M. Connell, C. L. Smith, and M. Somsel, Absence of effect of bran on blood-lipids, *Lancet* I (March 1975), pp. 496-497.

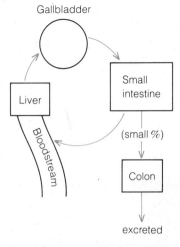

Gallbladder

Small intestine

Liver

Bloodstream

(small %)

Colon

excreted

Enterohepatic circulation of bile.

grains). Most effective is an as-yet-unidentified fiber found in legumes such as chickpeas.[12]

Once again, the lesson seems to be that foods, not purified nutrients or other food components, are mostly likely to offer the greatest benefits to those who seek good health—and not so much any particular foods as a variety of foods. You may recall that other nutrition knowledge points in the same direction (see pp. 4, 68, 163).

Practical Applications

We have described the anatomy of the digestive tract on several levels: the sequence of digestive organs, the structures of the villi and of the cells that compose them, and the selective machinery of the cell membranes. The intricate architecture of the GI tract makes it sensitive and responsive to conditions in its environment. Knowing what the optimal conditions are will help you to promote the best functioning of your system.

One indispensable condition is good health of the digestive tract itself. This health is affected by such factors of lifestyle as sleep, exercise, and state of mind. Adequate sleep allows for repair, maintenance of tissue, and removal of wastes that might impair efficient functioning. Exercise promotes healthy muscle tone. As for mental state: If you have read Highlight 5, you know that stress profoundly affects digestion and absorption. In a person under stress digestive secretions are reduced and the blood is routed to the skeletal muscles more than to the digestive tract, so that efficient absorption of nutrients is impaired. To digest and absorb food best, you should be relaxed and tranquil at mealtimes.

Another factor is the kind of diet you eat. Three characteristics of the diet promote optimal absorption of nutrients: balance, variety, and adequacy. Balance means having neither too much nor too little of any dietary component. For example, some fat is needed to stimulate the release of bile from the gallbladder, not only for its own emulsification but also to help absorb the fat-soluble vitamins. Fat also slows down intestinal motility, permitting time for some of the slower nutrients to be absorbed. Too much fat, however, can form an insoluble, soapy scum with calcium and so rob the body of this mineral. A well-planned meal presents you with perhaps 20 to 30 percent of its kcalories as fat.

Another example of diet balance is already familiar to you: Fiber stimulates intestinal motility. With too little fiber the intestines are

[12]E. M. N. Hamilton and E. N. Whitney, Controversy 5: Cholesterol, in *Nutrition: Concepts and Controversies* (St. Paul: West, 1979), pp. 109-114.

likely to be sluggish; they may then fail to mix their contents or fail to bring materials into contact with the sites on the walls where they can be absorbed. Too much fiber, however, causes the contents of the intestines to move so fast through the tract that they are not in contact with the walls long enough to be absorbed. A well-planned meal delivers a moderate amount of fiber along with a generous assortment of nutrients.

Variety is important for many reasons but partly because a peculiar interaction takes place between some food constituents and certain nutrients. Compounds known as binders combine chemically with certain nutrients so that the nutrients cannot be absorbed. For example, phytic acid and oxalic acid combine with iron and calcium to prevent their absorption. Phytic acid is found in oatmeal and other whole-grain cereals, and oxalic acid in rhubarb and spinach, rendering some of the calcium and iron in these foods "unavailable." This does not mean that oatmeal or spinach is an undesirable food; both are rightly praised for their nutrient contributions. But it does mean that a person who consumes oatmeal as his only grain food or spinach as his only dark-green vegetable may be deriving less calcium and iron from his diet than he would if he were to vary his choices.

As for adequacy—in a sense this entire book is about dietary adequacy. But here, at the end of this chapter, is a good place to underline the interdependence of the nutrients, which makes it necessary to supply them all in the amounts needed in order to achieve optimum health. It could almost be said that every nutrient depends on every other. Whimsically, we might attempt to sum up this notion in one overlong, oversimplified sentence. (Don't take this seriously; it is not for memorizing. Details we think you should learn are presented more systematically.) The sentence shows the needed nutrients in capital letters and those they interact with in italics.

You need PROTEIN to attract *water* into cells; to provide pumps and diffusion-mediators for *amino acids*, *monosaccharides*, *minerals*, and the *water-soluble vitamins*; to provide carriers for *iron*, the *lipids*, and the *fat-soluble vitamins*; and to provide hormone regulators for many of these; you need LIPID to stimulate the release of bile to emulsify *lipids* and *fat-soluble vitamins* and to slow down intestinal motility to allow time for absorption of certain *minerals*; you need CARBOHYDRATE as *glucose* to provide energy for the active transport of many nutrients into cells; as *lactose* to help calcium absorption (after being converted to an acid by bacteria in the intestines) and as *cellulose (fiber)* to stimulate the mixing and moving-along of *all* the nutrients; you need VITAMIN D for *calcium* absorption, VITAMIN C to help provide the acid environment needed for absorption of *iron* and *calcium*, and VITAMIN B_6 to help the

One long sentence

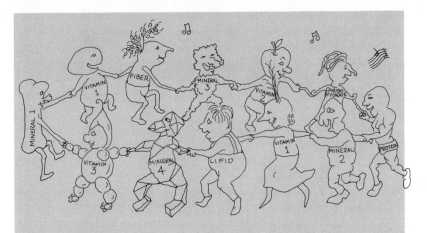

transport systems for *amino acids*; you need MINERALS such as *chlorine*, to make the hydrochloric acid that provides the stomach acidity that facilitates the digestion of *protein* and the absorption of *iron* and *calcium*; *sodium*, to provide the sodium bicarbonate secreted by the pancreas to neutralize stomach acid when it reaches the duodenum, to help with the withdrawal of *water* into cells, and to assist the transport system for *glucose*; and *phosphorus*, to assist *vitamin B₆*, which in turn assists the transport systems for *amino acids*; and you need WATER to suspend *all* of the above nutrients in a finely divided state so that they are accessible to the absorptive machinery.

You need not eat all of these nutrients at the same time in every meal, but they all work together and are all present in the cells of a healthy digestive tract. The point of all of this must be abundantly clear: To maintain health and promote the functions of the GI tract, adequacy, balance, and variety should be features of every day's menus.

Summing Up

Chapter 5 ended at the point where a hamburger or a piece of chocolate cake had been completely digested and the nutrients were ready for absorption. This chapter sums up the next part of the story. From carbohydrates, the monosaccharides—glucose, fructose, and galactose—are absorbed mostly from the small intestinal villi into the capillaries of the mesenteric membrane; the capillaries converge into veins, which in turn converge into the single large portal vein. The next stop is the liver.

From lipids, the medium- and short-chain fatty acids and glycerol follow the same route. The long-chain fatty acids and monoglycerides are reassembled into triglycerides and packaged, together with cholesterol and phospholipids, in protein to form chylomicrons, which leave the intestinal cells by way of the lymphatic system. These lipoproteins later join the general circulation through a vein from the lymphatic system into the heart, and ultimately most of them are cleared by the liver.

From proteins, the amino acids follow the same route as the monosaccharides, traveling through the mesenteric capillaries and veins and finally through the portal vein to the liver. The water-soluble B vitamins, vitamin C, and the minerals accompany the monosaccharides and amino acids; the fat-soluble vitamins (A, D, E, and K) are attached to carriers and follow the path of the larger fats. Some water moves with all of these nutrients; the water that remains is retrieved in the large intestine. Undigested fiber remains in the GI tract until it is excreted from the body.

The lipoproteins made in intestinal cells are mostly chylomicrons, and these are composed predominantly of triglycerides. These travel by way of the lymph and blood to the liver, which clears them and makes other lipoproteins—the VLDL and LDL. The VLDL and LDL transport lipids from the liver to the peripheral cells. The LDL may also deposit cholesterol in arterial plaques, contributing to atherosclerosis. Fats returning to the liver for dismantling and disposal are packaged in HDL; a raised HDL level correlates with a reduced risk of atherosclerosis.

In the process of absorption many compounds are interdependent. The absorption of many nutrients depends on protein; the absorption of many others, on minerals and vitamins. The whole picture is one of complex interrelationships, suggesting that for optimal functioning a mixture of nutrients should be taken together at each meal.

Atherosclerosis

The single most important approach to alleviating almost any disease is the reduction of stress. . . . Better still is the elimination of constant worry about your heart, plus the restoration of relaxation and pleasure to your mealtimes. Enjoy food rather than fear it.
EDWARD R. PINCKNEY AND
CATHEY PINCKNEY

As the eighth decade of the twentieth century was being ushered in, television commentators and newspaper reporters exulted over humanity's accomplishments during this remarkable century. They reminded us that the world had experienced its last case of smallpox, that we had conquered polio, that we could now have a new heart planted in us when the old one wore out. They even prophesied that it would soon be possible to wipe out starvation. However, the news media were surprisingly quiet about one event that had occurred in the last half of the 1970s: The rate of deaths from heart disease had declined. Until then, deaths from heart disease had been increasing so rapidly that the headline writers had been calling it an epidemic. But when statistics showed a downturn, the press became almost silent on the subject. It was as if they were saying, "Let's not publicize this good thing; our rejoicing may make it vanish."

The scientific-medical community was also quiet, but probably not because of a superstitious belief. Instead, scientists were arguing about the cause of the downturn. Was it due to changes in diet or to less cigarette smoking or to increased jogging? There were even some who showed that the downturn was not specific for heart disease but

reflected a decline in mortality from all causes.

This Highlight will pursue this controversy and also give some historical perspective so that you can understand the evolution of diet recommendations and be able to incorporate newer data as it unfolds. The focus is on atherosclerosis, which is the underlying cause of much heart disease and is central to the diet-heart argument.

The Formation of Plaques Atherosclerosis is characterized by soft lipid plaque, which accumulates in the intimal layer of the artery wall. Atherosclerosis has been known since the nineteenth century and was once thought to be an inevitable result of the aging process. However, autopsies performed on young U.S. soldiers during the Vietnam War revealed that the condition

was already in an advanced stage even in the 18-year-olds.[1] This finding gave new impetus to research into the causes of plaques and into ways that their progress could be halted.

The arteries carry blood away from the heart, and veins return blood to the heart. The arteries, then, are more responsive than veins to the beat of the heart as it pushes blood outward. They must expand as a large volume of blood rushes by and then contract so that a steady blood pressure is maintained. The space in the artery occupied by the blood is called the lumen. The inner surface of the artery, which touches the blood, contains a lining of cells that keeps the blood within the artery but allows the passage of necessary substances out into the surrounding tissues.

The artery wall has three layers—the intima, media, and adventitia. The composition of the intima varies with the type of artery and the age and sex of the person. For example, males have thicker intimas than females in the coronary arteries. (Coronary arteries branch off from the main artery where it leaves the heart and spread over the outside of the heart in a network, feeding the heart mus-

[1] J. E. Corey, Dietary factors and atherosclerosis prevention should begin early, *Journal of School Health* 44 (1974):511-513.

H	E	A	R	T

Everyone plays the game of health whether he wants to or not. What is your score? Add up the numbers in each category that most nearly describe you.*

	1	2	3	4	6
Heredity	No known history of heart disease	One relative with heart disease over 60 years	Two relatives with heart disease over 60 years	One relative with heart disease under 60 years	Two relatives with heart disease under 60 years
Exercise	**1** Intensive exercise, work, and recreation	**2** Moderate exercise, work, and recreation	**3** Sedentary work and intensive recreational exercise	**5** Sedentary work and moderate recreational exercise	**6** Sedentary work and light recreational exercise
Age	**1** 10-20	**2** 21-30	**3** 31-40	**4** 41-50	**6** 51-65
Lbs.	**0** More than 5 lbs below standard weight	**1** ± 5 lbs standard weight	**2** 6-20 lbs overweight	**4** 21-35 lbs overweight	**6** 36-50 lbs overweight
Tobacco	**0** Nonuser	**1** Cigar or pipe	**2** 10 cigarettes or fewer per day	**4** 20 cigarettes or more per day	**6** 30 cigarettes or more per day
Habits of eating fat	**1** 0% No animal or solid fats	**2** 10% Very little animal or solid fats	**3** 20% Little animal or solid fats	**4** 30% Much animal or solid fats	**5** 40% Very much animal or solid fats

Your risk of heart attack:

4-9	Very remote	16-20 Average	26-30 Dangerous
10-15	Below average	21-25 Moderate	31-35 Urgent danger—reduce score

Other conditions—such as stress, high blood pressure, and increased blood cholesterol—detract from heart health and should be evaluated by your physician.

*Courtesy of Loma Linda University

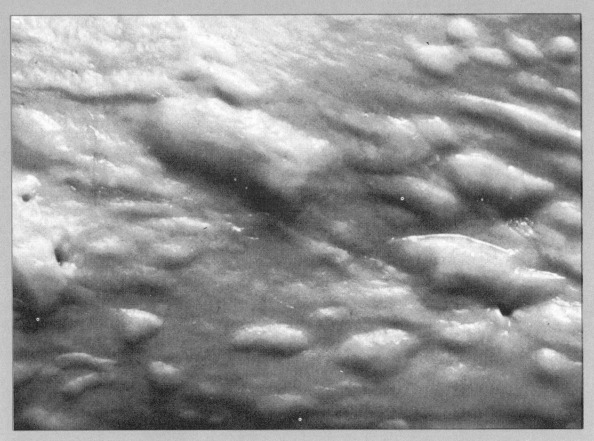

Atherosclerotic inner surface of a human artery that has been slit open—magnification 2.5X. The lumps are the plaques.

From *Scientific American* 236(1977):75. Reprinted by permission of Scientific American Inc.

cle.) The intima thickens with age and is the layer of the artery wall most affected by atherosclerosis. The media, composed of smooth-muscle cells, is an artery's principal supporting structure. The adventitia holds the capillaries that nourish the arteries and anchors the arteries in place.

As an atherosclerotic plaque invades the intima and enlarges, it narrows the lumen, thus increasing the pressure of the blood against the wall. (This consequence can be likened to the increased water pressure in a garden hose that has been pinched.) The increased pressure can damage the artery wall as well as all the organs of the body. In addition, the plaque causes the wall to lose its elasticity, so that it cannot respond to the beat of the heart by enlarging. This further raises the blood pressure.

If the plaque narrows the lumen enough, it can completely shut off the supply of blood. The result is the death of all tissues depending on that artery for nourishment and oxygen. However, in an advanced stage like this, it is more likely that a clot will form, plugging the artery. This event is known as a thrombosis.

The reason an atherosclerotic plaque begins is obscure, although there are a number of theories.[2] There seems to be general agreement that some type of injury to the lining of the artery allows the invasion of smooth-muscle cells, which then proliferate. For some reason these cells are unable to reach a balance between cholesterol coming into the cell and that being carried away. As a consequence, more and more free cholesterol accumulates at the place of the injury, and a plaque is born.

[2]D. M. Small, Cellular mechanisms for lipid deposition in atherosclerosis, part 2, *New England Journal of Medicine* 297 (1977):924-929; and E. P. Benditt, The origin of atherosclerosis, *Scientific American* 236 (1977):74-85.

Anatomy of an artery.

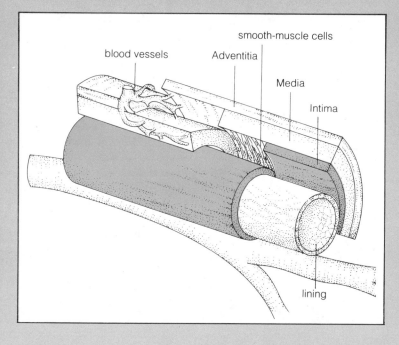

The Role of Cholesterol

In the early research on atherosclerosis, it was determined by chemical analysis that plaques are composed largely of lipid, particularly cholesterol. The conclusion was quickly drawn that cholesterol from food, and not the cholesterol made by the body, was the villain. Patients who had high levels of serum cholesterol or who had suffered heart attacks were advised to limit severely their intake of foods containing cholesterol. However, further research revealed that cholesterol from food is not the only source of serum cholesterol; the body synthesizes as much as 2,000 mg per day from any two-carbon fragments.

Food sources of two-carbon fragments are those containing nutrients that become the two-carbon compound acetyl CoA during metabolism. Thus glucose and amino acids, as well as fatty acids, contribute to the synthesis of cholesterol.

Saturated fats are excellent sources of two-carbon fragments, and it was soon shown that diets high in saturated fats would raise the serum cholesterol as much as 40 to 50 mg per 100 ml serum, whereas diets high in cholesterol would increase the serum cholesterol by only a few milligrams per 100 ml.[3] With this later knowledge, severe restrictions on foods containing cholesterol were eased, and it was recommended instead that total saturated fat in the diet be lowered.

As the search for dietary ways to lower serum cholesterol continued, a new idea was advanced: Polyunsaturated fatty acids seem to decrease serum cholesterol levels half as much per gram as saturated fatty acids raise these levels.[4] Thus diet recommendations began to shift from a mere restriction on saturated fats to a suggestion

[3]M. V. Krause and M. A. Hunscher, *Food, Nutrition and Diet Therapy* (Philadelphia: Saunders, 1972), p. 60

[4]A. Keys, J. Anderson, and F. Grande, Serum cholesterol response to dietary fat (a letter to the editor), *Lancet* I (1957):787.

to include polyunsaturated fats in their place.

In a joint policy statement of the American Medical Association (AMA) and the Food and Nutrition Board, it was stated that lowering serum cholesterol "can be achieved most practically by partial replacement of the dietary source of saturated fat with sources of unsaturated fat, especially those rich in polyunsaturated fatty acids, and by a reduction in the consumption of foods rich in cholesterol."[5]

This brief history of the evolution of dietary recommendations for lowering serum cholesterol has omitted much pertinent research and ignored the lively debate that accompanied each shift in diet emphasis. The policy statement just quoted is testimony to the fact that there was controversy. Whenever there is conflicting evidence, it is customary for an organization such as the AMA to form a committee whose job it is to sift through the evidence and to decide what is the fairest statement that can be made on the subject at that time. In

writing this Highlight, we have chosen to chronicle another more recent controversy and to ignore the conflict that surrounded this policy statement.

The idea that lowering total serum cholesterol might reduce the risk of heart disease came out of a study by Dawber and his associates, which has come to be known as the Framingham Study.[6] They found that men between the ages of 30 and 59 who had serum cholesterol levels below 200 mg per 100 ml of serum had half as many heart attacks as the total population. Men with serum cholesterol levels above 260 had almost twice as many heart attacks as the general population. This study provided the springboard for research into ways of lowering total serum cholesterol.

Diet: All Important, or Not Important?   The Framingham Study revealed that blood lipids are not the only factors related to heart disease. Other risk factors include high blood pressure, heavy cigarette smoking, obesity, and physical inactivity. It is interesting to note

that in the nineteenth century the causes of apoplexy, which we would class as a cerebrovascular disease, were listed as "corpulancy (obesity), a sedentary and luxurious mode of living, anxiety of mind, sex, and heredity."[7] Today we would have to add only cigarette smoking to this list (cigarettes had not been introduced at that time). Even in the nineteenth century, then, it was recognized that heart disease is multifactorial.

The war against atherosclerosis is being waged on a battleground littered with millions of numbers generated by study of thousands of human beings. Such a battle can be fought only with statistics and computers, not with paper-and-pencil calculations. When a number of factors operate to produce a human disease, it becomes nearly impossible to design a single study that will give clear-cut answers. In animal testing, all variables but one can be controlled, but the results are merely pointers and not valid for humans until they are tested in humans. In human testing on atherosclerosis, the interrelatedness of the variables forces reliance on sophisticated statistical and computer analyses. These analyses make it more

[5]Council on Foods and Nutrition, Diet and coronary heart disease, reprint from the *Journal of the American Medical Association* 222 (1972):1647.

[6]T. R. Dawber, F. E. Moore, and G. V. Mann, Coronary heart disease in the Framingham study, *American Journal of Public Health*, April 1957, pp. 4-23.

[7]R. A. Ahrens, Sucrose, hypertension, and heart disease: An historical perspective, *American Journal of Clinical Nutrition* 27 (1974):403-422.

difficult for you to judge the validity of what you read about atherosclerosis and add one more area for disagreement among the experts.

Such a disagreement took place between the covers of the *New England Journal of Medicine* in 1977 and 1978. Dr. George V. Mann of the Department of Biochemistry, Vanderbilt University, wrote an article titled "Diet-Heart: End of an Era."[8] Dr. Mann opened with the statement that "a generation of research on the diet-heart question has ended in disarray." He proceeded to back his thesis with data showing that all the work with diet had not lowered serum cholesterol or the coronary mortality rate. He chided the doctors: "A low fat, low cholesterol diet became as automatic in their treatment advice as a polite goodbye."

A flood of letters to the editor followed publication of this article. These letters and Dr. Mann's article make interesting reading, if only to show that doctors and scientists do not always write in dull, factual style. One critic said that Dr. Mann used a "distorted, dogmatic article to attack distortion and dogmatism."[9] Strong

rhetoric! Dr. Mann replied to those who disagreed with his data, "They want to argue and cite their bibliographies."[10] Good retort! Following are excerpts from the article and from some of the rebuttals.

"Diet-Heart: End of an Era"—Mann[11]

Diet-Heart Era: Premature Obituary?—Walker[12]

"The mortality trends since 1950 do not support the argument that the extensive dietary propaganda has had an effect on clinical events."—Mann[13]

The American Heart Association made its recommendations in 1964, not 1950. Since 65 percent of coronary deaths then occurred before patients reached any medical facility and few physicians recommended a change of diet for the others, it is not surprising that there was no decline in coronary mortality before 1964. There has been a steady decline since then.—Walker[14]

Vital statistics recently published in the Journal *and elsewhere have clearly indicated that the mortality rates have been declining ever since. Dr. Mann does not mention the fact of this dramatic decline but instead presents relatively flat, crude, total mortality rates as an argument that die-*

tary changes have done no good since 1950.—Hinds[15]

Atherosclerosis is known to be a multifactorial disease with many risk factors. To try to prove that diet is not one of these many factors by plotting crude death rates in the United States is highly irrelevant since such factors as widespread national immunization, the development of antibiotics, major wars, increasing cancer mortality and declining infant mortality all have a major effect on such trends. The subject of his discussion was coronary mortality. If Dr. Mann had plotted the overall age-specific or age-adjusted coronary mortality rates, the curve would have risen through 1963, followed by an early gradual decline with a later steeper decline that was still continuing in April, 1977. The overall magnitude of the decline now exceeds 25 percent. It is the first decline recorded in American history.—Walker[16]

"Neither is there evidence that cholesterolemia was diminished in the United States population during the interval 1962–1973, when the diet-heart propaganda was full blast."—Mann[17]

He [Mann himself] *then provides a graph clearly showing that cholesterol levels are lower in every adult age group in 1970-1974 than in 1960-1962, and that the reduction averages about 4 to 5 mg per 100 ml. Although the difference is small, it is highly consistent.*—Vogt[18]

[8]G. V. Mann, Diet-heart: End of an era, *New England Journal of Medicine* 297 (1977):644-650.

[9]T. M. Vogt, Letter to the editor, *New England Journal of Medicine* 298 (1978):107.

[10]G. V. Mann, Letter to the editor, *New England Journal of Medicine* 298 (1978):108.

[11]Mann, 1977, p. 644.

[12]W. J. Walker, Letter to the editor, *New England Journal of Medicine* 298 (1978):106-107.

[13]Mann, 1977, p. 645.

[14]Walker, 1978, p. 107.

[15]M. W. Hinds, Letter to the editor, *New England Journal of Medicine* 298 (1978):107.

[16]Walker, 1978, p. 106.

[17]Mann, 1977, p. 645.

[18]Vogt, 1978, p. 107.

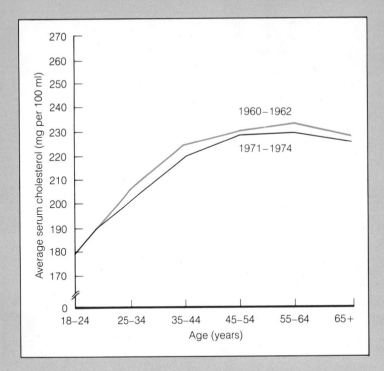

Cholesterolemia in U.S. men, as measured by two probability samples drawn 12 years apart. This graph from Dr. Mann's article is based on statistics from the U.S. Department of Health, Education, and Welfare.

"There is no doubt that these oily treatment diets double the incidence of cholelithiasis."—Mann[19]

This statement refers to reported increased cholelithiasis in a drug project study. None of the six groups included in the study were on any particular diet! — Walker[20]

"Whyte's . . . calculations [show] the futility of fussing with risk factors in men past 55 years of age."—Mann[21]

From 1963 to 1975, years of great emphasis on coronary risk factors, United States statistics showed a marked decline in

age-specific coronary mortality after the age of 55—for example, from 55 to 64, 23.7 percent, from 65 to 74, 25.3 percent, from 75 to 84, 12.8 percent, and after 85, 19.3 percent. —Walker[22]

"[An] impressive array of epidemiologic evidence suggests that . . . active people are spared the complications of athero-sclerosis."—Mann[23]

A review of 30 studies of physical inactivity as a risk factor for coronary heart disease concluded that the results are "contradic-tory and inconclusive."—Hinds[24]

Dr. Mann makes the errors he sees the diet-heart people making

in his assumption that the death rate from coronary heart diseases is declining because "the parks and streets are alive with joggers."—Vogt[25]

"No one has been able to prove that dietary treatments either prevent or modify the behavior of coronary heart disease."—Mann[26]

In the last two decades expert groups and responsible organi-zations have urged a serious ef-fort to control the factors re-peatedly identified by research as major coronary-risk factors: lipid-rich diet and hyper-cholesterolemia, cigarette smok-ing and high blood pressure. (Neither the American Heart As-sociation nor other informed sci-entific organizations ever named diet as the sole culprit.)—Vil et al.[27]

Above all, we must attempt to prevent the basic disease—atherosclerotic lesions. Both ex-perimental and clinical investiga-tions have produced strong evi-dence of a connection between hypercholesterolemia and ath-erosclerosis. Cholesterol deposits irritate the tissue of the vessel wall. Dietary saturated fats raise the blood cholesterol level in animals and in man. . . . It is not a question of dieting, but of using a more wholesome food readily acceptable to the entire family.—Malmros[28]

[19]Mann, 1977, p. 646.
[20]Walker, 1978, p. 106.
[21]Mann, 1977, p. 646.

[22]Walker, 1978, p. 106.
[23]Mann, 1977, p. 648.
[24]Hinds, 1978, p. 107.

[25]Vogt, 1978, p. 107.
[26]Mann, 1977, p. 644.
[27]C. S. Vil, K. H. Kohn, J. Last, M. H. Lepper, O. Paul, J. A. Schoenberger, J. M. Smith, and R. W. Wissler, Letter to the editor, New England Journal of Medicine 298 (1978):109.
[28]H. Malmros, Letter to the editor, New England Journal of Medicine 298 (1978):164.

These excerpts illustrate the point that research on a multifactorial disease such as atherosclerosis does not offer simple, clear-cut answers to our questions. The experts disagreed even when they were looking at the same graph. It may be that the decline in coronary mortality rates was temporary and that in the 1980s it will return to its earlier steep climb; judgment will have to be withheld on that. But viewing the entire debate, we agree with the critic who pointed out that no one has ever said diet is the only risk factor in heart disease. We also agree with Dr. Mann that it has not been proven that a change in diet will prevent heart disease. We do believe, however, there is strong evidence that diet is one of the risk factors and we recommend a low-fat, low-cholesterol diet for the general public. On the other points of contention, we urge you to study the original publications and to make your own judgments.

While this argument may seem to have degenerated to a schoolboys' stone throwing contest at times, it had two outstanding virtues. One is that it was aired. The *Journal* did not allow only one point of view to be expressed.

The other virtue of this argument arises from its having been published where it was, in a scien-

tific journal. When a scientist writes for a professional journal, he puts his reputation on the line. His colleagues read the article and rebuke him if they find errors in his reporting. Dr. Mann's article was roundly criticized—not for the view it espoused but for the weakness of the supporting data. It is risky to publish in a professional journal—and there is no pay. The writer's motivation is to get at and convey the truth as he sees it.

In contrast, someone who writes about science for popular newspapers, magazines, or books has no such restraints and gets paid. Some writers perform a valuable service by rooting out of the dull journals news of recent advances against heart disease or cancer. They translate the news into everyday language and enlarge it into a salable and helpful article. However, others may be allied with an organization that will profit by the promotion of a certain viewpoint. For instance, a writer may be employed by a tobacco growers' association, which would obviously be interested in widespread publication of any research that suggests cigarette smoking is not linked to atherosclerosis. It is difficult for the general

reader to detect a writer's motives. And the main criterion for acceptance of an article is all too often: Will it sell?

CAUTION WHEN YOU READ!

To weigh the reliability of nutrition information, ask yourself

Who wrote it?

Who published it?

Why was it published?

The Role of HDL   Cholesterol has not been the only constituent of blood to receive attention in heart disease research. As far back as the early 1950s, it was known that the level of the high-density lipoprotein (HDL) fraction (which carries about a fourth of the cholesterol[29]) has a negative correlation with coronary heart disease.[30] It was also known that levels of low-density lipoprotein (the LDL fraction, which carries most of the cholesterol) correlate directly with atherosclerosis. How-

[29]High blood lipid levels (Medical News), *Journal of the American Medical Association* 237 (1977):1066-1067, 1069-1070.

[30]W. B. Kannel, W. P. Castelli, and T. Gordon, Cholesterol in the prediction of atherosclerotic disease, *Annals of Internal Medicine* 90 (1979):85-91.

Mini-Glossary

Heart disease is so widely discussed that students often want to learn the meanings of the common terms. Not all are used in this book but here they are in case you are interested.

atherosclerosis, cholesterol, embolism, plaque, thrombosis: see Chapter 2.

lipoproteins, LDL, HDL: see Chapter 6.

adventitia (AD-ven-TISH-iuh): the outermost covering of an organ, especially of a blood vessel.

adventicious = coming from outside

aneurysm (AN-you-rism): the ballooning out of an artery wall where it has been weakened by deterioration.

ana = throughout
eurus = wide

angina (an-JIGH-nuh): pain in the heart region caused by lack of oxygen.

angere = to strangle

cardiovascular disease (CVD): heart and artery disease, ischemic heart disease.

cardium = heart
vascular = blood vessels

cerebrovascular accident (CVA): a disabling or fatal event in the brain, a stroke or aneurysm.

cerebro = brain

cholelithiasis (KOH-lee-lih-THIGH-uh-sis): gallstones.

chol = bile
lithos = stone

coronary artery disease (CAD): hardening of the arteries that feed the heart muscle, leading to heart attacks and other forms of heart damage. Also called **coronary heart disease (CHD).**

coronary = crowning (the heart)

hypercholesterolemia (HIGH-per-coh-LES-ter-ol-EEM-ee-uh): a high concentration of cholesterol in the blood.

intima (INT-ih-muh): the innermost layer of an organ, especially the wall of an artery or vein.

intimus = innermost

ischemic (ih-SKEE-mic) **heart disease (IHD):** formerly called arteriosclerosis, this general term means artery disease or "hardening of the arteries." Atherosclerosis is the principal form of IHD.

iskein = to keep back, restrain

lumen (LOO-men): the inner, open space of a tubular organ like a blood vessel.

media (MEE-dee-uh): the middle layer of an organ.

medium = middle

myocardial infarct (my-oh-CARD-ee-ul in-FARKT) **(MI):** a heart attack.

myo = muscle
infarct = blocking off

occlusion (ock-CLOO-zhun): shutting off the blood flow in an artery.

You might also like to know the meaning of two terms related to blood: **serum** (SEER-um) is the watery portion of the blood that remains after the cells and clot-forming material have been removed; **plasma** (PLAZ-muh) is unclotted blood with only the cells removed. In most instances, serum and plasma concentrations of substances are similar to those in whole blood.

A note on normal blood values: People sometimes ask about "high cholesterol": How high is too high? Normal blood cholesterol levels in the developed countries range from 140 to 260 mg per 100 ml plasma. Younger people should have lower values. Triglycerides range between 10 and 200 mg per 100 ml, depending on the individual and on the time since he ate his last fat-containing meal.

---

ever, the procedure for identifying LDL was so complicated and expensive that it was not used. Total serum cholesterol gave similar results and became the procedure of choice for studies of the relationship between plasma lipids and coronary heart disease.

Studies using animals have suggested that the LDLs supply cholesterol to the cells and that the HDLs remove it.[31] It may be that the controlling factor is how much

[31]D. M. Small, Cellular mechanisms for lipid deposition in atherosclerosis, part 1, *New England Journal of Medicine* 297 (1977):873-877.

free cholesterol there is in the cytoplasm of the cell. If the level is low, the cell is stimulated to do two things: to synthesize cholesterol and to manufacture new receptor sites for the LDLs that are circulating in the blood. If the level of free cholesterol in the cell is high, then the circulating LDLs would also be high, because the receptor sites would shut down.

In an attempt to see how these lipid fractions correlate with other known risk factors for heart disease, Williams and his associates in England studied 2,568 men.[32] They found that HDL levels were inversely related to cigarette smoking, relative weight, and serum triglyceride levels and directly related to physical activity, total cholesterol level, and alcohol consumption. They found that a better prediction of heart attack risk could be made by finding the ratio of HDL to total cholesterol. This was particularly true for older people, for whom cholesterol levels alone had proven poor predictors.

The problem now facing researchers and clinicians is to discover what elements of the diet will reduce total cholesterol and LDL and also those that will raise the HDL fraction. Truswell has reviewed the research on the effect of diet on plasma

lipids, citing 196 references.[33] He enumerates the foods that have shown promise and suggests some that should receive more attention. Some of his ideas are incorporated into the list below.

Here are some facts about foods and other risk factors in atherosclerosis, gleaned from all over. None of these are usable yet, and it could even be dangerous to take action based on them. They are presented here only to show how wide-ranging present research is.

● The level of circulating LDL is directly related to the consumption of cholesterol and saturated fats.[34]

● Men had lower HDL values than premenopausal women.[35]

● Long-lived families have high HDL levels.[36]

● A diet that resembles Asian and Mediterranean diets raises the HDL level. This means a diet of vegetables, cereals, fish, little if any meat, and "no 'junk' foods like hot dogs and potato

chips which are packed with saturated fat."[37]

● Residents of a Boston commune who ate a Zen macrobiotic diet had extremely low blood pressures and an average cholesterol level of 123 mg per 100 ml, as compared with the 185 mg per 100 ml average of the same-aged offspring of the Framingham men.[38]

● Those in the commune who ate fish had a slightly higher HDL concentration than the others.[39]

● Most oral contraceptives decrease HDL and increase LDL.[40]

● Dietary polyunsaturated fatty acids reduce the circulating LDL in some individuals.[41]

● Daily intake of 60 g of plant fiber is accompanied by a distinct reduction in serum LDL-cholesterol content and an elevation of HDL.[42]

[32]P. Williams, D. Robinson, and A. Bailey, High-density lipoprotein and coronary risk factors in normal men, *Lancet* I (1979):72-75.

[33]A. S. Truswell, Diet and plasma lipids: A reappraisal, *American Journal of Clinical Nutrition* 31 (1978):977-989.

[34]High blood lipid levels, 1977, p. 1066.

[35]High blood lipid levels, 1977, p. 1066.

[36]J. A. Kahn and C. J. Glueck, Familial hypobetalipoproteinemia, *Journal of the American Medical Association* 240 (1978):47-48.

[37]High blood lipid levels, 1977, p. 1069.

[38]High blood lipid levels, 1977, p. 1069.

[39]High blood lipid levels, 1977, p. 1069.

[40]High blood lipid levels, 1977, p. 1070.

[41]R. L. Jackson, O. D. Taunton, J. D. Morrisett, and A. M. Gotto, The role of dietary polyunsaturated fat in lowering blood cholesterol in man, *Circulation Research* 42 (4) (1978):447-452.

[42]J. W. Anderson and W. L. Chen, Plant fiber: Carbohydrate and lipid metabolism, *American Journal of Clinical Nutrition* 32 (1979):346-363.

● Dietary fat aids absorption of dietary cholesterol; plant sterols and fiber hinder absorption of cholesterol.[43]

● "Fortunately, most of the dietary modifications designed to lower serum total cholesterol have no adverse effect on the HDL. This is also true of other recommendations on control of coronary heart disease: reduction of overweight, decreased cigarette smoking and increased physical activity."[44]

● LDL-cholesterol levels were significantly higher among people who smoked cigarettes and consumed 5 or more cups of coffee per day than among nonsmokers who abstained from coffee.[45]

● Whole milk does not raise and may lower cholesterol.[46]

● Moderate amounts of eggs (up to one per day) seem not to be such a disadvantage in light of the valuable nutrients they contain.[47]

● Shellfish (which are high in cholesterol and are restricted on heart patients' diets) have not been tested on humans but only on rabbits, which are especially vulnerable to atherosclerosis.[48]

● Wheat fiber (bran) does not lower plasma cholesterol, but pectin does—and so does the pulp of two apples taken three times a day. Oatmeal may lower plasma cholesterol.[49]

● Whenever weight is lost, HDL levels increase.[50]

● Alcoholics have high HDL levels. People who die of cirrhosis are found to have arteries relatively free of atherosclerotic plaque.[51]

● Long-distance runners have elevated HDL levels.[52]

Some of these items may become hot news in the 1980s: Watch for them. (But remember to watch, not in the newspapers, but in the journals.)

This Highlight has followed the changing diet advice through the years. It has not yet been proven that a low-fat, low-cholesterol diet will prevent coronary heart disease, but most experts in the field seem to agree that diet plays a part. It will be interesting to watch the unfolding drama as exploration continues into the roles played by HDL and LDL. Lewis Thomas, in *The Lives of a Cell*, explains the communication network in science in these words:

> We like to think of exploring in science as a lonely, meditative business, and so it is in the first stages, but always, sooner or later, before the enterprise reaches completion, as we explore, we call to each other, communicate, publish, send letters to the editor, present papers, cry out on finding.[53]

We would add that we who merely read and enjoy also "cry out on finding."

To Explore Further

An interesting and optimistic view of people's responsiveness to changes in their lifestyles is Walker, W. J., Changing United States life-style and declining vascular mortality: Cause or coincidence? *New England Journal of Medicine* 297 (1977):163-165.

You may wish to read more about the relationship of exercise to heart attack risk:

Paffenbarger, R. S., Wing, A. L., and Hyde, R. T., Current exercise and heart attack risk, *Cardiac Rehabilitation* 10 (2) (1979):1-4.

The hypothesis that an atherosclerotic plaque arises from a single smooth muscle cell is discussed in Benditt, E. P., The origin of atherosclerosis, *Scientific American* 236 (1977):74-85.

[43]R. B. Alfin-Slater, Cholesterol, *Nutrition and the M.D.* 5 (1979):1-2.
[44]Kannel, Castelli, and Gordon, 1979, p. 90.
[45]S. Heyden, G. Heiss, C. Manegold, H. A. Tyroler, C. G. Hames, A. G. Bartel, and G. Cooper, The combined effect of smoking and coffee drinking on LDL and HDL cholesterol, *Circulation* 60 (1) (1979):22-25.
[46]Truswell, 1978, p. 979.
[47]Truswell, 1978, p. 979.

[48]Truswell, 1978, pp. 979-980.
[49]Truswell, 1978, p. 980.
[50]Truswell, 1978, p. 983.
[51]Truswell, 1978, p. 983.
[52]Truswell, 1978, p. 982.

[53]L. Thomas, *The Lives of a Cell: Notes of a Biology Watcher* (New York: Viking, 1974).

An entire issue of a monthly newsletter for physicians and nutritionists was devoted to an update on the diet-heart controversy: *Nutrition and the M.D.*, April 1979.

The following free pamphlet was recommended in the April 1979 issue of *Nutrition and the M.D.*:

Dietary Management of Hyperlipoproteinemia: A Handbook for Physicians and Dietitians, DHEW publication no. 73-110, available from the Office of Information, National Heart and Lung Institute, Bethesda, Maryland 20014.

The following pamphlet on dietary management of hyperlipidemia can be obtained free from your local Heart Association office:

Dietary Modification to Control Hyperlipidemia, Ad Hoc Committee for Medical and Community Programs, American Heart Association, reprinted from *Circulation* 58 (1978):381A.

Some 400 pages of controversy over the diet-heart issue were published in:

Proceedings of the Conference on the Decline in Coronary Heart Disease Mortality, U. S. Department of Health, Education and Welfare (NIH Publication No. 79-1610, May 1979).

CHAPTER 7

CONTENTS

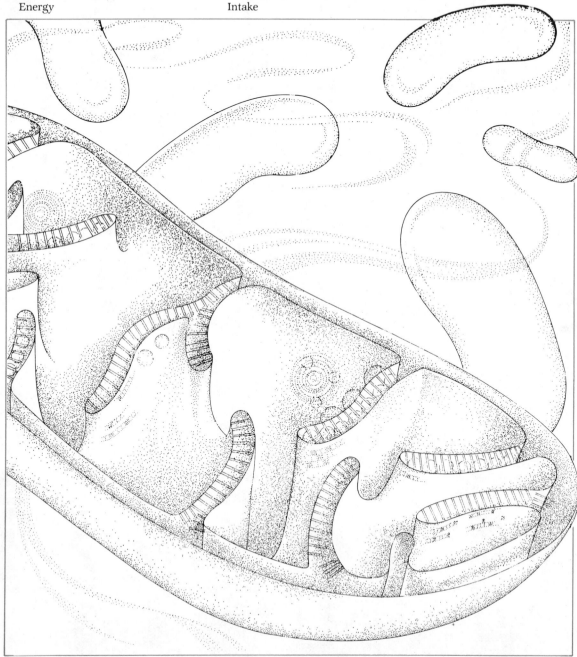

Much of the cell's metabolic activity takes place in structures like this one (a mitochondrion). A million enzyme-complexes are mounted on the membranes inside this particle, and there may be hundreds of such particles inside an active cell. Within each complex the enzymes are mounted in the order in which they perform their reactions.

METABOLISM:
Feasting, Fasting, and Energy Balance

The course of nature . . . seems delighted with transmutations . . .

SIR ISAAC NEWTON

When you eat too much you get fat; when you eat too little you get thin. Everybody knows these simple facts, but nobody knows exactly how to account for them. The mission of this chapter is to shed some light on what we do know and to provide answers to some of the questions people often ask about diets. What makes a person gain weight? Are carbohydrate-rich foods more fattening than other foods? What's the best way to lose weight: Is fasting dangerous? Are low-carbohydrate diets dangerous? The answers to these and many other questions lie in an understanding of metabolism.

Metabolism could be defined as the way the body handles the energy nutrients; a more precise definition appears in the margin. But before getting into the body cells to see metabolism in progress, a brief review of the energy nutrients themselves may be helpful.

metabolism: the sum total of all the chemical reactions that go on in living cells.

meta = among
bole = change

Starting Points

The first four chapters introduced the energy nutrients—carbohydrate, fat, and protein—as they are found in foods and in the human body. Chapters 5 and 6 followed the nutrients through digestion to the simpler units they are composed of and showed these units disappearing into the blood. Four of these units will be followed here.

(1) Carbohydrates come in several varieties in the diet: principally as the polysaccharide starch, the disaccharides, and the monosaccharides. During digestion, these units are all broken down to monosaccharides—glucose, fructose, and galactose—and are absorbed into the blood. The latter two are then taken into liver cells and converted to glucose or to very similar compounds. Thus to continue the story of what happens to carbohydrate thereafter, we will simply follow glucose.

(2 & 3) Lipids also come in several varieties, but 95 percent of those found in foods are triglycerides. The triglycerides undergo several transformations during digestion and absorption, but many of them

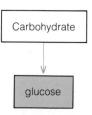

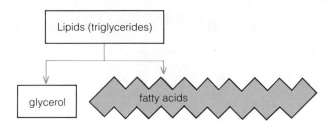

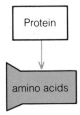

end up once again as triglycerides in body cells. There they can be dismantled to glycerol and fatty acids. Following the further transformations of glycerol and fatty acids will show the principal fates of dietary fat.

(4) Protein is digested to amino acids, absorbed into blood, and carried to the liver, where further transformations occur. Thus to follow protein through metabolism, we will trace the steps by which amino acids are further transformed.

Building Body Compounds

You already know what may happen to some of these basic units when their energy is not needed by the cells: They may be stored "as is," being used to build body compounds. Glucose units may be strung together to make glycogen chains. Glycerol and fatty acids may be assembled into triglycerides. Amino acids may be used to make proteins. These building reactions, in which simple compounds are put together to form larger, more complex structures, involve doing work—and so require energy. They are called anabolic reactions.

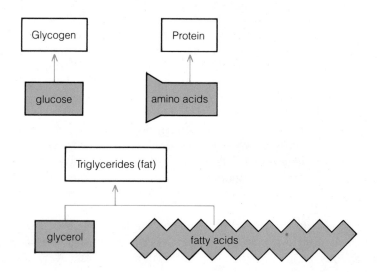

Breaking Down Nutrients for Energy

If the body does need energy, however, it may break apart any or all of these units into fragments. The breakdown reactions, which release energy, are called catabolic reactions.

At this point you must stop thinking about these compounds as the basic units of the nutrients and remember that they are composed of still more basic units, the atoms. During metabolism, the body goes to work with an "electron saw" and actually separates the atoms from one another. It will help if you recall the structures of these compounds (introduced in the first four chapters). There is no need to remember exactly how they are put together; it is enough to remember how many carbons are in their "backbones":

catabolism: reactions in which large molecules are broken down to smaller ones. Catabolic reactions involve oxidation and release energy.

kata = down

Arrows pointing down represent catabolic reactions. Much of the body's catabolic work is done in the liver cells, and all of the reactions described in this chapter can take place there.

Glucose = 6 carbons

Glycerol = 3 carbons

Fatty acids = even numbers of carbons (multiples of 2)

Amino acids = 2 or 3 or more carbons (to which nitrogen is always attached)

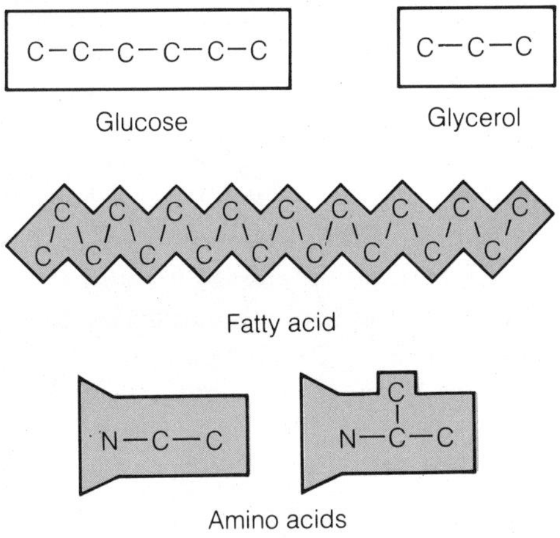

C—C—C—C—C—C

Glucose

C—C—C

Glycerol

Fatty acid

Amino acids

The main point to notice in the following discussion is that compounds that have a three-carbon skeleton can be used to make the vital nutrient glucose, but those that have two-carbon skeletons cannot.

The story of what happens to these compounds inside of cells can be told most simply by starting with glucose. Two new names appear—pyruvate (three carbons) and acetyl CoA (two carbons)—and once you have learned these, the rest of the story falls into place around them.

Glucose In breaking down, glucose first splits in half releasing energy. One product is the three-carbon compound pyruvate, and the other is converted into pyruvate, so that two identical halves result from this step.

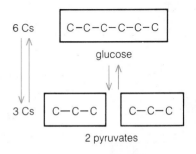

6 Cs

C—C—C—C—C—C

glucose

3 Cs

C—C—C   C—C—C

2 pyruvates

pyruvate (PIE-roo-vate): a salt of pyruvic acid. (Throughout this book the ending *ate* is used interchangeably with *ic acid*. Thus acetate is the same as acetic acid.)

Should a cell "change its mind" after splitting glucose to pyruvate, it could reverse this step. It could put the two halves back together to make glucose again.

If the cell still needs energy, however, it breaks the pyruvate molecules apart further, cleaving a carbon from each. The lone carbon is combined with oxygen to make carbon dioxide, which is released into the blood, circulated to the lungs, and excreted (breathed out). The two-carbon compound that remains is acetyl CoA. Should the cell "change its mind" at this point and want to retrieve the carbons and make glucose, it could not do so. The step from pyruvate to acetyl CoA is metabolically irreversible: It is a one-way step.

CoA (coh-AY): nickname for a compound described further in Chapter 9. As pyruvate loses a carbon and becomes a 2-carbon compound (acetate), a molecule of CoA is attached to it, making **acetyl CoA** (ASS-uh-teel co-AY).

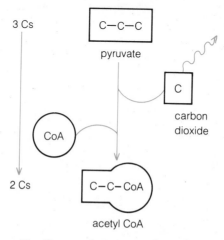

Finally acetyl CoA may be split, yielding two more carbon dioxide molecules. The energy released in this step powers most of the cell's activities. The process by which acetyl CoA splits and releases its energy is known as the TCA cycle; its details are not necessary to a basic understanding of nutrition but are given in Highlight 7 for those who are interested.

The reactions by which the complete oxidation of acetyl CoA is accomplished are those of the **TCA** (tricarboxylic acid) or **Krebs cycle** (named for the biochemist who elucidated them) and **oxidative phosphorylation.** Details are given in Highlight 7.

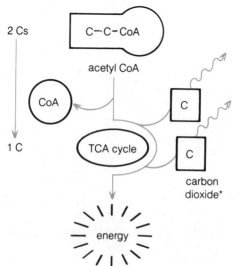

To sum up, then, the steps in the complete breakdown of glucose are:

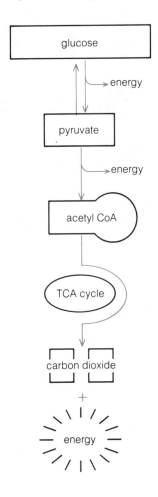

Only the first step is reversible. Energy is released at every step, but the breakdown of acetyl CoA provides most of the energy that powers the cell.

Why should you bother to learn about the intermediate compounds, pyruvate and acetyl CoA? What happens to these two compounds explains the most interesting and important aspects of nutrition and makes it possible to answer questions like those asked at the outset. The breakdown of protein and fat, as well as glucose, yields pyruvate and acetyl CoA. The parts of protein and fat that can be converted to pyruvate (3 carbons) *can* provide glucose for the body; those that are converted to acetyl CoA can *not* do so. And glucose is all-important to survival.

Glycerol and Fatty Acids   The typical triglyceride consists of a molecule of glycerol (3 carbons long) and three fatty acids (about 18 carbons each, or 54 carbons in all). When such a molecule is broken

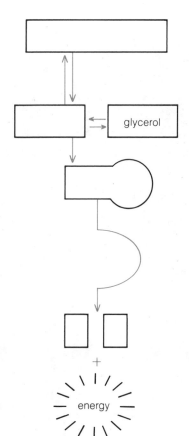

down inside a cell, these parts are first separated. The glycerol is easily converted to pyruvate (also three carbons long) and then may go either "up" to form glucose or "down" to form acetyl CoA and finally carbon dioxide. Thus one tiny piece of each fat molecule—about 5 percent of the total weight—can be used to meet the body's need for glucose.

But the three fatty acids are taken apart two carbons at a time to make acetyl CoA, and this cannot be used to make glucose. It is either broken down further, yielding energy, or put together to make compounds such as other fatty acids, cholesterol, or ketones. So fat is a very poor, inefficient source of glucose. About 95 percent of it cannot be converted to glucose at all.

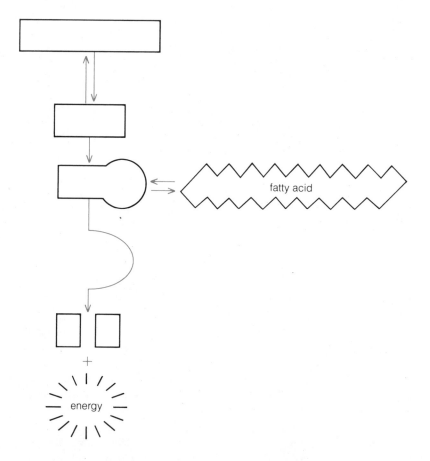

Amino Acids   Protein enters the body as an array of different amino acids. Ideally they will be used to build needed body proteins. But if energy needs are not met by carbohydrate and fat, then the amino acids will be sacrificed to provide energy. When this occurs, they are stripped of their nitrogen (see the next section) and then treated in a variety of

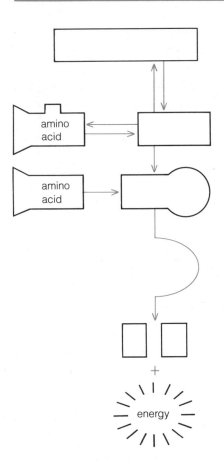

ways.[1] The net effect is that about half of amino acids can be converted to pyruvate; the other half go either to acetyl CoA or directly into the TCA cycle. Those that can be used to make pyruvate can provide glucose for the body. Thus protein, unlike fat, is a fairly good source of glucose when carbohydrate is not available.

Amino acids break down when energy needs are not met by carbohydrate and fat, as just described, but they also break down in the same way under another set of conditions: when surplus kcalories and protein are consumed. Surplus protein cannot be stored in the body as such; it has to be degraded. If you eat more protein than you can use at a given time, the excess amino acids quickly lose their nitrogens and most are converted to acetyl CoA either directly or indirectly (through pyruvate). But this acetyl CoA is not broken down further, because energy is not needed. Instead it is strung together into chains—fatty

The making of glucose from protein or fat is **gluconeogenesis** (gloo-co-nee-o-GEN-uh-sis). About 5 percent of fat (the glycerol portion of triglycerides) and about half of the amino acids (those that are glucogenic) can be converted to glucose.

gluco = glucose
neo = new
genesis = making

[1]Some are rearranged to form pyruvate. Others are four-carbon compounds that split into two acetyl CoA. One, which contains only two carbons after the nitrogen is removed, is rearranged directly to become acetyl CoA. Still others become compounds that enter the TCA cycle (see Highlight 7).

acids—and stored in body fat. Thus even the so-called "lean" nutrient, protein, can make you fat if you eat too much of it.

What Happens to the Nitrogen?   When amino acids are degraded for energy or to make fat, the first step is removal of their nitrogen-containing amino groups, a reaction called deamination. The product is ammonia, chemically identical to the ammonia in the bottled cleaning solutions used in hospitals and in industry. It is a strong-smelling and extremely potent poison.

deamination: removal of the amino (NH_2) group from a compound such as an amino acid.

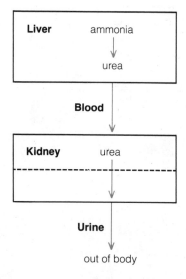

A small amount of ammonia is always being produced by liver deamination reactions. Some of this ammonia is captured by liver enzymes and used to synthesize other amino acids, but what cannot be used is quickly combined with a carbon-oxygen fragment to make urea, an inert and less toxic compound.

urea (yoo-REE-uh): the principal nitrogen-excretion product of metabolism. Two ammonia fragments are combined with a carbon-oxygen group to form urea. The diagram greatly oversimplifies the reactions.

The discovery of urea by Wöhler in 1828 was a momentous event in the history of science, technology, and agriculture. It represented the first synthesis in the laboratory of a body compound, laid a cornerstone for the science of organic chemistry, and made possible the beginnings of the fertilizer industry (see Appendix A).

Urea is released from the liver cells into the blood, where it circulates until it passes through the kidneys. One of the functions of the kidneys is to remove urea from the blood for excretion in the urine. Urea is the body's principal vehicle for excreting unused nitrogen; water is required to keep it in solution and excrete it. This explains why people who consume a high-protein diet must drink more water than usual.

(After excretion, urea may be converted spontaneously or by

bacterial action back to ammonia. This accounts for the ammonia odor of the diaper pail.)

Putting It All Together   After a normal mixed meal, if you do not overeat, the body handles the nutrients in all of the ways just described (see Figure 1).

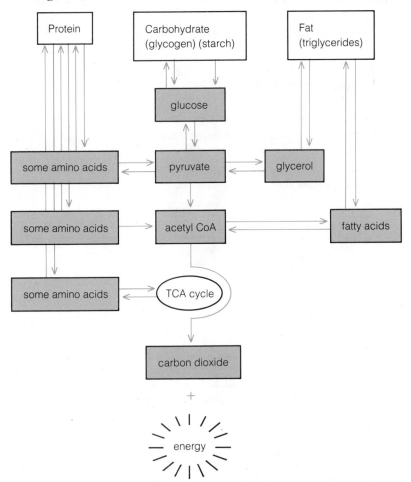

Figure 1   The central pathways of metabolism.

The carbohydrate yields glucose: Some is stored as glycogen, and some is taken into brain and other cells and broken down through pyruvate and acetyl CoA to provide energy. The protein yields amino acids: Some are used to build body protein, and (if there is a surplus) some are broken down through the same pathways as glucose to provide energy. The fat yields glycerol and fatty acids: Some are put together and stored as fat, and others are broken down through the same pathways as glucose to provide energy.

A few hours after the meal, the stored glycogen and fat begin to be released from storage to provide more glucose, glycerol, and fatty acids to keep the energy flow going. When all of the energy supplied from the last meal has been used up and reserves of these compounds are running low, it is time to eat again.

The average person consumes more than a million kcalories a year and expends more than 99 percent of them, maintaining a stable weight for years on end.[2] This remarkable achievement, which most people manage without even thinking about it, could be called the economy of maintenance: The body's energy budget is balanced. Some people, however, eat too little and get thin; others eat too much and get fat. The possible reasons for this are explored in Chapter 8; the metabolic consequences will be discussed here.

The Economy of Feasting

The pathways of metabolism just described make it clear why consuming too much of any energy nutrient can make you fat. Surplus carbohydrate (glucose) can be stored as glycogen, but there is a limit to

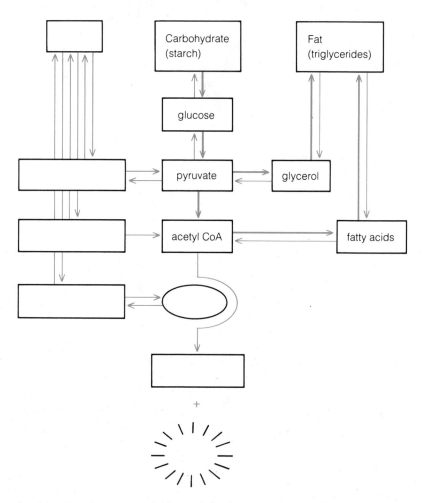

[2]G. A. Bray and L. A. Campfield, Metabolic factors in the control of energy stores, *Metabolism* 24 (1975):99-117.

the capacity of the glycogen-storing cells. Once glycogen stores are filled, the overflow is routed to fat (note the heavy arrows in the diagram below). Fat cells expand as they fill with fat, and they seem to be able to expand indefinitely. Thus excess carbohydrate, above and beyond the kcalorie need, can contribute to obesity.

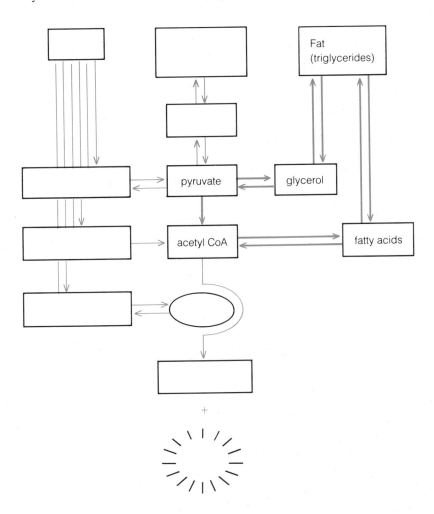

Of course, surplus fat in the diet can also contribute to the body's fat stores (note the heavy arrows in the adjacent diagram). It may break down to fragments such as acetyl CoA, but if energy flow is already rapid enough to meet the demand, these fragments will not enter the energy-yielding pathway. They will be diverted back again to the assembly of triglycerides and stored in the fat cells.

Finally, surplus protein may encounter the same fate (note the heavy arrows in this diagram). If not needed to build body protein or to meet present energy needs, amino acids will lose their nitrogens and be converted through the intermediates, pyruvate and acetyl CoA, to triglycerides. These, too, swell the fat cells and increase body weight.

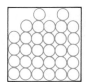

Fat cells enlarge.

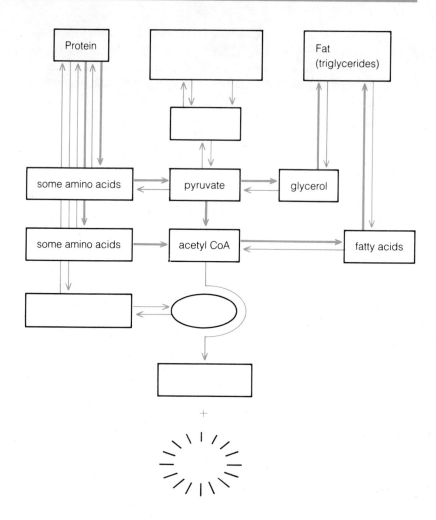

The Economy of Fasting

Even when you are asleep and totally relaxed, the cells of many organs are hard at work spending energy. In fact, the work that you are aware of, that you do with your muscles during waking hours, represents only about a third of the total energy you spend in a day. The rest is the metabolic work of the cells, for which they constantly require fuel.

The body's top priority is to meet these energy needs, and its normal way of doing so is by periodic refueling—that is, by eating. When food is withdrawn, the body must find other fuel sources in its own tissues. If people choose not to eat, we say they are fasting; if they have no choice (as in a famine), we say they are starving; but there is no metabolic difference between the two. In either case the body is forced to switch to a wasting metabolism, drawing on its stored reserves of carbohydrate and fat and within a day or so on its protein tissues as well.

Fuel must be delivered to every cell. As the fast begins, glucose and fatty acids are both flowing into cells, breaking down to yield acetyl CoA, and delivering energy to power the cells' work. Several hours later, however, most of the glucose is used up, the available glycogen has been withdrawn from storage to replenish it, and this source in turn is being exhausted.

At this point, most of the cells are depending on fatty acids to continue providing their fuel. But the brain cells cannot; they still need glucose. (The problem is that the only nutrient that can get through their membranes is glucose. Once inside, this glucose breaks down to acetyl CoA and is processed the same way as in other cells.) Normally the brain consumes about two-thirds of the total glucose used each day.

The brain's special requirement for glucose poses a problem for the fasting body. It can use its stores of fat, which may be quite generous, to furnish most of its cells with energy, but for the brain it must supply energy in the form of glucose. This is why body protein tissues, such as

The liver releases both fat and glucose to be used as fuel by the body's cells, but the brain can accept and use only the glucose.

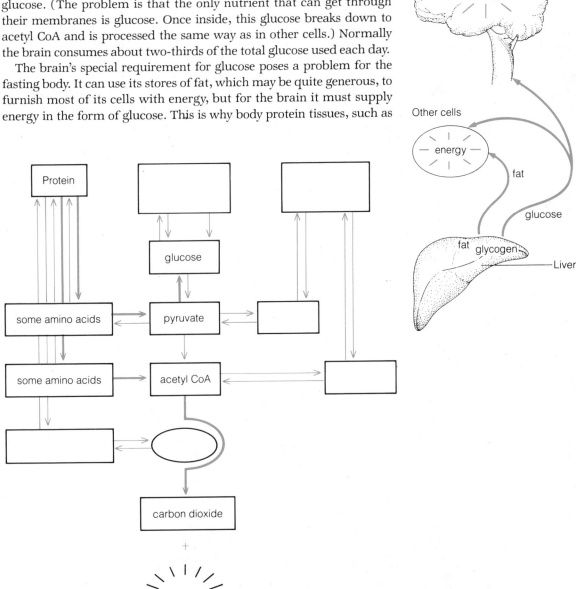

ketone (KEE-tone): a compound formed during the incomplete oxidation of fatty acids. Ketones contain a C=O group between other carbons; when they also contain a COOH, or acid group, they are called keto-acids. Small amounts of ketones are a normal part of the blood chemistry, but when their concentration rises, they spill into the urine. The combination of high blood ketones (ketonemia) and ketones in the urine (ketonuria) is termed **ketosis.**

muscle, always break down to some extent during fasting. Only those amino acids that yield three-carbon pyruvate can be used to make glucose, and to obtain them, whole proteins must be broken down and the other amino acids have to be disposed of. This is an expensive way to gain glucose. But to extract glycerol from fat is even more expensive: Every little three-carbon glycerol taken from fat obligates the body to dispose of some 50 or 60 carbons' worth of fatty acids. In the first few days of a fast, body protein provides about 90 percent of the needed glucose, and glycerol about 10 percent. If body protein loss were to continue at this rate, death would ensue within three weeks.

As the fast continues, the body adapts by producing an alternate energy source—ketones—by condensing together fragments derived from fatty acids. Normally produced and used in only small quantities, ketones can enter some brain cells and serve there as a fuel. Ketone production rises until, at the end of several weeks, it is meeting about half or more of the brain's energy needs. Still, many areas of the brain rely exclusively on glucose, and body protein continues to be sacrificed to produce it.[3]

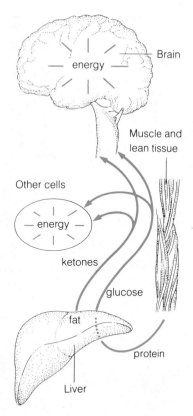

In fasting, muscle and lean tissue atrophy to supply protein for conversion to glucose. This glucose and the ketones produced from fat fuel the brain's activities.

2 acetyl CoA

A ketone (keto-acid)

This ketone may lose a molecule of carbon dioxide to become another ketone:

Acetone

Acetone (ASS-uh-tone) is familiar to some as the solvent used in nail polish remover. "Acetone breath" indicates that a person is in ketosis.

Simultaneously, the body drastically reduces its energy output in order to conserve both its fat and lean tissue. As the lean (protein-containing) organ tissue shrinks in mass, it performs less metabolic work, reducing energy needs. As the muscles waste, they do less work, enhancing this effect. Because of the slowed metabolism, the loss of fat falls to a bare minimum—less, in fact, than the fat that would be lost on a low-kcalorie diet.[4] Thus although weight loss during fasting may be quite dramatic, fat loss may be less than when at least some food is supplied.

[3] R. A. Hawkins and J. F. Biebuyck, Ketone bodies are selectively used by individual brain regions, *Science* 205 (1979):325-327.

[4] M. F. Ball, J. J. Canary, and L. H. Kyle, Comparative effects of calorie restriction and total starvation on body composition in obesity, *Annals of Internal Medicine* 67 (1967):60-67.

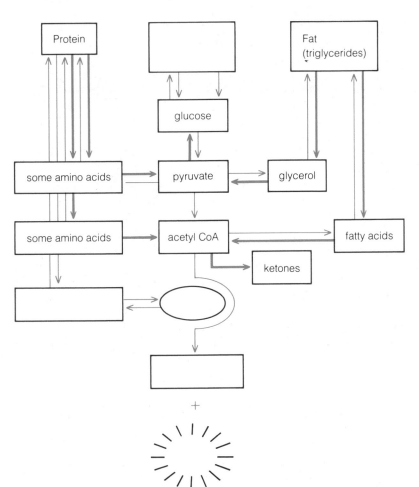

Figure 2 Metabolism during fasting. Protein breakdown supplies some glucose for the brain. Ketone production helps to support brain function. Darkened arrows show which pathways are speeded up during ketosis.

Marasmus   These adaptations also occur in the starving child and help to prolong its life. The severe malnutritional state resulting from starvation is termed marasmus. Together with protein deficiency, it is the most widespread malnutrition problem in the world. Children with marasmus suffer symptoms similar to those of children with the protein-deficiency disease kwashiorkor, due to the loss of body protein tissue; differences are that kwashiorkor children retain some of their stores of body fat, accumulate fat in their livers, and develop edema.

A marasmic child looks like a wizened little old person—just skin and bones. He is often sick, because his resistance to disease is low. All his muscles are wasted, including his heart muscle, and his heart is weak. His metabolism is so slow that his body temperature is subnormal. He has little or no fat under his skin to insulate against cold. The experience of hospital workers with victims of this disease is that their primary need is to be wrapped up and kept warm. They also need love, because they have often been deprived of maternal attention as well as food.

marasmus (ma-RAZ-mus): overt starvation due to a deficiency of kcalories from any source.

Kwashiorkor: see p. 138.

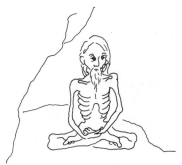

Unlike the kwashiorkor child, who is fed milk until weaning, the marasmic child may have been neglected from early infancy. The disease occurs most commonly in children from 6 to 18 months of age in all the overpopulated city slums of the world. Since the brain normally grows to almost its full adult size within the first two years of life, marasmus impairs brain development and so may have a permanent effect on learning ability.

For the effect of early malnutrition on brain development, see Highlight 4.

Marasmus also occurs in adults in countries where kcalorie deficiency is prevalent. The causes are manifold; Highlight 4 attempted to sort them out and put them in perspective. In recent years marasmus has also been seen to occur in many undernourished hospital patients.

Low-carbohydrate diet = eating protein and fat almost exclusively.

The Low-Carbohydrate Diet   A similar economy prevails if a low-carbohydrate diet is consumed. Advocates of the low-carbohydrate diet would have you believe that there is something magical about ketosis, which promotes faster weight loss than a regular low-kcalorie diet. In fact, the low-carbohydrate diet presents the same problem as a fast. Once the body's available glycogen reserves are spent, the only remaining source of energy in the form of glucose is protein. The low-carbohydrate diet provides a little protein from food, but some must still be taken from body tissue. The onset of ketosis is the signal that this wasting process has begun.

In a diet that provides fewer than about 900 kcal (for the average-size adult), it is pointless to supply any protein at all, because the protein will only be wasted to provide energy. Body protein is lost at the same rate in adults on such a diet whether or not they are given any food protein.[5]

One conclusion to draw from this is that a person who diets at the level of 900 kcal a day might as well eat carbohydrate and fat alone, without protein. This conclusion is valid: Carbohydrate-containing foods are less expensive than protein-rich foods, and both will serve the same purpose—supplying glucose. This is the choice made by the person on a juice fast, for juices contain only carbohydrate. But a wiser conclusion is that such a diet is unnecessarily low in kcalories, even dangerously so. The person who wishes to lose body *fat* will select a balanced diet of 1,200 or more kcalories, one containing carbohydrate, fat, *and* protein. At this level, body protein will be spared, ketosis need not occur, vital lean tissues (including both muscle and brain) will not starve, and only the unwanted *fat* will be lost.

Juice fast = eating only carbohydrate.

People are attracted to the low-carbohydrate diet because of the

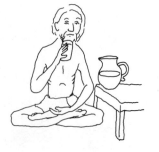

[5]A. A. Albanese and L. A. Orto, The proteins and amino acids, in *Modern Nutrition in Health and Disease*, 5th ed., eds. R. S. Goodhart and M. E. Shils (Philadelphia: Lea and Febiger, 1973), p. 56.

dramatic weight loss it brings about within the first few days. They would be disillusioned if they realized that much of this weight loss is a loss of protein, and with it, quantities of water and important minerals. A woman who boasts of losing seven pounds in two days on her diet may be unaware that at best, she has lost a pound or two of fat and five or six of lean tissue, water, and minerals. When she goes "off" her diet, her body will avidly devour and retain these needed materials, and her weight will zoom back to within two pounds of where she started.

CAUTION:

Beware of those who promote quick-weight-loss schemes. Learn to distinguish between loss of *fat* and loss of *weight*.

The Protein-Sparing Fast A variant on fasting is the technique of feeding the patient only protein. The hope is that the protein will spare lean tissue and that the patient will break down his own body fat at a maximal rate to meet his other energy needs. You may suspect that this is not so different from the low-kcalorie diet and will guess that this protein—together with the body's lean tissues—will be used to provide glucose. You are probably right. The idea sounded good when it was first advanced, but it has met with mixed results. It seems effective only after considerable lean tissue has already been lost, at which time the body may be conserving itself quite efficiently anyway, and the fast has not been shown more effective than a mixture of protein and carbohydrate.[6] Furthermore, it doesn't seem to "stick" very well; most patients regain the lost weight.[7] Thus the protein-sparing fast has to be judged at best a very moderate success and at worst a failure, for the ultimate criterion of success in any weight-loss program is maintenance of the new low weight.

Protein-sparing fast = eating only protein.

The idea of a protein-sparing fast originated with some responsible physicians who experimented carefully with it, using whole natural protein foods such as fish and lean beef. Unfortunately, the idea was then seized upon and began to be misused by the public with the publication of a popular book, *The Last Chance Diet*, in 1977.[8] Fad dieters, usually without any medical supervision, drank liquid protein potions prepared in questionable ways, and lost dramatic amounts of weight (including, of course, body lean tissue, water, and vital minerals). Within the year, 11 deaths had been ascribed to the fad and

[6]T. B. Van Itallie and M. U. Yang, Current concepts in nutrition: Diet and weight loss, *New England Journal of Medicine* 297 (1977):1158-1161.

[7]Morbid obesity: Long-term results of therapeutic fasting, *Nutrition Reviews* 36 (January 1978):6-7.

[8]R. Linn and S. L. Stuart, *The Last Chance Diet* (New York: Bantam Books, 1977).

the FDA had issued a stringent warning about liquid protein preparations.[9] Since then, many more have died on the fast, due to sudden stopping of the heart caused probably by mineral losses.[10]

The term *protein-sparing* has also been used in another connection. Malnourished hospital patients also lose body protein, and this is especially likely—and especially dangerous—if they are simultaneously fighting infection. The knowledgeable physician makes every effort to prevent the loss of vital lean tissue and supplies amino acids as well as glucose in some form—through a vein if the patient can't eat. The effort to provide protein-sparing *therapy* in these circumstances has met with notable success and has significantly reduced the death and disease rate in cases of severe hospital malnutrition. These praiseworthy efforts should not be confused with the profiteering efforts of faddists to sell the protein-sparing *fast*.

Moderate Weight Loss   The body's cells and the enzymes within them make it their task to convert the energy nutrients you eat into those you need. They are extraordinarily versatile and relieve you of having to compute exactly how much carbohydrate, fat, and protein to eat at each meal. As you have seen, they can convert either carbohydrate (glucose) or protein to fat. To some extent, they can convert protein to glucose. To a very limited extent, they can even convert fat (the glycerol portion) to glucose. But a grossly unbalanced diet or one that is severely limited in kcalories imposes hardships on the body. If kcalories are too low or if carbohydrate and protein kcalories are undersupplied, the body is forced to degrade its own lean tissue to meet its glucose need.

Someone who wants to lose body fat must reconcile himself to a hard fact: There is a limit to the rate at which this tissue will break down. The maximum rate, except for a very large person, is one to two pounds a week. To achieve this kind of weight loss, the sensible course is to adopt a balanced low-kcalorie diet supplying all three energy nutrients in reasonable amounts and possibly to increase energy expenditure by getting more exercise. In effect, this means adjusting the energy budget so that intake is 500 to 1,000 kcal per day less than output. A person who wants to gain weight needs to make the opposite adjustment. It might seem that both efforts would require tedious counting of kcalories, but the following sections show that shortcuts are possible.

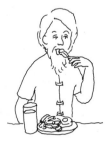

1 lb = 3,500 kcal   A pound of body fat (adipose tissue) is actually composed of a mixture of fat, protein, and water and yields 3,500 kcal on oxidation. A pound of pure fat (454 g) would yield 4,086 kcal (at 9 kcal per gram).

[9]"These liquid protein diets are made from hydrolyzed (predigested) collagen or gelatin obtained from animal hides, tendons, and bones. . . . None is nutritionally complete. . . . Liquid protein diets are neither registered nor approved by FDA. FDA is responsible for the labeling of such products, but generally the labeling does not give directions for weight-loss regimens. Such claims are made in books, by word of mouth, or in the media, which are beyond FDA's control. FDA can take action, such as seeking recall or seizing the product, only if the product has become adulterated." Predigested protein drinks and "modified fasting" diets, *Journal of the American Dietetic Association* 71 (1977): 609.

[10]T. B. Van Itallie, Liquid protein mayhem, *Journal of the American Medical Association* 240 (1978): 144-146.

The Energy in Food: kCalorie Intake

A bomb calorimeter is a device for measuring food energy by the heat given off when food is burned. The number of potential kcalories can be determined in a portion of any food. Researchers have found that the values produced by this method are higher than the number of kcalories the same food would give to an animal. This apparent discrepancy is explained by the fact that not all the food is metabolized by an animal all the way to carbon dioxide, as it is in a bomb calorimeter. Adjustments of bomb calorimeter values have resulted in tables showing the kcalorie content of foods and the values for kcalories in carbohydrate, protein, fat, and alcohol. If you want to balance your energy budget, you can rely on the kcalorie values given in Appendix H for the highest degree of accuracy available.

But looking up every food in kcalorie charts is boring and inconvenient, and only the most motivated will persist at it for a prolonged period of time. For the rest of us who may want to keep track of kcalories, some acquaintance with groups of foods, such as those described at the end of Chapter 1, provides a simpler method. The foods depicted below here could be found one by one in Appendix H, but it's quicker to translate them into exchanges and add up the kcalorie values to get a rough idea of the number. With some practice, you can look at any plate of food and "sense" the number of kcalories it represents. Some kcalorie amounts to remember are:

1 c skim milk (a milk exchange)   80 kcal
  (for whole milk, add 2 fat exchanges)

1 serving vegetable (a vegetable exchange)   25 kcal

1 serving fruit (a fruit exchange)   40 kcal

1 slice bread (a bread exchange)   70 kcal

1 oz lean meat (a meat exchange)   55 kcal
  (for medium-fat meat, add 1/2 fat exchange; for high-fat
  meat, add 1 fat exchange)

1 tsp fat or oil (a fat exchange)   45 kcal

In case you'd like to try guessing how many kcalories are in the meal depicted below, the answer is provided at the bottom of the next page.

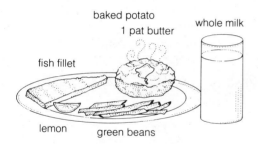

baked potato
1 pat butter
whole milk
fish fillet
lemon
green beans

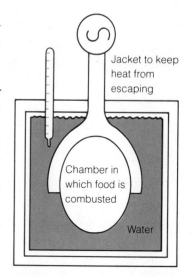

Jacket to keep heat from escaping

Chamber in which food is combusted

Water

Bomb calorimeter.

When an organic substance such as food is burned, the energy in the chemical bonds that held its carbons and hydrogens together is released in the form of heat. The amount of heat that is released can be measured; this direct measure of the amount of energy that was stored in the chemical bonds in the food is termed **direct calorimetry.**

As the chemical bonds in food are broken, the carbons (C) and hydrogens (H) combine with oxygen (O) to form carbon dioxide (CO_2) and water (H_2O). Measuring the amount of oxygen consumed in the process gives an indirect measure of the amount of energy released, termed **indirect calorimetry.**

calorimetry (cal-o-RIM-uh-tree): the measurement of energy.

calor = heat
metron = measure

The Body's Energy Needs: kCalorie Output

Counting the kcalories in your food tells you your energy income, but to balance your budget you also need to know your expenditure. How can you count the kcalories you expend in a day?

Government Recommendations   Government authorities such as the U.S. Committee on RDA and the Canadian Ministry of Health and Welfare have published recommended energy intakes for various age-sex groups in their populations. These are useful for population studies, but the range of energy needs for any one group is so broad that it would be impossible to guess an individual's needs without knowing more about his lifestyle. The U.S. recommendations shown in the accompanying material on pages 241-242 make this obvious: a 20-year-old woman, for example, may need about 2,100 kcal per day—if she is 5 feet 4 inches tall, if she weighs about 120 pounds, and if she typically engages in light activity. But very few 20-year-old women fit this description exactly.

We figure about 530 kcal for the meal below:

1 c milk (milk exchange plus 2 fat exchanges)	170 kcal
1/2 c beans (vegetable exchange)	25 kcal
1 small potato (bread exchange)	70 kcal
1 pat butter (fat exchange)	45 kcal
4 oz fish (4 lean-meat exchanges, assuming no fat is added)	220 kcal
1 lemon wedge	0 kcal
	530 kcal

   Appendix H values yield a total of about 500 kcalories, lower because these foods are low-kcalorie choices within the exchange groups. Any answer within about 50 to 100 kcalories of this is a good estimate.

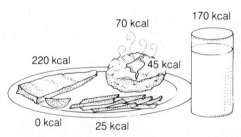

The Energy RDA for Adults (kcal)

Table 1. Recommended Daily Energy Intakes for Adults (kcal)

Age	Men	Women
19-22	2,900 (2,500-3,300)	2,100 (1,700-2,500)
23-50	2,700 (2,300-3,100)	2,000 (1,600-2,400)
51-75	2,400 (2,000-2,800)	1,800 (1,400-2,200)
76+	2,050 (1,650-2,450)	1,600 (1,200-2,000)

The recommendations in Table 1 are useful for population studies, but they are made for the "average person"—and no one, of course, is exactly average. The man used as a reference figure is 5 feet 10 inches tall and weighs 154 pounds (178 centimeters, 70 kilograms). The woman is 5 feet 4 inches tall and weighs 120 pounds (163 centimeters, 55 kilograms). Both engage in light activity: They sleep or lie down for eight hours a day, sit for seven hours, stand for five, walk for two, and spend two hours a day in light physical activity.

Very few people fit these descriptions exactly, although most fall close to the mean. The total span of needs is broad: For adults, it is believed that an 800-kcal range covers most individuals, but some are no doubt excluded at both the lower and upper ends of the range.

In setting the RDA for *protein*, the authorities considered two important facts: First, that the protein needs of individuals vary over a wide range; second, that the consequences of a protein deficiency are severe but that those of an excess of protein are not. In deciding what amount of protein to recommend for an individual of a given age-sex group, the Committee on RDA chose to set the recommendation rather high, so that it would cover the majority of the population. For an average person, whose protein needs fall near the mean, the RDA provides half again as much protein in a day as actually needed. For a vital nutrient such as protein, this recommendation makes sense, and it will do no harm to consume somewhat more than the actual need. kCalories, on the other hand, are harmful in excess, because they lead to obesity; a deficit (within reason) is not harmful.

Like protein needs, the energy needs of individuals vary, with most people needing some amount of energy near the middle of the range. In setting the RDA for energy, the Committee on RDA elected to draw the line right at the mean. This ensured (if all members of our population were to consume exactly the recommended intake) that half would be consuming somewhat less than they actually needed as individuals, and that half would be consuming somewhat more.

The nutrient RDAs are set so that only a few people's requirements will not be met by them. The energy RDAs are set so that half of the population's requirements will fall below and half above them.

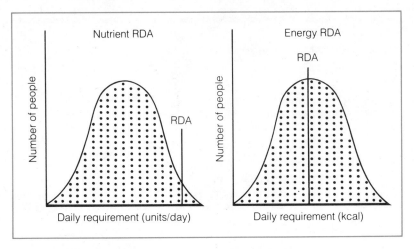

This choice minimizes the risk of encouraging excessive obesity or excessive thinness.

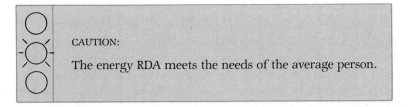

CAUTION:

The energy RDA meets the needs of the average person.

The Committee on RDA has made no recommendation for daily consumption of the energy nutrients (carbohydrate or fat)—only for total energy and protein. To understand the reason for this, recall that all three energy nutrients contribute kcalories, protein being unique among them because it also contributes nitrogen. You must therefore meet the RDA for protein to obtain the nitrogen you need. When you have consumed that amount of protein, you will have simultaneously consumed a certain number of kcalories. The remaining kcalories you need can come from carbohydrate and fat. It is left to you to choose how to balance these two nutrients in meeting your energy allowance.

The complete tables of heights and weights and recommended energy intakes for all age-sex groups are shown in Appendix O. The Canadian and FAO/WHO recommendations are also in Appendix O.

Diet Record Method   For an individualized estimate of your energy needs, the best indicator is the stability of your body weight over a period of time in which your activities are typical of your lifestyle. If you keep a strictly accurate record of all the food and beverages you consume for a week or two and if your weight does not change during that time, you can assume that your energy budget is balanced: kCalories-in equal kcalories-out. Records have to be kept for at least a week, however, because intakes fluctuate from day to day. (On about half the days you eat less, on the other half more kcalories than the average.) If during the week you gain a pound, you can assume that you expended 3,500 kcal less than you consumed, or an average of 500 kcal per day for seven days.

Laboratory Methods   Energy expenditures can also be accurately measured using laboratory equipment designed for this purpose. Two principles underlie the design of such machines. First, because heat is always a byproduct of energy expenditure, a device that measures escaping heat gives a direct measure of the kcalories being spent. Early efforts to accomplish this involved putting a person inside a large insulated, tightly sealed room with water circulating about it. The rise in the water's temperature indicated the number of kcalories being generated by the person's body. Inside the room, the person could be at rest or engaged in an activity such as studying or bicycle riding.

This clumsy and expensive method was replaced by a portable and much less expensive machine using the principle that the amount of oxygen consumed and carbon dioxide expelled is in direct proportion to the heat released. If twice as much heat is generated in one instance as in another, then twice as much oxygen will also be used. This advance made it possible to measure the kcalories expended during a wider range of physical activities. Laboratory studies of energy output by humans have been so extensive that tables are now available giving averages from which most people can estimate their own needs quite accurately. (An example appears in the Self-Study on Energy Output that follows Highlight 7.)

Estimating from Basal Metabolism and Activities   Human energy is spent in two major ways—on the basal metabolic processes and on voluntary activities. In order to calculate how much energy you spend in a day, you must obtain an estimate for the energy spent in each of these categories. A third way of spending energy, much smaller but still significant, is on digesting, absorbing, and metabolizing food. Let's take these up one by one.

● *Energy for basal metabolism.* Certain processes necessary for the maintenance of life proceed without your conscious awareness. The beating of the heart, the inhaling of oxygen and the exhaling of carbon dioxide, the ongoing metabolic activities of each cell, the maintenance of body temperature, and the sending of nerve impulses from the brain to direct these automatic activities are the basal metabolic processes that maintain life. Their minimum energy needs must be met before any kcalories can be used for physical activity or for the digestion of food.

The basal metabolic rate (BMR) is the rate at which kcalories are

basal metabolism: the total energy output of a body at rest after a 12-hour fast. Also called **basal metabolic rate** or **BMR.**

Shortcut for Estimating Energy Output

1. *Basal metabolism (BMR).* To get a rough approximation of the energy spent on BMR, use the factor 1.0 kcal per kilogram per hour (for men) or 0.9 kcal per kilogram per hour (for women). Example: for a 150-pound woman,

a. Change pounds to kilograms:

$$150 \text{ lb} \times \frac{1 \text{ kg}}{2.2 \text{ lb}} = 68 \text{ kg}$$

b. Multiply weight in kilograms by the BMR factor for women:

$$68 \text{ kg} \times \frac{0.9 \text{ kcal}}{\text{kg per hr}}$$
$$= 61 \text{ kcal per hr}$$

c. Multiply the kcalories used in one hour by the hours in a day:

$$61 \text{ kcal per hr} \times \frac{24 \text{ hr}}{1 \text{ day}}$$
$$= 1{,}464 \text{ kcal per day for BMR}$$

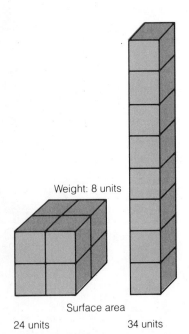

Weight: 8 units

Surface area

24 units   34 units

Both weigh the same, but the tall, thin structure will lose more heat to its surroundings.

spent for these maintenance activities, usually expressed as kcal per hour. The BMR varies from one person to another and may vary for one individual with a change in circumstance, physical condition, or age. The BMR is lowest when you are lying down in a room with a comfortable temperature and not digesting or metabolizing any food. In this relaxed state, few digestive juices are flowing, intestinal muscles are quiet, and other body muscles are just tense enough to keep them in good tone. At this time you need the least amount of oxygen and your cells are generating the least amount of heat. During sleep, you are probably more relaxed, but there is more muscular activity. That's why the basal metabolic rate is usually measured when the person is awake and can cooperate. She must be comfortable and relaxed and must have been without food or heavy exercise for at least 12 hours.

The BMR is surprisingly large. A woman whose total energy needs are 2,000 kcal a day may spend more than half of these, as much as 1,200 to 1,400 kcal, maintaining her basal metabolic processes. People often do not realize that so much of their energy is going to support the basic work of their bodies' cells, because they are unaware of all the work these cells do to maintain life.

The BMR is influenced by a number of factors. In general, the younger a person is, the higher the basal metabolic rate. This seems to be due to the increased activity of cells undergoing division, because it is most pronounced during the growth spurts that take place in infancy, puberty, and pregnancy. After growth stops, the BMR decreases by about 2 percent per decade throughout life.[11]

Body surface area also influences the BMR. Research has shown that it is indeed surface area, not weight, that is crucial. The greater the amount of body surface area, the higher the BMR. Thus of two people with different shapes who weigh the same amount, the short fat person will have a slower BMR than the tall thin person. The tall thin person has a greater skin surface from which heat is lost by radiation and so must run her metabolism faster to generate heat to replace it.

A third factor that influences BMR is gender. Males generally have a faster metabolic rate than females. It is thought that this may be due to the greater percentage of lean tissue in the male body. Muscle tissue is highly active even when it is resting, whereas fat tissue is comparatively inactive.

Fever also increases the energy needs of cells. Their increased activities to fight off infection require more energy and generate more heat than normal.

Fasting and constant malnutrition lower the BMR, in part because of the loss of lean tissues as well as the shutdown of functions the body can't afford to support. This lowering of BMR seems to be a protective mechanism to conserve energy when there is a shortage.

[11]Food and Nutrition Board, Committee on Recommended Allowances, *Recommended Dietary Allowances*, 8th ed. (Washington, D. C.: National Academy of Sciences, 1974).

Some glandular secretions influence the BMR. The adrenal glands secrete the hormone epinephrine into the blood in response to stress. The stress may be caused by as simple a situation as the command "Hurry, or you'll be late to work" or by as threatening a dilemma as the discovery of an intruder in the house. Whatever the cause, the body reacts by marshaling all its forces to meet the emergency. The increase in epinephrine increases the energy demands of every cell and thus temporarily raises the BMR.

The activity of the thyroid gland has a direct influence on basal metabolic rate. The less thyroxin secreted, the lower the energy requirement for maintenance of basal functions. Some people move about their tasks in a slow, deliberate fashion, due in part to the lower activity of their thyroid glands. Others race through the day, breaking dishes and becoming irritable, due to thyroid oversecretion. The difference in the two personalities may reflect a difference in their basal metabolic rates.

Contrary to what you might expect, physical training seems not to influence BMR. It might seem logical that athletes, with their greatly developed muscle tissue, would have a higher BMR than nonathletes of the same sex. Heavy exercise like jogging does speed up the basal metabolic rate, and it remains raised for several hours afterwards. However, research has revealed only a negligible difference in BMR between athletes and nonathletes under conditions of the BMR test—that is, after 12 hours of rest, when epinephrine secretion has returned to normal.

To sum up, basal metabolic rate is higher in the young, in people with a large surface area, in males, in people with fever or under stress, and in people with high thyroid gland activity. It is lowered by increasing age, fasting, and malnutrition, and it is unaffected by physical conditioning.

- *Energy for muscular activity.* The second of the three components of energy output is physical activity voluntarily undertaken and achieved by use of the skeletal muscles. The amount of energy needed for an activity like playing tennis or studying for an exam depends on the involvement of the muscles, on the amount of weight being moved, and on the length of time the activity is engaged in.

As disheartening as it may be for you to discover, mental activity requires very little energy, although it may make you very tired. Contraction of muscles, on the other hand, uses up a great many kcalories. In addition to the muscles involved in moving the body, the heart must beat faster to send nutrients and oxygen to the muscles, and the lungs must move faster to get rid of the carbon dioxide and bring in additional oxygen. The heavier person obviously needs more kcalories when performing the same task in the same time as a lighter person, because it takes extra effort to move her additional body weight. The longer the activity continues, the more kcalories will be used. The measurement of energy needed for a particular

thyroxin (thigh-ROX-in): a hormone secreted by the thyroid gland; regulates the basal metabolic rate.

2. *Activities.* To estimate the energy spent on muscular activities, classify the person's lifestyle as either sedentary, lightly active, moderately active, or very active and add the appropriate percentage to the BMR. The figures below are crude approximations based on the amount of muscular work performed. To select the one appropriate for you, remember to think in terms of the amount of *muscular* work you perform; don't confuse being busy with being active.

- For sedentary (mostly sitting) activity (a typist), add 20 percent of the BMR.
- For light activity (a teacher), add 30 percent.
- For moderate activity (a nurse), add 40 percent.
- For heavy work (a roofer), add 50 percent.

If the woman we're using as an example were a typist, we would estimate the energy she needs for physical activities by multiplying the BMR kcalories per day by 20 percent:

1,464 kcal per day × .20
= 293 kcal per day for physical activities

Energy for metabolizing food is called the **specific dynamic effect** (SDE), the specific dynamic energy, or the specific dynamic activity (SDA).

3. *SDE.* Energy spent by the body to deal with the food it receives represents a "tax" of about 10 percent of the kcalories in that food. If our woman ate 2,000 kcal in a day, the SDE "tax" would amount to

2,000 kcal × .10 = 200 kcal per day for the effect of food

4. *Total energy spent.* Now add items 1, 2, and 3 to obtain an estimate of the total energy spent in a day:

1,464 kcal + 293 kcal + 200 kcal = 1,957 kcal total per day (ANS.)

[If we didn't know how much she ate, we could guess. Assuming that her energy budget was balanced, we could reason that she ate about enough to meet her needs for items 1 and 2, and we could take 10 percent of that total to derive item 3:

1,464 kcal (BMR) + 293 kcal (activities) = 1,757 kcal
1,757 kcal × .10 = 176 kcal per day for the effect of food (SDE)
1,464 + 293 + 176 = 1,933 kcal per day (ANS.)]

Thus this woman's total energy needs for a day might be about 1,925 to 1,975 kcal. The exact figure is based on several estimates, so it's probably best to express her needs as falling within a 50-kcal range.

physical activity, then, is expressed in three units: kcalories per weight per unit of time.

As people age, their activities taper off somewhat. This slowing down varies greatly from one person to the next but averages out in such a way that people's total energy needs (including BMR) probably decrease by about 5 percent per decade after the age of 20.

● *Energy for metabolizing food.* The third component of energy expenditure has to do with processing food. When food is taken into the body, many cells that have been dormant begin to be active. The muscles that move the food through the intestinal tract speed up their rhythmic contractions; the cells that manufacture and secrete digestive juices begin their tasks. All these cells and others need extra energy as they "come alive" to participate in the digestion, absorption, and metabolism of food. In addition, the presence of food stimulates the general metabolism. This stimulation is the specific dynamic effect (SDE) of food, or the specific dynamic activity (SDA), and is generally thought to represent about 6 to 10 percent of the total food energy taken in. Because food energy taken in normally equals energy expended, the SDE is usually calculated by taking 10 percent of the total kcalories used for BMR and physical activity.

Food faddists make a big thing out of the specific dynamic effect, suggesting that a high-protein diet stimulates such tremendous energy losses that it will increase the rate of weight loss. Actually, high-protein and low-protein diets have the same effect.[12]

Weight Loss and Gain Rates

A deficit of 500 kcal a day brings about loss of body fat at the rate of a pound a week; of 1,000 kcal, two pounds a week. Extraordinarily active people, by virtue of their activities, or extremely obese persons, by virtue of the metabolic demands made by the sheer bulk of their body cells, can lose more. For those who are only moderately obese, the maximum possible rate of fat loss is one to two pounds a week, which for most people means an intake of about 1,000 to 1,500 kcal a day. Below 1,200, the dieter will be losing lean tissue, and at this restricted kcalorie level, the diet planner is hard put to achieve adequacy for all the vitamins and minerals.

The principles outlined in this chapter are simple, but putting them into practice is more difficult than you might imagine. Obesity and underweight are complex problems with social and psychological ramifications, as well as the metabolic ones just described. Chapter 8 provides some practical pointers for the dieter but deals first with all the factors that contribute to the problems of underweight and obesity.

[12]R. L. Pike and M. L. Brown, *Nutrition: An Integrated Approach*, 2nd ed. (New York: Wiley, 1975), p. 835.

Summing Up

Figure 1 summarizes the central pathways of metabolism. The principal compounds derived from carbohydrate, fat, and protein in the diet are glucose, glycerol and fatty acids, and amino acids. Glucose may be anabolized to glycogen or catabolized to pyruvate, which in turn yields acetyl CoA. Glycerol and fatty acids may be anabolized to triglycerides or catabolized (glycerol to pyruvate, fatty acids to acetyl CoA). Amino acids may be anabolized to protein or catabolized (after deamination) to pyruvate, acetyl CoA, or TCA cycle intermediates.

Pyruvate is reconvertible to glucose, but the reaction yielding acetyl CoA from pyruvate is irreversible. Hence fatty acids cannot serve as a source of glucose in the body. All three energy nutrients are convertible to acetyl CoA, however, and hence can be used to manufacture body fat.

If a person fasts or if carbohydrate is undersupplied, lean body tissue is catabolized to meet the brain's need for glucose. Within a day or so ketosis sets in: Fatty acids are metabolized to ketones, which can meet some of the brain's energy need. The nitrogen removed from protein is combined with carbon and oxygen in urea and excreted. Below about 900 kcal a day, a diet imposes lean tissue loss and ketosis, and the protein kcalories in such a diet are equivalent to carbohydrate kcalories in their protein-sparing effect. Weight loss may be dramatic, but fat loss may be slower than on a moderate, balanced low-kcalorie diet. To design such a diet requires adjusting energy balance so that the intake is reduced, the output is increased, or both.

Energy intake can be computed by adding up the kcalorie values of the foods consumed or can be estimated by using the averaged exchange system values for many foods. The energy available from food was originally determined by measuring the heat lost when the food was completely burned. Before tables of the kcaloric values of foods were published, adjustments were made for the incomplete breakdown of food in the body.

Energy output for various age-sex groups are provided by recommendations such as the RDA, but lifestyle has to be taken into account when estimating an individual's energy needs. Machines designed to measure energy expenditure work by measuring heat lost from the body or oxygen used. Data collected in this way have yielded tables from which you can estimate your energy needs quite accurately.

The body's total energy output falls into three categories: energy to support the basal metabolism, energy for muscular activity, and energy to digest, absorb, and metabolize food (SDE, the specific dynamic effect of food). Basal metabolic activities are estimated to require about 1.0 kcalorie per kilogram of body weight per hour (0.9 for women). Muscular activity requires an additional 20 to 50 percent above the basal metabolism. The effect of food adds another 10 percent to the total energy expenditure.

The basal metabolic rate is influenced primarily by age and growth rate, body shape, and sex (males have a higher BMR). It is also affected by fever, fasting, and hormonal secretions (especially epinephrine and thyroxin) but not by body conditioning.

An energy deficit of 3,500 kcal is necessary for the loss of a pound of body fat. Loss of body fat in excess of two pounds a week can rarely be sustained. A diet supplying fewer than 1,200 kcal per day can be made adequate in vitamins and minerals only with great difficulty.

To Explore Further

A brief and clear explanation in paperback of the ways energy flows through living things is Lehninger, A. L., *Bioenergetics: The Molecular Basis of Biological Energy Transformation* (New York: W. A. Benjamin, 1965).

What happens during fasting is clearly and completely explained in an article for the general reader:

Young, V. R., and Scrimshaw, N.S., The physiology of starvation, *Scientific American* 225 (1971):14-21.

An exploration of the parallels between modern science and Eastern mysticism is provided by Capra, F., *The Tao of Physics* (New York: Bantam Books, 1975).

HIGHLIGHT 7

AN OPTIONAL CHAPTER
Extracting Energy from
Carbohydrate, Fat, and Protein

It is through this structure, in the process of metabolism, that matter and energy flow. Entering in various forms and quantities, they are temporarily shaped exactly to the form and condition of the organism; they conform to the characteristics of the kingdom, class, order, family, genus, species, and variety to which it belongs, and they assume even the characteristics of the individual itself. Then they depart through the various channels of excretion.

LAWRENCE J. HENDERSON

When you were a student in the elementary grades, your teacher probably taught you that you ate food because it gave you energy to run and play. That is one level of understanding metabolism. Later you enlarged your knowledge to include the fact that when you ate meat you were receiving the energy of the sun, which had fallen on green plants to make glucose that was consumed by the grazing animal. Today you can embellish this fact with many chemical and biological details.

You do not need a deeper level of understanding of metabolism than the preceding chapters have given to master the remaining concepts in this book; however, metabolism is such a fascinating subject that we want to make the next level available to you. This optional chapter provides no more than a glimpse at the wonders of metabolism as seen by scientists, but we warn you that it may encourage you to pursue the subject further.

Energy

One of the strangest notions that human beings who study the nature of things have ever come up with is the idea of energy. Energy has no concrete existence; it weighs nothing. And yet it can move mountains and make itself felt over great distances. Energy is apparent to us sometimes as light, at other times as heat; one seems to turn into the other. Energy has no mass, and yet it possesses a characteristic that

energy: the capacity to do work.

Forms of energy: heat, light, electrical, mechanical, chemical.

249

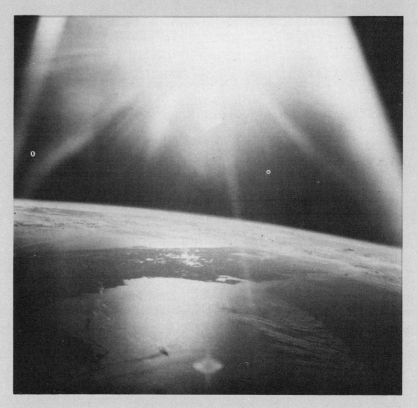

Sunlight provides the energy for life on earth. This photo, taken from an Apollo spacecraft, shows the Florida peninsula, with the Gulf of Mexico in the foreground. Courtesy of NASA.

work: the moving of a mass through a distance.

First Law of Thermodynamics: Energy is neither created nor destroyed during chemical or physical processes, but it may be transformed from one form to another.

physicists call charge—and so it can do the work of electricity. Physicists have measured energy and have satisfied themselves that energy is never created or destroyed. Instead, as it is converted from one form to another, energy is conserved. Wherever there is motion there is energy, and yet energy may seem to stand still, like the energy stored in a boulder at the edge of a mountain precipice. Wherever there is the power to move things there is also energy—like the energy in the storage battery of your car. If you like to ponder the mysteries of the universe, one of the most wonderful (wonder-full) is that energy is real. It exists; it has been measured; it works.

The energy in food, or more properly in the nutrients of which food is composed, is found in what we have somewhat imprecisely called the bonds that hold the atoms of those nutrients together. The glucose molecule, with which you are by now thoroughly familiar, possesses 24 atoms held together by 23 such bonds, each composed of a pair of electrons. As glucose is taken apart during catabolism, some of the electron energy that constitutes those bonds becomes available to form bonds between other atoms. As a glucose molecule is broken down from a six-carbon compound to two three-carbon compounds, your system can capture the energy that held the two three-carbon chains together and use that energy to combine two other molecules. Let's call the two molecules B and C and the new, larger compound B-C. Later, by breaking B-C, you can retrieve the energy and use it to put together two amino acids and begin forming a protein. The proteins of hair, for example, are formed by the addition of amino acids to a chain in a process fueled by energy released in the breaking of bonds like those in glucose.

Only living systems can perform this remarkable feat of transferring the energy from the breaking of bonds (catabolism) in one molecule to the synthesis of bonds (anabolism) between two other molecules without a significant rise in temperature or a shift in the acidity of the environment. Breaking of molecules also occurs in dead organic systems, but when such a breakdown occurs (for example, when firewood burns), the released energy is not captured in a usable form but is converted to heat and light energy, which radiate away from the object. The process by which the body breaks down glucose is ultimately similar to that by which the glucose (cellulose) in firewood is broken down when it burns: Oxygen is consumed and energy is released (along with carbon dioxide and water). But unlike burning firewood, the body doesn't go up in flames. Instead, it retains most of the energy in the chemical bonds of body compounds and releases only a little as heat.

In some ways, the metabolism of the nutrients is analogous to the transformations that can be performed with Tinker Toys. The wheels are atoms, the sticks electrons. A toy jungle gym built with these pieces, like a nutrient molecule, can be taken apart, and the same wheels and sticks can be used to build a toy crane (analogously, a body structure like hair). There are two important differences, however: A dismantled Tinker Toy can lie around for days before the pieces are used to build another one, but in chemical reactions, the electrons never stay still. They either escape or immediately become associated with atoms, holding them together. So in the body, electron energy removed from glucose and other nutrients is immediately used to form bonds in other compounds.

The other difference is that the sticks may be used over and over again without losing their binding ability, but in chemical reactions a little energy is lost (as heat) in each transfer. The loss of energy from your metabolic system literally heats you up; your body is maintained at 98.6° F by the rate of the metabolic reactions it performs. This continual loss of heat energy from the body makes it necessary for people to refuel periodically—that is, to obtain a new energy supply from food to continue their metabolic work.

Second Law of Thermodynamics: The natural tendency of any physical system consisting of a large number of individual units is to go from a state of order to a state of disorder, thus decreasing the usable energy.

Where does this heat energy go? The total amount of energy in the universe remains constant; in that sense this energy is not lost. But it is lost to you: You can only use energy in forms—such as chemical bonds—that can do your metabolic or mechanical work. Pondering this question has brought physicists to the brink of metaphysics and philosophy, areas outside our province as nutritionists. References at the end of this Highlight will carry you further in these directions should you choose to follow them.

As you try to put together your own mental picture of what happens to energy during metabolism, you may anticipate that a molecule B and a molecule C are available somewhere nearby while nutrients are being broken down. These molecules can be put together whenever energy becomes available. This is indeed the way the system works. Molecules B and C are floating around in all your body cells; wherever energy is made available to put them together, the compound B-C is formed. The energy is captured between them. B and C are brought together on the surface of an enzyme-complex that takes apart some other molecule, releasing energy.

The enzymes that can perform this energy transfer are those that catalyze coupled reactions. An example will illustrate. Picture an enzyme-complex (a cluster of giant molecules whose surfaces are bristling with positive and negative charges) that has on its surface a place for splitting glucose and elsewhere on its surface a place where B and C can be put together. A molecule of glucose approaches this enzyme-complex and begins to split in half. For the coupled reaction to occur, B and C must also be present at the other site. As the glucose splits, the electron energy that bonded it together is transferred to the bond between B and C (losing only a little energy as heat). At no time can the energy that bonded the glucose be freed or lost altogether as heat or light.

Loading Energy into Carriers

It is a strange paradox that even though energy weighs nothing, it still must be carried. When it is being held in the cells of animals for future use, it is carried in a compound like adenosine triphosphate (ATP). ATP is the compound B-C we have been using in our example of coupled reactions. Molecule B is adenosine diphosphate (ADP, containing two phosphates) and molecule C is another phosphate. When a molecule of any of the energy nutrients gives up some of its energy, ADP and P use that energy to combine into ATP, which has three phosphates.

coupled reaction: a chemical event in which an enzyme-complex catalyzes two reactions simultaneously; often involves the breakdown of one compound to two and the synthesis of another from two.

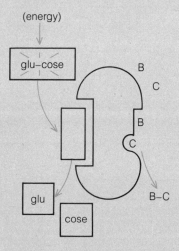

ATP or adenosine triphosphate (ad-DEN-o-sin try-FOS-fate): the commonest energy carrier in cells (structure is shown in Appendix C).

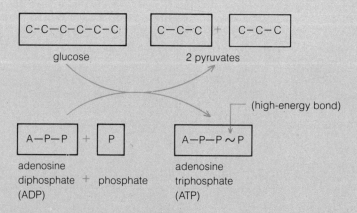

(It is not important to learn the structures of these compounds. ADP is merely another molecule like others you are familiar with, composed of C, H, O, and N and containing two phosphorus—P—atoms derived from the mineral phosphorus in the diet. Free phosphate, also derived from dietary phosphorus, abounds in cells too.)

Not all bonds in the nutrients possess enough energy to bind phosphate to ADP; there are high-energy bonds and low-energy bonds. Hence not every reaction in which a large molecule is broken down yields energy that can be captured in this way; many yield heat only. Then, too, some high-energy bonds cannot be used in the body because humans do not possess the necessary enzymes to make the transfer. This is why protein, fat, and carbohydrate (and alcohol) are the only molecules that serve as energy nutrients: During their breakdown your body cells can extract the energy from them in a usable form—high-energy compounds like ATP.

The metabolism of alcohol is described in Highlight 9.

There are billions and billions of molecules of ATP in your cells. When you use or spend this energy, the above reaction is reversed. ATP breaks down to ADP and P in a coupled reaction, using the energy to power the chemical work of the cell—whether that is the building of a protein or the contraction of a muscle. (The symbol for a coupled reaction is two arrows that first converge and then diverge, as illustrated in the margin.)

The symbol for a coupled reaction

The reversible reaction between ADP + P and ATP provides an energy-carrying system that is universal in animal organisms. Any other two molecules could be used in theory, and some are to a limited extent; the only requirement is that a high-energy bond be formed when they are put together. As it happens, animals have evolved to use the ATP system as a most convenient way of carrying and exchanging energy between molecules in their cells.

Other energy carriers in animal systems:

Guanosine (GWON-o-sine) diphosphate (GDP) + phosphate (P) → guanosine triphosphate (GTP) (used in protein synthesis).

Creatine (CREE-uh-tin) + P → creatine phosphate (used in muscle contraction).

Generating ATP: A Closer Look

Throughout this book we refer to glucose as a six-carbon compound that breaks apart into two molecules of pyruvate, yielding energy. This is true but not true enough for you who are studying this optional chapter. If you are to understand how the energy in nutrients is parceled out into ATPs, we must fill in the missing details. What happens between the time a molecule of glucose arrives in the cell and the time it is converted to pyruvate and then to acetyl CoA?

The conversion of a molecule of glucose to carbon dioxide and water yields a great deal of energy—far more than could be picked up by ADP all at once. Therefore, the release of this energy is accomplished by many small steps. This conversion takes place in two sets of reactions. The first of these, leading from glucose to pyruvate, is anaerobic (without oxygen) and is called glycolysis. The next set, leading from acetyl CoA to carbon dioxide, is aerobic (with oxygen) and involves the tricarboxylic acid (TCA) cycle.

anaerobic: taking place in the absence of oxygen.

  an = without
  aero = air (oxygen)

glycolysis (gligh-KOLL-ih-sis): the breakdown of glucose to pyruvate; an anaerobic process.

aerobic: taking place in the presence of oxygen.

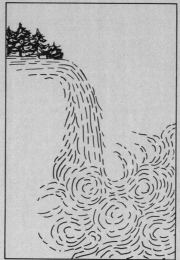

Energy of falling water too great to capture

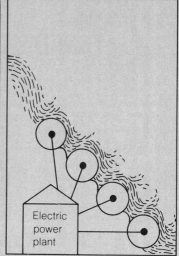

Energy of falling water captured by a series of water wheels

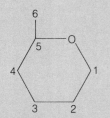

This is the way chemists number the carbons in a glucose molecule

NAD⁺: an organic ion. For a discussion of ions, see Appendix B. NAD^+ is further defined as a coenzyme in Chapter 9.

Glycolysis Glucose must be given some activation energy before it can proceed toward the release of its own energy, just as a log must be given some heat from twigs and paper before it will burn spontaneously. This activation of glucose is accomplished in a coupled reaction with ATP.

In the process of activation, a phosphate is attached to the carbon that chemists call number 6. The product is called, logically enough, glucose-6-phosphate. In the next step, glucose-6-phosphate is rearranged by an enzyme, and a phosphate is added in another coupled reaction with ATP. The product this time is fructose-1,6-diphosphate. At this point the six-carbon sugar has been activated. It has a phosphate group on its first and sixth carbons and enough energy to break apart. Two ATPs have been used to accomplish this.

(From this point to the production of pyruvate we will use letters in place of compound names. The names are in the drawing of the reactions on the next page, for those who wish to know them.)

When fructose-1,6-diphosphate breaks in half, the two three-carbon compounds (A and A′) are not identical. Each has a phosphate group attached, but only one converts directly to pyruvate. The other compound converts easily to the first. (Compound A′ is usually ignored, except for its role as the point of entry for glycerol; we say that two molecules of compound A are derived from one glucose.)

In the step from compound A to compound B, enough energy is released to convert NAD^+ to $NADH + H^+$. Also, in the steps from B to C and from E to pyruvate, ATP is regenerated. Remember that there are effectively two molecules of compound A coming from glucose;

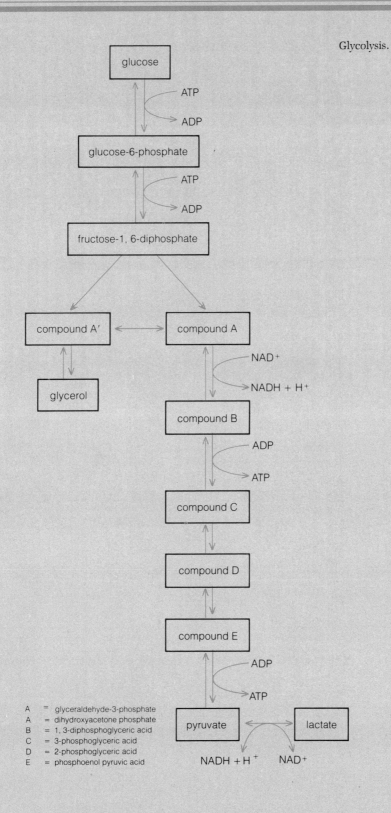

Glycolysis.

therefore, four ATP molecules are generated. Two ATPs were needed to get the sequence started, so the net gain at this point is two ATPs and two molecules of NADH + H$^+$.

So far, no oxygen has been used; the process has been anaerobic. But at this point, oxygen is needed. If oxygen is not immediately available, pyruvate converts to lactic acid, to soak up the hydrogens from the NADH + H$^+$ that was generated. Lactic acid accumulates until oxygen becomes available. However, in the energy path from glucose to carbon dioxide, this side step usually is not necessary. As you will see later, each NADH + H$^+$ moves to the electron transport chain to unload its hydrogens onto oxygen. The associated energy produces 2 ATPs, making the total yield 8 ATPs for the process from glucose to pyruvate.

The body's disposal of lactic acid is of great interest to the athlete who knows that its accumulation in his muscles will cause fatigue. The muscle cells draw their energy in the first burst of activity from the available high-energy compounds (similar to ATP) but soon exhaust this source. To replenish it, they then start breaking down their stored glycogen. So far, so good, but if the exertion is very severe, the heart cannot pump oxygen to them fast enough to permit aerobic metabolism to proceed at full speed. So lactic acid accumulates. At the end of the activity, the oxygen debt is repaid, and lactic acid is shunted back into the main stream of metabolism by being reconverted to pyruvate.

The muscles would be completely debilitated by the accumulation of lactic acid after a while, because they can't dispose of it. But they do have an alternative: They can release it into the bloodstream, and the liver can pick it up and reconvert it to glucose. To be well prepared for an endurance event, the athlete takes two steps based on these facts: He ensures that his muscles are well supplied with glycogen at the start (see page 22), and he warms up so that the cycling of lactate to the liver will already be underway when he enters the competition.

The Tricarboxylic Acid Cycle (TCA Cycle)   The TCA cycle is the name given to the set of reactions involving oxygen and leading from acetyl CoA to carbon dioxide (and water). To link glycolysis to the TCA cycle, pyruvate is converted to acetyl CoA. This set of aerobic reactions is not restricted to the metabolism of carbohydrate. It also includes fat and protein, as shown in the diagram that follows. Any substance that can be converted to acetyl CoA directly, or indirectly through pyruvate, may enter the cycle.

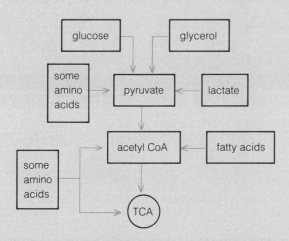

The step from pyruvate to acetyl CoA is an exceedingly complex one. We have included only those substances that will help you understand the transfer of energy from the nutrients. When pyruvate is in the presence of oxygen, it loses a carbon in the form of carbon dioxide, and CoA is attached. In the process NAD^+ picks up two hydrogens with their associated energy, becoming $NADH + H^+$.

As the acetyl CoA breaks down to carbon dioxide and water, its energy is captured in ATP. Let's follow the steps by which this occurs (see Figure 1):

1. Acetyl CoA combines with a four-carbon compound, oxaloacetate. The CoA comes off, and the product is a six-carbon compound, citrate.

2. The atoms of citrate are rearranged to form isocitrate.

3. Now NAD^+ reacts with isocitrate. Two Hs and two electrons are removed from the isocitrate. One H becomes attached to the NAD^+ with the two electrons; the other H is released as a free proton. Thus NAD^+ becomes $NADH + H^+$.

Remember this $NADH + H^+$. It is carrying the Hs and the energy from the last reaction. But let's follow the carbons first.

A carbon is removed and combined with oxygen, forming carbon dioxide (which diffuses away in the blood and is exhaled). What is left is the five-carbon compound alpha-ketoglutarate.

4. Now two compounds interact with alpha-ketoglutarate—a molecule of CoA and a molecule of NAD^+. In this complex reaction a carbon is removed and combined with oxygen (forming carbon dioxide); two Hs are removed and go to NAD^+ (forming $NADH + H^+$); and the CoA is attached to the remaining four-carbon compound, forming succinyl CoA.

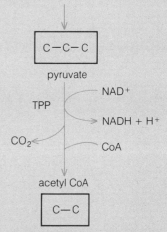

(TPP is a helper compound containing the B vitamin thiamin; see Chapter 9.)

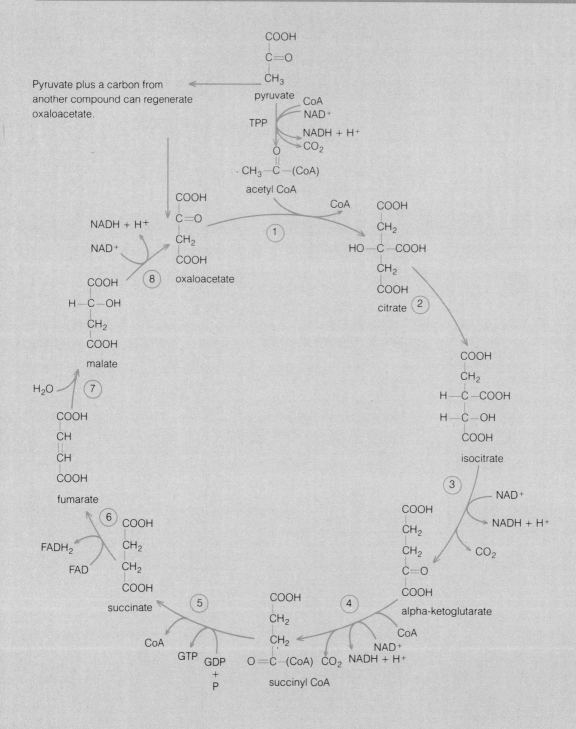

Figure 1 The TCA cycle.

Remember this NADH + H$^+$ also.
You will see later what happens to it.

5. Now two molecules react with succinyl CoA—a molecule called GDP and one of phosphate (P). The CoA comes off, the GDP and P combine to form the high-energy compound GTP, and succinate remains.

Remember this GTP.

6. In the next reaction two Hs with their energy are removed from succinate and are transferred to a molecule called FAD (an electron-hydrogen receiver like NAD$^+$) to form FADH$_2$. The product that remains is fumarate.

Remember this FADH$_2$.

7. Next a molecule of water is added to fumarate, forming malate.

8. A molecule of NAD$^+$ reacts with the malate; two Hs with their associated energy are removed from the malate and form NADH + H$^+$. The product that remains is the four-carbon compound oxaloacetate.

Remember this NADH + H$^+$.

We are back where we started. The oxaloacetate formed in this process can combine with another molecule of acetyl CoA (step 1), and the cycle can begin again. (The whole scheme is shown in Figure 1.)

So far, what you have seen is that two carbons are brought in with acetyl CoA and that two carbons end up in carbon dioxide. But where is the energy and the ATP we promised you?

Each time a pair of hydrogen atoms is removed from one of the compounds in the cycle, it carries a pair of electrons with it. This chemical bond energy is thus captured into the compound to which the Hs become attached. A review of the eight steps of the cycle shows that energy is thus transferred into other compounds in steps 3, 4, 6, and 8. In step 5, energy is harnessed to bind GDP and P together to form GTP. Thus the compounds NADH + H$^+$ (three molecules), FADH$_2$, and GTP are built with energy originally found in acetyl CoA. To see how this energy ends up in ATP, we must follow the electrons further. Let us take those attached to NAD$^+$ as an example.

The six reactions described here are those of the **electron transport chain.** Since oxygen is required for these reactions and ADP and P are combined to form ATP in several of them (ADP is phosphorylated), they are also called **oxidative phosphorylation.**

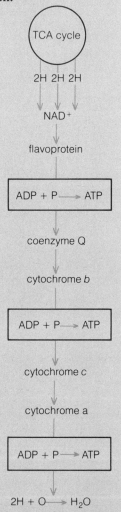

Electron transport. The electrons associated with the Hs move from compound to compound.

The Electron Transport Chain An important concept to remember at this point is that an electron is not a fixed amount of energy. The electrons that bond the H to NAD^+ in NADH have a relatively large amount of energy. In the series of reactions that follow, they lose this energy in small amounts, until at the end they are attached (with Hs) to oxygen (O) to make water (H_2O). In some of the steps, the energy they lose is captured into ATP in coupled reactions.

In the first step of the electron transport chain, NADH reacts with a molecule called a flavoprotein, losing its electrons (and their Hs). The products are NAD^+ and reduced flavoprotein. A little energy is lost as heat in this reaction.

The flavoprotein passes on the electrons to a molecule called coenzyme Q. Again they lose some energy as heat, but ADP and P participate in this reaction and gain much of the energy to bond together and form ATP. This is a coupled reaction.

$$ADP + P \rightarrow ATP$$

Coenzyme Q passes the electrons to cytochrome b. Again the electrons lose energy.

Cytochrome b passes the electrons to cytochrome c in a coupled reaction in which ATP is formed.

$$ADP + P \rightarrow ATP$$

Cytochrome c passes the electrons to cytochrome a.

Cytochrome a passes them (with their Hs) to an atom of oxygen (O), forming water (H_2O). This is a coupled reaction in which ATP is formed.

$$ADP + P \rightarrow ATP$$

The entire electron transport chain is diagramed in Figure 2. As you can see, each time NADH is oxidized (loses its electrons) by this means, the energy it loses is parceled out into three ATP molecules. When the electrons are passed on to water at the end, they have much less energy than they had to begin with. This completes the story of the electrons from NADH.

As for $FADH_2$, its electrons enter the electron transport chain at coenzyme Q. From coenzyme Q to water there are only two steps in which ATP is generated. Therefore, $FADH_2$ coming out of the TCA cycle yields just two ATP molecules.

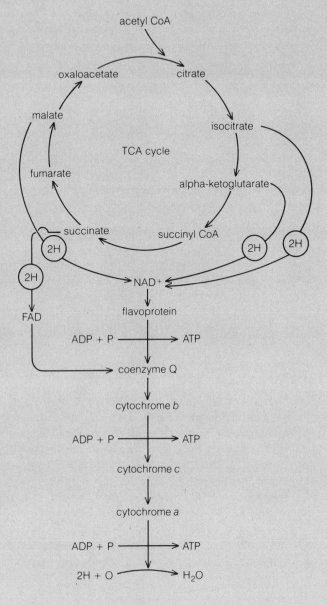

Figure 2   The electron transport chain.

One energy-receiving compound of the TCA cycle (GTP) does not enter the electron transport chain but gives its energy directly to ADP in a simple phosphorylation reaction.

You are now ready to look at the balance sheet of glucose metabolism (see table on p. 262). Glycolysis has yielded 4 NADH + H$^+$ and 4 ATP molecules and has spent 2 ATP. The 2 acetyl CoAs going through the TCA cycle have yielded 6 NADH + H$^+$, 2 FADH$_2$, and 2 GTP molecules. After the NADH + H$^+$ and FADH$_2$ have gone through the electron transport chain, there are 34 ATP. Added to these are the 4 ATP from

Table 1. Balance Sheet for Glucose Metabolism

	Expenditures	Income
Glycolysis:		
1 glucose	2 ATP	4 ATP
1 fructose-1,6-diphosphate		2 NADH + H^+
2 pyruvate		2 NADH + H^+
TCA cycle:		
2 isocitrate		2 NADH + H^+
2 alpha-ketoglutarate		2 NADH + H^+
2 succinyl CoA		2 GTP
2 succinate		2 $FADH_2$
2 malate		2 NADH + H^+
Total ATPs collected:		
From glycolysis	2 ATP	4 ATP
From 10 NADH + H^+		30 ATP
From 2 GTP		2 ATP
From 2 $FADH_2$		4 ATP
Totals:	2 ATP	40 ATP
Balance on hand from 1 molecule glucose:		38 ATP

glycolysis and the 2 ATP from GTP, making the total 40 ATP generated from one molecule of glucose. After the expense of 2 ATP is subtracted, there is a net gain of 38 ATP.

The TCA cycle and the electron transport chain are the body's major means of capturing the energy from nutrients in ATP molecules. There are other means that contribute (glycolysis is one), but these are the most efficient. Biologists and chemists understand much more about these processes than has been presented here. To Explore Further at the end of this Highlight suggests some readings that were selected for the clarity with which they present further details. Some considerations relating to the release of energy from ATP will complete this overview of the way in which energy from food does the body's work.

Unloading Energy from Carriers

Okay—so now you are full of energy. You have just eaten a meal and catabolized the carbohydrate, fat, and protein in it, making billions of molecules of ATP. What do you do with it? Fortunately, you don't have to make all of these decisions consciously. About two-thirds of your energy is spent automatically to maintain your vital functions, using a priority system that guarantees that the most important work is done first. The other third you are free to spend as you wish—contemplating the mysteries of nature, playing tennis, or doing whatever else you choose to do.

Two major classes of activities consume human energy each day. The first are the basal metabolic processes, which go on all the time, even during sleep. These are vital processes: the maintenance of the heartbeat, respiration, nerve function, glandular activity, generation of heat, and the like, without which you could not be said to be alive. The second are the voluntary activities, over which you have conscious control: sitting, standing, running, eating, playing the piano, and the like. The amount of energy spent on each of these types of activity can be measured, and their total (plus a little energy needed to metabolize food) represents the total amount of energy you must consume each day to stay in balance. These measurements and the concept of energy balance were the subjects of Chapter 7. But it seems worthwhile to give a few examples here of the way the energy taken from nutrients and transferred into ATP is used to power these activities.

Basal metabolism is defined and discussed further in Chapter 7.

● *ATP provides energy for catabolism.* A most vital need is to ensure that you have a continuous influx of energy to replace the energy you spend. At certain points during the catabolism of carbohydrate, fat, and protein, energy is needed to power a reaction that otherwise would not occur. At each of these points, a molecule of ATP is split into ADP + P to push the reaction.

   You can see that catabolism is not a cost-free process. Energy (ATP) must be spent at certain points to keep catabolism going. However, the amount of ATP generated during catabolism is greater than the amount consumed, so that in the end there is a net gain. The catabolism of acetyl CoA is the most efficient energy-yielding process in the body, estimated to capture about 66 percent of the total initial energy.

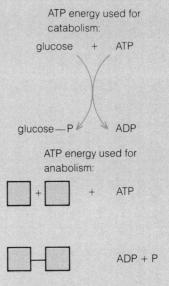

ATP energy used for catabolism:

glucose + ATP

glucose—P   ADP

ATP energy used for anabolism:

● *ATP provides energy for anabolism.* As already mentioned, anabolic processes require ATP. To make a protein chain, one ATP is split for each amino acid added to the chain; to make glycogen, one ATP provides the energy to add each glucose; to make fatty acids from acetyl CoA, ATP is needed at the rate of one for each acetate added; and so on. To keep the body's metabolic work going on, energy must continuously be supplied.

● *ATP provides energy for muscle movements.* A muscle cell is packed with an orderly array of long, thin protein molecules lined up side by side. To contract a muscle, molecule A and molecule B must combine chemically, moving closer together as they do so. They must then execute another chemical reaction that slides them even closer together. The reactions that make muscles move are powered by energy carriers similar to ATP. For peristalsis, for the beating of the heart muscle, for the inhalation of air into the lungs, and for many other automatic muscular actions, these reactions do the necessary work.

● *ATP provides energy for the transmission of nerve impulses.* Even during sleep, the brain and nerves are active. At the molecular level,

The contractile proteins of muscle are actin and myosin.

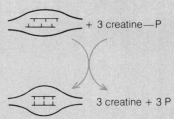

Creatine phosphate energy used for muscle contraction:

+ 3 creatine—P

3 creatine + 3 P

Lipid in muscle. The lipid droplets are stored close to the muscle fiber (bottom), and the mitochondria, which generate energy from fatty acids, crowd around these droplets. This was photographed under an electron microscope at a magnification of 47,000X.

From D. W. Fawcett, *An Atlas of Fine Structure*, (Philadelphia: Saunders, 1966), Fig. 60. Courtesy of the author and publisher.

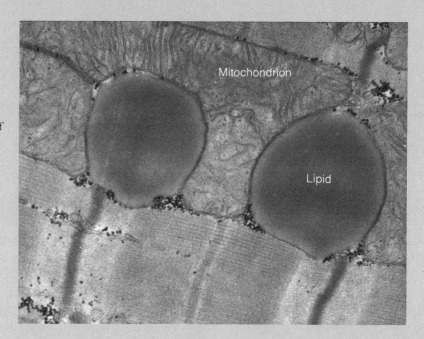

Mitochondrion

Lipid

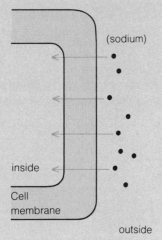

During the transmission of a nerve impulse, sodium rushes into the cell, depolarizing it. (Potassium rushes out: not shown.)

the membranes of the nerve cells, which contain protein pumps, maintain an electrical charge by pumping sodium ions out and potassium ions in. When a nerve impulse travels along these cells, they depolarize: Sodium rushes in and potassium out. To regain the readiness to fire, the membrane pumps go to work to repolarize the cell, sorting out the potassium and sodium ions again. Each protein pump splits one molecule of ATP each time it transfers an ion across the membrane.

These few examples show the uses of ATP-carried energy for basal metabolic activities. If you wish to use additional energy to compose a poem, knit a sweater, or jog a mile, additional ATP must be available for the extra nervous and muscular activities that are involved.

Completing the Picture

This Highlight concludes one of nutrition's major stories: how the four principal types of atoms found in food and the energy that bonds them flow into the body, undergo rearrangements there, and ultimately flow out again. It may be satisfying to you to realize that you can now follow any of these atoms, or the energy connecting them, through the complete cycle around which they flow. Just for fun, let's imagine painting a carbon atom red and watching it travel through its cycle. Let's begin at the point where the carbon atom forms part of a molecule of carbon dioxide in the air.

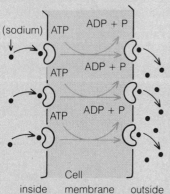

ATP energy is then used to repolarize the cell membrane.

This particular molecule of carbon dioxide enters a potato leaf. There, sparked by a photon from the sun, it is combined with water to become part of a molecule of glucose. This glucose then travels to the root, where it is attached to other glucose molecules to make starch. The starch is stored in the potato until you eat it. After you have swallowed it, the red carbon atom appears in your intestine, where the starch is hydrolyzed to glucose again; the glucose enters your bloodstream and is carried to a cell. Inside the cell, the glucose is broken down into two three-carbon compounds, and the red carbon atom finds itself in one of them.

Let's suppose that the three-carbon compound loses a carbon to carbon dioxide, leaving the red one in acetyl CoA. The acetyl CoA may be used to synthesize body fat, in which case the red carbon atom will be trapped in a fat cell for a while, or it may be used to synthesize an amino acid and become part of a protein such as hemoglobin and as such travel in a red blood cell throughout the circulatory system.

Now let's suppose that the body's primary need is for energy and that the acetyl CoA is further broken down to two molecules of carbon dioxide and water. Released in one of these carbon dioxide molecules, the red carbon atom finds its way back into the blood. Ultimately it is freed into air spaces in the lungs and breathed back into the atmosphere.

Around again the red carbon atom goes, possibly cycling back through another potato plant and into you again. But it is far more likely that it will go elsewhere next time—into an acorn on an oak tree, perhaps, and later into a chipmunk's cheek. And around again.

It may prove satisfying to you to follow the path of a hydrogen atom or an oxygen atom in the same way. There is also a nitrogen cycle, although the complete outlines are not apparent from the discussions of nitrogen that have been presented here. But let us take one more example of one of nature's shifting scenes—energy flow.

Energy is born in the sun. It enters a potato leaf and is captured into glucose. As part of the bonds in glucose, it enters your body. When the glucose is broken apart, energy is freed. It may be used to combine a molecule of ADP with phosphate to make ATP. Some energy therefore stays in your body when the carbon with which it was associated is breathed out. Later, the energy in the ATP is either spent or stored. Let's assume in this case that it is spent.

The ATP is broken apart, releasing some energy to help move a muscle or to transmit a nerve impulse. Some of the energy ends up as work accomplished and heat radiated away. You cannot say that this energy is lost; it is just no longer available to do work.

Energy changes forms, unlike atoms—which can cycle again and again through the atmosphere, to plants, and back to the atmosphere, always remaining recognizable. Originating in the sun, energy may exist for a while as part of a chemical bond and later as heat energy. This heat energy, although still in the same amount as when it came from the sun, cannot be used again by plants or animals to fuel their

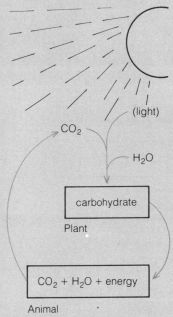

The carbon cycle.

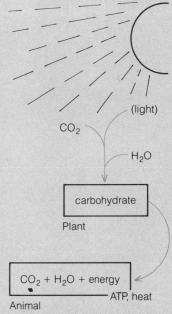

Energy flow.

The downhill flow of energy is not a cycle.

work. Thus life on earth can go on only for as long as the sun continues to burn and flood our plants with light.

This discussion has taken us far from the problems of nutrition, although you may agree that the concept of energy must be understood if the very real nutritional problems of underweight and obesity are to be dealt with. Ironically, although energy weighs almost nothing, you weigh more when you store energy. The reason this is so is clear from the Tinker Toy analogy, in which energy is represented by the sticks. The sticks weigh nothing but in order to keep them in place you must attach them to wheels, which do weigh something. To capture energy and store it in your body, you must trap it in molecules of fat. Thus the more energy you store, the heavier you become. Fat also takes up space, and so the more energy you store, the bulkier you become. The problems of energy excess, which causes overweight and obesity, and energy deficit, which causes underweight and kcalorie malnutrition, result from this arrangement. The practical considerations relating to these problems are taken up in Chapter 8.

Summing Up

The energy in food resides in the chemical bonds that hold nutrient molecules together. In the body, when these bonds are broken, some of this energy is released as heat; but much of the energy is captured through coupled reactions into energy-carrier molecules such as ATP. When ATP is broken down to ADP and phosphate, the energy is again released and used to anabolize body compounds. ATP-like compounds power all of the energy-requiring processes in the body.

The cell's most efficient means of generating ATP are the sequences of reactions known as the TCA cycle and the electron transport chain. In the TCA cycle, acetyl CoA (from carbohydrate, fat, or protein) is attached to oxaloacetate to form citrate, and citrate is processed in a series of reactions that convert it back to oxaloacetate. During these reactions, two carbon dioxide molecules are released, and energy is transferred into other carrier compounds. The major carrier is NAD^+. Each NAD^+ molecule receives two high-energy electrons to become $NADH + H^+$ and then transfers them to a series of other carriers. This is the electron transport chain. At each step the electrons lose energy. At several of these steps the energy is transferred, in a coupled reaction, to ATP. The electrons are finally donated to oxygen, yielding water.

The ATP generated in the electron transport chain carries a large amount of energy in its terminal phosphate group. Thus, it can participate in other coupled reactions to do the body's work. Among its contributions are energy to power the first step in the catabolism of glucose; energy to synthesize glycogen, fatty acids, and proteins; and energy for muscle movements and for repolarizing nerve cells after the transmission of nerve impulses. After the energy originally found in food has been transferred into ATP and used for these purposes, it leaves the body as heat or work accomplished and is no longer usable.

Thus although carbon and the other atoms present in nutrients cycle repeatedly through living things, energy flows downhill, being gradually dissipated as heat. Although no net energy is lost in this process, heat energy is not reconvertible to chemical bonds; hence a new supply of usable energy must flow constantly from the sun, through plants, and into animals and human beings. This explains the need for food to sustain life.

Energy storage involves the capture of energy that chemically binds organic molecules together and therefore entails storage of matter that occupies space and has weight. The problem of storing more energy than is needed therefore becomes a problem of storing more weight.

To Explore Further

A brief and clear explanation in paperback of the ways energy flows through living things is Lehninger, A. L., *Bioenergetics: The Basis of Biological Energy Transformations*, 2nd ed. (New York: Benjamin-Cummings, 1971).

A more technical but clear and highly accurate treatment of biochemical pathways, including the TCA cycle and the electron transport chain, is Lehninger, A. L., *Biochemistry*, 2nd ed. (New York: Worth, 1975).

An entire issue of *Scientific American* was devoted to energy flow from the sun through living systems and to its relevance to current human problems of pollution and the food supply:

The biosphere, *Scientific American*, September 1970.

Energy Output

This exercise provides a detailed method of determining your daily energy need. It has three main components: (1) energy for basal metabolism, (2) energy for muscular activities, and (3) energy for the specific dynamic effect of food.

1. You can determine the energy you need to support your basal metabolic rate (BMR) from your body surface area. First, use Figure 1 to determine your surface area. Draw a straight line from your height (left column) to your weight (right column). The point where that line crosses the middle column shows your surface area in square meters. For example, a person 5 feet 3 inches tall, weighing 110 pounds, has a surface area of 1.5 meters.

Next, use the BMR table (Table 1) to find the factor for your sex and age, and multiply your surface area by this factor. For a 19-year-old woman, the factor is 35.4 kcal per square meter per hour. This multiplied by 1.5 square meters equals 53 kcal per hour. (Notice that we round off at each step. Even this method is not so accurate that many decimal places are meaningful.)

Finally, multiply the product by 24 hours per day to find your BMR needs per day. Using our example, 53 kcal per hour times 24 hours per day equals 1,272 kcal per day.

2. Now determine the energy you need for your muscular activities. The following is an accurate method, provided that the day you select is typical. Keep a 24-hour diary of your activities. Record them on a form like Form 1, and specify the length of time that you spent at various energy levels in each activity. Refer to Table 2 for the levels and their energy cost. Every minute of your day should be accounted for (1,440 minutes in all).

Extra energy is spent running up and down stairs. Each time you go up or down a flight of stairs, consider the time spent to be walking time, and put it down as such

Table 1. Basal Metabolic Rate*

Age (yr)	Males (kcal/sq m/hr)	Females (kcal/sq m/hr)	Age (yr)	Males (kcal/sq m/hr)	Females (kcal/sq m/hr)
3	60.1	54.5	26	38.2	35.0
4	57.9	53.9	27	38.0	35.0
5	56.3	53.0			
6	54.0	51.2	28	37.8	35.0
7	52.3	49.7	29	37.7	35.0
			30	37.6	35.0
8	50.8	48.0	31	37.4	35.0
9	49.5	46.2	32	37.2	34.9
10	47.7	44.9			
11	46.5	43.5	33	37.1	34.9
12	45.3	42.0	34	37.0	34.9
			35	36.9	34.8
13	44.5	40.5	36	36.8	34.7
14	43.8	39.2	37	36.7	34.6
15	42.9	38.3			
16	42.0	37.2	38	36.7	34.5
17	41.5	36.4	39	36.6	34.4
			40-44	36.4	34.1
18	40.8	35.8	45-49	36.2	33.8
19	40.5	35.4	50-54	35.8	33.1
20	39.9	35.3			
21	39.5	35.2	55-59	35.1	32.8
22	39.2	35.2	60-64	34.5	32.0
			65-69	33.5	31.6
23	39.0	35.2	70-74	32.7	31.1
24	38.7	35.1	75+	31.8	
25	38.4	35.1			

*From W.M. Boothby, in *Handbook of Biological Data*, ed. W.S. Spector (1956), reprinted courtesy W.B. Saunders Company, Philadelphia.

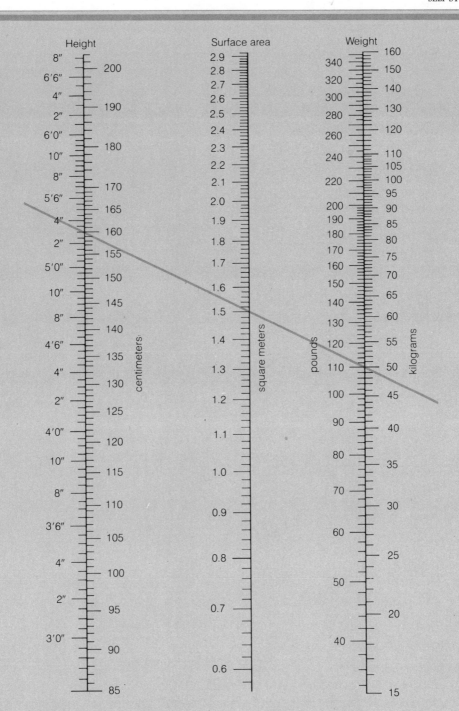

Figure 1 Chart for determination of surface area. A line is drawn between height (5 feet 3 inches) and weight (110 pounds) to yield 1.5 square meters as the surface area.

Adapted from W. M. Boothby, J. Berkson, and H. L. Dunn, Studies of the energy of normal individuals: a standard for basal metabolism, with a nomogram for clinical application, *American Journal of Physiology* 116(1936):468-484.

Form 1. Minutes Spent at Each Energy Level

Clock time	Total minutes	Activity	Energy level*							
			a	b	c	d	e	f	g	h
7:00–7:45	45	Dressing			23	14				
7:45–8:15	30	Eating		26	4					
8:15–9:00	45	Bike to School			4	25	16			
Total										

*See Table 2 for an explanation of these levels.

Table 2. Energy Levels and Their Energy Cost*

Energy level	Type of activity	Energy cost (kcal/kg/min)[†]
a	Sleep or lying still, relaxed[‡]	0.000
b	Sitting or standing still (includes activities like sewing, writing, eating)	0.010
c	Very light activity (includes driving a car, walking at moderate speed on level ground)	0.020
d	Light exercise (includes light housework such as sweeping the floor, walking at moderate speed on level ground carrying books)	0.025
e	Moderate exercise (includes activities like fast walking, dancing, bicycling at moderate speed)	0.040
f	Heavy exercise (includes activities like fast dancing, walking at almost a run, fast uphill walking)	0.070
g	Severe exercise (includes tennis, running)	0.110
h	Very severe exercise (includes wrestling, rowing, boxing, racing)	0.140

[†]Measured in kcalories per kilogram per minute above basal energy.

[‡]For purposes of this exercise, sleep is assumed to be the basal level of activity.

*Adapted from R. Passmore and J. V. G. A. Durnin, Human energy expenditure, *Physiological Reviews* 35 (1955):801-840.

on the form. But keep a separate record of the number of flights you climbed as well (count 14 to 15 steps as one flight of stairs).

For example, suppose you got up at 7:00 and spent the first 45 minutes of the day moving about quietly, dressing and getting ready for breakfast. You also went down a flight of stairs to get the newspaper, back up again, and then downstairs for breakfast. You might enter this 45-minute period on one line of the form as shown in Form 1, recording 8 minutes of it as activity at level b (sitting or standing still), 23 minutes as level c activity (very light), and 14 minutes as level d activity (light activity similar to housework). You would also note the stair climbing separately ("down twice, up once"). Continue until you have made a complete record for 24 hours.

The final step is to add up the number of minutes you spent at each energy level. These totals should add up to 1,440 minutes. Now compute the total energy spent for all activities in 24 hours, using Form 2. Notice that there is a place at the bottom of this form to record the extra energy spent climbing stairs. By completing this form, you will arrive at an estimate of your energy needs for muscular activities.

3. Now calculate the energy you spent on the digestion and metabolism of food (SDE). If you know how many kcalories you ingested that day, use 10 percent of the kcalories. Otherwise, add the energy you used for basal metabolism and for activities to obtain a subtotal. Assume that 10 percent of this subtotal is the energy for SDE.

4. Last, add all three figures—BMR needs per day, energy needs for activities, and energy for SDE—to obtain the total energy you spent in a 24-hour period. This figure represents the best estimate you can easily obtain of the number of kcalories you need to eat each day in order to maintain your weight. The RDA tables provide ranges of recommended energy intakes for people in your age-sex category (see Appendix O), but the figure you have arrived at here is your "personalized RDA" for energy. You will want to use this figure for the Self-Study on Diet Planning at the end of Highlight 8.

Form 2. Energy Cost for Activities (exclusive of basal metabolism and the effect of food)

Energy level	Total minutes spent	Energy cost per minute (kcal/kg/min)		Total energy cost per kg (kcal/kg)
a		× 0.000 =		0.000
b		× 0.010 =		
c		× 0.020 =		
d		× 0.025 =		
e		× 0.040 =		
f		× 0.070 =		
g		× 0.110 =		
h		× 0.140 =		
Subtotal	1,440			
Extra energy spent on stairs:				
flights down		× 0.012 =		
flights up		× 0.036 =		
Total kcal/kg/24 hours				
Now multiply by body weight (kg) to arrive at total energy spent on activities for the day:			×	kg
				kcal/ day

Optional Extras

● You can now classify your lifestyle as sedentary, lightly active, moderately active, or very active by the criteria described on p. 245. A sedentary person, for example, spends 20 percent as much energy on muscular activities as on basal metabolism. How much do you spend? For example:

My basal metabolic energy is 1,200 kcal/day.
My activity energy is 300 kcal/day.
300 is 25 percent of 1,200, so I would be classed as a lightly active person.

● Practice estimating kcalorie amounts in meals, using the exchange system as demonstrated in Chapter 7. List the foods you ate on one day of your record-taking (refer to p. 14) on a form like Form 3, and translate them into exchanges, using Appendix L. For foods not listed, estimate exchange groupings and kcalorie amounts.

Form 3. Foods Eaten in One Day

Food I ate	Serving size	Exchange group	Number of exchanges
Banana	1 medium	fruit	2

Now collect all similar exchanges into groups and add up the kcalorie amounts:

Form 4. kCalories Consumed in One Day (based on exchanges)*

Exchange group	Total exchanges	kCalories
Milk		
Vegetables		
Fruit		
Bread		
Meat		
Fat		
Total kcalories		

*If you used whole milk, add two fat exchanges for each milk exchange that you drank. If you used medium-
or high-fat meat, add fat exchanges as indicated in the exchange lists.

You will find that this system works well if you ate mostly protective foods (those listed in the exchange system), but it fails to take into account the less nutritious or empty-kcalorie foods, such as candy, cola beverages, alcoholic beverages, and the like. How closely does your kcalorie estimate agree with the calculated amount you have already arrived at? Would a greater familiarity with the exchange system be useful to you in estimating your nutrient and kcalorie intakes? If so, repeat this exercise using the second and third days' records of your Self-Study.

● Now that you know your "personalized RDA" for kcalories, you can estimate the number of kcalories you would have to consume daily in order to gain or lose weight. If you wanted to maintain your weight, how many kcalories would you have to consume each day, on the average (your "personalized RDA" for kcalories)? If you wanted to lose a pound a week, how many kcalories would you have to consume? To lose 1-1/2 pounds a week? If you wanted to gain a pound a week, how many kcalories would you have to consume? Remember that the number of kcalories in a pound of

body fat is estimated to be about 3,500.
● Denise, who spends 2,000 kcalories a day, is getting married six weeks from now, and she wants to lose 25 pounds so she can fit into a size 10 wedding dress. Advise her as to the number of kcalories she may consume per day in order to reach her goal by the deadline (assume no change in activity level).
● Discover why a fat person can lose weight faster at first than a thin person. Estimate the energy needs of a 300-pound woman. (Choose whatever height, age, and activity level you wish.) If she goes on a 1,000 kcal diet, how

much weight will she lose per week? Now estimate the energy needs of a 100-pound woman who is the same height and age and equally active or inactive. If she goes on a 1,000 kcal diet, how much weight will she lose per week? What factors account for the differences between these two women's energy needs?

● Discover the extent to which exercise affects energy output. Suppose a 70-kilogram man, age 20, sits around all day. How much energy does he spend? Now suppose he plays a game of tennis for an hour every day. How many kcalories does this add to his energy expenditure? Now suppose he gets a job operating a pneumatic hammer for eight hours a day (this costs three times as many kcalories as his basal metabolic rate does for 24 hours). How much additional energy will he spend?

● When a person has a fever, her energy needs for basal metabolism increase by 7 percent for each degree (Fahrenheit) of fever. Suppose you had a fever of 102.6° F. How many extra kcalories would this cost you in a day? Would there be enough compensating reduction in activity level to leave your total energy needs unchanged?

CHAPTER 8

CONTENTS

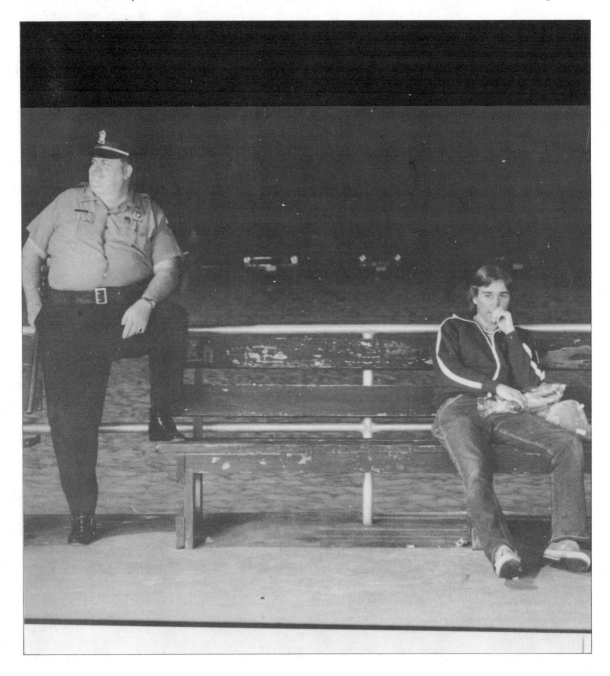

OVERWEIGHT AND UNDERWEIGHT

No matter how much you huff and puff, you can't just shake it off, rock it off, roll it off, knock it off or bake it off. . . . The only way is to eat less and exercise more.
AMERICAN MEDICAL ASSOCIATION

Obesity is a major malnutrition problem. It is simultaneously one of the most important and least understood areas in the science of nutrition. Everyone knows roughly what it is: If you are too fat, you are overweight; if much too fat, you are obese. But why and how obesity occurs and what can be done about it are matters for much speculation, debate, and frustration. For the obese person who has earnestly tried every known means of losing weight only to fail, frustration can turn to despair.

Less well recognized is the problem of underweight, which can be equally mysterious. A "skinny" person finds it as hard to gain a pound as a fat person does to lose one.

This chapter emphasizes the problems of overweight and obesity, partly because they have been more intensively studied and partly because they are a more widespread health problem in the developed countries. This does not imply that the underweight person faces a less difficult problem. The concluding section shows that what we know about the one extreme sometimes applies equally well to the other.

Overweight and underweight both result from unbalanced energy budgets. The overweight person has consumed more food energy (kcalories) than he has expended and has banked the surplus in his fat cells. The underweight person has not consumed enough and so has depleted his fat stores. Energy itself doesn't weigh anything and can't be seen, but when it exists in the form of chemical bonds in nutrients or body fat, the material that it holds together is both heavy and visible.

The amount of fat you might deposit or withdraw from "savings" on any given day depends on your energy balance for that day—the amount you consume (energy-in) versus the amount you expend (energy-out). And as Chapter 7 shows you can reduce your fat deposits by withdrawing more energy from them than you put in. A pound of body fat stores 3,500 kcal. To lose a pound (of body fat) you must experience a deficit: The kcalories you take in must be 3,500 less than the kcalories you expend. To lose that pound in a week, you would need to achieve an average deficit of 500 kcal a day. Repeat: Fat loss always obeys the rule that a person losing weight (fat) must experience a deficit of 3,500 kcal for every pound lost.

This cruel fact is one many of us would like to circumvent. Isn't there an easier way? No, the hard truth is that

> The only way to lose body fat is to cut kcalories.

Magical alternatives that have been offered time and again over the centuries—ways to "shrink the stomach," to eat "negative kcalories," to "eat all you want and lose weight"—prove to be born of wishful thinking. They are effective only when they indirectly affect the kcalorie balance. The success of these plans is not in achievement of their goals but in their popularity. They sell easily to susceptible people who want something for nothing, who become enthusiastic practitioners (but only briefly), and who pass on the word to the next person. This type of reaction reflects a human characteristic that for all our scientific rationality we have failed to outgrow: We love magic. Many writers of fallacious books on diets and sellers of fraudulent diet pills and formulas use this characteristic to their advantage.

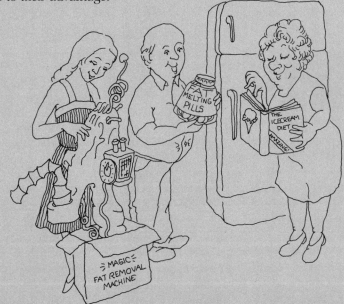

A FLAG SIGN OF A SPURIOUS CLAIM
IS THE USE OF:

Magical thinking
The promise of something for nothing

Ideal Weight and Body Fatness

How fat is too fat? And how thin is too thin? It isn't always possible to tell from the bathroom scales, because body weight says nothing about body composition. The relative amounts of lean and fat tissue vary widely from one person to the next. A dancer or an athlete, whose muscles are well developed and whose bones have become dense from constant stress, may weigh much more than a sedentary person with the same figure. What is needed is a measure of body fatness—not of body weight. Ideally, by a very rough approximation, fat makes up about 18 percent of a man's body weight and about 22 percent of a woman's, with the remainder being contributed by water (55 to 60 percent), muscle and other lean tissue (10 to 20 percent), and bone minerals (6 to 8 percent). But there is no easy way to look inside a person and see the bones and muscles.

Several laboratory techniques for estimating body fatness have been developed. One way is to determine the body's density (weight/volume). Lean tissue is denser than fat tissue, so the more dense a person's body is, the more lean tissue it must contain. Weight is easy to measure with a scale, but volume measurement involves submerging the whole body in water and measuring the amount of water displaced; this requires a large tank and takes up too much space to be practical for use in, say, a doctor's office. Another way is to inject a substance like radioactive potassium or heavy water (deuterium oxide) and allow it to penetrate into the lean tissues (these substances do not dissolve into the fat tissues). A blood sample will show the extent to which the substance has been diluted, providing an estimate of the amount of lean tissue.

A direct measure of the amount of body fat can be obtained by lifting a fold of skin from the back of the arm, from the back, or from other body surfaces and measuring its thickness with a caliper that applies a fixed amount of pressure. A skinfold over an inch thick indicates overfatness; under a half inch reflects underweight. The fat under the skin in these regions is roughly proportional to total body fat. This technique—the skinfold test—is a practical diagnostic tool in the hands of trained people and is in increasingly wide use.

A still simpler test is the mirror test: Undress and stand before a mirror. If you look too fat, you may be too fat. (A notoriously poor judge of this test, however, is the teenage girl who thinks any amount of fat, no matter how small, is a serious blemish. It may be that she needs to change her self-image—not to go on a diet.)

Even though the scales are not an accurate indicator of body fatness, they are most often used to estimate it, in conjunction with the so-called ideal weight tables. But these tables are not based on scientific determinations of the ideal weight; they are merely averages for the population. Their usefulness is mainly for the life insurance companies, which raise premiums for obese people. These tables indicate that a man 5 feet 11 inches tall (in shoes), for example, should weigh anywhere from 144 to 179 pounds. This range of values is divided into

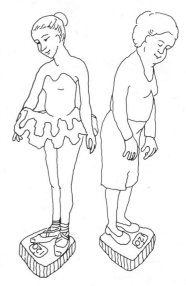

ideal weight: a misnomer, not the desirable but the average weight given in insurance tables for persons of a given sex and height in the United States—not necessarily ideal for a given individual.

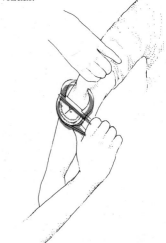

skinfold test: clinical test of body fatness in which the thickness of a fold of skin on the back of the arm (triceps), below the shoulder blade (subscapular), or in other places is measured using an instrument called a caliper. A new and better term for this is **fatfold test.**

frame size: the size of a person's bones and musculature. This is a vague term; frame-size standards have not been established.

overweight: body weight more than 10 percent above "ideal" weight.

obesity: excessive body fatness; often loosely defined as a condition of being overweight by 15 or 20 percent or more.

underweight: body weight more than 10 percent below normal or average ("ideal") weight.

juvenile-onset obesity: obesity arising in childhood; also called developmental obesity.

adult-onset obesity: obesity arising after adolescence; sometimes called reactive obesity if it appears to arise in response to a specific traumatic or stressful life event.

thirds—on the assumption that some of the differences in weight must be due to differences in skeletal type—and labeled small, medium, and large frame. But no standard is provided by which this man can determine his frame size.[1]

Choosing your own ideal weight is thus partly a matter of guesswork. To decide if you have "big bones," pick a bone you can see (for example, the wrist bone) and compare with several other people. Having decided on your frame size, you can look up the corresponding recommended weight range. For example, a man who is 5 feet 11 inches tall and has a medium frame should weigh, according to the tables, 150 to 165 pounds. You must then decide, on the basis of your own self-knowledge, whether this is the ideal weight for your body type and activity.

Ideal weight probably decreases with age. People typically become less active as they get older. Their muscles get smaller, and their bones decrease in density. Thus a man who is lean at 25 may be overfat at 65 without having gained a pound. Most of us should gradually lose weight once we have passed the age of 30. The fact that many people gain an average of 20 to 30 pounds during adulthood does not make it right.

With all their limitations, the ideal-weight tables are often used to draw arbitrary lines between too much and too little body weight. A person who is more than 10 percent above the weight on the table is considered overweight; if 20 percent or more, he is considered obese. (Some authorities say obesity is 15 percent above the ideal weight, some say 25 percent.) Similarly, a person who is more than 10 percent below the table weight is considered underweight. Obviously, for the reasons already given, these terms may be rejected in individual cases.

The Problem of Obesity

However you define it, obesity does occur to an alarming extent and is increasing in the developed countries. For example, in the United States some 10 to 25 percent of all teenagers and some 25 to 50 percent of all adults are obese.

Some people become fat in childhood and others later on. Few of either type lose the excess weight. There is no specific age that divides juvenile-onset obesity from adult-onset obesity, but as the terms imply, there is a distinction between the two types. A child who is obese will develop sturdy muscles and bones as she grows, to support her excess weight. Thus as an adult she will have more lean body mass and more

[1]A. Keys and F. Grande, Body weight, body composition and calorie status, in *Modern Nutrition in Health and Disease*, 5th ed., eds. R. S. Goodhart and M. E. Shils (Philadelphia: Lea and Febiger, 1973), pp. 1-27. A whole new method of estimating frame sizes from wrist measurements is available in Grant's *Nutritional Assessment Guidelines*, cited at the end of Chapter 9, but the validity of this method has not been determined.

body fat than the average person and will likely always be stocky, even after losing her excess fat. People who become obese as children are also less likely to be able to reduce successfully than people who become obese as adults.

Research on fat cells suggests a possible reason why early-onset obesity is especially resistant to treatment. Simply stated, early overfeeding stimulates fat cells to increase abnormally in *number*. The number of fat cells becomes fixed by adulthood. Thereafter, a gain in weight can take place only by increasing the *size* of the fat cells. The number of fat cells regulates hunger in some way, so a person with an abnormally large number of fat cells will be abnormally hungry and will always tend to overeat. On the other hand, a person who gains weight in adulthood has a normal number of fat cells and needs only to reduce the size of the cells.

This theory has been heavily criticized on several grounds.[2] But even the critics agree that there are certain periods in life when body fat increases more rapidly than lean tissue: early infancy (up to about two years), again during preadolescence (and throughout adolescence in girls), and possibly again during the third trimester of pregnancy. These are critical periods, in the sense that what happens at these times may be irreversible and crucial to the person's later physical fate. Prevention of obesity would thus be most important during these times. There is also agreement that fat is hard to lose no matter when it was gained.

Hazards of Obesity   Insurance companies report that fat people die younger from a host of causes including heart attacks, strokes, and complications of diabetes. In fact, gaining weight often appears to precipitate diabetes. Fat people more often suffer high levels of blood fat, hypertension, coronary heart disease, postsurgical complications, gynecological irregularities, and the toxemia of pregnancy. The burden of extra fat strains the skeletal system, causing arthritis—especially in the knees, hips, and lower spine. The muscles that support the belly may give way, resulting in abdominal hernias. When the leg muscles are abnormally fatty, they fail to contract efficiently to help blood return from the leg veins in the heart; blood collects in the leg veins, which swell, harden, and become varicose. Extra fat in and around the chest interferes with breathing, sometimes causing severe problems. Gout is more common and even the accident rate is greater for the severely obese.[3]

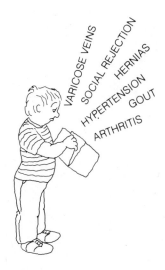

VARICOSE VEINS
SOCIAL REJECTION
HERNIAS
HYPERTENSION
GOUT
ARTHRITIS

[2]E. M. Widdowson and M. J. Dauncey, Obesity, in *Nutrition Reviews' Present Knowledge in Nutrition*, 4th ed. (Washington, D.C.: Nutrition Foundation, 1976), pp. 17-23.

[3]Keys and Grande, 1973; K. M. West, Prevention and therapy of diabetes mellitus, in *Nutrition Reviews' Present Knowledge in Nutrition*, 4th ed. (Washington, D.C.: Nutrition Foundation, 1976), pp. 356-364; B. B. Blouin, Diet and obesity (news digest), *Journal of the American Dietetic Association* 70 (1977):535; R. A. Seelig, Obesity: A review, reprint by United Fresh Fruit and Vegetable Association (Washington, D.C., 1976); and C. F. Gastineau, Obesity: Risks, causes, and treatment, *Medical Clinics of North America* 56 (July 1972):286-293.

A linear (straight-line) relationship:

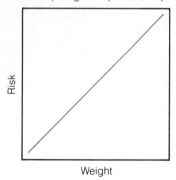

Weight

The actual relationship of risk to weight:

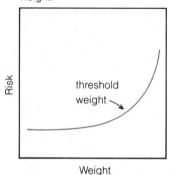

threshold weight

Weight

Adapted from C. C. Seltzer, Some re-evaluations of the *Build and Blood Pressure Study, 1959* as related to ponderal index, somatotype and mortality, *New England Journal of Medicine* 274 (1966):254-259.

As if all this were not enough, there are also social and economic disadvantages. A fat person is less often sought after for marriage, pays higher insurance premiums, meets discrimination when applying for a job, can't find attractive clothes so easily, and is limited in his choice of sports. Fat girls have only a third the chance of being accepted into college that lean girls have. The fat child often suffers ridicule from her classmates and the unbearable humiliation of having the captain of the team choose her last.

The many disadvantages justify our calling obesity a severe physical handicap. However, it is unlike other handicaps in two important ways. First, mortality risk is not linearly related to excess weight. Instead, there is a threshold at which risk dramatically increases. Being only a few pounds above this threshold weight may cause blood pressure, blood glucose, and blood lipids to zoom upwards. The concept of a danger zone of weight, which is relatively new, is illustrated in the margin. Second, obesity is reversible, and if it is corrected in time, some of its risks are too.[4] Mortality rates (from insurance data) are no higher for the formerly obese than for the never obese.[5]

Ideally a person would never have to struggle with the problem of obesity, because he would never have become obese to begin with. Preventive efforts are needed, especially in vulnerable groups: infants, preadolescents, adolescents, and women before they are pregnant. (This is in no way meant to imply that a woman who is pregnant should attempt to lose weight. Weight loss during pregnancy is even more hazardous than obesity.) Where prevention has failed, treatment is urgently needed. But how to treat? Before turning to the matters of diet, drugs, exercise, and other means of attacking the problem, it is necessary to try to figure out what causes it.

Causes of Obesity

kCalories are not stored in fat until the body's other energy needs have been met. Excess body fat can accumulate only when kcalories are eaten beyond those needed for the day's metabolic, muscular, and digestive activities. To put it bluntly, obesity results from overeating.

This fact, however, neither explains the cause of obesity nor indicates the cure. Why do people overeat? Is it a hunger problem? An appetite problem? A satiety problem? Is it genetic? Metabolic? Environmental? Is it a matter of habits learned in early childhood? Is it psychological? Would you believe that all of these factors may play a role? To tell the truth, we do not know the cause. The following paragraphs only offer ideas that are presently being considered.

[4]E. Eckholm and F. Record, *Worldwatch Paper 9: The Two Faces of Malnutrition* (Washington, D.C.: Worldwatch Institute, 1976).

[5]Gastineau, 1972.

Hunger, Appetite, and Satiety   The theories of how food intake is regulated could not be summarized in fewer than 50 pages.[6] It may be that the brain monitors blood glucose concentration and signals "eat" when glucose gets too low; the obese individual may have an insensitive monitor. Food intake may be regulated by fat cells, which send hormonal signals to the brain when they have been fed enough—and obese people may have too many fat cells. Then again, they may not.[7] Centers outside the brain may also initiate feeding behavior.[8] It may be that food tastes better to some people than to others, although recent experiments suggest there is no difference between the obese and nonobese in this respect.[9]

Hunger is said to be physiological—an inborn instinct—whereas appetite is psychological—a learned response to food. Possibly obese people have learned to enjoy eating for reasons other than to satisfy the hunger drive. We have all experienced appetite without hunger: "I'm not hungry, but I'd love to have a piece." The too-thin person may often experience the reverse, hunger without appetite: "I know I'm hungry, but I don't feel like eating."

The clue in some cases may lie in the fact that the obese person doesn't know when to stop: She goes on eating when she is full. One theory of food intake regulation states that feeding behavior is turned on all the time and that a neural or hormonal switch is supposed to turn it off whenever the body's physiological need has been met.[10] The stomach is known to be able to signal to the brain when nutrients have arrived. The satiety theory suggests that the obese person's "set point" is .oo high or is malfunctioning and that the underweight person's is too low. But the exact nature of the satiety signal is unknown.

External Cues   Some obese people are unconscious eaters. Rather than respond only to internal, visceral hunger cues, they respond helplessly to such external factors as the time of day ("It's time to eat") or the availability, sight, and taste of food.[11] This is the basis of the external cue theory.

hunger: the physiological need to eat.

appetite: the desire to eat, which normally accompanies hunger.

satiety (sat-EYE-uh-tee): the feeling of fullness or satisfaction at the end of a meal; it prompts a person to stop eating.

external cue theory: the theory that some people eat in response to such external factors as the presence of food or the time of day rather than to such internal factors as hunger.

[6]An example is S. Lepkovski, Regulation of food intake, *Advances in Food Research* 21 (1975):1-69.

[7]Widdowson and Dauncey, 1976.

[8]E. M. Stricker, N. Rowland, C. F. Saller, and M. I. Friedman, Homeostasis during hypoglycemia: Central control of adrenal secretion and peripheral control of feeding, *Science* 196 (1977):78-81.

[9]C. L. Hamilton, Physiologic control of food intake, *Journal of the American Dietetic Association* 62 (1973):35-40; and D. A. Thompson, H. R. Moskowitz, and R. G. Campbell, Taste and olfaction in human obesity, *Physiology and Behavior* 19 (1977):335-337.

[10]Keys and Grande, 1973; A. J. Stunkard, Eating patterns and obesity, *Psychiatric Quarterly* 33 (1959):284-295; P. H. Linton, M. Conley, C. Kuechenmeister, and H. McClusky, Satiety and obesity, *American Journal of Clinical Nutrition* 25 (1972):368-370; and M. Cabanac, R. Duclaux, and N. H. Spector, Sensory feedback in regulation of body weight: Is there a ponderostat? *Nature* 229 (1971): 125-127.

[11]J. F. Schumaker and M. K. Wagner, External-cue responsivity as a function of age at onset of obesity, *Journal of the American Dietetic Association* 70 (1977):275-279.

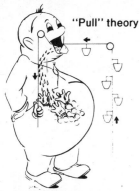

"Pull" theory

The "pull" theory of obesity proposes that a subtle metabolic disorder increases food intake either by affecting hunger-satiety signals transmitted to a "satiety center" or by altering the sensitivity of the satiety center to such signals.

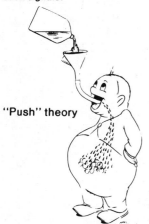

"Push" theory

The "push" theory proposes that the obese person "force-feeds" himself, overeating for nonphysiological reasons.

Adapted from T. B. Van Itallie and R. G. Campbell, Multidisciplinary approach to the problem of obesity, *Journal of the American Dietetic Association* 61(1972):385-390.

Of interest in this connection is the report of an experiment in which lean and fat people in a metabolic ward were offered their meals in monotonous liquid form from a feeding machine. The lean people ate enough to maintain their weight, but the fat people drastically reduced their food intake and lost weight. When kcalories were added to the formula, the lean people adjusted their intake to continue maintaining weight as if they had an internal, unconscious kcalorie counter. The obese people were insensitive to the change, continued drinking the same amount of formula as before, and stopped losing weight.[12]

For the person who responds to external cues, today's environment provides abundant cues to promote eating behavior. Restaurants, TV commercials, the display of food in our markets, vending machines in every office building and gas station—all prompt us to eat and drink high kcalorie foods. There are no "vegetable houses" on our main streets, only steakhouses. Kitchen appliances such as the hamburger cooker and the doughnut maker make high kcalorie foods easy to prepare and thus quickly available.

Psychology: Emotional Needs   The psychiatrist Dr. Hilde Bruch, who has devoted as much attention to the human hunger drive as Freud did to the sex drive, states that hunger and appetite are understandably mixed up together because both are intimately connected to deep emotional needs. Two factors that she finds most important in this connection are the fear of starvation and "the universal experience in the early life of every individual that food intake requires the cooperation of another person." Feeding behavior is a response not only to hunger or appetite but also to more complex human sensations, such as "yearning, craving, addiction, or compulsion."[13]

Others agree that food is widely used for non-nutritive purposes, especially in a culture like ours where food is abundant. An emotionally insecure person, who feels unsure of acceptance by other people, might eat as a substitute for seeking love or friendship. Eating is less threatening than calling a friend and risking rejection. Often, especially in adolescent girls, eating is used to relieve boredom. And one researcher has found that eating helps ward off depression.[14]

Obesity as a Response to Stress   Animals under stress have been observed to substitute one instinctive behavior for another. During a confrontation, for example, one animal may suddenly stop posturing

[12]T. B. Van Itallie and R. G. Campbell, Multidisciplinary approach to the problem of obesity, *Journal of the American Dietetic Association* 61 (1972):385-390.

[13]H. Bruch, Role of the emotions in hunger and appetite, *Annals of the New York Academy of Sciences* 63, part 1 (1955):68-75.

[14]R. I. Simon, Obesity as a depressive equivalent, *Journal of the American Medical Association* 183 (1963):208-210.

and begin to groom itself intensively. It is possible that people also displace one behavior with another when they are threatened. Rather than fight or flight, the activity they select may be eating.

The hormones secreted in response to physical stress favor the rapid metabolism of energy nutrients to fragments that can be used to fuel the muscular activity of fight or flight. Under emotional stress the same hormones are secreted. If a person fails to use the fuel in violent physical exertion, the body has no alternative but to turn these fragments to fat.[15] If blood glucose has been used this way, then the lowered glucose level will signal hunger, and the person will eat again soon after. Stress eating may appear in different patterns: Some people eat excessively at night when feeling anxious, others characteristically go on an eating binge during an emotional crisis.[16] The overly thin often react oppositely. Stress causes them to reject food and thus become thinner.

Metabolic Obesity   It may be that some people have inherited a greater tendency to accumulate body fat than others. One researcher speculates that some people might tend to use carbohydrate (from blood glucose and liver glycogen) more extensively to meet certain energy needs, whereas others might tend to use blood lipid. The glycogen users would experience lowered blood glucose more readily and so would be hungry more often.[17] A difference like this could be due to a difference in the amount of a particular hormone or enzyme involved in fat production and conceivably might imply that a low-carbohydrate diet is needed. Dozens of theories are presently being tested. Doubtless some will explain at least a few specific cases of obesity.

Insulin Insensitivity   Once a person has become obese, the situation tends to perpetuate itself. The enlarged fat cells become resistant to insulin, the hormone that promotes glucose uptake into cells and its conversion to fat. The excess glucose remains in the bloodstream and stimulates the insulin-producing cells of the pancreas to multiply and secrete more insulin. This promotes further fat storage.[18] As if this were not enough, the enlarged fat cells are also less sensitive to other

Insulin: see also Chapter 1.

[15]This response to stress has been studied in animals. An example of such a study is C. D. Berdanier, R. Wurdeman, and R. B. Tobin, Further studies on the role of the adrenal hormones in the responses of rats to meal-feeding, *Journal of Nutrition* 106 (1976):1791-1800.

[16]Stunkard, 1959.

[17]W. H. Griffith, Food as a regulator of metabolism, *American Journal of Clinical Nutrition* 17 (1965):391-398.

[18]J. Mayer, as quoted by M. Kernan, Inactivity places burden of obesity on America's youth, *St. Petersburg Times*, 12 August 1973.

hormones that promote fat breakdown.[19] Weight loss restores insulin levels to normal, but it first has to be achieved against these odds.

Heredity versus Environment   Hormones and enzymes are under the control of genes, and genes are inherited. In some animal strains, obesity is inherited as predictably as hair or eye color. Is human obesity inherited? One way to test this possibility is to study identical twins raised in different families, one family fat and the other thin. If genes determine fatness, then both twins will become equally fat or thin. But if the environment is responsible, the twins will resemble their respective families. Another approach is to study adopted children, to see whether they resemble their natural or adoptive parents. Studies of both kinds suggest that the tendency to obesity is inherited.[20] But the environment is permissive; that is, it can allow obesity to develop when the potential is there.

Inheritance of the tendency to obesity is probably very complex and governed by many different genes. To complicate the situation further, these genes probably occur with different frequencies in different populations.[21]

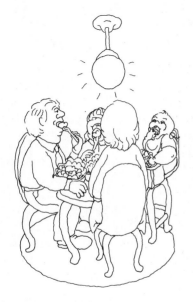

Habits: Learned Responses to Food   If a person can inherit the potential to become obese, the environment can doubtless help it become real. Food-centered families encourage such behaviors as overeating at mealtimes, rapid eating, excessive snacking, and eating to meet needs other than hunger. Children readily imitate overeating parents, and their behavior at the table persists outside the home. Obese children have been observed to take more bites of food per interval of time and to chew them less thoroughly than their nonobese schoolmates.[22]

People who eat small but frequent meals may tend to store less fat than those who eat large meals at irregular intervals.[23] Thus families that allow their children to skip meals may be promoting obesity.

Inactivity   The many possible causes of obesity mentioned so far all relate to the input side of the energy equation. What about output? A

[19]*Obesity '73: A Report from the Geigy Symposium on Obesity, Its Problems and Prognosis* (New York: Ardsley, 1973).

[20]J. Mayer, Obesity, in *Modern Nutrition in Health and Disease*, 5th ed., eds. R. S. Goodhart and M. E. Shils (Philadelphia: Lea and Febiger, 1973), pp. 625-644.

[21]A. Montagu, Obesity and the evolution of man, *Journal of the American Medical Association* 195 (1966):105-107.

[22]R. S. Drabman, D. Hammer, and G. J. Jarvie, Eating rates of elementary school children, *Journal of Nutrition Education* 9 (1977):80-82.

[23]P. Fabry, Metabolic consequences of the pattern of food intake, in *Handbook of Physiology*, section 6, ed. C. F. Code (Washington, D.C.: American Physiological Society, 1967), pp. 31-49; and G. A. Leveille and D. R. Romsos, Meal eating and obesity, *Nutrition Today*, November/December 1974, pp. 4-9.

person may be obese because he eats too much, but another possibility is that he spends too little energy. It is probable that the most important single contributor to the obesity problem in our country is under-activity.[24] The control of hunger/appetite actually works quite well in active people and only fails when activity falls below a certain minimum level.[25] Obese people under close observation are often seen to eat less than lean people, but they are sometimes so extraordinarily inactive that they still manage to have a kcalorie surplus. One authority has noted that normal people actually swim 35 minutes during "an hour of swimming," whereas obese people swim only 7 minutes. Most of their time is spent sitting, standing, or lying in the sun.[26]

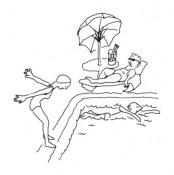

Individuality   No two people are like either physically or psychologi-cally, and no doubt the causes of obesity are as varied as the people who are obese. Many causes may contribute to the problem in a single person. Given this complexity, it is obvious that there is no panacea. The top priority should be prevention, but where prevention has failed the treatment of obesity must involve a simultaneous attack on many fronts.

Treatments of Obesity: Poor Choices

The only means of reducing body fat is to shift the energy budget so that energy-in is less than energy-out. This is most effectively done by eating less and exercising more. A later section of this chapter addresses these strategies, but because rumors of other means fly about, they will first be dispensed with briefly.

Water Pills   For the obese person, the idea that excess weight is due to water accumulation may be an attractive one. Indeed, temporary water retention, seen in many women around the time of the menstrual period, may make a difference of several pounds on the scale. Oral contraceptives may have the same effect. (They may also promote actual fat gain in some women. A woman who has this problem should consult her physician about switching brands.) In cases of severe swelling of the belly, as much as 20 pounds of excess body water may accumulate.[27]

If water retention is a problem, it can be diagnosed by a physician, who will prescribe a diuretic (water pill) and possibly a mild degree of

[24]Keys and Grande, 1973.

[25]J. Yudkin, Prevention of obesity, *Royal Society of Health Journal* (July 1961), pp. 221-224.

[26]Mayer as quoted by Kernan, 1973; B. Bullen, as quoted in R. A. Seelig, 1976.

[27]Keys and Grande, 1973.

salt restriction. But the obese—that is, overfat—subject has a smaller percentage of body water than the person of normal weight. If she takes a self-prescribed diuretic, she has done nothing to solve her fat problem, although she may lose a few pounds on the scale for half a day and suffer from dehydration.

Diet Pills   Some doctors prescribe amphetamines ("speed") to help with weight loss (the best known are dexedrine and benzedrine). These reduce appetite—but only temporarily. Typically the appetite returns to normal after a week or two, the lost weight is regained, and the user then has the problem of trying to get off the drug without gaining more weight. It is generally agreed that these drugs cause a dangerous dependency and are of little or no usefulness in treating obesity.[28] No known drug is both safe and effective, and many are hazardous. The only effective appetite-reducing agent to which tolerance does not develop in time is cigarette smoking, which of course entails hazards of its own too numerous to mention.[29]

Health Spas   One of the biggest money-making schemes that profits from people's desires to lose weight the easy way is the health spa. Equipped with hot baths, massaging machines, health drinks, and the like, these places provide programs for the unsuspecting public to improve their figures while putting forth a minimum of effort. They can be used to advantage. People who really exercise there reap the expected benefits. But health spas can be extremely costly, and most of the gimmicks offer no real health advantage other than the psychological boost the consumer herself supplies. Hot baths do not speed up the basal metabolic rate so that pounds can be lost in hours. Steam and sauna baths do not melt the fat off the body, although they may dehydrate a person so that his weight on the scales changes dramatically. Machines intended to jiggle parts of the body while the person leans passively on them provide pleasant stimulation but no exercise and so no expenditure of kcalories.

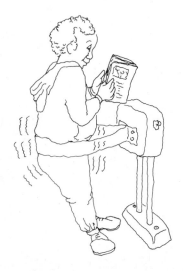

Some people believe there are two kinds of body fat: regular fat and "cellulite." Cellulite is supposed to be a hard and lumpy fat that yields to being "burned up" only if it is first broken up by methods like the massage or the machine typical of the health spa. The notion that there is such a thing as cellulite received wide publicity with the publication of a book by a certain Madam R of Paris, which sold widely during the 1970s. The American Medical Association reviewed the evidence on cellulite (there was none) and concluded that cellulite was a hoax.

[28]L. Eisenberg, The clinical use of stimulant drugs in children, *Pediatrics* 49 (1972):709-715; G. R. Edison, Amphetamines: A dangerous illusion, *Annals of Internal Medicine* 74 (1971):605-610; and B. Lucas and C. J. Sells, Nutrient intake and stimulant drugs in hyperactive children, *Journal of the American Dietetic Association* 70 (1970):373-377.

[29]*Geigy Symposium*, 1973.

Books like the one by Madam R are often written to make money, and they vary widely in reliability. Madame R probably earns a sizable income from the proceeds of her spa, and her book has enticed many people to spend their money there. She is under no legal obligation to publish only confirmed research findings, and she has not done so: She has published misinformation. Yet she can't be sued unless a customer of hers can prove that her book has caused him bodily harm.

The First Amendment, which guarantees freedom of the press, makes it possible for people like Madame R to express whatever views they like, whether sound or unsound or even dangerous. This freedom is a cornerstone of the U.S. Constitution, and to deny it would be to move hazardously near to totalitarianism. But it puts the burden on consumers to read books skeptically and critically and to use their own judgment in evaluating them. Quacks may hesitate to sell *products* that are outright frauds, because they can readily be punished for misrepresentation, but they do not hesitate to sell *books*.

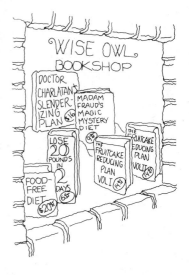

CAUTION WHEN YOU READ!

Seeing a statement in the pages of a book is no guarantee that it is a fact.

The public is not generally aware that books on nutrition are so unreliable that most professional organizations have had to form committees to combat the misinformation they publish. An example is the Committee on Nutritional Misinformation of the Food and Nutrition Board, National Academy of Sciences/National Research Council. If there is a reward for working on these committees, it is not a dollar reward. On the contrary, it costs time and energy for people to serve on them and money to the organizations to publish their statements.

What about textbooks? Perhaps we, the authors, stand too close to the subject to speak without bias about them, but it is our impression that they sell better if other professors find them factual and reliable. We also stand close enough to know that science professors who write textbooks welcome, even seek, criticism from others in the field. One of the sources of our motivation is plain curiosity, which drives us to keep reading and studying in the hope of getting satisfactory answers to our own and our students' questions.

By far the most reliable of all publications on nutrition are the scientific journals. But even among these there are differences. Those that we rely on most heavily are what we call reputable journals. They are the publications of such organizations as the American Medical Association and the American Dietetic Association, which require confirmed credentials and training for membership. Articles are published in them only after a rigorous review by peers of the authors, people who know how to do research and who are familiar with the area under study. The general reader may find journal articles unspeakably dull and boring, but the motivated reader finds them a gold mine of information. Once the purposes and methods are understood, a journal article can be more exciting than a detective story.

Hormones Because hormones are powerful body chemicals and many affect fat metabolism, it has long been hoped that a hormone might be found that would promote weight loss. Several have been tried. With testing, all have proven ineffective and often hazardous as well. Thyroid hormone, in particular, causes loss of lean body mass and heart problems except when medically prescribed for the correction of a thyroid deficiency—and thyroid deficiency is very seldom the cause of obesity.[30]

human chorionic gonadotropin (core-ee-ON-ic go-nad-o-TROPE-in) **(HCG):** a hormone extracted from the urine of pregnant women; believed (incorrectly) to promote fat breakdown.

Among the hormones advertised as promoting weight loss is HCG (human chorionic gonadotropin), a hormone extracted from the urine of pregnant women. HCG has legitimate uses; for example, it can stimulate ovulation in a woman who has had difficulty becoming pregnant. But it has no effect on weight loss and does not reduce hunger.[31] A rash of "clinics" run by "doctors" that sprang up on the West Coast during 1976 and 1977 advertised tremendous success using HCG in the treatment of obesity. These outfits seem to have had one element in common: They prescribed an extremely rigid low-kcalorie diet, which accounted for their apparent effectiveness. The American Medical Association and the California Medical Association have concluded that the claims made for HCG are groundless and that the side effects are unknown and probably dangerous.[32]

Surgery Sheer desperation prompts some obese patients to request bypass surgery, an operation in which a portion of the small intestine is

[30]Current concepts of obesity, reviewed by M. R. C. Greenwood and J. Hirsch, *Dairy Council Digest* 46 (1975).

[31]U.S. Department of Health, Education, and Welfare, Food and Drug Administration, *FDA Consumer Memo*, HEW publication no. (FDA) 77-3035 (Washington, D.C.: Government Printing Office, 1977).

[32]HEW, 1977.

removed or disconnected. Then the patient can continue overeating but will absorb considerably fewer kcalories. Side effects from this procedure are many and highly undesirable, including liver failure, massive and frequent diarrhea, urinary stones, intestinal infection, and malnutrition. Reports of mortality range from 2 to 10 percent. Still, in the United States surgery has been reported to be effective more than half the time for treating the massively obese where all other methods have failed.[33] It should probably be attempted only in otherwise healthy and cooperative patients under 30 who weigh more than 300 pounds and who have tried everything else.[34]

The Successful Treatment of Obesity

It seems that the only realistic and sensible way for the obese person to achieve and maintain ideal weight is to cut kcalories, to increase activity, and to maintain this changed lifestyle to the end of his life. This is a tall order. Fewer than a third of those who lose weight manage to keep it off over the long run. To succeed means modifying all of the attitudes and behaviors that have contributed to the problem in the first place, sometimes against physiological pressures that can't be changed. Still, it can be and has been done successfully, as many former "fatties" can attest. A three-pronged approach usually accounts for their success: diet, exercise, and behavior modification.

The way a particular person loses weight is a highly individual matter. Two weight-loss plans may both be successful and yet have little or nothing in common. To heighten the sense of individuality, the following sections are written in terms of advice to "you." This is not intended to put you under pressure to take it personally but to give you the illusion of listening in on a conversation in which an obese person (with, say, 50 pounds to lose) is being competently counseled by someone familiar with the techniques known to be effective. Notes in the margin highlight the principles involved.

Diet   No particular diet is magical, and no particular food must either be included or avoided. You are the one who will have to live with the diet, so you had better be involved in its planning. Don't think of it as a diet you are going "on"—because then you may be tempted to go "off." The diet can be called successful only if the pounds do not return. Think of it as an eating plan that you will adopt for life. It must consist of foods that you like, that are available to you, and that are within your means.

Diet Counseling Principles:

Involve the person.

---

[33]*American Journal of Clinical Nutrition*, January 1977. This entire issue was devoted to surgery for the obese.

[34]*Geigy Symposium*, 1973.

Planning a Weight Loss Diet

When you are maintaining weight on, say, 2,400 kcalories a day, the following balance is suggested:

15 percent of kcalories from protein
30 percent or less from fat
55 percent or more from carbohydrate

These kcalorie amounts translate into grams as follows:

Protein, 360 kcal or 90 g
Fat, 720 kcal or about 80 g
Carbohydrate, 1,320 kcal or 330 g

Now suppose you want to reduce weight. You could cut your kcalorie amount in half, to 1,200 kcal per day. To avoid getting too hungry, for "satiety value," you must have ample protein and fat. But for health reasons, fat should not supply more than about a third of your kcalories. You must therefore cut the fat grams in half. For maximum satiety, then, leave the protein amount as is. (Protein intake, of course, should never be cut much below the recommended intake.)

So far, you have:
Protein, 90 g or 360 kcal
Fat, 40 g or 360 kcal

This gives a total of 720 kcal and therefore leaves only 480 to be supplied by carbohydrate. This means:

Carbohydrate, 120 g or 480 kcal

Thus you have had to cut your carbohydrate down to about a third of what it was formerly. This balance is typical of successful, nutritious weight-loss plans.[35] The protein may even be raised and the carbohydrate lowered a little more to deliver a nearly perfect 1/3-1/3-1/3 balance of kcalories from the three energy nutrients. In terms of exchanges, such a plan might be designed as follows:

Adopt a realistic plan.

Choose a kcalorie level you can live with. If you maintain your weight on 2,000 kcal a day, then you can certainly lose at least a pound a week on a 1,200 kcal diet. A deficit of 500 kcal a day for seven days is a 3,500-kcal deficit—enough to lose a pound of body fat. But let's make a larger deficit, just to be sure. There is no point in hurrying, because you will never go off the diet—and nutritional adequacy can't be achieved on fewer than about 1,200 kcal—1,000 at the very least.

Make the diet adequate.

Put diet adequacy high on your list of priorities. This is a way of putting yourself first. "I like me, and I'm going to take good care of me"

[35]A. J. Vergroesen, Physiological effects of dietary linoleic acid, *Nutrition Reviews* 35 (January 1977):1-5.

Table 1   A Sample Balanced Weight-Loss Diet*

Exchange group	Number of exchanges	Carbohydrate (g)	Protein (g)	Fat (g)
Milk (skim)	2	24	16	0
Vegetables	4	20	8	0
Fruit	3	30	0	0
Bread	2	30	4	0
Meat (lean)	11	0	77	33
Fat	2	0	0	10
Total		104	105	43

*In this diet, carbohydrate supplies 34 percent of the kcalories, protein 34 percent, and fat 32 percent. The protein kcalories are higher than needed for maintenance. When the dieter returns to a maintenance plan by adding (mostly) carbohydrate foods, the ratio will resemble the recommended 15 percent protein, 30 percent fat, 55 percent carbohydrate.

This diet is one of many that offers the needed balance. Another could be higher in bread and fat and lower in meat exchanges.

The design of a weight-reduction diet—with all the protein, half the fat, and only a third the carbohydrate of a regular diet—may be responsible for many people's belief that cutting carbohydrate is necessary for weight loss. In a sound weight-loss diet, however, carbohydrate kcalories are not cut below about a third of the total. To eliminate carbohydrate altogether would be to invite a host of health hazards. Nor should you fast, except under a doctor's supervision.

is the attitude to adopt. This means including low-kcalorie foods that are rich in valuable nutrients—tasty vegetables and fruits, whole-grain breads and cereals, and a limited amount of lean protein-rich foods like poultry, fish, eggs, cottage cheese, and skim milk. Within these categories, learn what foods you like and use them often. If you plan resolutely to include a certain number of servings of food from each of these groups each day, you may be so busy making sure you get what you need that you will have little time or appetite left for high-kcalorie or empty-kcalorie foods.

Emphasize high nutrient density.

Individualize: Use foods you like.

Stress do's, not don'ts.

About a third of the kcalories in your diet should come from fat, to make your meals more satisfying. At least a third of the fat should be polyunsaturated fat—soft margarine, salad dressing, mayonnaise, or the like. Read the label to be sure of the kind of fat. And measure your fat with extra caution: A slip of the butterknife adds even more kcalories than a slip of the sugar spoon. And speaking of empty kcalories, omit sugar, pure fat/oil, and alcohol altogether—if you are willing. Let your carbohydrate come from starchy foods and your fat from protein-rich foods. Table 1 shows how you can plan a diet using the exchange system.

If at all possible, give up alcohol altogether until you have reached your goal, then add a conservative amount to your daily maintenance plan. If you insist on including alcohol in your diet plan, limit it strictly to no more than 150 kcal a day (see Table 2). Add this amount on top of your diet plan and reconcile yourself to a slower rate of weight loss. On no account should the empty kcalories of alcohol be allowed to displace the nutritious kcalories of the foods in the plan.

Eat regular meals, no skipping—at least 3 a day.

Eat regularly, and if at all possible, eat before you are very hungry. When you do decide to eat, eat the entire meal you have planned for yourself. Then don't eat again until the next meal. Save "free" or favorite foods or beverages for the end of the day, in case you are hungry once more.

Take a positive view of yourself.

You may have blamed yourself for eating compulsively in the past. That very character trait can work to your advantage: Compulsive people finish what they have started. So diet compulsively. Keep a record of what you have eaten each day for at least a week or two until your habits are beginning to be automatic.

It may seem at first as if you have to spend all your waking hours thinking about and planning your meals. Such a massive effort is

Table 2.   kCalories in Alcoholic Beverages and Mixers

Beverage	Amount (oz)	kCalories
Beer	12	150
Gin, rum, vodka, whiskey (86 proof)	1 1/2	105
Dessert wine	3 1/2	140
Table wine	3 1/2	85
Tonic, ginger ale, other sweetened carbonated waters	8	80
Cola, root beer	8	100
Fruit-flavored soda, Tom Collins mix	8	115
Club soda, diet drinks	8	1

100 proof means 50 percent alcohol; 86 proof means 43 percent.

One oz is 28 g, 1 1/2 oz is 42 g.

One gram alcohol = 7 kcal.

always required when a new skill is being learned. (You spent hours practicing writing the alphabet when you were in the first grade.) But after about three weeks, it will be much easier. Your new eating pattern will become a habit. Many sound and helpful books and booklets are available to help you get started, some of which are listed in this chapter's To Explore Further.

Visualize a changed future self.

Weigh yourself only once every week or two and always on the same scale, so that you can see clearly the progress you are making. Although 3,500 kcal roughly equals a pound of body fat, there is no simple relationship between kcalorie balance and weight loss over short intervals. Gains or losses of a pound or more in a matter of days reverse themselves quickly; the smoothed-out average is what is real. Don't expect to lose continuously as fast as you did at first. A sizable water loss is common in the first week, but it will not happen again.

Take well-spaced weighings to avoid discouragement.

If you see a gain in weight and you know you have strictly followed your diet, this probably represents a shift in water weight. Many dieters experience a temporary plateau after about three weeks—not because they are slipping but because they have gained water weight temporarily while they are still losing body fat. The fat you are hoping to lose must be combined with oxygen (oxidized) to make carbon dioxide and water if it is to leave the body. The oxygen you breath in combines with the carbons of the fat to make carbon dioxide and with the hydrogens to make water. The carbon dioxide will be breathed out quickly. But the water stays in the body for a longer time. The water takes a while to leave the cell, then enters the spaces between the cells, then works its way into the lymph system, and finally enters the bloodstream. Only after the water arrives in the blood will the kidneys "see" it and send it to the bladder for excretion. While water is making its way into the blood, you have a weight gain, because the water weighs more than the fat that was oxidized.[36] If you faithfully follow your diet plan, one day the plateau will break. You can tell from your frequent urination.

Anticipate a plateau (realistic expectations from the start).

You may find it helpful to control your environment, to avoid situations that prompt you to eat. Begin at the grocery store. Shop when you aren't hungry, and buy only the foods you plan to use on your diet. Purge from your pantry all forbidden items. If you must keep them on hand for other members of your family, surrender them into someone else's possession and ask that they be kept out of your sight as much as possible. Have low-kcalorie foods ready to eat; prepare ahead. To help further with your motivation, mount a mirror on the refrigerator door.

Control external cues.

It is easier to exclude a food than to exercise away its kcalories. To remind yourself of the reality that kcalories eaten must be spent in physical activity, post the following table conspicuously in a place where you might otherwise be tempted to eat:

Discourage magical thinking.

---

[36]Water weight accumulates during fat oxidation because one fatty acid weighing 284 units leaves behind water weighing 324 units, 14 percent more.

Table 3. Activity Equivalents of Food kCalorie Values*

Food	kCalories	Activity equivalent to work off the kcalories (minutes)		
		Walk[†]	Jog[‡]	Wait[§]
Apple, large	101	19	5	78
Beer, 1 glass	114	22	6	88
Cookie, chocolate chip	51	10	3	39
Ice cream, 1/6 qt	193	37	10	148
Steak, T-bone	235	45	12	181

*Adapted from M. V. Krause and M. A. Hunscher, *Food, Nutrition and Diet Therapy*, 5th ed. (Philadelphia: Saunders, 1972), p. 431.

[†]Energy cost of walking at 3.5 mph, for a 70-kilogram person is 5.2 kcal per minute.

[‡]Energy cost of running is 19.4 kcal per minute.

[§]Energy cost of reclining is 1.3 kcal per minute.

After losing 20 to 30 pounds, expect to reach a stable plateau.[37] Take this as a good sign. It means that you have lost so much weight that you now require fewer kcalories to maintain your weight. Take a deep breath (you knew this was coming and you are courageous) and institute a change: Increase your activity, cut your kcalories further, or both.

Use positive reinforcement. Never blame, never punish.

If you slip, don't punish yourself. Positive reinforcement is very effective at changing behavior, but punishment seldom works. If you ate an extra 1,000 kcal yesterday, don't try to eat 1,000 fewer kcalories today. Just go back to your diet. On the other hand, you can plan ahead and budget for binges. If you want to celebrate your birthday with cake and ice cream, cut the necessary kcalories from your bread and milk allowance for several days *beforehand*. Again, if you do this compulsively, your weight loss will be as smooth as if you had stayed with the daily plan.

Identify your problem and correct it.
Watch serving sizes.

You may have to get tough with yourself if you stop losing weight or start gaining unexpectedly. You may be slipping on serving sizes. Many a dieter has let herself, in time, measure out her meat exchanges too carelessly—and added an extra 500 kcal to the day's intake. Equally common is the "just this once" substitution of high-fat meat like steak for a fish fillet that was in the plan. You can get away with this only if

Learn kcaloric values and fat contents of foods.

you scrupulously omit the right amount of fat from other foods the same day. Ask yourself honestly (no one is listening in), "What am I doing wrong?" Very, very seldom does an unpredicted weight plateau of any duration have no explanation in the dieter's own choices.

[37]Keys and Grande, 1973; and L. Haimes, E. Harrison, H. A. Jordan, P. G. Lindner, and J. Rodin, Applying behavioral techniques in a bariatric practice, part 1, *Obesity and Bariatric Medicine* 6 (January/February 1977):10-16.

Finally, if you stop losing weight or begin to gain, be aware that you may be choosing to stop. Your weight is under your control, and you are entirely free to gain if you wish. You may find you are choosing to take a break, to go into a holding pattern, and to get adjusted before going on. Rather than letting yourself suffer from guilt feelings and feelings of failure, hold your head high and take the attitude, "This is me, and this is the way I am choosing to be right now."

Stress personal responsibility.

Honor the individual.

Exercise Weight loss is possible without exercise. Obese people often—and very understandably—do not enjoy moving their bodies very much. They feel heavy, clumsy, even ridiculous. The choice of whether to exercise regularly, informally, or not at all is a strictly individual matter. But even if you choose not to alter your habits at first, let your mind be open to the possibility that you will want to take up sports, dancing, or another activity later on. As the pounds come off, moving your body becomes a pleasure, as does letting others see you move. And the health advantages of regular exercise are well documented. It can truly make you look, feel, and be healthier.

Pave the way for later changes.

You must keep in mind that if exercise is to help with weight loss, it must be active exercise—voluntary moving of muscles. Being moved passively, as by a machine at a health spa or by a massage, does not increase kcaloric expenditure. The more muscles you move, the more kcalories you spend.

If you are very inactive, you may find yourself stuck at a plateau after a while unless you undertake some form of regular muscular activity. As with foods, let the activity be one that you enjoy—or that you feel you can most likely learn to enjoy in time. What fits best with your self-image: Rapid walking? Bicycling? Running errands for friends? Many people find that after two or three weeks of effort, exercise becomes as habitual as binge eating was before: You can get addicted to it.

Behavior Modification Everybody is different, but people who overeat are often seen to behave in certain ways at the table. Hence the need for behavior modification. Most of us are only faintly aware of our eating behavior and can find it interesting, even funny, to observe ourselves. Notice your own table style and compare it to someone else's. How often do you put down your fork (if at all)? How often do you interrupt your eating to converse with a friend? How fast do you chew your food? Do you always clean your plate? Several good books and other resources (check To Explore Further) can help you not only to observe yourself closely but also to set about systematically and effectively retraining yourself to eat like a thin person.

For many people, learning to eat slowly is one of the most important behavior changes to adopt. The satiety signal indicating that you are full is sent after a 20-minute lag. You may eat a great deal more than you need before the signal reaches your brain. Conversely, underweight people need to learn to eat more food within the first 20 minutes of a meal.

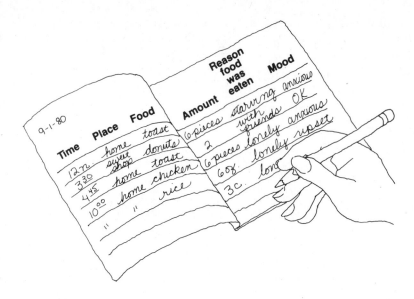

You may find it helpful to join a group such as TOPS (Take Off Pounds Sensibly) or Weight Watchers. A modest expenditure for your own health and well-being is well worth while (but avoid expensive, quick-weight-loss, "magical" ripoffs, of course). Many dieters find it helpful to form their own self-help groups structured around some of the resources already mentioned.[38] Sometimes it also helps to enlist a family member's participation and cooperation.[39] Correspondence groups are also available.[40]

Keep records to increase your personal investment in success.

In case you are a person who eats in response to external cues rather than internally felt hunger, you may need to keep a record for a while of all the circumstances surrounding your eating—the time, the place, the person you are with, the emotions you have at the time, the physical sensations, and other things. An example of such a record is shown above. Looking back, you can see what stimulates you to eat and learn to control these stimuli. If you find that you are indeed eating for the "wrong" reasons—for example, boredom—this discovery will pave the way for adopting behaviors better suited to your needs than compulsive eating. You can begin to make rules for yourself, like "Never eat when you're upset."

If you are especially sensitive to pressure from your family or friends or hosts (can't say no), it will help to have some assertiveness training. Learning not to clean your plate might be one of your first objectives.

[38]H. A. Jordan and L. S. Levitz, Behavior modification in a self-help group, *Journal of the American Dietetic Association* 62 (1973):27-29.

[39]L. S. Levitz, Behavior therapy in treating obesity, *Journal of the American Dietetic Association* 62 (1973):22-26.

[40]An example is described in A. R. Marston, M. R. Marston, and J. Ross, A correspondence course behavioral program for weight reduction, *Obesity and Bariatric Medicine* 6 (July/August 1977):140. Abstract cited in *Journal of the American Dietetic Association* 71 (1977):462.

From all the behavior changes available to you, you can choose the ones to begin with. Don't try to master them all at once. No one who attempts too many changes at one time is successful. Set your own priorities: Pick one trouble area that you think you can handle, start with that, practice your strategy until it is habitual and automatic. Then you can select another trouble area to work on.

Enjoy your new, emerging self. Inside of every fat person a thin person is struggling to be freed. Get in touch with—reach out your hand to—your thin self, and help that self to feel welcome in the light of day.

Use small-step modification.

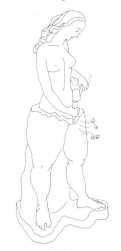

The Problem of Underweight

Much of what has been said about obesity applies to underweight as well, although its hazards are not so great. In fact, the only causes of death seen more often in thin people than in normal-weight people are infections such as tuberculosis. (Suicide is more common among underweight people, but the underweight is not thought to be a cause. The severe depression probably came first and caused anorexia, or lack of appetite.)

The causes of underweight may be as diverse as those of overeating. Hunger, appetite, and satiety irregularities may exist; there may be contributory psychological factors in some cases and metabolic ones in others. Clearly there is a genetic component as well. Early underfeeding may limit the number of fat cells in the same way overfeeding may increase it—although an episode of undernutrition sometimes precipitates later overeating and obesity. Habits learned early in childhood, especially food aversions, may perpetuate the problem. The demand for kcalories to support physical activity and growth often contributes: An extremely active boy during his adolescent growth spurt may need more than 4,000 kcal a day to maintain his weight. Such a boy may be too busy to take the time to eat that much. The underweight person states with justification that it is as hard for him to gain a pound as for an obese person to lose one. So much energy may be spent adapting to a higher food intake that it may take as many as 750 to 800 extra kcalories a day for the underweight person to gain a pound a week.[41]

Strategies recommended for weight gain center mostly on increasing food intake, using foods that provide as many kcalories in as small a volume as possible so as not to get uncomfortably full. Recommended are nutritious, high-kcalorie milkshakes; liberal servings of meat, bread, and starchy vegetables; and desserts. Whereas the weight loser is urged to select the lowest kcalorie items from each food group, the gainer is encouraged to pick the highest-kcalorie items from those same

anorexia (an-o-REX-ee-uh): lack of appetite.

an = not
orexis = appetite

[41]Questions doctors ask . . . , *Nutrition and the MD*, June 1978.

groups. Often she may need to resort to systematic between-meal snacking in addition to regular meals. No known pill, shot, hormone, or surgical procedure will increase weight safely, and a reduction in activity is not recommended unless the condition is associated with illness or is so severe as to threaten overall health.

As with weight loss, the person attempting a weight gain must anticipate a plateau, at which time a further increase in food intake will be necessary to continue the gain.[42] A mild degree of underweight is probably desirable, because it increases life expectancy.

anorexia nervosa (nerv-OH-sah): a severe self-imposed limitation of food intake sometimes seen in adolescents; a dangerous condition requiring skilled professional treatment.

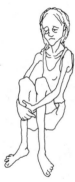

Anorexia Nervosa An extreme underweight condition is sometimes seen, usually in young women who claim to be exercising self-denial in order to control their weight. They actually go to such an extreme that they become severely undernourished, finally achieving a body weight of 70 pounds or even less. The distinguishing feature of the anorexic, as opposed to other very thin people, is that she intentionally starves herself. Often there is a whole cluster of accompanying "typical" characteristics of the family and the girl's attitudes.[43]

Anorexia nervosa is a serious condition that demands treatment by an experienced doctor or clinic. Even if temporarily reversed by forced feeding, it can reappear. If the underlying cause is not successfully dealt with, this illness can result in permanent brain damage or death. Strategies for successful treatment are well worked out, and recent advances have been encouraging.[44]

Summing Up

People of the same sex, age, and height may differ in weight due to differing densities of their bones and muscles. The weight compatible with good health depends on the individual. A person whose body fat contributes significantly more than about 10 percent of body weight is considered overweight. Weight tables based on height give an approximation of the weight ranges found to be average for the population as a whole. Body fatness, and therefore body weight, should normally decline with age as metabolism and activity decline.

Obesity is sometimes defined as body weight more than 20 percent above desirable weight. More precisely, obesity is excessive body fatness, which can be accurately diagnosed using the skinfold test. Some 10 to

[42]Keys and Grande, 1973.

[43]H. Bruch, ed., Anorexia nervosa: A review, *Dietetic Currents, Ross Timesaver* 4 (March/April 1977).

[44]Articles describing successful recovery are Bruch, 1977; B. J. Stordy, V. Marks, F. R. C. Path, R. S. Kalucy, and A. H. Crisp, Weight gain, thermic effect of glucose and resting metabolic rate during recovery from anorexia nervosa, *American Journal of Clinical Nutrition* 30 (1977):138-146; and K. C. Fox and N. M. James, Anorexia nervosa: A study of 44 strictly defined cases, *New Zealand Medical Journal* 84 (27 October 1976):309. Abstract cited in *Journal of the American Dietetic Association* 70 (1977):660-661.

25 percent of the young people in the United States and some 25 to 50 percent of its adults are obese by these standards.

Obesity sometimes arises in early life (juvenile onset) and sometimes later (adult onset); the former is harder to correct and both need to be prevented. Possible reasons for the irreversibility of juvenile-onset obesity include overmultiplication of fat cells in response to overfeeding and establishment of the wrong metabolic set-point for hunger or satiety.

Obesity entails a host of health hazards, including heart and blood vessel disease, diabetes, complications in pregnancy or after surgery, arthritis, abdominal hernias, varicose veins, respiratory problems, and gout, in addition to social and economic disadvantages. By contrast, underweight (weight more than 10 percent below desirable weight) is associated with an increased risk of infection. Mortality risk in obesity is not linear and is reversible.

Causes of obesity are a matter for much speculation and may include abnormalities in hunger or satiety regulation, in fat-cell number, in responsiveness to external cues that prompt eating behavior, in reactions to emotions and stress, in metabolism, in heredity, or in learned eating habits. An important contributor to obesity in this country is the extreme physical passivity and inactivity that characterize a sedentary lifestyle. However, causes differ widely among different people; treatment must therefore be individualized and multifaceted.

Ineffective and dangerous treatments include the use of diuretics ("water pills"), amphetamines ("diet pills"), hormones, and—except as a last resort for the intractably and morbidly obese—surgery. The most important step in successful treatment is the adoption of a balanced and nourishing low-kcalorie diet, and fat loss is greatly enhanced by regular exercise and behavior modification. Major criteria for success are a permanent change in eating habits and maintenance of the goal weight over the long term.

Diet can also help the underweight person. Behavior modification and other strategies that facilitate weight loss can be adapted to promote weight gain. But the special case of anorexia nervosa requires skilled professional attention. In all weight-control problems—obesity, underweight, and anorexia—real success is achieved only when new, adaptive eating and coping behaviors have permanently replaced the old ones.

To Explore Further

Recommended references on all nutrition topics are listed in Appendix J. In addition, we selected many to cite in this chapter's notes.

A brief review of the concepts of hunger, appetite, drive, and satiety and of the roles of fat cells and the hypothalamus in controlling food intake appears in Lepkovski, S., Regulation of food intake, *Advances in Food Research* 21 (1975):1-69.

The following are among the more popular behavior modification guides for the do-it-yourself dieter. The two Ferguson books and the Stuart and Davis book come in paperback.

Ferguson, J. M., *Habits, Not Diets: The Real Way to Weight Control* (Palo Alto, Calif.: Bull Publishing, 1976).

Ferguson, J. M., *Learning to Eat: Behavior Modification for Weight Control* (Palo Alto, Calif.: Bull Publishing, 1975).

Jordan, H. A., Levitz, L. S., and Kimbrell, G. M., *Eating Is Okay! A Radical Approach to Successful Weight Loss*, ed. S. Gelman (New York: Rawson Associates, 1976).

Mahoney, M. J., and Mahoney, K., *Permanent Weight Control* (New York: Norton, 1976).

Stuart, R. B., and Davis, B., *Slim Chance in a Fat World: Behavioral Control of Obesity* (Champaign, Ill.: Research Press, 1977).

One of many recent popular books to help people learn to be more assertive (in paperback):

Smith, M. J., *When I Say No, I Feel Guilty* (New York: Bantam Books, 1975).

Free from Metropolitan Life Insurance Company offices in many cities are three pamphlets:

Exercise Guide for Men and Women, 1976.
New Metropolitan Cookbook, 1973.
Four Steps to Weight Control, 1969.

Weight Watchers, Inc. publishes several cookbooks, all based on the exchange system, that present a very sensible, nutritious, balanced diet for weight loss.

Among other cookbooks useful for dieters is this paperback:

Jones, J., *The Calculating Cook: A Gourmet Cookbook for Diabetics and Dieters* (San Francisco: 101 Productions, 1977).

On anorexia nervosa, H. Bruch is the most authoritative speaker for the general reader. She has written an excellent book on the subject:

Bruch, H., *The Golden Cage: The Enigma of Anorexia Nervosa* (Cambridge, Mass.: Harvard University Press, 1978).

Diet Fallacies

In the long run, shortcuts are likely to be only self deceptions.

RONALD M. DEUTSCH

The North American public is obsessed with youthfulness and sexiness. It frequently equates these characteristics with a slim and feminine or a powerful and masculine figure. People who seek these physical attributes often begin by searching for an easy way to lose weight—and thus become willing victims of the diet con artist.

Criminologists tell us that the con game is unique in that its victims are active participants in the crime. The victims want something for nothing so badly that they become blind to the possibility that they may lose their life savings. It is often this way for those who long for a slim figure. They do not want to make the effort to change poor eating habits, to give up favorite foods, to count kcalories, or to study nutrition. So instead they fall for the advertising of a book or a mail-order diet that promises "quick, easy weight loss while you eat all your favorite foods" and do not realize that they may lose their good health.

The following are direct quotations from some of this type of advertising in popular magazines:

CRASH DIET ONLY $1.00—LOSE UP TO 5 POUNDS OVERNIGHT—NO PILLS, NO EXERCISE, ONE-DAY REDUCING FORMULA. EAT YOUR FILL! GO TO SLEEP, WAKE UP AND YOU HAVE LOST UP TO FIVE POUNDS.

TAKE THAT UGLY FAT OFF THIGHS, NECK, LEGS, WAISTLINE, ALL OVER, WITHOUT PUTTING DOWN YOUR KNIFE AND FORK—EAT THE FOODS YOU LIKE—LIKE VEAL SCALLOPINI, ROAST CHICKEN, STEAK AND LAMB, ROAST BEEF.

NEW FAT-BURNING SYSTEM SLIMS YOU DOWN POUNDS IN JUST 10 DAYS.

What scintillating promises to those who want fervently to lose those ugly bulges!

There is nothing magical about weight reduction, despite the promises implied in these ads. From your study of the first eight chapters, you know that the human body has evolved a system whereby kcalories are given top priority. kCalories are never thrown away frivolously just because they are in good supply. Relatively few kcalories are lost through excretion, few are used for keeping the body warm or to digest food, more are used to fuel the body's vital organs, and many are used to move the body. If some extra kcalories are taken in and not spent on these activities, they are stored in the liver and muscle as glycogen, ready for quick withdrawal when needed. If there is a larger surplus of kcalories than can be stored as glycogen, these extra kcalories are converted to fat and stored in the adipose tissue. When kcalories are in short supply the stored fat is withdrawn from the adipose tissue and metabolized for energy. This is the fundamental principle that the willing victims of diet con artists do not understand (or refuse to acknowledge).

The Low-Carbohydrate Diet A student tells the story: "I attended a dinner meeting the other day and saw an old friend there. I hardly recognized her, she had lost so much weight. I was delighted at how pretty she looked and asked her how she had done it. She had been attending a weight-loss clinic. When she described

---

Mini-Glossary

fallacy: an argument that fails to satisfy the conditions of valid or correct reasoning from evidence.

fallacia = deceit

---

the regimen, I realized she was on a high-protein, high-fat diet. She told me she had more to eat than she could consume, she was checked regularly by a doctor, and she was receiving vitamin and mineral supplements." This was a low-carbohydrate diet, and it appeared to be working well. (Stay tuned; there's more to come.)

One of the oldest and most popular reducing diets is the low-carbohydrate diet, currently being advertised as "new" and "revolutionary." However, it is a very old regimen that resurfaces every decade or so under a new name: the Air Force diet, the drinking man's diet, the Scarsdale diet, the calories-don't-count diet, for instance. The low-carbohydrate diet consists of cutting carbohydrate intake to 60 g a day or less while allowing all the protein or fat foods a dieter wants to eat: "Unlimited food intake while you lose weight!" As you might suspect, there are a number of fallacies in this method of losing weight.

The most striking indictment of the low-carbohydrate diet lies in the fact that it is dangerous. It is ketogenic (see page 234); its high fat content would tend to contribute to atherosclerosis (see Highlight 6). Since this type of diet is often promoted by physicians, the public assumes that it will not only result in weight loss but will also be medically safe to follow. That it is *not* considered medically safe by the majority of the medical profession is evidenced by the statement of the AMA Council on Food and Nutrition, which presents experimental proof of its fallacies and dangers.[1] Also, a number of prominent nutritionists have spoken out against it. One of these is Dr. Frederick Stare, chairman of the Nutrition Department of Harvard University, who testified before a Senate committee investigating fad diets:[2]

Since coronary heart disease is the principal cause of death in the United States, and any diet which tends to be high in saturated fats and cholesterol tends to elevate the chance that the individual will get heart disease, any book that recommends unlimited amounts of meat, butter, and eggs, as this one does, in my opinion is dangerous. The author [a doctor] who makes the suggestion is guilty of malpractice.

[1] A critique of low-carbohydrate ketogenic weight reduction regimens, *Journal of the American Medical Association* 224 (1973):1415-1419.

[2] U.S. Senate, Select Committee on Nutrition and Human Needs, Obesity and Fad Diets, *Nutrition and Disease (Hearings)* (Washington, D.C.: Government Printing Office, 1973), part 1.

As you read this and the following paragraphs exploding the low-carbohydrate diet fallacy, you should be aware that many tools useful for sifting fact from fancy are being used here. You have been urged to ask yourself who wrote a source of nutrition information, who published it, and why it was published. In the case of many of these diets, "who wrote it" and "who published it" were people or companies whose major goal was not to further the advancement of science but to earn fame and fortune for themselves. It has also been pointed out that claims based on logic alone must stand the test of experimentation. The rationale for many of these diets seems logical enough but proves false on experimental testing, as a scrutiny of the AMA statement will show you. In fact, a perusal of the scientific literature shows that *none* of the claims made by promoters of these diets stands up to testing.

In attempting to sort out fact from fancy, you will find an additional guideline helpful. If the promoters refer to scientific reports in journals such as those referred to in this and other Highlights, you can check them for yourself; if they make no reference to evidence substantiating their claims, you must suspect their word. Also, every creditable institution seems to have a fake counterpart. Watch out for "doctors" without an MD, "universities" with only a PO box address, "nutrition organizations" with no recognized standing, and the like.

A FLAG SIGN OF A SPURIOUS CLAIM IS ASSERTIONS LIKE:

"Doctors agree"— when the identity of the "doctors" is not revealed.

"Authorities agree"—when no reference to an authoritative publication is provided.

One of the reasons that warnings about the low-carbohydrate diet by prominent groups like the AMA have fallen on deaf ears is that restricting carbohydrates can produce a dramatic loss of weight. However, there is no experimental evidence that *fat* loss occurs while the dieters are consuming more kcalories than they are expending, and there is abun-

dant experimental evidence that the diet is damaging to the body. Remember that a dieter must seek oxidation of his own body fat. There is no magic in the combination of protein and fat that allows you to eat more energy foods than you need and at the same time oxidize your own body fat.

The fat loss that occurs in the low-carbohydrate diet appears to come from the toxic effects of the ketones, which produce nausea and thus suppress the appetite, and through self-restriction of kcalories. It seems nearly impossible to shift from a mixed diet to one totally devoid of carbohydrates and then to eat enough protein and fat to make up the kcalorie deficit. For example, Yudkin and Corey studied the normal diets of six obese people and then placed them on a carbohydrate-restricted diet in which they could eat all the protein and fat they wanted.[3] When the low-carbohydrate diets were studied, it was found that none of the subjects had increased his intake of fat foods and that there had been a reduction of kcalories ranging from 13 to 55 percent. With reduction in kcalories came fat loss.

The low-carbohydrate diet also produces weight loss due

[3]J. Yudkin and M. Carey, The treatment of obesity by the "high-fat" diet: The inevitability of calories, *Lancet* ii (1960):939-941.

to excretion of salt, according to the AMA statement.[4] Since water follows salt, much of the drop in pounds seen on the bathroom scales may be due to the excretion of salt and water. Not only is it dangerous to upset the water and electrolyte balance, but also this weight will be regained rapidly when the person resumes carbohydrate ingestion.

In judging any weight-reduction program, it is imperative to speak of the weight loss in terms of a change in body composition rather than in terms of the change in the reading on the bathroom scales. If on Tuesday you weigh five pounds less than you did on Monday, the next question is, Was that a loss of fat, which is desirable, or just a loss of water, which is usually undesirable? A change in body composition, a shift to a lower percentage of body weight in the adipose tissue, is the goal of a valid reducing diet regimen. (There is, however, a form of water loss that is desirable and that represents a change in body composition: loss of the water that is generated by the oxidation of body fat; see p. 295.)

The student mentioned earlier had more to say about her friend at the weight-loss clinic: "When the meeting was breaking up, I passed by my friend, and I overheard

[4]Critique of ketogenic regimens, 1973.

her telling someone that she hadn't completed some work over the weekend. She had been nauseated and had had double vision. She complained that 'I just couldn't get my mind to working right. I was so confused, I finally just gave up and went to bed for the entire weekend.' That's when I realized the diet wasn't working so well after all."

Health professionals have universally condemned the low-carbohydrate diet as hazardous in a number of ways. It raises blood uric acid, disposing the dieter to gout.[5] It lowers blood potassium, causing irregular heartbeats.[6] It increases the acidity of the blood, because ketones are acid. It causes sodium loss and consequent dehydration.[7] It causes fatigue and blood pressure abnormalities[8] and aggravates kidney problems. It causes pronounced elevation of serum cholesterol, a known risk factor for heart disease.[9]

[5]Critique of ketogenic regimens, 1973.

[6]*Obesity '73: A Report from the Geigy Symposium on Obesity, Its Problems and Prognosis* (New York: Ardsley, 1973).

[7]H. T. Randall, Water, electrolytes and acid-base balance, in *Modern Nutrition in Health and Disease*, 5th ed., eds. R. S. Goodhart and M. E. Shils (Philadelphia: Lea and Febiger, 1973) pp. 324-361.

[8]Critique of ketogenic regimens, 1973.

Following any of the fad diets can be especially dangerous to vulnerable groups, such as people with a tendency towards diabetes, hyperlipidemia, or heart disease. Of particular interest in this regard is the danger of ketosis to the developing fetus in the pregnant woman on a low-carbohydrate diet. Dr. Karlis Adamsons, professor of obstetrics and gynecology, City University, New York City, testified before the Senate committee investigating fad diets.[10] He stated that although the fetus is very well protected from harm and generally gets the nutrients it needs from the mother's blood supply, two substances critical to its development—glucose and oxygen—are not stored in the mother's body. Cellular glucose deprivation occurs in the state of ketosis, which accompanies some diseases (diabetes) and diets lacking carbohydrate foods. The mother may be able to tolerate glucose starvation temporarily, but the fetus may suffer permanent brain damage during such starvation, because glucose is the only fuel that the developing central nervous system can use. Even an adult's brain

[9]F. Rickman, N. Mitchell, J. Dingman, and J. E. Dalen, Changes in serum cholesterol during the Stillman diet, *Journal of the American Medical Association* 228 (1974):54-58.

[10]Senate Select Committee, 1973.

suffers, however, as the student's story shows. Her friend could not think, and had to go to bed for the whole weekend. She probably could have done her work if she had just drunk a glass of orange juice.

A number of persons and organizations are being quoted here. How are you to know that a person or organization is one whose opinion you can trust?

The American Dietetic Association, the Canadian Dietetic Association, the American Medical Association, and the Canadian Medical Association are professional organizations. Membership in these associations is limited to people who have qualified for membership by their education and experience (graduate dietitians or medical doctors). The journals of these organizations are the vehicles by which scientific information is disseminated to the membership. These journals constitute the arena in which professional arguments can be resolved. If one of these professional journals speaks out editorially on a controversial topic, you can safely assume that the editorial reflects a consensus of member opinions.

There are also scientific organizations that any person can join simply by paying the fees. The membership is composed of people who have a common interest or viewpoint. The journals of these organizations do not necessarily publish incorrect scientific information; they just do not have the checks and balances of the journals of the professional organizations. You cannot rely on the educational background of the writers or assume that the articles have been screened by competent professionals before publication, nor can you trust the purpose for which the articles were written.

CAUTION WHEN YOU READ!

When an organization's journal speaks out on a controversial topic, ask yourself:

Is the organization back of this statement an association of professionals, or can anyone join?

A reputable nutritionist is one who is educated in nutrition or a closely allied field. Usually such nutritionists are associated with a fairly large university or medical center, where they are able to engage in teaching or research assignments. When you examine the qualifications of a nutritionist, pay no attention to such advertising adjectives as *famous*, or *well-known* or even *reputable*. Look instead at the educational background or present affiliations of the person.

It is relatively easy to judge the lack of qualifications of, say, movie stars who speak on nutrition, but it is much more difficult to make a valid judgment when medical doctors or scientists outside the nutritional field speak on the subject. A careful writer will help you make these judgments. For example, on p. 304 Dr. Stare is quoted on a nutrition topic. You will note that you were told he is chairman of the Nutrition Department at Harvard University. On p. 306 Dr. Adamsons is quoted on a nutritional topic also. He is a professor of obstetrics and gynecology at City University, New York. Is he then qualified to testify on nutrition? In this case yes, because the topic is concerned with conditions affecting the unborn—the nutrition of the mother.

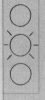

CAUTION WHEN YOU READ!

When an "authority" gives an opinion on a topic, ask yourself:

Does this person have the educational and experiential background to speak on this topic?

In the face of today's precarious food situation, authors of diet schemes like the low-carbohydrate diet are acting irresponsibly. They are intimating to the public that the only way to be slim and healthy is to avoid carbohydrate (plant) foods and to eat meat. But plant foods generally cost less than meat and use much less of the available land to grow. They contribute to the diet many important nutrients in addition to carbohydrates: protein, vitamins, minerals, fiber, and perhaps as-yet-undiscovered substances present in unrefined complex-carbohydrate foods.

When you are told (by a doctor on television or in a book) that you must avoid carbohydrates to regain your lost figure, you may interpret this to mean that carbohydrates are fattening. But you know from your study of Chapters 1 to 3 that carbohydrate kcalories are no more fattening than any other kcalories. Gram for gram, carbohydrate produces the same number of kcalories as protein and less than half as many kcalories as fat. You may be enthusiastic about losing some "excess baggage," but you should use that enthusiasm to start an eating program that you can follow for life, without danger.

Many diets are variations of the low-carbohydrate diet. For instance, if you are advised to eat a high-protein diet, you are being asked to limit carbohydrates. You have learned that one of the functions of the carbohydrates is to spare the valuable amino acids. Amino acids taken in excess of the need to build or repair tissues are used for energy; amino acids eaten when there is an absolute energy deficit are also used for energy. Since you are extracting energy from the protein, you might as well eat a less expensive source— carbohydrate. Athletes are often urged to eat high-protein diets in the hope that this will stimulate muscle growth. What they really need is high kcalories to support the extra expenditure of energy during games and enough protein for repair and maintenance of tissue.[11]

Some Other Diets Other diets are based on equally fallacious reasoning. The "Mayo Diet," which is not and never has been advocated by the highly reputable Mayo Clinic of Rochester, Minnesota,[12] has many variations—but may include as many as nine eggs a day. This diet is a high-cholesterol diet and therefore may present a danger to vulnerable persons (see Highlight 6). If it results in weight loss, it is probably because dieters become bored with the few foods allowed them and stop eating. Certainly this diet would not be conducive to learning good eating habits.

The "grapefruit diet" claims that grapefruit burns up other foods. Thus grapefruit is to be eaten before every meal. The meals themselves are composed mostly of low-kcalorie vegetables and fruit. However, no food burns up another food. The diet probably is based on an erroneous understanding of the specific dynamic effect of foods (a few kcalories are used to fuel the digestive processes; see Chapter 7).

One of the oldest ways of reducing is total fasting, which allows only non-kcaloric liquids. The physical hazards of fasting have already been described (Chapter 7); there is also

mental anguish associated with it because lean body tissue is restored at the very first intake of protein. With each pound of protein replaced, three pounds of water must be provided for the intracellular spaces of the protein mass.[13] The obese person, who deprives himself totally of food to lose weight, then sees his weight zoom back up again at his very first little snack. No wonder he thinks that he will gain weight no matter how little he eats.

Up to this point we have been discussing weight-reduction diets. However, there is another type of diet that is receiving a great deal of emphasis today, especially among young people.[14] The Zen macrobiotic diet is promoted as a means of awakening a spiritual rebirth. This diet actually consists of ten diets. The lowest includes cereals, vegetables, animal products, and fruit; the highest includes only cereals. According to the AMA Council on Foods and Nutrition,

> To merely brand as food faddists those individuals whose dietary beliefs are not in accord with what is ordinarily considered sound nutritional practice serves no useful pur-

[11]Position paper on food and nutrition misinformation on selected topics, *Journal of the American Dietetic Association* 66 (1975):277-279.

[12]Committee on Dietetics, *Mayo Clinic Diet Manual*, 4th ed. (Philadelphia: Saunders, 1971).

[13]S. K. Fineberg, The realities of obesity and fad diets, *Nutrition Today*, July/August 1972, pp. 23-26.

[14]U. D. Register and L. M. Sonnenberg, The vegetarian diet, *Journal of the American Dietetic Association* 62 (1973):253-261.

pose. . . .But, when a diet has been shown to cause irreversible damage to health and ultimately lead to death, it should be roundly condemned as a threat to human health. The Council . . . believes that such is the case with the rigid dietary restrictions placed on the followers of the Zen macrobiotic philosophy.[15]

In summary, you should always suspect a claim if it is couched in terms that sound like magical thinking. Be wary when a scientist resorts to writing on technical matters in the public arena, unless you can find corroborating testimony in the scientific journals. And suspect that

[15]Zen macrobiotic diets, *Journal of the American Medical Association* 218 (1971):397.

the claims for any diet are probably unsound if entire classes of food are either eliminated or overemphasized.

To Explore Further

A help in understanding the problem of obesity and why some diets do not contribute to permanent loss of weight:

Leveille, G. A., and Romsos, D. R., Meal eating and obesity, *Nutrition Today,* November/December 1974, pp. 4-9.

Fineberg, S. K., The realities of obesity and fad diets, *Nutrition Today,* July/August 1972, pp. 23-26.

Lewis, S. B., Wallin, J. D., Kane, J. P., and Gerich, J. E., Effect of diet composition on metabolic adaptations to hy-

pocaloric nutrition: Comparison of high carbohydrate and high fat isocaloric diets. *American Journal of Clinical Nutrition* 30 (1977):160-169.

Margolius's book is very well written and very interesting; Deutsch's book has become a classic exposé of popular food fads:

Deutsch, R. M., *The New Nuts Among the Berries: How Nutrition Nonsense Captured America* (Palo Alto, Calif.: Bull Publishing, 1977).

Margolius, S., *Health Foods: Facts and Fakes* (New York: Walker, 1974).

The Healthy Way to Weigh Less and *Critique of Low-Carbohydrate Ketogenic Weight Reduction Regimens,* a pamphlet and a reprint, can be ordered from the American Medical Association (address in Appendix J).

Diet Planning

Diets can be planned using the exchange system to gain weight, lose weight, or stay the same. For practice in the use of this convenient system, try planning two diets, one for weight maintenance or gain, the other for weight loss. Use your own "personalized RDA for energy," derived in the Self-Study on Energy Output (p. 268), as a baseline for planning.

Diet for Weight Maintenance or Gain

1. Set your daily kcalorie level. If you choose to maintain weight, it should be equal to your "personalized RDA." If you wish to gain weight, it should be at least 500 kcal above your "RDA" (see Chapter 7 Self-Study).

2. Decide on the ratio of protein:fat:carbohydrate kcalories to be delivered by the diet. A suggested ratio is: about 10 to 15 percent of the kcalories from protein, not more than 30 percent from fat, and the rest from carbohydrate. Given the daily kcalorie level you chose, how many kcalories will you allot to each nutrient?

3. Translate these kcalorie amounts into grams. (Remember, 1 g protein or carbohydrate = 4 kcal; 1 g fat = 9 kcal.) Enter these gram amounts at the top of Form 1.

4. Now decide how many exchanges of milk, vegetables, and fruit you'd like to have each day; enter these numbers in the form; and compute the number of grams of carbohydrate, protein, and fat they will deliver (don't compute kcalories yet). See p. 41 or Appendix L for the exchange system values. (Caution: Use pencil. You'll want to change these numbers several times before you finalize your plan.)

Form 1. Diet Planning by Exchange Groups

Exchange group	Number of exchanges*	Amounts to be delivered[†]			
		Carbohydrate (g)	Protein (g)	Fat (g)	Energy[‡] (kcal)
Milk					
Vegetable					
Fruit					
Bread					
Meat					
Fat					
	Total actually delivered				

*From steps 4, 5, 6.
†From step 3.
‡From step 7.

Only one more group of foods—the bread exchanges—contribute any carbohydrate to the diet. Select the number of bread exchanges that will bring your total carbohydrate intake close to the amount you want. Adjust the numbers of these four exchanges until they seem reasonable to you.

(Suggestions: Diets for adults should include two to three milk exchanges daily, two or more vegetable exchanges, and at least two and preferably more fruit exchanges. The number of bread exchanges is variable, but the bread list includes many nutritious foods containing complex carbohydrates. It is not unusual for women's diets to include four to six bread exchanges and for men's to include twice as many or even more. High-kcalorie diets can have many more of all of these carbohydrate-containing exchanges.)

If you have a special fondness for sugar or sugar-containing foods, add a line to Form 1 under Bread, and allow yourself some "sugar exchanges" (see p. 42). At the end of this step, you should have a carbohydrate gram total within about 10 percent of the number you planned in step 3.

5. Subtotal the protein grams delivered by these four groups of foods. Only one more group of foods—the meat exchanges—will con-

tribute any protein to the diet. Select the number of meat exchanges you need to bring your total protein intake close to what you planned in step 3.

Note: The recommended intake of carbohydrate is high compared to what many people are used to. Planners often find that once they have completed step 4 of this procedure they have almost used up their protein allowance and must therefore drastically limit their meat consumption. If it works out this way for you, you have two choices. You can accept the dictates of this pattern and resolve to limit your meat intake accordingly. Or you can increase the number of protein grams you will allow yourself (step 3) and reduce carbohydrate and/or fat to keep the kcalorie level within bounds.

At the end of this step, you should have a protein gram total that agrees (within 10 percent) with your plan of step 3.

6. Subtotal the fat grams delivered by these five groups of foods. Now use the fat exchanges to bring your total fat intake up to the level planned in step 3.

7. Fill in the kcalorie amounts contributed by the exchanges you have selected, and check to see that the total agrees (within 10 percent) with the kcalorie level you set in step 1. The completed form now indicates

the total exchanges of each type that you will consume on each day of your diet.

8. Distribute the exchanges you have selected into a meal pattern like that of Form 2. You may want to plan four to six meals a day or to have only one snack; if so, or if you have other preferences, make your own form.

9. Finally, to see how your diet plan might work out on an actual day, make a sample menu. Look over the exchange groups and choose foods you would like to eat in each category that fit the pattern you worked out in step 8. For example:

My meal pattern for breakfast specifies:

  1 fruit
  2 bread
  1 milk
  1 sugar
  1 fat

So I might choose:

  1/2 c orange juice
  3/4 oz dry cereal and
    1 slice bread, toasted
  1/2 c milk on the cereal,
    1/2 c milk in a glass
  1 tsp sugar on the cereal
  1 pat margarine on the
    toast

Diet for Weight Loss

1. Set your daily kcalorie level. If you wish to lose a pound a week, set it 500 kcal per day below your "personalized RDA." You could

Form 2. Meal Patterns

Exchange group	Total exchanges consumed daily*	Exchanges consumed at each meal				
		Breakfast	Lunch	Snack	Dinner	Snack
Milk						
Vegetable						
Fruit						
Bread						
Meat						
Fat						

*From Form 1, column 2.

set it higher or lower than this, but on no account should you set it below 1,000 kcal per day.

2. Decide on the ratio of protein:fat:carbohydrate kcalories to be delivered by the diet. A suggested ratio is that offered in Table 1 of Chapter 8: about 33 percent of the kcalories from each energy nutrient.

3. Translate these kcalorie amounts into grams, as in the previous diet plan.

4. Now decide on the number of carbohydrate-containing exchanges you'll have, as in step 4 of the first plan. Try to include two milk, two vegetable, and at least two fruit exchanges, and make up the rest of your carbohydrate intake with bread exchanges. Allow no

sugar unless you really can't do without it. At the end of this step you should have a carbohydrate gram total within about 10 percent of the number you planned in step 3.

5. Now subtotal the protein grams you have so far, and bring your total protein intake up to the level of your plan by adding meat exchanges. At the end of this step, you should have a protein gram total that agrees (within 10 percent) with your plan of step 3.

6. Now subtotal the fat grams you have so far, and add fat exchanges to bring your total fat intake up to the level planned in step 3.

7. Fill in the kcalorie amounts contributed by the exchanges you have selected,

and check to see that the total agrees (within 10 percent) with the kcalorie level you set in step 1.

8. Distribute the exchanges into a meal pattern, using Form 2 or your own form based on your own preferences.

9. Make a day's sample menus, as in step 9 of the first plan.

Optional Extra

● Spot the fallacies in crash-diet ads. The following are direct quotes from advertisements in a magazine for teenagers. What can you find in them to criticize, in light of what you have read in Chapter 8 and Highlight 8?

CRASH DIET ONLY $1. LOSE UP TO 5 POUNDS OVERNIGHT! LEARN THE SECRET OF TV'S FANTASTIC NO-PILL, NO-EXERCISE ONE-DAY REDUCING FORMULA! EAT YOUR FILL! GO TO SLEEP! WAKE UP!—AND YOU HAVE LOST UP TO 5 POUNDS. AMAZING? SURE! BUT GUARANTEED TO WORK OR YOUR MONEY BACK! SEND ONLY $1.00. SORRY, NO C.O.D.'S.

WEIGHT LOSS BY THE HOUR! 8 AM . . . 126 POUNDS! 8 PM . . . 124 POUNDS! 8 AM . . . TOMORROW 122 POUNDS! . . . IMAGINE LOSING A FULL POUND IN THE FIRST 6 HOURS! 2 POUNDS BETWEEN MORNING AND NIGHT! UP TO 5 POUNDS IN AS LITTLE AS 24 HOURS! IF THAT SOUNDS UN-BELIEVABLE, GET THE ENTIRE PROGRAM NOW AND READ WHAN AN EMINENT DOCTOR SAYS ABOUT IT. READ WHAT PEOPLE WHO HAVE TRIED IT SAY HAPPENED TO THEM! READ THE SCIENTIFIC AND

MEDICAL REASONS WHY IT MAY VERY WELL BE THE FAST-EST, MOST EFFECTIVE, SAFEST WAY TO LOSE WEIGHT THAT HAS EVER BEEN DISCOVERED.

"THERE'S NO MORE HEALTH-FUL WAY TO LOSE SO MUCH WEIGHT SO FAST!"—DR. FRANK R. RICARDO, M.D.

16 TIMES MORE POTENT THAN THE FAMOUS "GRAPEFRUIT DIET." 10 TIMES MORE EFFEC-TIVE THAN THE POPULAR "HI-PROTEIN" DIET— ABSOLUTELY NO DRUGS OF ANY KIND. NO EXHAUSTIVE EXERCISES, AND NO HUNGER PAINS—EVER. POUNDS AND INCHES BEGIN TO DISAPPEAR WITH YOUR FIRST HEARTY BREAKFAST OF EGGS, HAM, JUICE, TOAST AND COFFEE. WORD OF MOUTH IS SPREAD-ING THE "MEGA-VITAMIN" DIET LIKE UNCONTROLLED WILDFIRE! A NEWLY DE-VELOPED SUPER PROTEIN TAB-LET. CREATED ESPECIALLY FOR THIS DIET. CONTAINS A WHOP-

PING 570 MILLIGRAMS OF SOLID NATURAL PROTEIN. EACH TINY MILLIGRAM ZEROS IN ON FATTY TISSUES TO BREAK DOWN AND BURN OFF MANY TIMES ITS EQUIVALENT WEIGHT. A DOZEN T-BONE STEAKS COULD NOT PROVIDE AS MUCH UNDILUTED, FAT-FREE, NATURAL PROTEIN AS THIS ONE, TINY, SUPER PRO-TEIN TABLET. THE QUARTER-BACK OF THE SUPER SUCCESS-FUL TEAM, "ULTRA-IRON" CONTAINS THE EXACT AND REQUIRED DOSAGES OF MAN-GANESE TO ACTIVATE YOUR ENZYMES AND MAINTAIN GOOD GLANDULAR FUNC-TIONS, BETAINE TO PREVENT ANY ACCUMULATION OF FAT, ZINC, THE ESSENTIAL INGRE-DIENT RELATED TO CARBOHY-DRATE METABOLISM, AND COPPER, TO PROVIDE CON-TINUAL BODY ENERGY, PLUS 25 MICROGRAMS OF THE HIGHLY DESIRABLE B-12 COMPLEX.

PART TWO

VITAMINS, MINERALS, AND WATER

INTRODUCTION

CONTENTS

SUPPORTING ACTORS

The introduction to Part One identified the nutrients: carbohydrate, lipid, protein, vitamins, minerals, and water. The eight chapters in Part One were devoted entirely to the first three of these—the principal actors—whose presence in the body accounts for what you are (you are literally made of these three materials and compounds derived from them) and for what you do (because they supply the energy for all your activities).

As you saw, each of those three nutrients is a giant by molecular standards. A single molecule of carbohydrate may be composed of 300 glucose units, each containing 24 atoms, for a total of some 7,000 atoms. Lipids and proteins are similar in size. Even when they are broken down during digestion, they are absorbed as sizable units—and these are often reassembled in the cells back into macromolecules. Only if they are oxidized for fuel do they diminish in size to tiny molecules of carbon dioxide and water (three atoms each). If this occurs, they release tremendous quantities of energy for your use.

Furthermore, you eat (by molecular standards) tremendous quantities of these three nutrients: a hundred or so grams a day of each. If you could purify the carbohydrate, lipid, and protein in your daily diet, they would fill two or three cups.

The second three nutrients—vitamins, minerals, and water—differ profoundly from the first three in almost every way: in their size and shape, in the roles they play in the body, in the amounts you consume. Perhaps the only characteristics they share with the first three are that they are vital to life and that they are available in food.

Chapters 9 to 14 are devoted to these nutrients: three to the vitamins, two to the minerals, and one to water. A few generalizations presented here will help you put these supporting actors in perspective.

Carbohydrate, fat, and protein: large organic molecules.

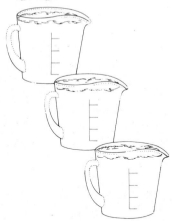

Amount of energy nutrients eaten daily

Carbohydrate, fat, and protein: 50-200 g a day of each.

Vitamins: small organic molecules.

Vitamins: yield no energy.

vitamin: an organic compound vital to life, needed in minute amounts. (The first vitamins discovered were amines.)

vita = life
amine = containing nitrogen

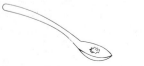

Amount of vitamins eaten daily

Organic: see p. 5.

Vitamins

The vitamins are organic compounds generally much smaller than the energy nutrients. A molecule of vitamin C, for example, is comparable in size to a single glucose unit. Vitamins are never strung together to make body compounds (although each may be attached to a protein), and if they are broken down they yield no usable energy. You consume minute amounts of vitamins daily—a few micrograms (millionths of a gram) or milligrams (thousandths of a gram) or, at the very most, a few grams. Yet they are vital; in fact, they were named for this characteristic. As you will see in Chapters 9 to 11, they serve as helpers, making possible the processes by which the first three nutrients are digested, absorbed, and metabolized in the body. There are some 15 different vitamins, each with its own special roles to play.

Vitamins as Organic Substances   The fact that vitamins are organic has several consequences. For one, vitamins are destructible. They can be broken down, oxidized, altered in shape. They must therefore be handled with care. Your body makes special provisions to absorb them, providing several of them with custom-made protein carriers like those provided for the lipids. A vitamin may be useful in one form here and another there, so special enzymes are also provided that can slightly alter the form of a vitamin to make it active in a given role.

> Many vitamins exist in several related forms.

The destructibility of vitamins also has implications for their handling outside the body. Food handlers and cooks are well-advised to be aware of the vulnerability of the vitamins in foods and to treat them with respect.

> Vitamins are destructible.

Fat-Soluble and Water-Soluble Vitamins   As you may recall, some organic compounds are hydrophilic (water-loving), because positive and negative charges abound on their surfaces and so attract them to the positive (H^+) and negative (OH^-) ions of water. Others are hydrophobic (water-avoiding) and are attracted into the neighborhood of the uncharged, fat-loving compounds. Carbohydrates and proteins are in the first and lipids in the second category. The vitamins are divided between these classes: some are water-soluble (the B vitamins and vitamin C) and others are fat-soluble (vitamins A, D, E, and K).

> Water-soluble vitamins: B complex and C.
> Fat-soluble vitamins: A, D, E, K.

This fact has several implications for vitamin absorption, transport, storage, and excretion.

Absorption of Vitamins The digestive system absorbs these two types of substances differently. Water-soluble substances cross the intestinal and vascular walls directly into the blood, but fat-soluble substances are handled laboriously. Except for the short-chain fatty acids, fat-soluble substances must be emulsified and carried across the membranes of the intestinal cells associated with fat and often with bile. They cannot cross the blood vessel walls to enter the bloodstream directly but must be transported by way of the lymph, from which they later enter the bloodstream.

Lymphatic system: see pp. 190-191.

> Water-soluble vitamins: absorbed into blood.
> Fat-soluble vitamins: absorbed into lymph with fat.

Transport of Vitamins The body's principal transportation system — the bloodstream — is a system of waterways. Water-soluble vitamins travel freely dissolved in blood; fat-soluble vitamins must be made soluble in water by being attached to protein carriers.

> Water-soluble vitamins: free in blood.
> Fat-soluble vitamins: carried by proteins.

Storage and Excretion of Vitamins Once the fat-soluble vitamins have been absorbed and transported to cells of the body, they tend to become sequestered there, associated with fat. The water-soluble vitamins, on the other hand, are not held so firmly in place. If they are not in use, they circulate freely among all organs of the body, including the kidneys.

The body's principal excretion medium is also water. The kidneys are sensitive to high concentrations of substances in the blood that flows through them. They selectively remove those substances in excess and pass them into the urine. The kidneys detect and remove excess water-soluble vitamins, but they less readily detect excess fat-soluble vitamins, because these do not accumulate in the blood; they tend to be hidden away in fat-storage places in the body.

> Water-soluble vitamins: excesses excreted.
> Fat-soluble vitamins: excesses stored.

This difference has two implications. First, excess vitamin A eaten today may be stored to meet next month's needs, and blood levels will remain normal. But if too much vitamin C is in the blood, the kidneys respond by excreting the excess, and tomorrow's needs will be met by depleting the vitamin C pool in the blood. Thus vitamin A can be eaten in large amounts once in a while and still meet your body's needs over the interval. But vitamin C must be eaten in smaller amounts more frequently.

> Water-soluble vitamins: needed in frequent small doses.
> Fat-soluble vitamins: can be taken in larger doses less often.

The B vitamin riboflavin is a yellow compound so bright that it is easy to see in a water solution. Since excesses of the B vitamins are excreted, bright yellow urine may signify the presence of this vitamin. If you are in the habit of taking a multivitamin supplement "to avoid deficiencies" and your diet is otherwise adequate, you may notice this effect.

Some vitamin supplements are inexpensive, but others entail costs far above the value they confer on you in preventing possible deficiencies. As you read on, you may discover that it is easy to make your diet adequate by eating nutritious foods alone and that you do not need a vitamin supplement. If you do consume an adequate diet, the following statement may apply to you:

> Overdosing with B vitamins may not hurt you, but it will do nothing for you except to increase the dollar value of your urine.

The difference in the body's handling of excess fat-soluble and water-soluble vitamins has a second implication: Because the water-soluble vitamins are excreted almost as rapidly as they are taken in, toxicity from overdoses occurs transiently if at all. The fat-soluble vitamins, however, can accumulate and reach toxic levels in body stores. This is known to occur with vitamins A and D in particular.

If you help yourself to a second piece of pecan pie at dinner, you are aware that you are eating more food. The sheer bulk of the energy nutrients and water in the pie makes you feel full. You know, too, that you are eating more kcalories. But excess vitamin intakes can be undetectable. The amount of vitamin A you need, in pure form, is but a droplet a day. Ten times as much is still only a few drops. This means that it is far easier to take an overdose of vitamins, especially in pure form (pills or drops), than of energy nutrients.

> Water-soluble vitamins: toxicity unlikely.
> Fat-soluble vitamins: toxicity likely.

Vitamins and the Four Food Group Plan   Throughout Part One, we made frequent reference to the exchange system of grouping foods, because that system is based on the carbohydrate-fat-protein composition of foods. Now that the vitamins are under consideration, the Four Food Group Plan becomes more useful. The grouping of foods in this plan is based largely on their protein, vitamin, and mineral contents. The first group, milk and milk products, includes the foods that make outstanding contributions of the vitamin riboflavin and the mineral calcium, as well as protein. The second group, meats and meat substitutes, is notable for its contributions of several B vitamins and the mineral iron, besides protein. Because of their high concentrations of riboflavin and calcium and their low concentrations of iron, the cheeses (which in the exchange system were treated as meat substitutes) are classified with milk and milk products in this plan. The third group, the vegetable and fruit group, is notable for its vitamin A and C contents, and the fourth, the grain products, adds important B vitamins and iron to the total. A review of the description of the Four Food Group Plan in Chapter 1 is recommended before you proceed with the chapters to come.

Minerals

As Chapters 12 and 13 will explain, the minerals are inorganic compounds, smaller than vitamins and found in still more simple forms in foods. Table salt, for example, is the principal source of the minerals sodium and chlorine; it enters the body as a two-atom pair (NaCl). Some minerals may be put together into building blocks for structures such as bones and teeth—but only with the help of the lively enzymes, which arrange them in orderly arrays. When minerals are withdrawn from bone and excreted, they yield no energy. They may also float about in the fluids of the body, by their presence giving the fluids certain characteristics, but they are not metabolized—arranged and rearranged—in the complicated ways or to the same extent as the energy nutrients are. You consume only small amounts of minerals daily, comparable to the amounts of vitamins in your diet. There are some 20 or 30 different minerals important in nutrition.

Minerals: small inorganic molecules.

Na and Cl: symbols for sodium and chlorine (see Appendix B).

Minerals: yield no energy.

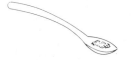

Amount of minerals eaten daily

Minerals as Inorganic Substances   The minerals are elements— like carbon, hydrogen, oxygen, and nitrogen of which the energy nutrients are composed—and so are simpler than the vitamins, which are compounds. Because they contain no carbon, minerals are inorganic; they need never have been part of a living thing. This means that the variety of forms they may take is more limited than for the vitamins; that is, minerals cannot have different chemical structures. Calcium, for example, enters the body as an ion with two positive charges. It may be combined with any of a number of negative ions

Element and compound: see Appendix B.

Ion: see Appendix B.

salt: a compound composed of two ions other than H^+ and OH^-, such as $CaCl_2$ or NaCl ($Ca^{++}Cl_2^-$ or Na^+Cl^-), held together by an ionic bond (electrostatic attraction). See Chapter 14 and Appendix B.

ionic state: the number of positive or negative charges that an ion may carry. The two states of iron are explained in Appendix B.

(phosphate, sulfate, and the like) to form salts in foods. The calcium may be more absorbable in these combinations, but in the body these dissociate, and the calcium ion itself is what is used. Some minerals, however, do play key roles as part of large organic complexes. For example, the iron in hemoglobin is responsible for that protein's oxygen-carrying function, and many minerals are responsible for the specificity of enzymes. Still, even in these associations, the minerals remain distinct.

Minerals exist as inorganic ions.

The Indestructibility of Minerals   An atom of iron may exist in two different ionic states, and it may be combined with a variety of other ions in salts, but it never loses its identity. It is always iron. Cooking it, exposing it to air or acid, or mixing it with other substances has no effect on it. In fact, if you burn a food until only the ash is left and eat the ash, you will be eating all the minerals that were in the food before it was burned. Once they have entered your body they are there until excreted; they cannot be changed into anything else.

Minerals retain their chemical identity.

Because they are indestructible, minerals in food need no special handling to preserve them. You need only make sure that you don't soak them out of the food or throw them away in cooking water. As long as they are kept in the food, they may be handled in any way whatever without any effect on the amount of the mineral present.

Minerals and Water   By virtue of being ionic, minerals tend to associate with water and thus tend to form either acidic or basic solutions.

Mineral ions are water-soluble.

Acid-base balance: see p. 133 and Chapter 14.

Water balance: see p. 131 and Chapter 14.

Because minerals are water-soluble, they influence the acid-base balance of the body. In associating with other ions in the body fluids, they affect the distribution of water into the various body compartments.

Absorption, Transport, and Excretion of Minerals   Like the water-soluble vitamins, some minerals are readily absorbed into the blood, transported freely, and readily excreted by the kidneys. There are exceptions, however. Each mineral differs in the amounts the body can absorb and in the extent to which it must be handled specially and transported by protein or other organic carriers.

Minerals vary in the amounts absorbed and in the routes and ease of excretion.

Like fat-soluble vitamins, some minerals must have carriers to be absorbed and to travel in the blood. Others travel freely as ions.

Some minerals require carriers.

Some are stored like the fat-soluble vitamins and like them are therefore toxic if taken in excess. Because their presence is not obvious in foods, overdosing with toxic minerals is a real possibility.

Some minerals are toxic in excess.

Toxic in excess: iron, copper, chlorine, magnesium, manganese, iodine, fluorine, and others.

Other minerals do not accumulate in the body but are readily excreted; toxicity with these is not a risk.

Minerals in the Diet   The amount of minerals needed in the daily diet varies from a few micrograms for minerals like cobalt to a million times as much, a gram or more, for minerals like calcium, phosphorus, and sodium. The amount of each mineral found in the body varies equally widely. Thus many authorities divide them into two categories: the major minerals (Chapter 12) and the trace minerals (Chapter 13). A diet made up of a wide variety of foods is certain to provide enough minerals in both categories.

In publishing its 1980 recommendations, the U.S. Committee on RDA gave ranges of safe intakes for many of the trace minerals and made a point of saying that the upper limits should not habitually be exceeded.

Water

Water is abundant, indispensable, and often ignored—because like air, it is everywhere and we take it for granted. Water is inorganic, a single molecule being composed of three atoms (H_2O).[1] The amounts you must consume relative to the other nutrients are enormous: 2 to 3 l a day. That's 2,000 to 3,000 grams, about ten times the amount of energy nutrients you need. Of course, you need not drink water as such in these quantities; it comes abundantly in foods and beverages. The specific ways that the body uses water are described in Chapter 14.

Water: small inorganic molecule.

Water: yields no energy.

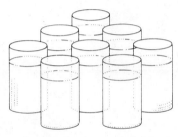

Amount of water needed daily

[1]A more accurate way to describe how water is organized would be to say that, although we know that the ratio of hydrogen atoms to oxygen atoms is 2:1, we do not know that water exists as discrete molecules.

CHAPTER 9

CONTENTS

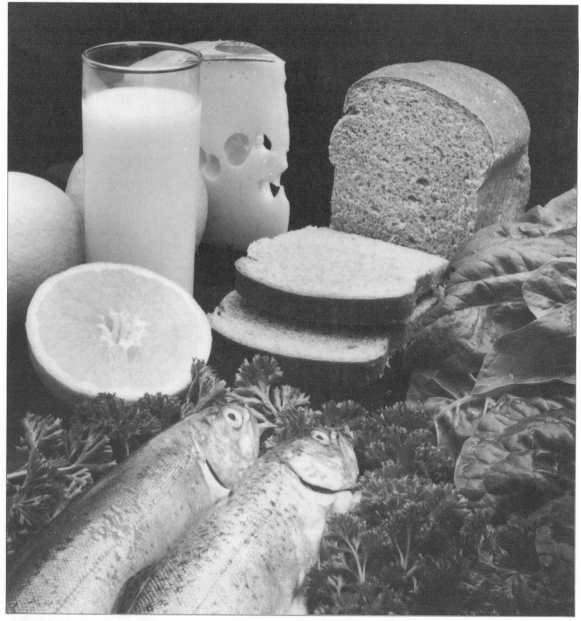

Foods rich in B vitamins.

THE B VITAMINS

Tests were initiated by the results of my studies on a chicken disease similar to beriberi. I was able to establish that that disease is caused by feeding certain grains, especially rice. Only polished rice (raw or boiled) proved to be harmful; unpolished rice was tolerated quite well by the chickens. . . . From these experiments I drew the conclusion that the cuticles probably contain a substance or substances which neutralize the harmful influence of the starchy nutriment. . . .

C. EIJKMAN, 1897

A television commercial broadcast widely some years ago shows a middle-aged businessman shuffling weakly out of his bedroom with his bathrobe slung loosely around his sagging paunch. He sinks into his chair at the breakfast table and wearily lifts the morning paper to screen his face from the daylight and from his bright-eyed, energetic wife. As she places his coffee cup before him, she observes sympathetically, "Sweetie, you look so tired. Did you forget to take your vitamin pill today?" (Fadeout, with the voice of the announcer saying, "Are you tired in the morning? Do you hate to face the day? What you need is Brand A Vitamins.") Repeat: The same man, transformed, trim and bouncy, waltzes into the breakfast nook, pirouettes gaily around the table, kisses his sweet wife affectionately, takes two hasty sips of coffee, and strides humming out the door. She turns cheerfully to the camera and smiles, "Brand A Vitamins have done wonders for my Harry."

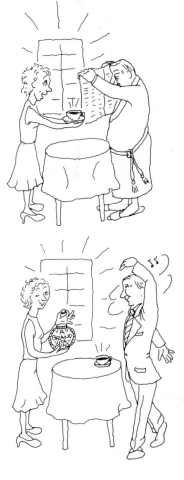

True? No. Poor Harry. If he tries to live on only coffee and vitamins, he will remain a wreck. Like all of the organic nutrients found in foods, the B vitamins are composed of carbon, hydrogen, oxygen, and other atoms linked together by chemical bonds. Of course, these bonds contain energy, but that energy cannot be used to fuel activities or to do the body's work. The energy Harry needs comes from carbohydrate, fat, and protein; the vitamins will only help him burn the fuel if he has the fuel to burn.

It is true, however, that without B vitamins you would certainly feel tired. You would lack energy. Why is this? Some of the B vitamins serve as helpers to the enzymes that release energy from the three energy nutrients—carbohydrate, fat, and protein. The B vitamins stand alongside the metabolic pathways and help to keep the disassembly lines moving. In an industrial plant they would be called expediters. Some of them help manufacture the red blood cells, which carry oxygen to the body's tissues; the oxygen must be present for oxidation and energy release to occur.

325

So long as B vitamins are present, their presence is not felt. Only when they are missing does their absence manifest itself as a lack of energy. A child who learned this defined vitamins on a test as "what if you don't eat you get sick." The definition is one of the most insightful we've seen.

Coenzymes

coenzyme (co-EN-zime): small molecule that works with an enzyme to promote the enzyme's activity. Many coenzymes have B vitamins as part of their structure.

co = with

prosthetic (pros-THET-ic) **group:** a coenzyme that is physically part of (attached to) its enzyme.

prosth = in addition to

active site: that part of the enzyme surface on which the reaction takes place.

To review the structures and functions of enzymes, see Chapter 3.

The B vitamins are entitled to individual attention, but the whole array of them is presented here first to show you the "forest" in which they are the trees. They come together in foods, they work together in the body, and there is much to be learned from viewing them as a group.

Each of the B vitamins is part of an enzyme helper known as a coenzyme. A coenzyme is a small nonprotein molecule that associates closely with an enzyme. Some coenzymes form part of the enzyme structure, in which case they are known as prosthetic groups; others are associated more loosely with the enzyme. Some participate in the reaction being performed and are chemically altered in the process, but they are always regenerated sooner or later. Others are unaltered but form part of the active site of the enzyme. Thus although there are differences in details, one thing is true of all: Without the coenzymes, the enzymes cannot function.

The consequences of a failure of metabolic enzymes can be catastrophic, as you will realize if you restudy the central pathway of metabolism by which glucose is broken down. The nicknames for some of the coenzymes that keep the processes going (NAD^+, TPP, FAD, and CoA) are listed beside the reactions they facilitate.

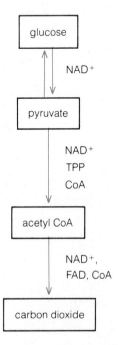

B-Vitamin Terminology

Many of the vitamins have both names and numbers, a mixture of terminologies that confuses newcomers to the study of nutrition. As of 1979, a single set of names for the vitamins had been agreed on and was published,[1] and those names are used in this book. Still, to read the many worthwhile writings published prior to 1979, you have to be aware of the alternative names:

Correct name	Other names commonly used (see also Appendix C)
thiamin	vitamin B_1
riboflavin	vitamin B_2
niacin	nicotinic acid, nicotinamide, niacinamide
vitamin B_6	pyridoxine, pyridoxal, pyridoxamine
folacin	folate, folic acid
vitamin B_{12}	cobalamin
pantothenic acid	(none)
biotin	(none)

(These examples of coenzyme functions are intended to illustrate the way these little molecules work to facilitate enzymatic reactions. It is not necessary to memorize the details in order to understand this principle. The full names and structures of these coenzymes are presented in Appendix C.)

Look at the first step. Some of the enzymes involved in the breakdown of glucose to pyruvate require the coenzyme NAD^+. Part of this molecule is a structure the body cannot make, hence it must be obtained from the diet; it is an *essential nutrient*. This essential part is the B vitamin called niacin.

In other words, to take glucose apart the cells must have certain enzymes. For the enzymes to work, they must have the coenzyme NAD^+. To make NAD^+, the cells must be supplied with niacin (or a closely related compound they can alter to make niacin). The rest of the coenzyme they can make without outside help.

The next step in glucose catabolism is the breakdown of pyruvate to acetyl CoA. The enzymes involved in this step require NAD^+ plus another coenzyme, TPP. The cells can manufacture the TPP they need from thiamin, but thiamin is a compound they cannot synthesize, so it must be supplied in the diet. Thiamin is the vitamin part.

Another coenzyme needed for this step is coenzyme A, or CoA for short. As you have probably guessed, the cells can make CoA except for an essential part of it that must be obtained in the diet. This essential part—the vitamin part—is pantothenic acid.

niacin (NIGH-uh-sin): a B vitamin. Niacin can be eaten preformed or can be made in the body from one of the amino acids (see pp. 340-342).

thiamin (THIGH-uh-min): a B vitamin.

pantothenic (PAN-to-THEN-ic) **acid:** a B vitamin.

[1] The vitamin names used here are those agreed on and published in 1979 by the Committee on Nomenclature, American Institute of Nutrition, in Nomenclature policy: Generic descriptors and trivial names for vitamins and related compounds, *Journal of Nutrition* 109 (1979):8-15.

riboflavin (RIBE-o-flay-vin): a B vitamin.

The above 4 B vitamins are parts of coenzymes in the glucose-to-energy pathway. Some of these coenzymes have other functions too (see Appendix C).

For want of a nail, a horseshoe
was lost.
For want of a horseshoe, a horse
was lost.
For want of a horse, a soldier was
lost.
For want of a soldier, a battle
was lost.
For want of a battle, the war was
lost,
And all for the want of a horse-
shoe nail!
—Mother Goose

The next step in glucose catabolism is breakdown of acetyl CoA to carbon dioxide. The enzymes involved in this process require two of the three coenzymes mentioned above—NAD$^+$ and coenzyme A—and, in addition, another—FAD. Again, FAD is synthesized in the body, but part of its structure, the vitamin riboflavin, must be obtained in the diet.

Now suppose the body's cells lack one of these B vitamins—niacin, for example. Without niacin, the cells cannot make NAD$^+$. Without NAD$^+$, the enzymes involved in every step of the glucose-to-energy pathway will fail to function. Since it is from these steps that energy is made available for all of the body's activities, everything will begin to grind to a halt. This is no exaggeration. The symptoms of niacin deficiency are the devastating "four Ds": dermatitis, which reflects a failure of the skin to maintain itself; dementia (insanity), a failure of the nervous system; diarrhea, a failure of digestion and absorption; and death. These are only the most obvious, observable symptoms. Every organ in the body, being dependent on the energy pathways, is profoundly affected by niacin deficiency. As you can see, niacin is a little like the horseshoe nail for want of which a war was lost.

The complete breakdown of amino acids and fat, as well as that of glucose, depends on the coenzymes just described. You may remember that a major product of the breakdown of amino acids and fat is acetyl

Coenzyme action. Each coenzyme is specialized for certain kinds of chemical reactions. NAD$^+$ (containing niacin), for example, can accept hydrogen atoms removed from other compounds and can lose them to compounds that ultimately pass them to oxygen (see Highlight 7). There are many steps during the catabolism of glucose in which hydrogens are removed and NAD$^+$ participates in this way. A model of the way NAD$^+$ works with an enzyme to remove hydrogens is shown here.

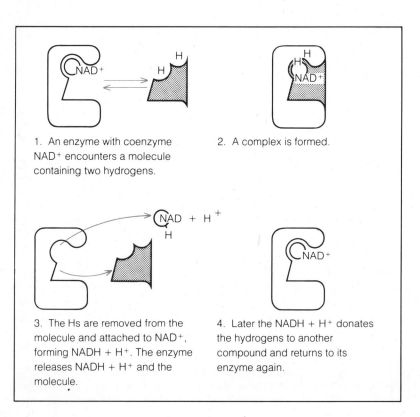

1. An enzyme with coenzyme NAD$^+$ encounters a molecule containing two hydrogens.

2. A complex is formed.

3. The Hs are removed from the molecule and attached to NAD$^+$, forming NADH + H$^+$. The enzyme releases NADH + H$^+$ and the molecule.

4. Later the NADH + H$^+$ donates the hydrogens to another compound and returns to its enzyme again.

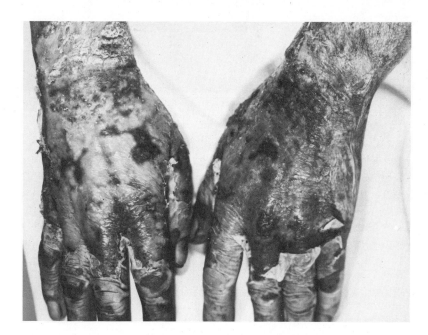

The dermatitis of pellagra. The skin darkens and flakes away as if it were sunburned. In kwashiorkor there is also a "flaky paint" dermatitis but the two are easily distinguishable. The dermatitis of pellagra is bilateral and symmetrical, and occurs only on those parts of the body exposed to the sun.

Courtesy of Dr. Samuel Dreizen, D.D.S., M.D.

CoA and that this product is processed in exactly the same way as the acetyl CoA from glucose. Thus the release of energy from all foods depends on the same vitamins.

Not only the breakdown (catabolism) but also the building (anabolism) of compounds in the body requires coenzymes. For example, one step in the manufacture of a nonessential amino acid is the step in which the nitrogen-containing amino group is attached to a carbon skeleton—a process called transamination. Enzymes performing this function require a coenzyme made from the essential nutrient vitamin B$_6$.

Two other B vitamins—folacin and vitamin B$_{12}$—are involved in building the units that form part of DNA and RNA. Whenever a cell divides, it must make a whole new copy of its DNA; thus these two coenzymes are necessary for making all new cells. They also serve other functions. (Folacin, for example, is a coenzyme in the reaction shown on p. 104, in which one amino acid is converted to another by removing a CH$_2$OH group.)

Finally, biotin, another B vitamin, serves as helper in many reactions in which acid groups are shifted from one structure to another. This activity is needed in making fatty acids.

In summary, these eight B vitamins play many specific roles in helping the enzymes to perform thousands of different molecular conversions in your body. They are active in carbohydrate, fat, and protein metabolism and in the making of DNA and thus new cells. They are found in every cell and must be present continuously for the cells to function as they should. It must now be abundantly clear why

transamination: the transfer of an amino group from one compound to another, as when nonessential amino acids are manufactured in the body.

vitamin B$_6$: a family of compounds that act as part of the coenzymes in amino acid metabolism. The step that begins the breakdown of stored glycogen to glucose also depends on these coenzymes.

folacin (FOLL-uh-sin) and **vitamin B$_{12}$:** two B vitamins that act as part of the coenzymes in the manufacture of new DNA and new cells.

biotin (BY-o-tin): a B vitamin; a coenzyme involved in fat synthesis.

poor Harry needs the B vitamins to make him feel well, even though by themselves they do nothing for him. No matter what he eats, he needs B vitamins to help him process it.

B Vitamins and Prescription Drugs

Like the coenzymes, drugs are small but potent molecules, and they often work in the body by altering the actions of its proteins. However, although the body is equipped by eons of evolutionary time to accommodate the vitamins and to use them appropriately, it has had no such long experience with drugs. Most of the prescription drugs are new compounds, synthesized in the laboratory, which by chance have effects on body functions that may be useful when disease threatens. But many drugs have side effects: While they work in one area to counteract the disease process or to correct an abnormality, they may also work in other areas to interfere with normal body processes. Sometimes they interfere with the action of the B vitamins.

For example, a potent drug that blocks the action of the tuberculosis bacterium, nicknamed INH,[2] has saved countless lives because of its efficacy against tuberculosis. But INH is also a vitamin B_6 antagonist: It binds and inactivates the vitamin, inducing a deficiency. Whenever INH is used to treat tuberculosis, supplements of vitamin B_6 are given as a precautionary measure.

Another example is aspirin, the most frequently prescribed pain reliever. It is very effective against pain, but it also interferes with the absorption of folacin from the GI tract and so can cause a deficiency. (It has similar effects on vitamin C and iron.) This doesn't imply that aspirin should never be used but rather that people using drugs and physicians prescribing them should be aware that they may have nutritional consequences and take the appropriate measures to find out and correct them.

It is important for someone new to the study of nutrition to be reminded at this point that this is a book about healthy people only. The nutrient needs of people who are ill or who are using large amounts of drugs—including nonprescription drugs like alcohol—are not discussed here. Nor are the special needs of people with inborn genetic defects that may greatly increase their individual needs for certain nutrients. The recommended intakes and the statements about foods that provide the recommended amounts apply to most people, normally, but there are exceptions that are outside our province. To Explore Further at the end of this chapter points the way toward learning more about nutrition in disease, and Highlight 9 is devoted to the special effects of alcohol.

---

[2]Isonicotinic acid hydrazide, or isoniazid.

B-Vitamin Deficiency

Removing a number of "horseshoe nails" can have such disastrous and far-reaching effects that it is difficult to imagine or predict the results. Oddly enough, although we know a great deal about their individual molecular functions, we are unable to say precisely why a deficiency of one B vitamin produces the disease beriberi whereas the deficiency of another produces pellagra. We do know, however, that with the deficiency of any B vitamin, many body systems become deranged, and similar symptoms may appear.

A B-vitamin deficiency seldom shows up in isolation. After all, people do not eat nutrients singly; they eat foods, which contain mixtures of nutrients. If a major class of foods is missing from the diet, the nutrients contributed by that class of foods will all be lacking to varying extents. In only two cases have dietary deficiencies associated with

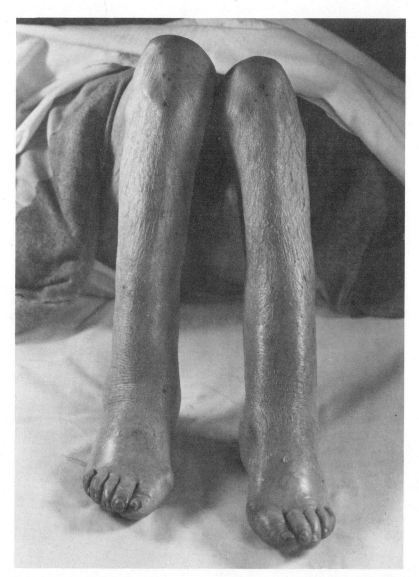

The edema of beriberi. Thiamin deficiency also sometimes produces a "dry" beriberi, without edema, for reasons not well understood. Another marked symptom is inability to walk, manifested by collapse of the lower limbs when the person tries to stand.

Courtesy of Dr. Samuel Dreizen, D.D.S., M.D.

beriberi: the thiamin-deficiency disease; pointed the way to discovery of the first vitamin, thiamin.

For a history of discoveries of the vitamins, see Appendix A.

pellagra (pell-AY-gra): the niacin-deficiency disease.

pellis = skin
agra = seizure

single B vitamins been observed on a large scale in human populations, and deficiency diseases have been named for them. One of these diseases, beriberi, was first observed in the Far East when the custom of polishing rice became widespread. Rice contributed 80 percent of the kcalories consumed by the people of those areas, and rice hulls were their principal source of thiamin. When the hulls were removed, beriberi spread like wildfire. It was believed to be an epidemic, and medical researchers wasted much time and energy seeking a microbial cause before they realized that the problem was not what was present but what was absent.

The other disease, pellagra, became widespread in the U.S. South in the early part of this century, when people subsisted on a low-protein diet whose staple grain was corn. This diet was unusual in that it supplied neither enough niacin nor enough of its amino acid precursor to make up the deficiency.

Even in these cases, the deficiencies were not pure. When foods were provided containing the one vitamin known to be needed, the other needed vitamins that may have been in short supply came as part of the package.

Significantly, these deficiency diseases were eliminated by supplying foods—not pills. Although both diseases were attributed to single B vitamins, both were likely to have been B-complex deficiencies in which one vitamin stood out above the rest. Giving one B vitamin to patients with a B-complex deficiency may make overt latent deficiencies of other B vitamins.

Pushers of vitamin pills make much of the fact that vitamins are vital and indispensable to life. But life went on long before there were vitamin pills, and human beings thrived on exactly the same kinds of foods as are available now. If your diet lacks a vitamin, the natural solution is to adjust it so that food supplies that vitamin.

Pushers of so-called natural vitamins would have you believe that their pills are the best of all because they are purified from real foods rather than synthesized in a laboratory. But if you think back on the course of human evolution, you may conclude that it really is not natural to take any kind of pills at all. In reality, the finest, most complete vitamin "supplements" available are meat, legumes, milk and milk products, vegetables, fruits, and grain products.

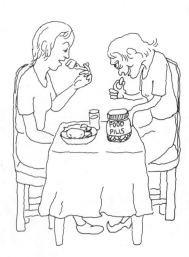

A FLAG SIGN OF A SPURIOUS CLAIM
IS THE IMPLICATION THAT:

Vitamin needs should be met by taking pills.

Once vitamin research was well under way and other B vitamins had been discovered, the clarification of their function was often greatly helped by laboratory experiments in which animals or human volunteers were fed diets devoid of one vitamin. The effects of the deficiency of that vitamin could then be studied to determine what functions it normally performed. Other deficiency diseases were discovered in this way and have since been observed to occur outside the laboratory.

Table 1 sums up a few of the better-established facts about vitamin B deficiency. A look at the table will make another generalization possible. Different body systems depend to different extents on these vitamins. Processes in nerves and in their responding tissues, the muscles, depend heavily on glucose metabolism, and hence on thiamin; thus paralysis sets in when this nutrient is lacking. The replacement of old red blood cells with new ones occurs at a rapid pace, and the making of new cells depends on folacin and vitamin B_{12}, so one of the first symptoms of a deficiency of either of these nutrients is a type of anemia. But again, each nutrient is important in all systems, and these lists of symptoms are far from complete.

The skin and the tongue appear to be especially sensitive to vitamin B deficiencies, although the listing of these items in Table 1 may give them undue emphasis. Remember that in a medical examination these are two body parts that the doctor can easily observe. The skin is a visible body tissue, and if it is degenerating, there may well be other tissues beneath it that are also manifesting ill effects. Similarly, the

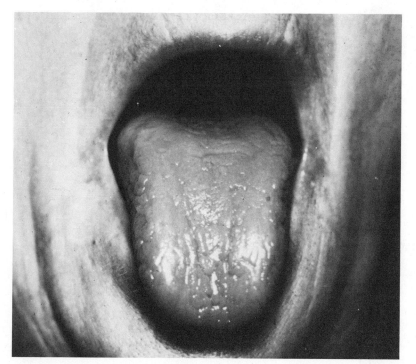

Tongue symptom of B-vitamin deficiency. The tongue is smooth due to atrophy of the tissues (glossitis). This person has a folacin deficiency.

Courtesy of Dr. Samuel Dreizen, D.D.S., M.D.

Table 1. Vitamin B-Deficiency Symptoms

Vitamin	Disease	Deficiency syndrome		Technical terms for symptoms
		Area affected	**Main effects**	
Thiamin	beriberi	nervous system	mental confusion peripheral paralysis	
		muscles	weakness wasting painful calf muscles	
		cardiovascular system	edema enlarged heart death from cardiac failure	
Riboflavin	ariboflavinosis	facial skin	dermatitis around nose and lips cracking of corners of mouth	**cheilosis** (kee-LOH-sis)
		eyes	hypersensitivity to light reddening of cornea	**photophobia**
Niacin	pellagra	skin	bilateral symmetrical dermatitis, especially on body parts exposed to sun	
		tongue	smoothness (atrophy of surface structures)	**glossitis** (gloss-EYE-tis)
		GI tract	diarrhea	
		nervous system	irritability mental confusion, progressing to psychosis or delirium	
Vitamin B_6	(no name)	skin	dermatitis cracking of corners of mouth irritation of sweat glands	**cheilosis**
		tongue	smoothness (atrophy of surface structures)	**glossitis**
		nervous system	abnormal brain wave pattern convulsions	
Folacin	(no name)	tongue	smoothness (atrophy of surface structures)	**glossitis**
		GI tract	diarrhea	
		blood	anemia (characterized by large cells)	**macrocytic anemia**
Vitamin B_{12}	pernicious anemia	blood	anemia (characterized by large cells)	**macrocytic anemia**
		nervous system	degeneration of peripheral nerves	
Pantothenic acid	(Deficiency observed only in animals)			
Biotin	(Deficiency observed in humans only under experimental conditions)			

mouth and tongue are the visible parts of the digestive system; if they are abnormal, there may well be an abnormality throughout the GI tract. What is really happening in a vitamin deficiency happens inside the cells of the body; what the doctor sees and reports are its outward manifestations.

It is more and more apparent that you cannot observe a symptom and automatically jump to a conclusion regarding its cause. This warning was given earlier (in Chapter 2) about dermatitis: A symptom is not a disease. As you have seen, deficiencies of linoleic acid, riboflavin, niacin, and vitamin B_6 can all cause dermatitis. A deficiency of vitamin A can too. Because skin is on the outside, where you and your doctor can easily look at it, it is a useful indicator of things-going-wrong-in-cells. But by itself a skin symptom tells you nothing about its possible cause.

The same is true of anemia. We often think of anemia as being caused by an iron deficiency, and often it is. But anemia can also be caused by a folacin or vitamin B_{12} deficiency, by digestive tract failure to absorb any of these nutrients, or by such nonnutritional causes as infections, parasites, or loss of blood. So caution: A little knowledge is a dangerous thing.

A FLAG SIGN OF A SPURIOUS CLAIM
IS THE IMPLICATION THAT:

A specific nutrient will cure a given symptom.

A person who feels chronically tired may be tempted to diagnose herself as having anemia. Knowing only enough to associate iron deficiency with this condition, she may decide to take an iron supplement. But the iron supplement will relieve her tiredness only if the symptom is caused by iron-deficiency anemia. If she has a folacin deficiency (and folacin deficiency may be the most widespread vitamin deficiency in the world), taking iron will only prolong the period in which she receives no relief. If she is better informed, she may decide to take a vitamin supplement with iron, covering the possibility of a vitamin deficiency. But now she is forgetting that there may be a nonnutritional cause of her symptom. If the cause of her tiredness is actually hidden blood loss due to cancer, the postponement of a diagnosis may be equivalent to suicide.

fortification: the addition of nutrients to a food, often in amounts much larger than might be found naturally in that food.

enrichment: now considered synonymous with fortification but previously referred to the addition of specific nutrients to refined breads and cereals in the United States.

whole-grain products: grain products made from the whole grain, including the bran, the germ, and the endosperm.

bran: the nutrient-rich coat of a wheat grain.

germ: the nutrient-rich part of the wheat grain, which provides nutrients for the plant's growth.

endosperm: the starchy, relatively nutrient-free bulk of the wheat grain.

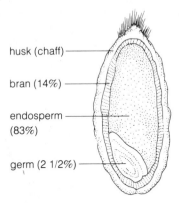

A kernel of wheat.

husk (chaff)

bran (14%)

endosperm (83%)

germ (2 1/2%)

refined grain products: products made of grain that has been milled, losing most of the bran and the germ in the process and containing only the endosperm.

Major, epidemic-like deficiency diseases such as pellagra and beriberi are no longer seen in the United States and Canada, but lesser deficiencies of nutrients, including the B vitamins, sometimes are observed. They occur in people whose food choices are poor because of poverty, ignorance, illness, or poor health habits like alcohol abuse. They are especially likely if the staple grain food is refined, as were most bread and cereal products chosen by U.S. consumers during the 1930s. One way to protect these people is to add nutrients to their staple food, a process known as fortification or enrichment. The enrichment of refined breads and cereals, required by law in the United States since the early 1940s, has increased many people's B-vitamin intakes. Thus before noting which foods are the richest sources of the individual B vitamins, you need to know what enrichment means.

Refined, Enriched, and Whole-Grain Bread

The part of the wheat plant that is made into flour and then into bread and other baked goods is the kernel. About 50 kernels cluster in the head of the plant, on top of the stem, where they stick tightly until fully ripe. In the milling process these kernels are first separated from the stem and then further broken apart.

The wheat kernel (whole grain) has three main parts: the germ, the bran, and the endosperm. The germ is the part that reproduces when planted, and so it contains concentrated food to support the new life. It is especially rich in iron, vitamin E, and the B vitamins thiamin, riboflavin, and niacin. The bran, a protective coating around the kernel similar to the shell of a nut, is also rich in nutrients. In addition, the bran is a source of valuable fiber. The endosperm is the soft inside portion of the kernel containing starch and proteins (including gluten, which is used for making white flour). The husk, commonly called chaff, is unusable for most purposes.

People interested in nutrition are concerned about the loss of nutrients from the wheat kernel during the milling process. In earlier times the kernel was milled by grinding it between two stones to expose the endosperm and then blowing or sifting out the inedible chaff. Much of the bran and germ were included in the final product.

As improvements were made in the machinery for milling, a whiter, smoother-textured flour resulted. Consumers liked this flour better than the former crunchy, dark brown, "old-fashioned" flour. But to produce white flour, millers use only the endosperm. (To produce whole-wheat flour, millers grind the entire kernel.) Thus during the further processing of refined, white flour for the market, additional nutrients are lost. The bran layers and other parts of the kernel that remain after white flour is milled are used as livestock and poultry feed. These parts of the grain actually contain more protein, minerals, and vitamins than the endosperm does.

As white flour became more popular for making breads, bread eaters suffered a tragic loss of needed nutrients. A survey conducted in the United States in 1936 revealed that people were suffering from the loss of the nutrients iron, thiamin, riboflavin, and niacin, which they had formerly received from their unrefined bread. The Enrichment Act of 1942 required that these lost nutrients be returned to the flour. Thus enriched bread restores iron and the vitamins thiamin and niacin to the level of whole wheat; riboflavin is added to a level about twice that in whole grain.

To a great extent, the enrichment of white flour eliminated the deficiency problems that had been observed in people who depended on bread for most of their kcalories but who were unwilling to use the whole-grain product. Today you can almost take it for granted that all refined bread, grains like rice, wheat products like macaroni and spaghetti, and cereals like farina have been enriched. The law provides that all grain products that cross state lines must be enriched. A look at Table 2 shows to what levels whole-grain bread, unenriched white bread, and enriched white bread contains these four nutrients.

enrichment: with respect to breads and cereals in particular, this term refers to the process by which four specific nutrients lost during refinement are added back to refined grain products at levels specified by law: thiamin, niacin, and iron at levels about equal to those in the original whole grain; riboflavin at a level about twice that in the original whole grain.

A wheat plant.

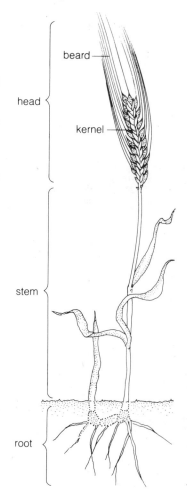

Table 2.   Nutrient Levels of 1-lb Loaves of Bread

Item number*	Type of bread	Iron (mg)	Thiamin (mg)	Riboflavin (mg)	Niacin (mg)
368	Whole-wheat	13.6	1.36	0.45	12.7
346	Italian, unenriched	3.2	0.41	0.27	3.6
345	Italian, enriched	10.0	1.32	0.91	11.8

*As listed in Appendix H.

But the food composition tables don't tell the whole story. When the grain is refined, many nutrients not listed in the tables are also lost. As more and more foods are refined and processed, other nutrients may begin to be lost from our diet. Evidence is piling up that fiber needs are increasing as fiber is lost from many refined foods, not just from bread and cereal. Some experts have attributed the new cases of chromium-deficiency diabetes to the increased use of processed foods. Therefore, although the enrichment of wheat and other cereal products restores four of the lost nutrients, there is increasing evidence that we should return to the use of the whole grain in order to restore trace minerals and fiber to our diet. *Nutrition and the MD* reports: "Whole grain items are preferred over enriched products because they contain more magnesium, zinc, folacin, and vitamin B_6 than enriched bread and cereals."[3]

[3]Improving on the basic four, *Nutrition and the MD*, October 1977.

The B Vitamins in Food

The preceding sections have shown both the great importance of the B vitamins in promoting normal, healthy functioning of all body systems and the severe consequences of deficiency. Now you may want to know how to be sure you are getting enough of these vital nutrients. This chapter concludes with some practical pointers regarding food intake.

First, a Caution One way to discover whether your intake of a vitamin is sufficient is to calculate the amount you are consuming each day in the foods you eat and to compare your intake with the recommended intake (RDA or Canadian Dietary Standard. See the Self-Study that follows Highlight 9). This is an informative exercise, and some 15 nutrients can be studied this way. However, there are more accurate means of determining whether a deficiency exists, and there are other distinct limitations on the dietary record method. First, you have to assume that the recommended intake applies to you. People's needs for nutrients vary over a wide range; you may not be typical. Of course, you may need much less, but you may also need more. Second, you have to assume that your body's handling and absorption of the vitamin is normal. If your digestive system is disturbed, if you are ill (especially with diarrhea), or if you are emotionally upset, your absorption of certain nutrients may be impaired. Third, when you look

The table of food composition most often used is given in Appendix H.

up the foods you eat in a table of food composition, you have to assume that the food you ate contained the amount of the nutrient listed in the table. But foods vary too. Not all 200-g tomatoes contain exactly 1.3 mg of niacin. The nutrient contents of foods are averages. Furthermore, the professionals who make up the tables make still a fourth assumption—that the foods are stored and prepared in a way that minimizes losses of vitamins. So there are at least four possible sources of error in assuming that your nutrient intakes compared with your nutrient needs this way are meaningful.

Still, the dietary record is the simplest way to check on a person's nutrient status and is the way most often used by the average person. Some more-precise means of assessing nutritional status (physical examination, body measurements, and biochemical tests) are described at the beginning of Highlight 15.

With the above cautions in mind, let us examine the foods for their B-vitamin content. Only six of the B vitamins are discussed in detail here—those for which the contents of foods have been relatively well analyzed and for which the Canadian and U.S. governments have set dietary standards. Once a diet has been planned to meet the needs for these vitamins, it meets the general description of "a balanced and varied diet" and is therefore likely to ensure adequacy for other nutrients not considered here.

Thiamin The recommended daily thiamin intake for adults is about 1.5 mg for men and about 1.0 mg for women (plus an extra half milligram during pregnancy). Infants require about half a milligram and children about three-fourths.

Because thiamin is used for energy production, more is needed when energy expenditure is high. (In fact, the thiamin requirement can be stated in terms of milligrams per 1,000 kcal.) Provided that you are consuming enough kcalories to meet your energy needs—and obtaining those kcalories from thiamin-containing foods—your thiamin intake will adjust automatically to your need. However, people who derive a large proportion of their kcalories from empty-kcalorie items like sugar or alcohol may suffer thiamin deficiency. A person who is fasting or who has adopted a very low-kcalorie diet needs the same amount of thiamin as he did when he was eating more; needs remain unchanged during fasting because they are proportional to energy expenditure, not to energy intake.[4]

Table 3 shows the thiamin contents of 50 common foods. If you study the table while thinking about your own food habits, you will probably conclude that many of the foods you like and eat daily contribute some thiamin, but none by itself can meet your total need for a day. A useful guideline is to eliminate empty-kcalorie foods from your diet and to include ten or more different servings of nutritious foods each day, assuming that on the average each serving will contribute about 10 percent of your need. Foods chosen from the bread and cereal group should be either whole-grain or enriched. Thiamin is not stored in the body to any great extent, so daily intake is best.

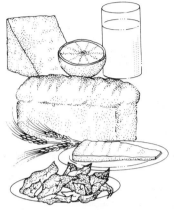

Thiamin: Most nutritious foods contribute about 10 percent of daily need per serving.

Riboflavin The recommended daily riboflavin intake for adults is about 1.4 to 1.8 mg for men and about 1.1 to 1.3 mg for women (plus about 0.3 mg during pregnancy), depending on how much energy they expend daily. (Like thiamin, riboflavin needs can be stated in terms of milligrams per 1,000 kcal.) Young children's needs begin at about 1 mg a day and rise rapidly during their growing years. Teenagers, because they are very active, need more riboflavin than adults.

Unlike thiamin, riboflavin is not evenly distributed among the food groups. Table 4 shows the riboflavin contents of 50 common foods; the concentration of 1s and 5s in the left-hand column shows that the major contributors are milk and meat. The need for riboflavin provides a major reason for including milk in some form in every day's meals; no other food that is commonly eaten can make such a substantial contribution toward meeting the day's needs. People who don't use milk products can substitute generous servings of dark-green leafy vegetables, because a cup of greens—collards, for example—provides about the same amount of riboflavin as a cup of milk. Among the meats, liver and heart are the richest sources, but all lean meats, as well as eggs, provide some riboflavin. Most people derive about half their riboflavin from milk and milk products, about a fourth from meats,

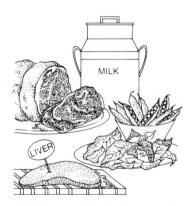

Riboflavin: Milk contributes about 50 percent, meat about 25 percent, enriched breads and cereals additional amounts. The person who does not drink milk should substitute greens.

[4]M. Brin and J. C. Bauernfeind, Vitamin needs of the elderly, *Postgraduate Medicine* 63 (3) (1978):155-163.

Table 3. Thiamin Contents of 50 Common Foods*

Exchange group[†]	Food	Serving size[‡]	Thiamin (mg)	Exchange group[†]	Food	Serving size[‡]	Thiamin (mg)
5L	Lean pork roast	3 oz	.91	1	Whole milk	1 c	.07
5L	Ham	3 oz	.40	1	Yogurt (from whole milk)	1 c	.07
5L	Oysters	3/4 c	.25	4	Corn muffin	1	.07
5M	Liver, beef	3 oz	.23	4	Bran flakes	1/2 c	.07
4	Green peas	1/2 c	.22	4	Puffed rice	1 c	.07
5M	Beef heart	3 oz	.21	4	Muffin	1	.07
4	Lima beans	1/2 c	.16[§]	5M	Hamburger	3 oz	.07
2	Collard greens	1/2 c	.14	2	Cooked tomatoes	1/2 c	.06
3	Orange	1	.13	2	Tomato juice	1/2 c	.06
4	Dried beans	1/2 c	.13	2	Brussels sprouts	1/2 c	.06
5L	Lamb, leg	3 oz	.13	3	Pineapple	1/2 c	.06
2	Dandelion greens	1/2 c	.12	4	White bread	1 slice	.06
4	Rice, enriched	1/2 c	.12	4	Whole-wheat bread	1 slice	.06
2	Asparagus	1/2 c	.12	4	Hamburger bun	1/2	.06
3	Orange juice	1/2 c	.11	4	Potato chips	15	.06
5L	Veal roast	3 oz	.11	4	French fried potatoes	8	.06
1	2% fat fortified milk	1 c	.10	5L	Chipped beef	3 oz	.06
4	Spaghetti, enriched	1/2 c	.10	2	Mustard greens	1/2 c	.06
4	Macaroni, enriched	1/2 c	.10	2	Broccoli	1/2 c	.06
4	Cooked cereal	1/2 c	.10	5M	Egg	1	.05
4	Corn on cob	1 small	.09	3	Pink grapefruit	1/2	.05
1	Skim milk	1 c	.09	2	Summer squash	1/2 c	.05
4	Potato	1 small	.08	2	Green beans	1/2 c	.05
4	Mashed potato	1/2 c	.08	5L	Chicken, meat only	3 oz	.05
1	Powdered skim milk	1/3 c	.08	5L	Lean beef roast	3 oz	.05

*These are not necessarily the best food sources but are selected to show a range of thiamin contents. Note the presence of all food groups except fat in the left-hand column.

†The numbers refer to the exchange lists: 1 is milk; 2, vegetables; 3, fruit; 4, bread; 5L, lean meat; 5M, medium-fat meat.

‡Serving sizes are the sizes listed in the exchange lists, except for meat.

§One serving of any of the first six foods contains at least 10 percent of the RDA (for an adult male) of 1.5 mg.

and most of the rest from leafy green vegetables and whole-grain or enriched bread and cereal products.

Riboflavin is light-sensitive; it can be destroyed by the ultraviolet rays of the sun or of fluorescent lamps. For this reason milk is seldom sold and should not be stored in transparent glass containers. Cardboard or plastic containers protect the riboflavin in the milk from ultraviolet rays.

niacin equivalents: the amount of niacin present in food, including the niacin that can theoretically be made from the tryptophan present in the food.

Niacin Recommended niacin intakes are stated in "equivalents," a term that requires explanation. Niacin is unique among the B vitamins because it can be obtained from another nutrient source—protein. The amino acid tryptophan can be converted to niacin in the body: 60 mg of

Table 4. Riboflavin Contents of 50 Common Foods*

Ex-change group[†]	Food	Serving size[‡]	Ribo-flavin (mg)	Ex-change group[†]	Food	Serving size[‡]	Ribo-flavin (mg)
5M	Beef liver	3 oz	3.60	2	Brussels sprouts	1/2 c	.11
5M	Beef heart	3 oz	1.04	2	Spinach	1/2 c	.11
1	2% fat fortified milk[§]	1 c	.52	5L	Canned tuna	3 oz	.10
1	Skim milk	1 c	.44	2	Mustard greens	1/2 c	.10
1	Canned evaporated milk	1/2 c	.43	4	Lima beans	1/2 c	.09
1	Whole milk	1 c	.41	4	Green peas	1/2 c	.09
1	Dry skim milk	1/3 c	.40	4	Pumpkin	3/4 c	.09
1	Yogurt (whole milk)	1 c	.39	4	Muffin	1	.09
5L	Oysters	3/4 c	.30	4	Corn muffin	1	.08
5L	Chipped beef	3 oz	.30	3	Strawberries	3/4 c	.08
5L	Veal roast	3 oz	.26	2	Summer squash	1/2 c	.08
5L	Leg of lamb	3 oz	.23	4	Corn on cob	1 small	.08
5L	Lean roast beef	3 oz	.19	4	Dried beans	1/2 c	.07
2	Collard greens	1/2 c	.19	3	Pear	1	.07
5M	Hamburger	3 oz	.18°	4	Spaghetti, enriched	1/2 c	.06
5L	Sardines	3 oz	.17	4	Macaroni, enriched	1/2 c	.06
5L	Ham	3 oz	.16	3	Raspberries	1/2 c	.06
5L	Chicken, meat only	3 oz	.16	4	Pancake	1	.06
5L	Canned salmon	3 oz	.16	2	Green beans	1/2 c	.06
2	Dandelion greens	1/2 c	.15	4	White bread	1 slice	.05
5M	Egg	1	.15	2	Cauliflower	1/2 c	.05
5M	Cheese, creamed cottage	1/4 c	.15	4	Mashed potatoes	1/2 c	.05
4	Winter squash	1/2 c	.14	3	Orange	1	.05
2	Asparagus	1/2 c	.13	3	Peach	1	.05
2	Broccoli	1/2 c	.12	4	Hamburger bun	1/2	.04

*These are not necessarily the best food sources but are selected to show a range of riboflavin contents. Note in the left-hand column that the 1s and 5s cluster at the top and that the 2s near the top all represent 1/2-c servings of dark-green leafy vegetables.

†The numbers refer to the exchange lists: 1 is milk; 2, vegetables; 3, fruit; 4, bread; 5L, lean meat; 5M, medium-fat meat.

‡Serving sizes are the sizes listed in the exchange lists, except for meat.

§2% milk appears above skim milk because it is fortified with dry powdered milk, not because of the fat in it (riboflavin is water-soluble). Canadian 2% milk has only vitamin D added.

°One serving of any of the foods to this point contains at least 10 percent of the RDA (for an adult male) of 1.7 mg.

tryptophan yields 1 mg of niacin. Thus a food containing 1 mg niacin and 60 mg tryptophan contains the equivalent of 2 mg niacin, or 2 mg equivalents.

Recommended daily intakes for men are about 15 to 20 mg equivalents and for women about 12 to 15 (plus 2 to 5 mg equivalents during pregnancy and lactation). Infants', children's, and teenagers' needs are proportional not to their size but to their energy output.

Tables of food composition list only the preformed niacin in foods, although people actually derive the vitamin from both niacin itself and dietary tryptophan. However, tryptophan is also used to build needed

A compound that can be converted to a nutrient in the body is known as a **precursor** of that nutrient. Thus tryptophan is a precursor of niacin.

To obtain a rough approximation of your niacin intake:

1. Calculate total protein consumed (g).
2. Subtract your protein requirement to obtain "leftover" protein usable to make niacin (g).
3. Divide by 100 to obtain the amount of tryptophan in this protein (g).
4. Multiply by 1,000 to express this amount of tryptophan in milligrams (mg).
5. Divide by 60 to get niacin equivalents (mg).
6. Finally, add the amount of niacin obtained preformed in the diet (mg).

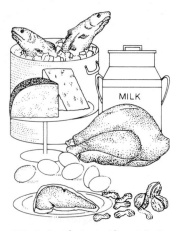

MILK

Niacin is adequate if protein is adequate.

schizophrenia (skitz-oh-FREN-ee-uh): a kind of mental illness.

schizo = split
phren = mind

orthomolecular psychiatry: a branch of psychiatry that attempts to treat mental illness by correcting nutrient imbalances and deficiencies.

ortho = right

body proteins, so not all of it is available for making niacin. Thus calculating the amount of niacin available from the diet is a complicated matter. A means of obtaining a rough approximation is shown in the margin, but the simplest assumption is that if the diet is adequate in complete protein, it will supply enough niacin equivalents to meet the daily need.

Milk, eggs, meat, poultry, and fish contribute about half the niacin equivalents consumed by most people, and about a fourth come from enriched breads and cereals. Vegetarians are well advised to emphasize nuts and legumes in their diets, as these are good sources of niacin and protein. A look at the nutrient contents of foods (in Appendix H) will reveal other good sources.

Most people in Canada and the United States presently consume a lot of animal protein, so niacin deficiency is a problem only where protein deficiency occurs. The widespread pellagra that was seen during the early part of this century in the U.S. South was due to the fact that the predominantly cornmeal-salt pork-molasses diet of the people of that area was lacking in both niacin and protein; what little protein they consumed was unusually low in tryptophan. Symptoms of niacin deficiency are no longer observed very often, except in people like alcoholics and undernourished hospital patients, whose protein intakes are unacceptably low.

At the time that pellagra was widespread in the South, half the cases in insane asylums were caused by niacin deficiency.[5] Unfortunately, not all insanity is caused by a lack of niacin; if it were, it would be wonderfully easy to cure. Insanity induced by niacin deficiency has symptoms very like those of schizophrenia, but it clears up miraculously when niacin or tryptophan is given. The hope that large doses of niacin would also cure schizophrenia has led to some important research and a whole new area of study—orthomolecular psychiatry—but the results so far have been disappointing. There is no evidence that large doses of niacin have any effect whatever on mental disease other than the dementia of pellagra.[6]

Large doses of niacin have been observed, however, to lower blood cholesterol levels in some cases, and for a while interest ran high in exploring the possible value of niacin therapy in the prevention of atherosclerosis. Both niacin and niacinamide (an alternative form of the vitamin) have been extensively tested for their cholesterol-lowering effects, but both have been found disappointing. Niacin causes irritation of the intestines and possibly liver damage, and niacinamide

[5]H. N. Munro, Impact of nutritional research on human health and survival, *Federation Proceedings* 30 (July/August 1971), reprinted in *The Nutrition Crisis: A Reader*, ed. T. P. Labuza (St. Paul: West, 1975), pp. 5-13.

[6]Task Force on Vitamin Therapy in Psychiatry, American Psychiatric Association, Megavitamin and orthomolecular therapy in psychiatry, pp. 44-47. Excerpts reprinted in *Nutrition Reviews/Supplement: Nutrition Misinformation and Food Faddism*, July 1974, pp. 67-70.

is ineffective altogether.[7] Research into the possible benefits of niacin therapy for atherosclerosis has largely given way to other, more promising approaches.

One problem with large therapeutic doses of niacin (ten times the normal intake) is that they produce flushed skin and a painful, stinging sensation that may be alarming, although megadoses seem to cause no permanent harm if taken only a few times. Some people who believe in the therapeutic power of niacin even like this "niacin flush." Those who don't like the reaction can take niacinamide.

Vitamin B$_6$ Because the vitamin B$_6$ coenzymes play many roles in amino acid metabolism, dietary needs are roughly proportional to protein intakes. Adults need about 2 mg of vitamin B$_6$ a day; this is enough to handle 100 g of protein. Pregnant and lactating women need about half a milligram more. Infants probably receive enough B$_6$ either from breast milk or cow's milk formula. There is some possibility that older people have a greater need for vitamin B$_6$ than young adults.

Pregnant women often show low blood concentrations of B$_6$ even though their diets are ample in the vitamin. It is thought that this is due to the high demand for B$_6$ by the fetus, whose blood normally has about five times more B$_6$ than the mother's. Vitamin B$_6$ is often prescribed for relief of the nausea and vomiting of pregnancy as well as for depression felt by women taking oral contraceptives.[8]

Convenient reference tables showing vitamin B$_6$ contents of foods are not available. However, by this time you must have realized that the B vitamins are found for the most part in the same groups of foods. Thus the only workable strategy for meeting B-vitamin needs is to eat a variety of nutritious foods. In the case of vitamin B$_6$, the richest food sources seem to be muscle meats, liver, vegetables, and whole-grain cereals.

Folacin   Folacin occurs in foods in both bound and free forms; the free form is better absorbed. Canada's recommendation for daily intake, stated in terms of "free folate (folacin)," is 200 μg a day for adults, with 50 μg added for pregnancy. The U.S. recommendation for adults is stated in terms of all forms of folacin and is 400 μg a day. The need for folacin rises dramatically during pregnancy, more than the need for any other nutrient, even protein; the RDA doubles the folacin intake to 800 μg a day during pregnancy. This increased need reflects the role folacin plays in cell multiplication. The blood volume in a pregnant woman nearly doubles, for example, and the folacin

megavitamin therapy: the administration of huge doses of vitamins in the attempt to cure disease.

mega = huge

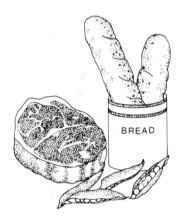

Vitamin B$_6$ is found in meats, vegetables, and whole-grain cereals.

Note: Recommended folacin intakes are stated in micrograms (μg). A microgram is a thousandth of a milligram or a millionth of a gram. The RDA for folacin, 400 μg, can also be stated as 0.4 mg.

[7]M. K. Horwitt, The Vitamins, Section G: Niacin, in *Modern Nutrition in Health and Disease*, 5th ed., eds. R. S. Goodhart and M. E. Shils (Philadelphia: Lea and Febiger, 1973), pp. 198-202.

[8]B. S. Worthington, J. Vermeersch, and S. R. Williams, *Nutrition in Pregnancy and Lactation* (St. Louis: Mosby, 1977), p. 185.

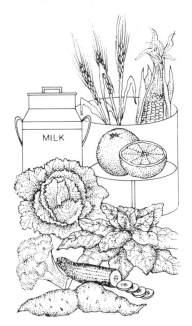

Folacin is the "foliage" vitamin.

coenzymes are used to manufacture the new blood cells. The typical diet in the United States probably delivers about 600 μg daily.

Tables of the folacin contents of foods are now being developed and probably soon will be incorporated into the standard table of food composition. The best food sources of this vitamin are organ meats (such as liver), green, leafy vegetables (the name of the vitamin is related to the word *foliage*), beets, and members of the cabbage family (such as cauliflower, broccoli, and brussels sprouts). Among the fruits, oranges, orange juice, and cantaloupe are the best sources; among the starchy vegetables, corn, lima beans, parsnips, green peas, pumpkin, and sweet potato are good sources. Whole-wheat bread, wheat germ, and milk also supply folacin.

The presence of folacin in dark-green leafy vegetables is one reason for the Four Food Group Plan recommendation that these vegetables be included in the diet at least every other day. Some forms of folacin are readily destroyed by cooking, hence the advisability of including raw vegetables like salad greens and fruits like citrus fruits in daily menus.

Folacin deficiency may result from an inadequate intake, impaired absorption, or unusual metabolic need for the vitamin. A significant number of cases of anemia develop from these causes, especially among pregnant women. Among the poor and in other parts of the world, folacin deficiency due to inadequate intake is probably the most common vitamin deficiency.

The risks of overdosing with folacin are greater than those for the other B vitamins discussed so far. They arise from the close relationship between folacin and vitamin B_{12} (see next section).

Note: Recommended vitamin B_{12} intakes are stated in micrograms.

Vitamin B_{12} is adequate if animal foods are included in the diet. Among vegetable products only a few (those that include microorganisms) contain B_{12}, most notably yeast and fermented soy products.

Lacto-ovo-vegetarians: see p. 121.

intrinsic: inside the system. The intrinsic factor necessary to prevent pernicious anemia is now known to be a mucopolysaccharide, made in the stomach, that aids in the absorption of vitamin B_{12}.

Vitamin B_{12}   According to both the U.S. and Canadian recommendations, adults need about 3 μg of vitamin B_{12} a day (plus 1 μg during pregnancy). This is the tiniest amount imaginable—three-millionths of a gram, and a gram would not even fill a quarter-teaspoon. The ink in the period at the end of this sentence probably weighs about 3 μg. But what seems like such a tiny amount to the human eye contains billions of molecules of vitamin B_{12}, enough to provide coenzymes for all the enzymes that need its help.

Vitamin B_{12} is unique among the nutrients in being found almost exclusively in animal flesh and animal products. Anyone who eats meat is guaranteed an adequate intake, and lacto-ovo-vegetarians (who use milk, cheese, and eggs) are also protected from deficiency. But strict vegetarians must use vitamin B_{12}-fortified soy milk or other such products or take B_{12} supplements.

A second special characteristic of vitamin B_{12} is that it requires an "intrinsic factor"—a compound made inside the body—for absorption from the intestinal tract into the bloodstream. The design for this factor is carried in the genes. The intrinsic factor is now known to be synthesized in the stomach, where it attaches to the vitamin; the complex then passes to the small intestine and is gradually absorbed.

Certain people have in their genetic makeup a defective gene for the intrinsic factor and so cannot make it; this defect usually becomes manifest in midlife. Without the intrinsic factor, they can't absorb the vitamin even though they are taking enough in their diets, and so they develop deficiency symptoms. In such a case, or when the stomach has been injured and cannot produce enough of the intrinsic factor, vitamin B_{12} must be supplied to the body by injection, thus bypassing the block in the intestinal tract.

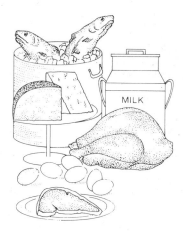

One of the most obvious B_{12}-deficiency symptoms is the kind of anemia characterized by large, immature red blood cells identical to those seen in folacin deficiency. Either vitamin B_{12} or folacin will clear up this condition. However, vitamin B_{12} also functions in maintaining the sheath that surrounds and protects nerve fibers and in promoting their normal growth, as well as in producing mature red blood cells. Thus a deficiency of vitamin B_{12} also causes a creeping paralysis of the nerves and muscles, which begins at the extremities and works inward and up the spine. This paralysis cannot be remedied by administering folacin, so early detection and correction of the B_{12} deficiency is necessary if permanent nerve damage and paralysis are to be avoided. Hence the name "pernicious" anemia: The vitamin B_{12} deficiency has a hidden, sneaky, and frightening symptom. Because of the danger of a high level of folacin masking a lack of B_{12}, the amount of folacin in over-the-counter vitamin preparations is limited by law to 400 μg, an amount too low to have this effect.[9]

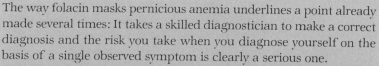

The way folacin masks pernicious anemia underlines a point already made several times: It takes a skilled diagnostician to make a correct diagnosis and the risk you take when you diagnose yourself on the basis of a single observed symptom is clearly a serious one.

A second point should also be underlined here. Since B_{12} deficiency in the body may be caused by either a lack of B_{12} in the diet or a genetically caused inability to absorb the vitamin, a change in diet alone may not correct it. You might wish to think about this in relation to the cautions offered on p. 67 and 335.

Strict vegetarians are at special risk for unchecked B_{12} deficiency for two reasons: first, because they receive none in their diets; and second, because they consume large amounts of folacin from the vegetables they eat. The amount of vitamin B_{12} that can be stored in the body is 1,000 times the amount used each day, so it may take years for a deficiency to develop in a new vegetarian. When it does, it may be masked by the high folacin intake. Sometimes the damage is first seen in the breast-fed infant of a vegan mother.[10]

Vegan: see p. 121.

[9]Committee on Safety, Toxicity, and Misuse of Vitamins and Trace Minerals, National Nutrition Consortium, *Vitamin-Mineral Safety, Toxicity, and Misuse* (Chicago: The American Dietetic Association, 1978).

[10]Vitamin B_{12} deficiency in the breast-fed infant of a strict vegetarian, *Nutrition Reviews* 37 (May 1979):142-144.

extrinsic: outside the system. The extrinsic factor first detected in raw liver and found necessary to prevent pernicious anemia is now known to be vitamin B_{12}.

The history of the discovery of vitamin B_{12} makes an intriguing story and epitomizes the fascination of vitamin research. In the early years, all that was known about pernicious anemia was that it could be controlled but not cured by eating large amounts of calf liver. (Researchers concluded that liver contained a factor—the "extrinsic factor"—needed to prevent the disease, and later they identified the factor as vitamin B_{12}.) The concentration of B_{12} in liver was so great that some was absorbed even without the help of the intrinsic factor. At one time people suffering from pernicious anemia had no choice but to eat several pounds of liver a day, but now they can be cured by the injection of a few micrograms of the purified vitamin every three weeks.

Pantothenic acid and biotin: deficiencies not seen in humans.

The photograph on this book's cover shows crystals of purified pantothenic acid.

Other B Vitamins   The six best-known B vitamins have already been discussed. Two other B vitamins—pantothenic acid and biotin—are needed for the synthesis of coenzymes that are active in a multitude of body systems. These are just as important for normal body function as the vitamins discussed so far, but little is known about the human requirements for them. Both pantothenic acid and biotin are widespread in foods, and there seems to be no danger that people who consume a variety of foods will suffer deficiencies. Claims that they are needed in pill form to prevent or cure disease conditions are at best unfounded and at worst intentionally misleading.

Possible B vitamins:

inositol (eye-NOSS-i-tall)
choline (KO-leen)

Another pair of compounds sometimes called B vitamins are inositol and choline. These are probably not essential nutrients for humans, although deficiencies can be induced in laboratory animals in order to study their functions. Like the B vitamins described above, they serve as coenzymes in metabolism. Even if they were essential for humans, supplements would be unnecessary, because they are abundant in foods.

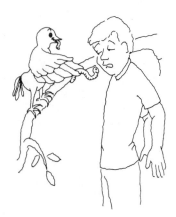

Health food purveyors make much of inositol and choline, insisting that we must supplement our diets with them. This incorrect notion arises from an unjustified application of findings from animal studies to human beings.

CAUTION WHEN YOU READ!

To weigh the reliability of nutrition information, ask yourself, Has the finding been proved applicable to human beings?

Highlight 11 enlarges on this theme, which has been a major problem with recent publicity about vitamin E.

B Vitamins That Are Not   A newcomer among vitamin frauds is "vitamin B_{15}," pangamic acid. First isolated in 1951 from rice bran, brewer's yeast, and horse liver, pangamic acid was thought to be a B vitamin because of its presence in common foods. Many physiological functions were attributed to it. It is not known, however, whether humans or animals can synthesize pangamic acid, and no specific disease state can be attributed to a deficiency of it. No person who eats a balanced and varied diet need fear a deficiency, and no person who does not eat a balanced and varied diet will benefit significantly by adding purified pangamic acid to her vitamin pill collection.

Preparations sold as vitamin B_{15} may contain any mixture of chemicals; their contents are not controlled by the governments of either the United States or Canada because in both nations vitamin B_{15} is considered an illegal drug.[11] *Nutrition and the MD* has nominated B_{15} for the title "quack nutrient of the year."[12]

Two other compounds deserve mention here, if only to say that they are not vitamins: the bioflavonoids and laetrile. The bioflavonoids are natural body constituents to which vitaminlike characteristics have been attributed. Sold in some stores in purified form as "vitamin P," they have made much money for store owners. However, despite much work, no bioflavonoid deficiency has been induced in animals or discovered in humans, and there is therefore no need to make special efforts to include them in the diet. They were disqualified as vitamins by the American Institute of Nutrition and the American Society of Biological Chemists in 1950.[13] As for laetrile (also called amygdalin and dubbed "vitamin B_{17}" by its enthusiasts), it has been proclaimed a cancer cure by the general public. However, it has never been shown by any kind of reliable testing to cure cancer.[14] Thus the FDA labels laetrile a hoax.

Not vitamins:

vitamin B_{15} (pangamic acid)

vitamin P (bioflavonoids)

vitamin B_{17} (laetrile, amygdalin)

Much of the success of products like vitamin P and vitamin B_{17} is due to their emotional appeal. We have called the trick of inducing people to believe in miracle cures magical thinking. In the case of laetrile, another kind of emotional appeal is also used: scare tactics. People fear cancer, perhaps more than they fear any other disease. Laetrile proponents have capitalized on this fear by scaring the public into believing that the medical establishment frowns on

[11]K. McNutt, Vitamin B_{15}—pangamic acid—what is it?, unpublished statement from the National Nutrition Consortium, June 1978.

[12]Pangamic acid . . . "vitamin B_{15}," *Nutrition and the MD*, December 1978.

[13]R. S. Goodhart, The vitamins, Section M: Miscellany, in *Modern Nutrition in Health and Disease*, 5th ed., eds. R. S. Goodhart and M. E. Shils (Philadelphia: Lea and Febiger, 1973), pp. 259-267.

[14]Controversy 15: The FDA, in E. M. N. Hamilton and E. N. Whitney, *Nutrition: Concepts and Controversies* (St. Paul: West, 1979), pp. 362-364.

laetrile for dishonest reasons. "The doctors don't care if you die," they say, "so long as you pay huge sums for their services." Wanting to trust someone, wanting to hope that a cure is possible, the victim of cancer and her friends and relatives fall easy prey to this deception. The deception is all the more cruel because the victim yields to it out of love of life, and her relatives go along because they care about her and are willing to try anything to help her get well.

A FLAG SIGN OF A SPURIOUS CLAIM IS:

Scare tactics.

Putting It All Together   If you wanted to plan a diet that was adequate for the six B vitamins discussed above, you would be well advised to consume daily 2c or more of milk or dairy products (for riboflavin and niacin equivalents); two or more servings of meat, fish, poultry, or eggs, including liver and pork occasionally (for thiamin, riboflavin, niacin, and vitamin B_6); whole-grain breads and cereals (for thiamin, riboflavin, niacin, and vitamin B_6); and green, leafy vegetables (for folacin). The animal products would supply vitamin B_{12}, and all would supply thiamin. What foods would then be missing? Other vegetables, fruits, and fats—but as you will see in the following chapters, these latter foods are rich in vitamins A, C, D, E, and K. The conclusion is unavoidable: A balanced and varied diet is the best guarantee of adequacy for the essential nutrients. Such a diet would include selections from all the food groups.

Minimizing Losses in Food Handling

The B vitamins are all water-soluble. Whenever a vegetable is soaked or cooked in water and the water is thrown away, significant losses of these vitamins occur. In addition, each of the B vitamins is sensitive to heat to some extent, and riboflavin can be destroyed by light.

Bad advice

Moralizing is tiresome. For fun, we will play the devil's advocate instead and tell you how to maximize *losses* of the B vitamins. First, cook meats at high temperatures for long periods of time and throw away the juices that leak out of them. Leave milk in a transparent container on the countertop in the sunlight for several hours to destroy the riboflavin before storing it in the refrigerator. When baking, bake at high temperatures for long periods of time, using unenriched refined flour for your recipes. Buy unenriched bread and cereal products. When buying vegetables, select those that are several days old and that have been sitting at room temperature in the market since they came in. On bringing them home, put them in the sink, cover them with water, and let them soak for half a day before washing them. When cooking them, slice them thinly, cover them completely with water, bring the water slowly to a boil, and cook them for a long time. Discard the cooking water. If leftover vegetables are to be reheated, pour off the old water and add fresh water. Up to 50 or 60 percent of the B-vitamin content of foods can be lost in this way.

Lest you fear that we will offer no practical, positive suggestions about storing and cooking foods containing water-soluble vitamins, you may be reassured to learn that we provide these at the end of Chapter 10. Of all the water-soluble vitamins, vitamin C is the most vulnerable—to losses in cooking water, to heat, and to several other agents as well. Recommendations for the preservation of this most sensitive of the vitamins apply to the B vitamins too.

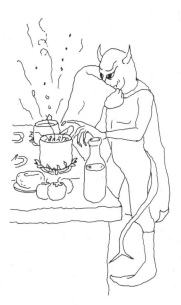

Summing Up

The B vitamins serve as coenzymes assisting many enzymes in the body. Thiamin, riboflavin, niacin, and pantothenic acid are especially important in the glucose-to-energy pathway; they are active in the coenzymes TPP, FAD, NAD^+, and CoA respectively. Vitamin B_6 facilitates amino acid transformations and thus protein metabolism; folacin and vitamin B_{12} are involved in pathways leading to the synthesis of new cells, and biotin is involved in lipid synthesis. These are only examples of the coenzymes' roles; there are many others.

B-vitamin deficiencies seldom occur in isolation; all have multiple symptoms affecting each body organ and tissue in proportion to the roles they play there. A lack of thiamin causes beriberi; a lack of niacin (unless compensated for by its amino acid precursor tryptophan) causes pellagra; a lack of vitamin B_{12} causes pernicious anemia. Human deficiencies of the other B vitamins, although not given names, have been observed for riboflavin, vitamin B_6, and folacin. The anemia of folacin deficiency resembles that of B_{12} deficiency because it produces large immature red blood cells; a key difference between the two, however, is that B_{12} deficiency also causes nerve damage and paralysis.

Vitamin deficiencies cannot be confirmed by inspection of an individual's food intake alone, although food intake provides some clues. The comparison of calculated nutrient intakes with recommendations rests on several assumptions: (1) that the individual is average (that the recommendations are applicable), (2) that body absorption is normal, (3) that the foods consumed are typical (that nutrient values found in tables of food composition are accurate), and (4) that the food has been prepared with reasonable care. Biochemical assessments of nutritional status are more accurate means of pinpointing nutritional problems. These cautions are meant to provide you with a context for considering food sources and nutrient intakes.

Thiamin is widely distributed in foods, but no food contributes a very great amount of it; a balanced and varied diet of nutritious food will best assure an adequate amount of this nutrient. Riboflavin is primarily concentrated in milk and secondarily in meats, which makes eating members of these two food groups advisable. Niacin is found wherever protein is found and can also be made from the amino acid tryptophan; it is therefore supplied in proportion to the amounts of protein in all common foods, except corn (which is low in tryptophan). These three vitamins (and iron) are added to all enriched breads and cereals. Vitamin B_6 is most abundant in meats, vitamin B_{12} is found only in animal products, and folacin is supplied best by green, leafy vegetables. Any diet plan that includes moderate amounts of all these foods assures probable adequacy for these nutrients.

To Explore Further

The complete terminology for the vitamins, together with their popular names and the correct chemical structures, were agreed on by the relevant scientific societies and published in Nomenclature policy: Generic descriptors and trivial names for vitamins and related compounds, *Journal of Nutrition* 109 (1979):8-15.

The most authoritative (and still readable) book on the interactions of drugs with nutrients, including the vitamins, is Roe, D. A., *Drug-Induced Nutritional Deficiencies* (Westport, N.Y.: Avi Publishing, 1976).

Another useful book for detecting the influence of drugs on nutritional status, which should be on every clinical nutritionist's desk, is Grant, A., *Nutritional Assessment Guidelines*, 2nd ed., 1979. It is available from Anne Grant, Box 25057, Northgate Station, Seattle, WA 98125 ($7.50 plus $1.00 for postage and handling).

The altered nutritional needs of people with illnesses are the subject of whole textbooks for dietitians and physicians. Two of the best:

Krause, M. V., and Mahan, L. K., *Food, Nutrition and Diet Therapy*, 6th ed. (Philadelphia: Saunders, 1979).

Schneider, H. A., Anderson, C. E., and Coursin, D. B., eds., *Nutritional Support of Medical Practice* (Hagerstown, Md.: Harper & Row, 1977).

The principal hazards of overdosing with vitamins and minerals have been reviewed and published by the National Nutrition Consortium in a 1978 booklet, *Vitamin-Mineral Safety, Toxicity, and Misuse*, which is available from the American Dietetic Association, 430 North Michigan Avenue, Chicago, IL 60611.

Those who are interested in the history of nutritional discoveries may want to read the original report on the treatment of pernicious anemia using liver, which has been republished from the 1926 *Journal of the American Medical Association:*

Minot, G. R., and Murphy, W. P., Treatment of pernicious anemia by a special diet (Nutrition Classics), *Nutrition Reviews* 36 (February 1978):50-52.

Other references of interest appear in this chapter's footnotes.

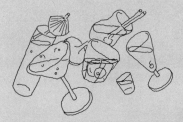

Alcohol and the B Vitamins

If liver cells could talk, they would describe the alcohol of intoxicating beverages as demanding, egocentric, and disruptive of the liver's normally efficient way of running its business. For example, liver cells prefer fatty acids as their fuel, but when alcohol is present, they are forced to use alcohol and let the fatty acids accumulate in huge stockpiles.[1]

Brain cells would make the same criticisms. They are tooled to use glucose for fuel and need niacin and thiamin to convert glucose energy to ATP energy. When alcohol enters the body it grabs all the available supply of these two B vitamins, so that the glucose remains idle and unused. The work of the brain cells thus slows down for lack of glucose energy.

The most dramatic evidence of alcohol's disruptive behavior appears in the liver. This is the only organ whose cells can burn alcohol for fuel. All other cells are affected by the presence of alcohol but can do nothing about getting rid of it. What

[1]C. S. Lieber, Liver adaptation and injury in alcoholism, *New England Journal of Medicine* 288 (1973):356-361.

Glucose, the typical physiological sugar, is urgently important to the brain. The brain draws it from the blood . . . to use at once. . . . Narcotics diminish the oxidation of sugar by the brain. When the quantity of sugar supplied to the brain by the blood is less the oxidative turn-over is less owing to the lack of oxidative food. Without vitamin B the brain cannot make proper use of glucose as a food. Thought and behavior alter. If the conditions be prolonged, unconsciousness ensues, and if prolonged further the brain-cells are permanently damaged.

SIR CHARLES SHERRINGTON

liver cells have that other cells do not have is the ability to make an enzyme, alcohol dehydrogenase. This enzyme can convert alcohol to acetaldehyde, which can in turn be converted to acetyl CoA, the compound that all energy nutrients become on their way to being used as fuel. But we are getting ahead of our story. Let's start at the beginning, when alcohol first enters the body in a beverage, and follow it until it leaves or is made into useful acetyl CoA.

Alcohol Enters the Body

To the chemist, *alcohol* refers to a class of compounds with reactive hydroxyl (OH) groups on them. The glycerol to which fatty acids are attached in triglycerides is an example of a chemist's alcohol. But to the average person, *alcohol* refers to the intoxicating ingredient in beer, wine, and hard liquor (distilled spirits). The chemist's name for this particular alcohol is *ethanol*. Glycerol has

$$
\begin{array}{c}
H \\
| \\
H-C-OH \\
| \\
H-C-OH \\
| \\
H-C-OH \\
| \\
H
\end{array}
$$

Glycerol is an alcohol.

$$
\begin{array}{c}
H \\
| \\
H-C-H \\
| \\
H-C-H \\
| \\
OH
\end{array}
$$

Ethanol is the alcohol in beer, wine, and distilled spirits.

three carbons with three hydroxyl groups attached; ethanol has only two carbons and one hydroxyl group. For the remainder of this Highlight we will be discussing "alcohol," but you will know that we are really talking about a particular alcohol—ethanol.

From the moment alcohol enters the body in a beverage, it is treated as if it has special privileges.[2] Foods sit around in the stomach for a while, but not alcohol. Alcohol molecules are so small that they can diffuse right through the walls of the stomach. The euphoric effects of a drink can be felt so quickly because no time is needed for digestion before absorption. It also explains why the effects of a drink are felt more quickly when the stomach is empty. If you don't want to become inebriated at parties, eat the high-fat snacks provided by the host. When your stomach is full of food, the molecules of alcohol have less chance of touching the walls and diffusing through.

When the stomach contents are emptied into the duodenum, it doesn't matter that plenty of food is mixed with the alcohol. The alcohol is absorbed rapidly, "as if it were a V. I. P."[3] Here again, the high-fat snacks help moderate the effects of alcohol. Fat slows down peristalsis and thus delays the emptying of the stomach, which keeps the alcohol from rapidly entering the bloodstream.

Alcohol Arrives in the Liver The capillaries that surround the digestive tract merge into the veins that carry the alcohol-laden blood

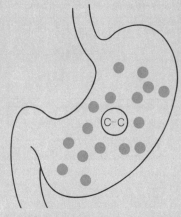

The alcohol (C-C) in a stomach filled with food has a low probability of touching the walls and diffusing through.

to the liver. Here the veins branch and rebranch into capillaries that touch every liver cell. Liver cells are the only cells in the body that know how to make alcohol dehydrogenase, the enzyme that can convert alcohol to a compound the body can use.

Alcohol dehydrogenase converts alcohol to acetaldehyde. Simultaneously it converts a molecule of NAD^+ to $NADH + H^+$. (You may recall that the N in NAD^+ is a form of niacin, one of the B vitamins.) Acetaldehyde uses another NAD^+ and TPP (the T stands for thiamin) to be converted to acetyl CoA, the compound that enters the TCA cycle to become carbon dioxide, water, and most importantly ATP.

For every molecule of alcohol that enters the capillaries of the liver, then, two molecules of niacin and one of

thiamin are needed. A well-nourished person probably has enough niacin and thiamin to take care of a moderate amount of alcohol, but the liver only makes a limited amount of alcohol dehydrogenase, so the rate at which the alcohol is disposed of is limited. If more molecules of alcohol arrive at the liver cells than the enzymes can handle, the molecules of alcohol that are left stranded continue on by and re-enter the general circulation. From the liver they are carried to all parts of the body, circulating again and again through the liver until enzymes are free to convert them to acetaldehyde.

The amount of alcohol dehydrogenase, then, is the rate-limiting factor in the body's handling of alcohol.

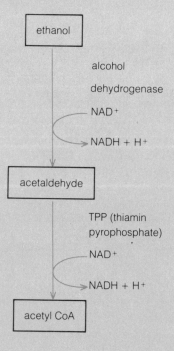

[2]F. Iber, In alcoholism, the liver sets the pace, *Nutrition Today,* January/February 1971, pp. 2-9.
[3]Iber, 1971.

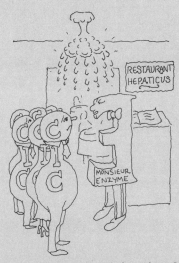

"I have places for only four of you."

The amount of enzyme that is produced varies with individuals and is controlled by heredity. Some racial groups, particularly Orientals and Native Americans, do not have the genetic information for producing alcohol dehydrogenase. This difference has been offered as an explanation for some persons, particularly Orientals, not becoming heavy drinkers; they are made too uncomfortable to become addicted. In those who can produce the enzyme, production is increased (up to the inherited limits) the more frequently it is stimulated. Thus an experienced drinker has an abundant supply of alcohol dehydrogenase, which causes him to recover from the effect of a drink very quickly. (This may be how addiction occurs: A person consumes ever more alcohol to achieve the same euphoria.)

The amount of alcohol dehydrogenase is also affected by whether you eat or not. Fasting for as little as a day causes degradation of the enzyme (protein) within the cells, and can reduce the rate of alcohol metabolism by half. Drinking on an empty stomach thus brings about higher blood alcohol levels for longer periods of time and increases the effect of alcohol in anesthetizing the brain.

As more and more alcohol is converted first to acetaldehyde and then to acetyl CoA, the supply of niacin and thiamin is depleted. This has a profound effect on every cell in the entire body. There may be abundant glucose going past the cells to fuel their work, but cells need niacin and thiamin to make use of the glucose. Brain cells are especially vulnerable to a deficit of niacin and thiamin since they rely solely on glucose for their energy.

Figure 1 is a drawing of the pathway from glucose to ATP, showing the many places along the way that require niacin (NAD^+) and thiamin (TPP). The drawing of pathways like this one seems to be a favorite pastime of chemists and a most unfavorite kind of activity for beginning nutrition students. If you are such a student, take a moment with us to look carefully at this map, which shows how to get from here to there chemically.

Maps can be simple or complex, according to need. Sometimes when you ask for directions, the directing person will say simply, "At the second stoplight, turn left." He knows, and you do too, that there is no need to know the names of the streets you are passing and certainly no need to be told of possible obstacles. In Figure 1, we have named only the "streets" that are crucial to your understanding, but we have drawn in places where there may be a "drawbridge" open or "street construction" that will cause traffic to back up or necessitate an alternate route.

This map is intended to show you that to get from "here to there," niacin and/or thiamin must be present. If they are not (and when alcohol is present they may not be), the road will be blocked and traffic will back up—or an alternate route will be taken. There are physical consequences to such changes in the normal flow of traffic from glucose to ATP. Think about some of these as you follow the diagram.

Figure 1 A simplified version of the glucose-to-energy pathway, showing the entry of ethanol into the pathway. The coenzymes that are the active forms of thiamin and niacin are the only ones included. (For a more detailed diagram, see the figure on p. 258).

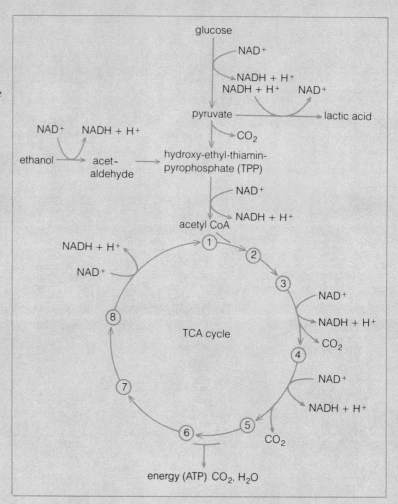

Acetyl CoAs are blocked from getting into the TCA cycle by the high level of NADH. Instead of being used for energy, they become building blocks for fatty acids.

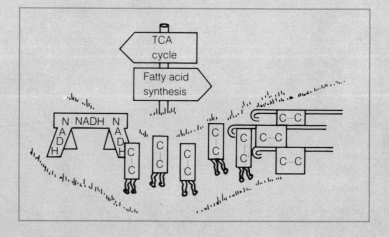

If all the body's niacin and thiamin are depleted, no energy will be produced even if there is plenty of glucose. (A shortage of glucose affects the brain, creating confusion and a change in behavior.) In each step where NAD$^+$ is converted to NADH + H$^+$, hydrogen builds up. (As a result, the acid base balance shifts toward acid; this is dangerous.) If there is some niacin and thiamin but not enough niacin to carry the compounds through the TCA cycle, acetyl CoA will build up. The excess acetyl CoA then takes the route to the synthesis of fatty acids. (Fat clogs the liver so it cannot function.[4]) As thiamin is depleted, more and more pyruvate builds up; it is converted to lactic acid, because there is a surplus of NADH + H$^+$, which this reaction uses. The conversion of pyruvate to lactic acid relieves the accumulation of NADH + H$^+$, but creates new problems: A lactic acid buildup has serious consequences of its own (it adds to the body's acid burden and interferes with the excretion of uric acid, causing goutlike symptoms).

If you need to know the names of the compounds involved in this pathway

[4]Lieber, 1973.

or their structures, you will find a more complete map in Highlight 7.

When the liver lays aside important functions to attend to alcohol, there are other consequences. Protein synthesis nearly halts, because the liver cells use all the available resources to make alcohol dehydrogenase. As a result there is no protein for wrapping up the triglycerides to be carried through the blood. Some important antibodies and other enzymes essential to the health

Pyruvate is converted to lactic acid if the pathway to acetyl CoA is blocked.

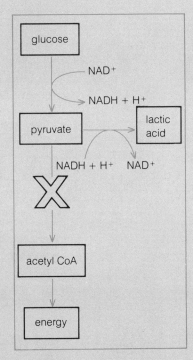

of the body are not synthesized either.

The synthesis of fatty acids is stepped up, because none of the acetyl CoA from the energy nutrients can get into the TCA cycle. This event, combined with the lack of protein carriers, increases the amount of fat stuck in the liver. Fatty liver, so often seen in heavy drinkers, interferes with the distribution of nutrients and oxygen to the liver cells. If the condition lasts long enough, the liver cells will die and the area will be invaded by fibrous scar tissue—another stage of liver deterioration called fibrosis. Fibrosis is reversible with good nutrition and abstinence from alcohol, but the next stage—cirrhosis—is not.

Ethanol Arrives in the Brain Alcohol is a narcotic. It was used for centuries as an anesthetic because of its ability to deaden pain. But it wasn't a very good one, because one could never be sure how much a person would need or how much would be a lethal dose. As new, more predictable anesthetics were discovered, they quickly replaced alcohol. However, alcohol continues to be used today as a kind of anesthetic in social situations, to help people relax or to relieve anxiety.

When alcohol flows to the brain it reaches the frontal lobe first. Thus as the alcohol molecules diffuse into the brain cells, they first anesthetize the cells of this lobe, the reasoning part. If additional molecules continue to enter the bloodstream from the digestive tract before the liver has had time to oxidize the first ones, then the speech and vision centers of the brain become narcotized, and the area that governs reasoning becomes more incapacitated. Later the cells of the brain responsible for large-muscle control are affected; at this point, people "under the influence" stagger or weave when they try to walk.

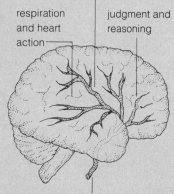

muscular control

respiration and heart action

judgment and reasoning

Blood carrying alcohol enters here.

Liver cells are not the only cells that die with excessive exposure to alcohol; brain cells are particularly sensitive. When liver cells have died, others may later multiply to replace them, but there is no regeneration of nerve cells. Hence the permanent brain damage observed in some heavy drinkers.

With these changes in mind, it is time to take a look at alcohol consumption from the social view and at the malnutrition that results from excessive drinking.

Drinking and Drunkenness If you want to drink socially, you should drink with food and should sip, not gulp, your drinks. If you drink this way, the alcohol molecules will dribble into the liver cells, and the enzymes will be able to handle the load. Spacing of drinks is important too: It takes about 1-1/2 hours to metabolize one drink, depending on your body size, on previous drinking experience, and on how you are feeling at the time.

If a friend has drunk too much and you want to help him sober up, there is no reason to wear yourself out walking him around the block. The muscles have to work harder, but since they can't metabolize alcohol, they can't help clear the blood. Time is the only thing that will do the job; each person has a particular level of the enzyme alcohol dehydrogenase, and it clears the blood at a steady rate. This is not true for most nutrients. If you bring in more of a nutrient, generally the body steps up its metabolism. But not with alcohol.

Nor will it help your friend to give him a cup of coffee. Caffeine is a stimulant, but it won't speed up the metabolism of alcohol. The police say ruefully, "If you give a drunk a cup of coffee you won't make him sober, but you'll make him an awake drunk."

So far we have mentioned only one way that the blood is cleared of alcohol—metabolism by the liver. However, about 10 percent of the alcohol is excreted through the breath and in the urine. This fact is the basis for the breathalyzer test for drunkenness administered by police. The amount of alcohol in the breath is in proportion to that still in the bloodstream. In most states legal drunkenness is set at 0.15 percent, although many states are lowering the criterion to 0.10 percent—especially as statistics ac-

Alcohol Doses and Brain Responses

Number of drinks	Blood alcohol	Effect on brain
2 drinks	.05%	judgment impaired
4 drinks	.10%	control impaired
6 drinks	.15%	muscle coordination and reflexes impaired
8 drinks	.20%	vision impaired
12 drinks	.30%	drunk, out of control
14 drinks or more	.50-.60%	amnesia, finally death

cumulate that show a relationship between alcohol use and industrial and traffic accidents.

The lack of glucose for the brain's function and the length of time needed to clear the blood of alcohol are responsible for some diverse consequences of drinking alcohol. You may occasionally read in the newspaper of the death of a person, often a young college student, during a drinking contest. Coma and death are brought on in these cases by the lack of glucose to fuel the brain and by the anesthetizing of the respiratory center deep in the brain.[5] Responsible aircraft pilots know that they must allow 24 hours for their bodies to clear alcohol completely and refuse to fly any sooner.[6] Major airlines enforce this rule. Finally, women who may become pregnant are warned to abstain from the use of alcohol because the lack of glucose may interrupt the development of the fetus's central nervous system.[7] This could occur even before the woman is aware that she is pregnant.

You may have heard the story of the country woman who kept saying "Amen!" as

[5]Lieber, 1973.

[6]Private communication from Captain Francis J. Black, senior Eastern Airlines pilot, retired after 35 years' service, now residing in Tallahassee, Florida.

[7]Fetal alcohol syndrome, *Nutrition and the MD*, July 1978.

Mini-Glossary

alcohol dehydrogenase: an enzyme found in the liver that converts ethanol to **acetaldehyde** (ass-et-AL-duh-hide).

antidiuretic hormone (ADH): a hormone produced by the pituitary gland in response to dehydration (or a high sodium concentration in the blood); stimulates the kidneys to reabsorb more water and so excrete less. This ADH should not be confused with the enzyme alcohol dehydrogenase, which is sometimes also abbreviated ADH.

cirrhosis (seer-OH-sis): irreversible hardening of liver tissue. The cirrhotic liver is nodular and orange in color (see also p. 140).

cirrhos = orange

fibrosis: the invasion of scar tissue into a necrotic area.

gout (gowt): a disease in which uric acid and salts are deposited around joints. It causes swelling and severe pain, especially in the big toe.

narcotic (nar-KOT-ic): any drug that dulls the senses, induces sleep, and becomes addictive with prolonged use.

necrosis (neck-RO-sis): death of tissue.

---

the preacher ranted about one sin after another; but when he got to her favorite sin, she whispered to her husband that the preacher had "quit preachin' and gone to meddlin'." We've tried to stick to scientific facts, so the only "meddlin'" that we will do is to urge you to look again at the drawing of the brain on p. 356 and note that judgment is affected first. When you hear someone say he is a better driver or a better salesman when he has had one drink, you can be sure he is ignorant of alcohol's action in the brain. What has really happened is that his judgment has been altered by one drink so that he *thinks* he is a better driver or salesman. If he really did perform better, it was because the alcohol released his inhibitions or muted his self-criticisms or tensions. He needs to look for a more healthful way of solving those problems.

Drinking and Malnutrition It has been estimated that more than 9 million people in the United States abuse alcohol to the point that their personal relationships, their jobs, or their health are impaired. One of the health hazards is malnutrition. Alcohol depresses appetite by the euphoria it produces as well as by its attack on the mucosa of the stomach, so that heavy drinkers usually eat poorly if at all. With a large portion of their kcalories coming from the empty kcalories of alcohol, it is difficult for them to obtain the essential nutrients. Thus some of their malnutrition is due to lack of food. If they eat well during the times they are not drinking, they may survive for many years without clinical evidence of deficiencies. Another cause of malnutrition, as already mentioned, is the B-vitamin depletion that plagues the long-time drinker.

Protein deficiency would be expected to develop, partly from the poor diet but also from the depression of protein synthesis in the cells, which would ordinarily use the amino acids that happen to be eaten by the drinker. Instead, the drinker's liver deaminates the amino acids and channels their carbon backbones into fat or into the TCA cycle to be used for energy. Alcohol's interference with glucose metabolism tends to increase the body's use of amino acids for energy.

Two additional deficiencies that research has uncovered even in well-nourished alcoholics are iron deficiency[8] and folic acid deficiency.[9] Abstaining from alcohol cures both deficiencies very quickly; at the most it takes only two or three days eating ordinary hospital diets. But with continued use of alcohol, even with extra supple-

mentation, the deficiencies continue.[10]

Alcohol depresses the anti-diuretic hormone (ADH). All people who drink have observed the increase in urination that accompanies drinking, but they may not realize that they are eliminating more than just water and some alcohol. With water loss there is a loss of such important minerals as magnesium, potassium, and zinc. These minerals are vital to the maintenance of fluid balance and to many chemical reactions in the cells, including muscle contraction. Repletion therapy is often instituted in the recovering alcoholic to bring magnesium and potassium levels back to normal as quickly as possible.

In summary, ethanol—the two-carbon alcohol present in beer, wine, and distilled alcoholic beverages—interferes with many chemical and hormonal reactions in the body. In particular, this disruptive molecule depresses protein synthesis, increases fatty acid synthesis, increases mineral loss through increased urinary excretion, and interferes with the metabolism of glucose to energy by grabbing all the niacin and thiamin for its own metabolism. Its kcalories are available only to the liver cells, and it effectively blocks the utilization of glucose by the rest of the

body. Protein, the B vitamins, and minerals (especially magnesium and potassium), are the principal nutritional deficiences found in heavy drinkers.

To Explore Further

In both of the following articles, the metabolism of alcohol in the body is clearly enunciated. Iber's article is especially well suited for the general reader.

Lieber, C. S., The metabolism of alcohol, *Scientific American* 234 (1976):25-33.

Iber, F., In alcoholism, the liver sets the pace, *Nutrition Today*, January/February 1971, pp. 2-9.

A clear, advanced, and up-to-date description of alcohol's metabolic and nutritional effects is presented in Shaw, S. and Lieber, C.S., Nutrition and alcoholism, in *Modern Nutrition in Health and Disease*, 6th ed., Goodhart, R. S., and Shils, M. E., eds. (Philadelphia: Lea and Febiger, 1980), pp. 1220-1243.

One of the possible explanations for the fact that some people do not become alcoholic while others with seemingly similar backgrounds do is studied in Wolff, P. H., Ethnic differences in alcohol sensitivity, *Science* 175 (1972):449.

A teaching aid, *Alcoholic Malnutrition* by F. Iber, is a set of 16 slides illustrating the way the liver sets the pace in the nutritional troubles that beset the alcoholic. This aid can be ordered from the Nutrition Today Society (address in Appendix J).

---

[8] E. R. Eichner, The hematologic disorders of alcoholism, *American Journal of Medicine* 54 (1973):621-630.

[9] E. B. Southmayd, The role of the dietitian in team therapy for chronic alcoholism, *Journal of the American Dietetic Association* 64 (1974):184-186.

[10] Eichner, 1973.

Exercises 1 to 3 make use of the information you recorded on Forms 1 to 3 in the Self-Study at the end of the introduction to Part One.

1. Look up and record your recommended intake of thiamin (from the RDA tables on the inside front cover or from the Canadian Dietary Standard in Appendix O). Also record your actual intake, from the average derived on Form 2 (p. 16). What percentage of your recommended intake did you consume? Was this enough? What foods contribute the greatest amount of thiamin to your diet? If you consumed more than the recommendation, was this too much? Why or why not? In what ways would you change your diet to improve thiamin intake?

2. Repeat Exercise 1 using riboflavin as the subject.

3. Estimate your niacin intake using the method outlined on p. 342. Did you consume enough niacin preformed in foods to meet your recommended intake? If not, did you consume enough extra protein to bring your intake up to the recommendation? What do you suppose are the limitations on this means of estimating niacin intake?

Optional Extras

● Find alternative sources of B vitamins for the person who doesn't drink milk. Many nonwhites avoid milk products because of lactose intolerance or personal preference. How can these people meet their riboflavin needs without drinking milk? Plan a day's menus around the favorite foods of the U.S. South (pork, fish, chicken, greens, corn bread, hominy grits, and sweet potatoes) to provide adequacy for thiamin and riboflavin. Be sure not to exceed the appropriate kcalorie level. Is it necessary to eat enriched corn bread and grits in order to get enough of these nutrients? Show your calculations.

You could also plan a day's menus around your own favorite foods (if you avoid milk) or around the favorite foods of a friend of yours who dislikes milk. Is it necessary for you or your friend to eat enriched or whole-grain breads and cereals in order to get enough thiamin and riboflavin? Show your calculations.

● Explode some of the myths surrounding the vitamins. Go to a health food store and interview the owner or salesperson about the virtues of the products being sold there. Jot down these claims and the evidence cited to substantiate them. Which claims would you be inclined to believe on the basis of the evidence? Which are examples of the spurious claims that we have identified with flag signs?

CHAPTER 10

CONTENTS

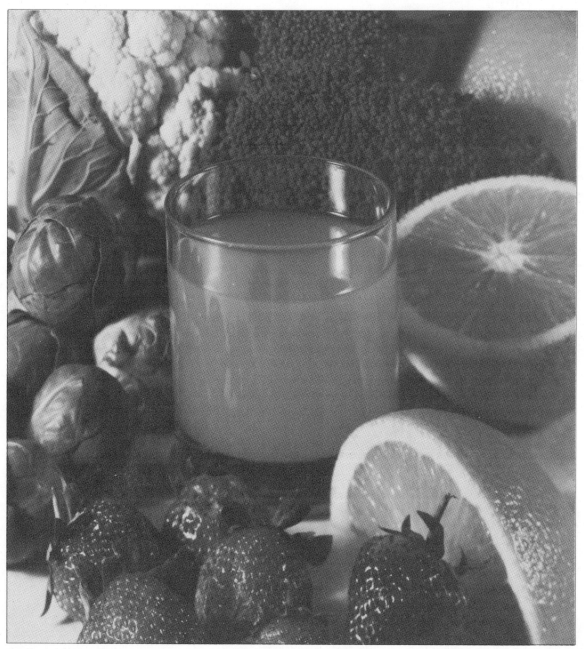

Foods rich in C vitamins.

VITAMIN C: Ascorbic Acid

It is often felt that only the discovery of a microtheory affords real scientific understanding of any type of phenomenon, because only it gives us insight into the inner mechanism of the phenomenon, so to speak.

C. G. HEMPEL and P. OPPENHEIM

Two hundred years ago, any man who joined the crew of a seagoing ship knew he had only half a chance of returning alive—not because he might be slain by pirates or die in a storm but because he might contract the dread disease scurvy. As many as two-thirds of a ship's men might die of scurvy on a long voyage. Only ships that sailed on short voyages, especially around the Mediterranean Sea, were safe from this disease. It was not known at the time that the special hazard of long ocean voyages was that the ship's cook used up his provisions of fresh fruits and vegetables early and relied for the duration of the voyage on cereals and live animals brought along as provisions.

The first nutrition experiment conducted on human beings was devised in 1747 to find a cure for scurvy. Dr. James Lind, a British physician, divided 12 sailors with scurvy into six pairs. Each pair received a different supplemental ration: vinegar, sulfuric acid, sea water, orange, lemon, or none. The ones receiving the citrus fruits were cured within a short time. Sadly, it was 50 years before the British Navy made use of Lind's experiment by requiring all vessels to carry sufficient limes for every sailor to have lime juice daily. British sailors are still derisively called "limeys" as a result of this tradition.

The anti-scurvy "something" in limes and other foods was dubbed the antiscorbutic factor. Nearly 200 years later, the factor was isolated from lemon juice and found to be a six-carbon compound similar to glucose. It was named ascorbic acid.[1] Shortly thereafter it was synthesized, and today hundreds of millions of vitamin C pills are produced in pharmaceutical laboratories each year and sold for a few dollars a bottle.

Human needs for vitamin C are the subject of much disagreement among experts. The publication of Linus Pauling's controversial book *Vitamin C and the Common Cold* thrust this vitamin into the limelight in 1970 and persuaded thousands of readers that they should be taking

scurvy: the vitamin C-deficiency disease.

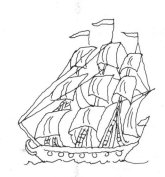

For more history of the discovery of the vitamins, see Appendix A.

antiscorbutic factor: the original name for vitamin C.

anti = against
scorbutic = causing scurvy

ascorbic acid: one of the two active forms of vitamin C (see Figure 1). Many people consistently refer to all vitamin C by this name.

a = without
scorbic = having scurvy

---

[1]The agreed-on term for this vitamin, which has often been referred to as ascorbic acid, is vitamin C: American Institute of Nutrition, Committee on Nomenclature, Nomenclature policy: Generic descriptors and trivial names for vitamins and related compounds, *Journal of Nutrition* 109 (1979):8-15.

Doses of 10 to 20 or more times the recommended intake of a nutrient are termed **megadoses**. In the case of vitamin C, any amount over 1 g (1,000 mg) is considered a megadose.

doses much higher than the 30 or so milligrams a day cited as adequate in published recommended intakes. Highly respected nutritionists and other scientists have taken positions at both extremes on this issue. The controversy over the common cold has largely died down in the popular press (see Highlight 10), but the question of how much is enough is still being hotly debated.

There is also a controversy over the risks of taking large doses of vitamin C. Some argue for megadoses on the grounds that the risks are negligible but the risks of deficiency are great. Others argue against megadoses because the risk of deficiency is negligible but the risks of toxicity are great. Both positions are based on reasoning from small amounts of evidence and large numbers of words.

We face a difficult task in trying to sort out what is known about vitamin C, what is possible, and what claims are clearly unfounded. This chapter deals with the vitamin's known roles and debunks the obvious myths, leaving matters that are in the realm of uncertainty to Highlight 10.

Metabolic Roles of Vitamin C

Vitamin C is a mysterious vitamin. Like all the vitamins, it is a small organic compound needed by human beings in minute amounts daily. Being organic, it is convertible to several different forms, two of which are active (see Figure 1). Like the B vitamins, it is water-soluble, and so it is excreted rapidly when excesses are taken and is not stored for long in the body. But unlike the B vitamins (which for the most part have clearly defined metabolic roles as coenzymes), vitamin C acts in ways that are imperfectly understood. It plays many different important roles in the body, and the secret may be that its mode of action is different in each case. In some settings it may act as a coenzyme or cofactor, assisting a specific enzyme in the performance of its job. In others, it may act in a more general way—for example, as an antioxidant. Often the conclusion reached by investigators researching vitamin C is that it has to "be present" for certain reactions to occur but that the mechanism of its action will require further research.

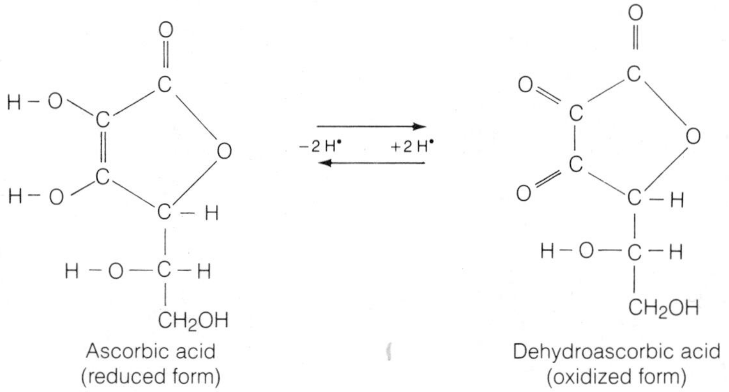

Figure 1 Active forms of vitamin C. The reduced form can lose two hydrogens with their electrons, becoming oxidized. The electrons may then reduce some other compound.

Ascorbic acid
(reduced form)

−2 H·   +2 H·

Dehydroascorbic acid
(oxidized form)

Collagen Formation   The best-understood metabolic role of vitamin C is its function in helping to form the protein collagen. Brief mention was made of this protein in Chapter 4; it is the single most important protein of connective tissue. It serves as the matrix on which bone is formed and is the material of scars. When you have been wounded, collagen forms, and glues the separated tissue faces together, making a scar. The cement that holds cells together is largely made of collagen (and calcium); this function is especially important in the artery walls, which must expand and contract with each beat of the heart, and in the walls of the capillaries, which are thin and fragile and must withstand a pulse of blood every second or so without giving way.

Collagen, like all proteins, is formed by stringing together a chain of amino acids. An unusual amino acid found in abundance in collagen is hydroxyproline. After the amino acid proline has been added to the chain, an enzyme adds an OH group to it, making hydroxyproline. This step, which completes the manufacture of collagen, requires oxygen and a special form of iron—the ferrous ion. This iron has a tendency to convert to another form (ferric ion), which the enzyme can't use. Vitamin C stands by to catch ferric ions and reconvert them to the

collagen: a water-insoluble protein; the characteristic protein of connective tissue.

kolla = glue
gennan = to produce

Collagen is unique among body proteins, because it contains large amounts of the amino acid proline and has OH groups attached to this amino acid. (For the structure of proline, see Appendix C.)

Ion: see Appendix B. Iron is an atom that can exist in two ionic states, ferric (Fe^{+++}, lacking 3 electrons) or ferrous (Fe^{++}, lacking 2).

1. Amino acids are strung together in a chain that includes many prolines.

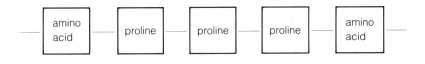

Figure 2   How vitamin C helps form collagen.

2. An enzyme, with the help of iron (Fe^{++}), adds OH groups to the prolines. Vitamin C stabilizes the iron in the ferrous form.

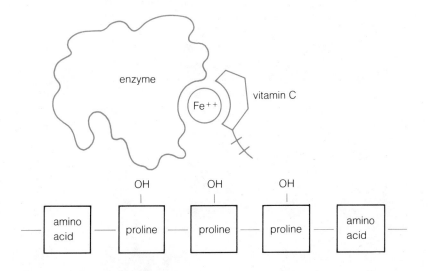

3. The completed collagen molecule contains many hydroxyproline units.

ferrous form so that the enzyme can keep on working.[2] Figure 2 shows how this process is believed to occur.

Antioxidant Action Chemists call the two forms of iron just described oxidized and reduced iron. The oxidized (ferric) form has lost electrons (see Appendix B); the reduced (ferrous) form has regained them. Any substance that can donate electrons to another is a reducing agent; when it donates its electrons it reduces another compound and simultaneously becomes oxidized itself. Vitamin C is such a compound.

The technicalities of oxidation-reduction reactions are not within our province, and the object of mentioning them is only to make one point clear: Many substances found in foods and important in the body can be altered or even destroyed by oxidation. (An example in Chapter 2 was oils that turn rancid when exposed to air.) Vitamin C—because it can be oxidized itself—can protect other substances from this destruction. Vitamin C is like a bodyguard for oxidizable substances: It stands ready to sacrifice its own life to save the life of another. Unemotionally, the chemists call such a bodyguard an antioxidant.

Because of its antioxidant property, vitamin C is sometimes added to food products, not only to improve their nutritional value but also to protect important constituents from oxidation. In the intestines, it protects ferrous iron in this way. In the cells and body fluids, it probably helps to protect other molecules, including the fat-soluble compounds vitamin A, vitamin E, and the polyunsaturated fatty acids, by maintaining their watery neighborhood in the appropriately reduced state.[3] Vitamin E and the polyunsaturated fatty acids are very important constituents of cell membranes, and these membranes house much of the cells' machinery. This machinery must be meticulously maintained so that the cells can live and work and so that they will discriminate successfully among the things that should enter them (cross their membranes) and those that should be excluded. Vitamin C—perhaps by way of its ability to alternate between the oxidized and the reduced state—helps maintain these vital functions.

The Absorption of Iron Vitamin C eaten at the same time as iron helps to promote the absorption of this mineral. It is not yet known how the vitamin performs this service, but one intriguing possibility is entitled to a paragraph of explanation.

You can't pick up a screw with a screwdriver—unless the screwdriver is magnetic. Even then, the screw may fall off at the slightest jolt. You can pick up a screw with a pair of pliers, but then you have to hold it tightly or it will fall out of their grip. But if you have a magnetic pair

For a picture of the way oxygen destroys the double bonds in an unsaturated fatty acid, see p. 68.

antioxidant: a compound that protects others from oxidation by being oxidized itself.

Chemists describe this action of vitamin C as maintaining the "oxidation-reduction equilibrium" or "redox state" and as participating in "electron transport."

[2]The role of ascorbic acid in the hydroxylation of peptide-bound proline, *Nutrition Reviews* 37 (January 1979):26-28.

[3]R. E. Hodges and E. M. Baker, The vitamins, Section K: Ascorbic acid, in *Modern Nutrition in Health and Disease*, 5th ed., eds. R. S. Goodhart and M. E. Shils (Philadelphia: Lea and Febiger, 1973), pp. 245-255.

of pliers, you can hold the screw so securely that the only problem may be that you can't let it go. A chelating agent is the molecular equivalent of a magnetized pair of pliers, and vitamin C is an outstanding example of such a molecule. These molecules are especially good at holding onto ions that have two positive charges, like ferrous iron (Fe^{++}). Vitamin C can grab and hold such an ion because it has two arms with negative charges on them (see the diagram in the margin). Thus vitamin C can not only reduce iron but can also stabilize it in the reduced form. The complex, iron-chelated-by-vitamin-C, may be much more easily absorbed by the intestinal cells than iron alone.[4]

Whatever the mechanism, it is now well known that eating foods containing vitamin C at the same meal with foods containing iron can double the absorption of iron. This strategy is highly recommended for women and for children, whose kcalorie intakes are not large enough to guarantee that they will get enough iron from the foods they typically eat.

chelating (KEE-late-ing) **agent:** a molecule that can assume a form suitable for trapping ions with two positive charges.

The typical U.S. diet supplies only 5-6 mg iron in every 1,000 kcal. Children need 10 mg per day, and women need 18 mg (see Chapter 13).

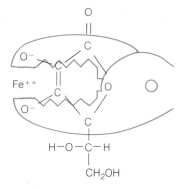

Chelation. The negatively charged "arms" of the chelating agent stabilize the two positive charges of the ferrous ion and hold the ion in place.

The Chinese have for centuries employed the strategy of serving vitamin C-rich fruits or vegetables and iron-rich meats in the very same dishes: loquat chicken, beef with broccoli, sweet-and-sour pork (including pineapple), chop suey (meat with cabbage), and dozens of others. Westerners are more likely to serve foods singly, although it is traditional to accompany certain meats with certain fruits: turkey with cranberries or pork with applesauce. These combinations are especially desirable if you choose to reduce your meat consumption in line with recent recommendations. To get the maximum iron value from small servings of iron-rich foods, serve a vitamin C-rich food at every meal.[5]

Some people try to protect the body from overwork by serving it different foods separately so that it can concentrate on handling those foods one at a time. Some evidence against this notion is presented in Chapter 5. The cooperation between vitamin C and iron, which seldom appear together in any one food, provides another argument against this simplistic notion.

A FLAG SIGN OF A SPURIOUS CLAIM
IS THE NOTION THAT:

Foods should be ingested singly to ease the body's work.

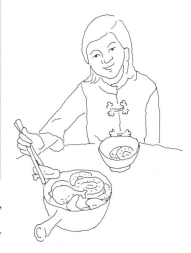

[4]We are indebted to Professor Stanley Winter of Golden West College, Huntington Beach, California, for pointing out this possible role of vitamin C to us.

[5]M. Balsley, Soon to come: 1978 Recommended Dietary Allowances, *Journal of the American Dietetic Association* 71 (1977): 149-151.

On the contrary: Multicolored, mixed dishes are probably those to which the body, as well as the eye and the palate, responds most gratefully.

Amino Acid Metabolism   Vitamin C is involved in the metabolism of several amino acids. In at least some instances it probably functions as it does during collagen formation, by keeping iron or copper in a reduced state to aid an enzyme in adding OH groups to other compounds. Some of these amino acids may end up being converted to hormones of great importance in body functioning, among them norepinephrine and thyroxin.

The adrenal gland contains a higher concentration of vitamin C than any other organ in the body, and during stress it releases large quantities of the vitamin together with the stress hormones epinephrine and norepinephrine. What the vitamin has to do with the stress reaction is unclear, but it is known that stress increases vitamin C needs.

Vitamin C is also needed for the synthesis of the thyroid hormone, thyroxin, which regulates the rate of metabolism. The metabolic rate speeds up under extreme stress and also when you need to produce more heat—for example, when you have a fever or when you are in a very cold climate. Thus infections and exposure to cold increase your needs for vitamin C. Perhaps its involvement in the fever response to infection explains the vitamin's possible effects on cold prevention and symptoms, although there are other possibilities (see Highlight 10).

In scurvy, protein metabolism may be altered, incurring a negative nitrogen balance.[6] No one knows why this occurs, but the involvement of vitamin C with amino acids provides a notable example of the way nutrients of different classes cooperate with one another to maintain health.

Vitamin C and Other Nutrients   Some evidence suggests that vitamin C in some way aids the body in using folic acid and vitamin B_{12}. It also interacts with calcium. Bones and teeth were long believed to be inert, like stones, but they are actually very active. Calcium is continuously being withdrawn and redeposited in these structures, another process for which vitamin C is essential. In scurvy, the teeth become loose in the jawbone and fillings may become loose in the teeth, reflecting loss of tooth material faster than it can be replaced.

Epinephrine and norepinephrine were formerly called adrenaline and noradrenaline.

[6]Hodges and Baker, 1973.

Vitamin C Deficiency

In both the United States and Canada, vitamin C deficiency is still seen despite the past century's explosion of nutritional knowledge. In the United States, the Ten-State Survey (see Highlight 15) showed evidence of unacceptable serum levels of vitamin C in about 15 percent of all age groups studied, with symptoms of outright scurvy showing up in 4 percent. Especially in infants, teenagers, and people over 60 years of age, intakes of vitamin C were much lower than the RDA (less than 50 percent). In Canada, many Eskimos and Indians and some members of the general population have deficiency symptoms. Evidently all we need is to be alerted to the symptoms that can result and to make efforts to obtain enough of this vitamin.

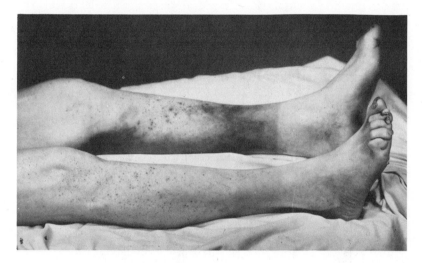

Early skin symptom of scurvy. There is a tiny hemorrhage around each hair follicle. These pinpoint hemorrhages are called **petechiae** (pet-EEK-ee-eye).

Photo courtesy of Dr. Samuel Dreizen, D.D.S., M.D.

With an adequate intake, the body maintains a fixed pool of vitamin C and rapidly excretes any excess in the urine. With an inadequate intake, the pool becomes depleted at the rate of about 3 percent a day. Obvious deficiency symptoms don't begin to appear until the pool has been reduced to about a fifth of its optimal size, and this may take two months or more to occur. Thus the first sign of an incipient vitamin C deficiency is a lowered serum or plasma vitamin C concentration.[7] A low intake as revealed by the diet history is the cue that prompts the diagnostician to request a clinical test to measure the body's vitamin C levels.

Clinical tests: see discussion on p. 567.

As the pool size continues to fall, latent scurvy appears. Two of the earliest signs have to do with the role of the vitamin in maintaining

latent: the period in disease when the conditions are present but before the symptoms have begun to appear.

latens = lying hidden

overt: out in the open, full-blown.

ouvrire = to open

[7]Vitamin C shifts unpredictably between the plasma and the white blood cells known as leukocytes; thus a plasma or serum determination may not accurately reflect the body's pool. The appropriate clinical test may be a measurement of leukocyte vitamin C. A combination of both tests may be more reliable than either one alone.

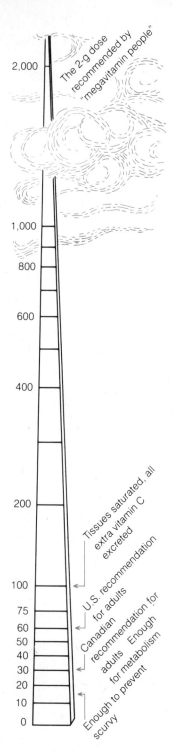

The 2-g dose recommended by "megavitamin people"

2,000

1,000

800

600

400

200

Tissues saturated, all extra vitamin C excreted

U.S. recommendation for adults

100

75
60
50
40
30
20
10
0

Canadian recommendation for adults

Enough for metabolism

Enough to prevent scurvy

Recommendations for vitamin C intake (mg).

capillary integrity: The gums bleed easily, and spontaneous breakage of capillaries under the skin produces pinpoint hemorrhages. If the vitamin levels continue to fall, the full set of symptoms of overt scurvy appears. Failure to promote normal collagen synthesis causes further hemorrhaging. Muscles, including the heart muscle, may degenerate. The skin becomes rough, brown, scaly, and dry. Wounds fail to heal because scar tissue will not form. Bone rebuilding is not maintained; the ends of the long bones become softened, malformed, and painful, and fractures appear. The teeth soften, and may become loose in the jawbone. Anemia is frequently seen, and infections are common. There are also characteristic psychological signs, including hysteria and depression. Sudden death is likely, perhaps because of massive bleeding into the joints and body cavities.

Once diagnosed, scurvy is readily reversed by giving vitamin C. It can be cured within about five days. Moderate doses in the neighborhood of 100 mg per day are all that are needed.[8]

Recommended Intakes of Vitamin C

How much vitamin C is enough? Allowances recommended by different nations vary from as low as 30 mg per day in Britain and Canada to 60 mg per day in the United States and 75 mg in Germany. The requirement—the amount needed to prevent the appearance of the overt deficiency symptoms of scurvy—is well known to be only 10 mg, but larger intakes raise the pool size. At about 60 mg per day the pool size becomes stable and does not respond to further increases. At an intake of 100 mg per day, 95 percent of the population probably reach the maximum pool size.[9]

It may seem strange that of the United States and Canada, two similar industrialized nations, one should recommend twice the vitamin C intake of the other. In view of the wide range of possible intakes, however, the Canadian and U.S. recommendations are not so far apart. Both are generously above the minimum requirement, and both are well below the level at which toxicity symptoms might appear. The range of possible intakes, illustrated in the margin from the perspective of people who espouse megadoses, shows that the Canadian and U.S. allowances are in the same ballpark. In contrast, the recommendation by Pauling and others that people should take 2 to 4 g a day (or even 10 g!) is clearly 'way up in the clouds.

It is important to remember that recommended allowances for vitamin C, like those for all the nutrients, are amounts intended to maintain health in healthy people, not to restore health in sick people.

[8]Hodges and Baker, 1973.

[9]A. Kallner, D. Hartmann, and D. Hornig, Steady-state turnover and body pool of ascorbic acid in man, *American Journal of Clinical Nutrition* 32 (1979):530-539.

Unusual circumstances may increase nutrient needs. In the case of vitamin C, a variety of stresses deplete the body pool and may make intakes higher than 50 or so mg desirable. Among the stresses known to increase vitamin C needs are infections; burns; extremely high or low temperatures; cigarette smoking; toxic levels of heavy metals such as lead, mercury, and cadmium; and the chronic use of certain medications, including aspirin, barbiturates, and oral contraceptives.[10] After a major operation (such as removal of a breast) or extensive burns, when a tremendous amount of scar tissue must form during healing, the amount needed may be as high as 1,000 mg (1 g) a day or even more.

Remember the distinction between the *requirement* and the recommended *allowance* or *standard* (see pp. 110-112).

Vitamin C Toxicity

The easy availability of vitamin C in pill form and the publication of Pauling's book recommending intakes of over 2 g a day have led thousands of people to take vitamin C megadoses. Not surprisingly, instances have surfaced of vitamin C causing harm.

Some of the suspected toxic effects of megadoses have not been confirmed for doses up to 3 g or more per day. Among these are formation of stones in the kidneys, upset of the body's acid-base balance, and destruction of vitamin B_{12} resulting in a deficiency. Research and reasoning have demonstrated that these effects are theoretically possible, but no cases of their actual occurrence in human beings have yet been seen.

When vitamin C is inactivated and degraded, a product along the way is oxalate. People sometimes have oxalate crystals in their kidneys that are not due to vitamin C overdoses.[11]

Other toxic effects, however, have been seen often enough to warrant concern. Nausea, abdominal cramps, and diarrhea are often reported. Several instances of interference with medical regimens are known. The large amounts of vitamin C excreted in the urine obscure the results of tests used to detect diabetes, giving a false positive result in some instances and a false negative result in others. Patients taking medications to prevent their blood from clotting may unwittingly abolish the effect of these medicines if they also take massive doses of vitamin C.

The anti-clotting agents with which vitamin C interferes are such anticoagulants as warfarin and dicoumarol.

People of certain genetic backgrounds are more likely to be harmed by vitamin C megadoses than others. Some black Americans, Sephardic Jews, Orientals, and certain other ethnic groups have an inherited enzyme deficiency that makes them susceptible to any strong reducing agent. Megadoses of vitamin C can make their red blood cells burst, causing hemolytic anemia. At least one person has died from this

[10]F. Clark, Drugs and vitamin deficiency, *Journal of Human Nutrition* 30 (1976):333-337; and Committee on Safety, Toxicity, and Misuse of Vitamins and Trace Minerals, National Nutrition Consortium, *Vitamin-Mineral Safety, Toxicity, and Misuse* (Chicago: The American Dietetic Association, 1978).

[11]*Vitamin-Mineral Safety*, 1978.

sequence of events. Those with the sickle-cell trait may also be more vulnerable to megadoses of vitamin C. In sickle-cell anemia, the hemoglobin protein is abnormal; it responds to a reducing agent by assuming a shape that distorts the red blood cells, making them clump, and clog capillaries. A case of this kind has also been reported. Those who have a tendency toward gout and those who have a genetic abnormality that alters the way they break down vitamin C to its excretion products are theoretically more prone to forming stones if they take megadoses of C, although no instances of either of these two events have yet been reported.

gout (gowt): a metabolic disease in which crystals of uric acid precipitate in the joints.

The proponents of vitamin C megadoses argue that these conditions are very rare and that the "normal" person need not worry about them. Opponents angrily retort that they are *not* rare and that nobody is "normal." The enzyme abnormality mentioned in the paragraph above is found in about 13 percent of black Americans and in a higher percentage of Sephardic Jews and Orientals.[12] If you have few acquaintances among these ethnic groups, then this condition may seem rare to you, but if you know more than ten such people, or if you are a member of any of these ethnic groups yourself, the risks of taking massive doses of vitamin C may apply directly to you or to one of your friends.

No two people have the same genetic heritage. Nobody has a complete set of "normal" genes and enzymes. No two people's nutritional needs—or risks—are exactly alike. There are doubtless some whose needs for vitamin C are much higher than the average, and there are also some for whom the risks of taking large doses are much more severe than they are for others. Perhaps the greatest risk in speculating about megadosing with C or any other nutrient is the risk of generalizing. What is safe for your friend may not be safe for you.

CAUTION WHEN YOU READ!

A statement that applies to nearly all people does not apply to all people.

[12]The risks of vitamin C overdosing for special genetic types are spelled out by V. Herbert, Facts and fictions about megavitamin therapy, *Journal of the Florida Medical Association* 66 (April 1979):475-481.

The body of a person who has taken large doses of vitamin C for a long time adjusts by destroying and excreting more of the vitamin than usual. If the person then suddenly reduces her intake to normal, the accelerated disposal system can't put on its brakes fast enough to avoid causing a deficiency: It destroys too much. Some case histories have shown that adults who discontinue megadosing develop scurvy on intakes that would protect a normal adult. They have developed a temporary vitamin C dependency. An innocent victim of this kind of error is the newborn baby of a megadoser. In his mother's womb he has adjusted to high levels of vitamin C; once born into an environment providing much smaller amounts, he develops scurvy.[13]

vitamin C dependency: a temporary condition manifested by the withdrawal symptoms experienced by the person who stops overdosing; the body has adjusted to a high intake and so "needs" a high intake until it can readjust.

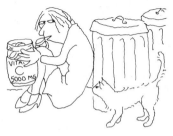

The experience of a person who stops megadosing and then experiences a vitamin C deficiency on a normal intake may lead him to the wrong conclusion. "I took 3 g a day," he may say, "and then when I stopped my gums started to bleed and I knew I was vitamin C-deficient. Don't you see, that proves that I need very high doses? The recommended 30 to 60 mg are not nearly enough for me."

In reality, this person has deceived himself. To see whether the recommended, moderate intake of vitamin C is sufficient, he will have to taper off, reducing his large intakes gradually and allowing his body to adjust back to the normal condition. The emergence of withdrawal symptoms from drug doses of vitamin C does not prove a need any more than the emergence of withdrawal symptoms in a person using heroin or alcohol proves that he needs heroin or alcohol. The addict's body appears to need the drug only because it has adapted in order to cope with the drug, not because the drug is an essential nutrient. In these cases, as in hundreds of others, the consequences of drug abuse cannot be used to justify continued drug use. And in these cases, as in hundreds of others, medical help may be needed to assist in withdrawal.

A pharmacological dose is higher than the intake needed to prevent deficiency symptoms and may have unexpected effects, as it may be working by a different mechanism than that by which the preventive or physiological dose works. See the discussion on pp. 467–468.

withdrawal reaction: a reaction to withdrawal (usually of a drug) that reveals that the user has become dependent, as for example when an infant born of a mother who took massive doses of vitamin C develops scurvy on an intake that would be adequate for the average infant, or when an infant born of an alcoholic mother suffers from the symptoms of withdrawal from alcohol (fetal alcohol syndrome).

After reviewing the published research on large doses of vitamin C, the National Nutrition Consortium reported in 1978 that there are probably very few instances in which taking more than 100 to 300 mg a day is beneficial. Adults may not be exposing themselves to very severe risks if they choose to dose themselves with 1 to 2 g a day, but above 2 g "genuine caution should be exercised," and amounts above 8 g per day may be "distinctly harmful. It is irresponsible and inexcusable to

[13]Two cases of this kind have been reported: *Vitamin-Mineral Safety*, 1978.

proclaim that ascorbic acid is safe in any amounts that may be ingested."[14]

In conclusion, the range of safe vitamin C intakes seems to be broad, as is typical for the other water-soluble vitamins. Between the absolute minimum of 10 mg a day and the reasonable maximum of 1,000 mg, nearly everyone should be able to find a suitable intake. People who venture outside these limits do so at their own risk.

Vitamin C in Fruits and Vegetables

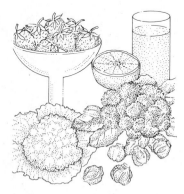

The inclusion of intelligently selected fruits and vegetables in the daily diet guarantees a generous intake of vitamin C. Even those who wish to ingest amounts well above the recommended 30 to 60 mg can easily meet their goals. If you drink a cup of orange juice at breakfast, choose a salad for lunch, and include a stalk of broccoli and a potato on your dinner plate, you will exceed 300 mg even before counting the contributions made by incidental other sources. Clearly, then, you would have no need for vitamin C pills unless you wanted to join the ranks of the megadosers.

Table 1 shows the vitamin C contents of 50 common foods and reveals that the citrus fruits are rightly famous for their C-rich nature. But certain vegetables and some other fruits are in the same league: broccoli, brussels sprouts, cantaloupe, and strawberries. A single serving of any of these provides more than 30 mg of the vitamin.

The humble potato is an important source of vitamin C in Western countries, not because a potato by itself meets the daily needs but because potatoes are such a popular staple and are eaten so frequently that overall they make substantial contributions. They provide about 20 percent of all the vitamin C in the U.S. diet. Some young men report french fries as their only regular source of vitamin C, and yet because they eat so many, they receive the recommended amounts.

Foods that contain vitamin C are sometimes classified as "excellent," "good," or "fair" sources. The "excellent" category includes several dark-green vegetables and sweet peppers, as well as some of the foods already mentioned. The "good" category includes cauliflower and several more varieties of greens. The "fair" group includes asparagus, green peas, lima beans, turnip, tomatoes, lettuce, and many other plant foods. You might want to skim the fruit and vegetable sections of Appendix H to see which of your favorite foods are the best vitamin C contributors. Some of the items may prove a pleasant surprise.

Vitamin C contents of individual foods vary widely, as a look at various types of oranges (Appendix H) will show. One factor influencing the amount of vitamin C found in a fruit or vegetable is the

staple: a food kept on hand at all times and used daily or almost daily in meal preparation.

[14]*Vitamin-Mineral Safety*, 1978.

Table 1.   Vitamin C Contents of 50 Common Foods*

Exchange group†	Food	Serving size‡	Vitamin C (mg)	Exchange group†	Food	Serving size‡	Vitamin C (mg)
2	Brussels sprouts	1/2 c	68	4	Winter squash	1/2 c	14
3	Strawberries	3/4 c	66	3	Pineapple	1/2 c	12
3	Orange	1	66	2	Spinach	1/2 c	12
3	Orange juice	1/2 c	60	2	Summer squash	1/2 c	11
2	Broccoli	1/2 c	52	4	French-fried potatoes	8	10
3	Grapefruit juice	1/2 c	48	2	Radishes	4	10
3	White grapefruit	1/2	44	4	Mashed potatoes	1/2 c	10
3	Pink grapefruit	1/2	44	3	Blueberries	1/2 c	10
2	Collard greens	1/2 c	44	4	Pumpkin	3/4 c	9
2	Mustard greens	1/2 c	34	2	Green beans	1/2 c	8
2	Cauliflower	1/2 c	33	4	Sweet potato	1/4 c	8
3	Cantaloupe	1/4	32§	4	Corn on cob	1 small	7
3	Tangerine	1	27	3	Pear	1	7
2	Cabbage	1/2 c	24	3	Peach	1	7
5M	Beef liver	3 oz	23	2	Onions	1/2 c	7
2	Cooked tomatoes	1/2 c	21	3	Pineapple juice	1/3 c	7
2	Tomato juice	1/2 c	20	3	Banana	1/2 med	6
2	Asparagus	1/2 c	19	4	Potato chips	15	5
4	Green peas	1/2 c	17	2	Beets	1/2 c	5
2	Turnips	1/2 c	17	2	Carrots	1/2 c	5
2	Dandelion greens	1/2 c	16	4	Corn	1/3 c	4
3	Raspberries	1/2 c	16	1	2% fat fortified milk	1 c	2
4	Potato	1 small	15	1	Skim milk	1 c	2
3	Blackberries	1/2 c	15	1	Whole milk	1 c	2
4	Lima beans	1/2 c	15	1	Yogurt	1 c	2

*These are not necessarily the best food sources but are selected to show a range of vitamin C contents. Note in the left-hand column the clustering of 2s and 3s at the top and 1s and 4s at the bottom. No grains appear among the 4s, and there is a marked lack of 5s (meats) and a total absence of 6s (fats).

†The numbers refer to the exchange lists: 1 is milk; 2, vegetables; 3, fruit; 4, bread; 5L, lean meat; 5M, medium-fat meat.

‡Serving sizes are the sizes listed in the exchange lists, except for meat.

§One serving of any of the foods to this point contains the Canadian standard of 30 mg vitamin C, equal to half the RDA for adults (60 mg).

amount of sun it is exposed to. The reason for this may be clear to you if you recall that the vitamin, being a hexose, is a member of the carbohydrate family and that carbohydrates are produced by photosynthesis. No vitamin C is found in seeds, only in growing plants. Thus grains (breads and cereals) contain negligible amounts of the vitamin. Milk is also a notoriously poor source, and this is why orange juice is added early to an infant's diet.

Hexose: see p. 26.

No animal foods other than the organ meats contain vitamin C. For this reason, if for no other, fruits and vegetables must be included in any diet to make it nutritionally adequate.

Protecting Vitamin C

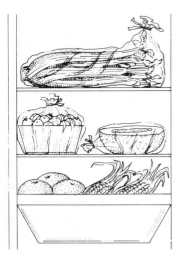

Vitamin C is an organic compound synthesized and broken down by enzymes found in the fruits and vegetables that contain it. Like all enzymes, these have a temperature optimum: They work best at temperatures at which the plants grow, normally about 70° F (25°C), which is also the room temperature in most homes. When a fruit has been picked, synthesizing activity (which has depended on a continued influx of energy from sunlight) largely stops; degradative activity, which releases energy, continues. Chilling the fruit slows down these processes. To maximize and protect vitamin C content, fruits and vegetables should be sun-ripened, chilled immediately after picking, and kept cold until they are used.

Because it is an acid and antioxidant, vitamin C is most stable in an acid solution, away from air. Citrus fruits, tomatoes, and many fruit beverages containing the vitamin are acid enough to favor its stability. As long as the skin is uncut or the can is unopened, the vitamin is protected from air. If you store a cut vegetable or fruit or an opened container of juice, you should cover it tightly with a wrapper that excludes air and store it in the refrigerator.

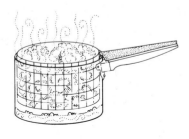

Being water-soluble, vitamin C readily dissolves into water that vegetables are washed or boiled in. If the water is discarded, the vitamin is poured down the drain with it. Cooking methods that minimize this kind of loss are steaming vegetables over water rather than in it or boiling them in a volume of water small enough to be reabsorbed into the vegetables by the time they are cooked. Of course, if the water soaks back into the food, as in making preserves or fruit pies, a larger volume of water can be used.

High temperatures and long cooking times should be avoided, to minimize the exposure of vitamin C to oxygen. Iron destroys vitamin C by catalyzing its oxidation, but perhaps the benefits of cooking with iron utensils outweigh this disadvantage (see Chapter 12). Another agent that destroys C is copper.

All of these factors represent legitimate concerns to which industrial food processors rightly pay attention. Awareness of them has brought about changes in many commercial products: fortification of instant mashed potatoes with vitamin C to replace that lost during processing, quick freezing of vegetables to minimize losses, and display of fresh produce in crushed-ice cases in grocery stores. Saving a small percentage of the vitamin C activity in foods can mean saving several hundred pounds of the vitamin a day; when some of it goes to people whose intakes are otherwise marginal, this can make a crucial difference.

Meanwhile, in your own kitchen, a law of diminishing returns operates. Vitamin C losses under reasonable conditions are not catastrophic. (For example, reconstituted orange juice typically retains 80 percent of its original vitamin C activity after eight days of storage.) You have other things to do besides hovering over your precious ascorbic acid, shielding it from all harm. If you turn the devil loose in your kitchen, as suggested in Chapter 9, you can indeed suffer undesirably high losses of this nutrient, but you can tolerate some losses if you make sure to start with plenty of foods containing ample amounts of vitamin C. To be on the side of the angels, perhaps all you need is a little common sense.

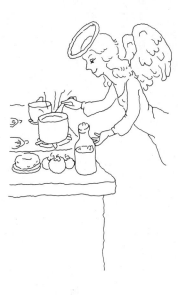

Summing Up

Vitamin C acts as an antioxidant in the body, helping to maintain iron in its reduced (ferrous ion) form and thus cooperating with enzymes that require this form of iron as a cofactor. The vitamin also helps regulate the overall oxidation-reduction state of the body cells and fluids, probably protecting vitamins A and E and the polyunsaturated fatty acids in this manner. In cooperation with iron it promotes the formation of the protein collagen, which is needed for scar tissue, intercellular cement, connective tissues (especially those of capillaries and other blood vessels), and the matrix of bones and teeth. It is involved in the metabolism of several amino acids, including the amino acid precursors of the hormones norepinephrine and thyroxin. It may also be involved in the absorption and utilization of folic acid and vitamin B_{12}, and it aids in the absorption of the mineral calcium.

Deficiency of vitamin C causes scurvy, characterized by bleeding from capillaries in the gums and under the skin, degeneration of muscles, failure of wounds to heal, malformations of bones and teeth, anemia, and ultimately death. Scurvy is prevented by the daily intake of only 10 mg of vitamin C and can be cured by a few days of 100-mg doses.

Recommended daily intakes of vitamin C range from 30 mg (Canada) to 60 mg (United States) or slightly higher (Germany). Stresses such as cigarette smoking or chronic aspirin use increase needs somewhat. Therapeutic doses used to aid recovery from scurvy, major operations, burns, or fractures range from 100 mg to not more than 1,000 mg (1 g). Toxic effects of megadoses (3 to 10 g) have been reported. The sudden discontinuance of megadoses may unveil an induced dependency, and scurvy may occur when intake is reduced to normal.

The best food sources of vitamin C are the citrus fruits, strawberries and cantaloupe, broccoli and other members of the cabbage family, and greens. Important "fair" sources include tomatoes, green peas, and (because they are eaten frequently by many people) potatoes. Preparation of foods to protect their vitamin C contents is best done away from air and alkaline solutions and without the use of large volumes of water. The inclusion of intelligently selected fruits and vegetables in the daily diet makes it easy to ingest well over 100 mg of vitamin C and unnecessary for healthy people to take any kind of vitamin C supplements.

To Explore Further

The American Dietetic Association has made available a cassette on vitamin C, Cassette-a-Month 7-78. The Association's address is in Appendix J.

A thoughtful and informative 1978 update on vitamin C appears in a publication by the National Nutrition Consortium, *Vitamin-Mineral Safety, Toxicity, and Misuse*. This also is available from the American Dietetic Association.

The entire September 1975 issue of the *Annals of the New York Academy of Sciences* (volume 258) was devoted to vitamin C; it contains 51 important articles reviewing recent research. Even the general reader might take this volume off the shelf and skim through it just to see how involved and extensive the work on this little vitamin really is.

Vitamin C: Rumors versus Research

When Dr. Linus Pauling published his book *Vitamin C and the Common Cold* in 1970, he started a storm of controversy that raged for a decade.[1] Newspaper headlines screamed VITAMIN C CURES COLDS; others yelled back VITAMIN C NO EFFECT. One "famous scientist" said this, another that. Meanwhile, behind the scenes, teams of researchers in laboratories and hospitals across the world went to work designing and executing experiments to determine whether in fact vitamin C has any therapeutic or preventive effect against the viruses that cause the myriad disorders collectively called the cold.

Since then some hundreds of articles have been published in the research journals, numbering several thousands of pages. Hundreds of people have been tested in a variety of experimental designs and still the answer is not completely clear.

The purpose of this Highlight is twofold. First, it is intended to make you aware of the difficulties inherent in attempting to discover whether a nutrient (or any therapeutic approach) remediates symptoms or cures a disease. The second purpose—because vitamin C may actu-

I have seen a paper with some writing on it strung round the neck heal such illness of the whole body and in a single night. I have seen a fever banished by pronouncing a few ceremonial words. But such remedies do not cure for long. We have to be on the watch. Illness can be fictitious, so also can cure. Human nature is perverse.

PLATO

ally be involved in some way with cures of colds and cancer—is to show you the kinds of research questions that will have to be answered before we can know what it does.

In most studies on the efficacy of vitamin C, two groups of people were selected. Only one group was given vitamin C; both were followed to determine whether the vitamin C group had fewer or less-severe colds than the control group. A number of pitfalls are inherent in an experiment of this kind; they must be avoided if the results are to be believed.

[1]L. C. Pauling, *Vitamin C and the Common Cold* (San Francisco: W. H. Freeman, 1970).

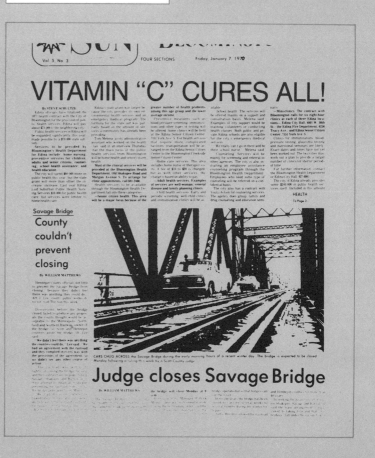

Controls First, the two groups must be similar in all respects except for vitamin C dosages. Most important, both must be equally susceptible to colds to rule out the possibility that an observed difference might have occurred anyway. (If group A gets twice as many colds as group B anyway, then the fact that group B received the vitamin proves nothing.) Also, in experiments involving a nutrient it is imperative that the diets of both groups be similar, especially with respect to that nutrient. (If those in group B were receiving less vitamin C from their diet, this fact might cancel the effects of the supplement.) Similarity of the experimental and control groups is one of the characteristics of a well-controlled experiment.

Sample Size To ensure that chance variation between the two groups does not influence the results, the groups must be large. (If one member of a group of five people catches a bad cold by chance, the whole group will have a spuriously high "cold severity," but if one member of a group of 500 catches a bad cold, it will not unduly affect the group average.) In reviewing the results of experiments of this kind, a question to ask is always, Was the number of people tested large enough to rule out chance variation? Statistical methods are useful for determining the significance of differences between groups of various sizes.

Placebos If a person takes vitamin C for a cold and believes it will cure him, his chances of recovery are greatly improved. The administration of any pill that the taker believes is medicine hastens recovery in about half of all cases.[2] This phenomenon, the effect of faith on healing, is known as the placebo effect. In experiments designed to find out whether vitamin C actually affects prevention of or recovery from colds, this mind-body effect must rigorously be ruled out.

To control for this effect, the experimenters must give pills to all participants, some containing vitamin C and others, of similar appearance and taste, containing an inert ingredient (placebos). All subjects must believe they are receiving the vitamin so that the effects of faith will work equally in both groups.

As the public has become more sophisticated and better acquainted with research designs of this kind, more and more people have learned about the use of placebos and have become suspicious when they are offered pills that purport to contain a certain substance. If it is not possible to convince all subjects that they are receiving vitamin C, then the extent of unbelief must be the same in both groups. An experiment conducted under these conditions is called blind.

Double Blind With all of these precautions, a further pitfall exists in experiments of this kind: The expectations of the experimenters can also influence the results. They too must not know which subjects are receiving the placebo and which are receiving the vitamin C. Being fallible human beings and having an emotional investment in a successful outcome, they tend to hear what they want to hear and so to interpret and record results with a bias in the expected direction. This is not dishonest but is an unconscious shifting of the experimenters' perception of reality to agree with their expectations. To avoid it, the pills given to the subjects must be coded by a third party, who does not reveal to the experimenters which subjects received which medication until all results have been recorded quantitatively.

[2]This finding is widely agreed on; it is discussed, among other places, in the debate on vitamin C in *Nutrition Today* (March/April 1978). See To Explore Further at the end of this Highlight.

In discussing all of these subtleties of experimental design, our intent is not to make a research scientist out of you but to show you what a far cry real scientific validity is from the experience of your neighbor Mary (sample size, one, no control group), who says she takes vitamin C when she feels a cold coming on and "it works every time." (She knows what she is taking, and she has faith in its efficacy.)

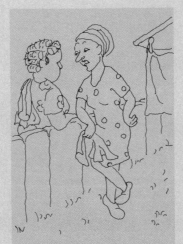

CAUTION WHEN YOU READ!

Before concluding that an experiment has shown that a nutrient cures a disease or alleviates a sympton, ask yourself:

Was there a control group similar in all important ways to the experimental group?

Was the sample size large enough to rule out chance variation?

Was a placebo effectively administered (blind)?

Was the experiment double blind?

These are a few but not all of the important variables involved in researching a "cure." With them in mind, let us review the literature to see how suc-

cessfully Dr. Pauling's vitamin C theory has stood the test of experimentation.

Reviewing the Evidence

Thomas C. Chalmers, a physician at Mount Sinai Medical Center, New York City, reviewed the data from 14 clinical trials of vitamin C in the treatment and prevention of the common cold in the April 1975 issue of the *American Journal of Medicine.*[3] Of the 14 clinical trials reviewed, 5 were poorly controlled, in Chalmers's judgment, and 8 were reasonably well controlled in that the subjects given vitamin C and those given placebos were randomly chosen. In addition, these 8 studies were double blind.

When the data from these 8 studies were pooled, there was a difference of 1/10 of a cold per year and an average difference in duration of 1/10 of a day per cold in those subjects taking vitamin C over those taking the placebo. In two studies, the effects of vitamin C seemed to be more striking in girls than in boys.

In one study, a questionnaire given at the conclusion revealed that a number of the subjects had correctly guessed the contents of their capsules. A reanalysis of the results showed that those who received the placebo *who thought they were receiving vitamin C* had fewer colds than the group receiving vitamin C *who thought they were receiving placebos!* In this study there were no differences in duration of colds among those who did not know which medication they were taking.

Other reviewers who have assembled and looked at all the evidence, as Chalmers did, have reached the same conclusions.[4] At the end of the 1970s, reports of additional experiments were still

[3]T. C. Chalmers, Effects of ascorbic acid on the common cold, *American Journal of Medicine* 58 (1975):532-536.

[4]An independent 1975 review that covered the same experiments and reached the same conclusions was M. H. M. Dykes and P. Meier, Ascorbic acid and the common cold: Evaluation of its efficacy and toxicity, *Journal of the American Medical Association* 231 (1975):1073-1079.

coming out, and most were consistent with previous findings. The balanced picture emerging from the reviews seems to indicate that the effects of the vitamin, if any, are small.

The writer of popular science articles rarely reports on these reviews of literature because they are cold, objective, and give many viewpoints, rarely stressing one. They are not, therefore, sensational enough to sell in the marketplace. Who wants to read a scholarly, conservative, textbooklike report in a newspaper? What usually appears in the newspaper or in the TV news is the report of one experiment that obtained a significant result. "Professor So-and-So of the Such-and-Such Lab at the Etcetera University," the commentator may say, "has found that vitamin C does make a difference after all, at least for little girls. In a double-blind, co-twin study, in which one of each pair of twins received vitamin C and the other a placebo, the youngest girls receiving vitamin C had significantly shorter and less severe illnesses than their twins. . . ."

If you chose to look up the source of this report, you would probably find that the study had been conducted as described and that this result had been obtained.[5] But the researchers themselves did not jump to the conclusion that vitamin C does make a difference. They pointed out very carefully that they had seen such a difference in *their* experiment, and in an admirable effort to put their finding in perspective, they went on to say: "One should be aware that, as the number of tests increases, the possibility of obtaining a 'significant' result by chance alone is also increased." In other words, the experiment would have to be repeated and the same result seen several times more before it could be accepted as real. The general public may be made uneasy by scientists who admit that their results are inconclusive, but the scientific community prefers total honesty to dogmatic statements.

The scientist who reports a "significant" finding from a single experiment is not being dishonest. Her purpose is simply to tell how she did it and what she saw, adding a piece to the total picture. To get the total picture, you must look at many experiments. Another kind of scientific reporting is useful for this purpose: reviews of literature, such as Chalmers's review referred to in this Highlight. These articles are just what their name implies—candid, objective reviews of all or nearly all of the experimental work on a theory that has been reported in the professional journals. The purpose of a review is to present a balanced picture of the research in an area. The reviewers are scientists first and writers second. They put their knowledge and skill to work in analyzing the various reports of research. They analyze the reports, then make judgments as to the validity of the data and of the conclusions drawn from the data. Sometimes they gather together several studies that have comparable designs in order to pool the data to form a larger sample. Their work makes a valuable contribution because it compiles the critical points from a number of reports, allowing the busy person to gain an overview of what is being written on a subject. Probably the

[5] J. Z. Miller, W. E. Nance, J. A. Norton, R. L. Wolen, R. S. Griffith, and R. J. Rose, Therapeutic effect of vitamin C: A co-twin control study, *Journal of the American Medical Association* 237 (1977):248-251.

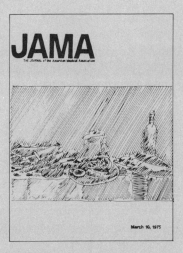

Journals

Reports of single experiments are presented in journals like the *Journal of the American Medical Association*.

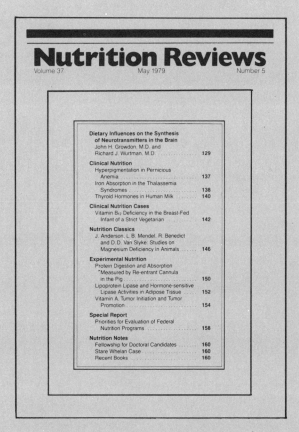

Reviews

To find a critique of all the important work on a subject, you can turn to a journal of reviews like the one shown here. One major review appears in *Nutrition Reviews* every month. It is followed by a bibliography that provides references to all of the original work reviewed.

Index

You can look up a large number of experiments on a single topic in an index of abstracts. The part of a page shown here, from *Biological Abstracts*, lists all recently published titles containing the word *vitamin C* and gives each one a reference number. The number refers to a short summary of the reported work, which also tells exactly where it was published. The indexes will lead you to reports of experiments in many different journals. New volumes of *Biological Abstracts* come out semimonthly. *Nutrition Abstracts and Reviews*, a monthly publication, would also contain titles including the word *vitamin C*.

Subject Context	▼ Keyword	Ref. No.
HABILITY/ INFLUENCE OF	VITAMIN B-6 UPON REPRODUCTION AND	50647
VITAMIN B-1 VITAMIN B-2	B-6 VITAMIN A VITAMIN C VITA	18486
AGNESIUM COPPER ZINC	B-6 VITAMIN A VITAMIN C	69163
ASTIC-DRUG VITAMIN B-1	B-6 VITAMIN B-12 DIAGNOSIS L	23040
E CHANGES VITAMIN B-1	B-6 VITAMIN B-12 METABOLIC-D	49852
M VITAMIN A VITAMIN B-1	B-6 VITAMIN B-12 VITAMIN C P	7317
ITAMIN K FOLACIN NIACIN	B-6 VITAMIN B-12 VITAMIN C P	24026
VITAMIN B-1 VITAMIN B-2	B-6 VITAMIN B-12 VITAMIN C/	24030
VITAMIN B-1 VITAMIN B-2	B-6 VITAMIN C VITAMIN P EPIN	43638
E METABOLIC-DRUG ANTI	B-6 4 AMINO BUTYRATE 2 OXO	62889
ROL BILE ACID VITAMIN C	B-6/ EFFECT OF THE ALIMENTAR	42968
LORIDE IN RAT JEJUNUM	B-6/ IN-VIVO ABSORPTION AND	7806
BROMINE THEOPHYLLINE	BIOGENIC AMINE PSYCHOTROPIC	75520
UCTIVITY IN COWS GRASS	BUTTER FAT/ EFFECT OF A MICR	51809
SYNERGISTIC EFFECT OF	C AND ASPIRIN ON GASTRIC LES	12698
ENTATION OF DIETS WITH	C AND ASPIRIN TO IMPROVE THE	57020
T FOOD/ NITRATE NITRITE	C AND IN-VITRO MET HEMO GLO	25613
TH ON PECTIN ESTERASE	C AND PROTEIN CONTENTS OF T	63379
ATURAL COMPOUNDS OF	C AND THE POSSIBILITY OF ITS	71403
NTENTS OF DRY MATTER	C AND VITAMIN B-1 THERMOLABI	8724
M/ INHIBITING EFFECT OF	C AND VITAMIN B-12 ON THE MI	62091
PONSE TO A MIXTURE OF	C AND VITAMIN E AND CHOLINE	69403
LOVECH BULGARIA WITH	C AND VITAMIN P BY THE METH	57246
IN B-2 VITAMIN D-3 AND	C BY DENSITOMETRY OF THIN LA	24199
RATE CALCIUM THIAMINE	C CALORIC VALUE/ NUTRIENT C	53439
FLAVINE PYRIDOXINE AND	C CHILD VITAMIN K VITAMIN D	43033
RMONE DRUG VITAMIN A	C COENZYME Q-10 ZYMOSAN P	4081
TION ON VITAMIN A AND	C CONTENT OF WHEY SOY DRIN	30295
NEY HYDROXY PROLINE/	C DEFICIENCY IN GUINEA-PIGS	62414
YPER CHOLESTEROLEMIA	C DEFICIENCY/ FUNCTION OF VI	68530
SED CONDITIONS HUMAN	C DEFICIENT GUINEA-PIGS INFL	32645
ISEASE CZECHOSLOVAKIA	C DRY MATTER SPECIFIC GRAVIT	22052

Figure 1   Sources of reliable nutrition information.

section of a review of literature that students most appreciate is the list of references. Without having to research the indexes on a topic, they can find a large number of references (perhaps as many as 50 or 60) listed in one place and in addition may read a critique of each (see Figure 1).

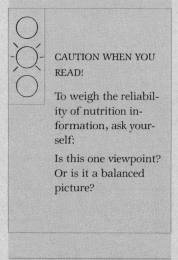

CAUTION WHEN YOU READ!

To weigh the reliability of nutrition information, ask yourself:

Is this one viewpoint? Or is it a balanced picture?

The reviews and experiments on vitamin C and the cold have provided one answer that still has to be cautiously phrased: The statistical effect of vitamin C on colds in the kinds of populations studied has been small. The questions that remain are important, and they haven't been answered. They have to do with individual differences in need, with the recommended intakes of vitamin C, and with the risks of overdoses.

Individual Differences in Need   The populations studied and reported on have mostly been people under normal amounts of stress whose intakes of vitamin C from their diets were generous to begin with—around 50 to 150 mg per day. It is safe to say that larger doses of vitamin C have little effect on the incidence or severity of colds in most such people under these conditions. But we still do not know what protective effect the vitamin might have in people whose vitamin C intakes are lower to begin with—or in people under extraordinary stress. Chapter 10 named some stresses—including extremes of temperature, medications, toxins, burns, and others— that increase vitamin C needs. Stress is hard to measure, and little research relating degrees of stress to needs for added vitamin C has been reported. Nor do we know very much about individual people's responses to stress: What may induce a violent stress reaction in one person may evoke a much milder reaction in another. Consequently, vitamin C needs might become much more varied in people under stress, and some might be quite high.

Recommended Intakes of Vitamin C   The problem of individual differences in the need for vitamin C has made it difficult for authorities to reach agreement on the levels

at which recommended intakes should be set. The problem of possible differences in people's stress reactions, which would increase their needs, makes it even more difficult. The present Canadian and U.S. recommendations, 30 and 60 mg per day, respectively, are well above the levels needed to prevent scurvy but shy of the level at which 95 percent of the population would show evidence of tissue saturation by excreting all added vitamin C in their urine (100 mg per day). And at 100 mg per day, 1 out of every 20 people would still not have arrived at "tissue saturation," even without the added complication of stress. No one knows whether tissue saturation is the ideal to aim for or whether this level is undesirably high—but if it is a desirable state, then some normal, healthy U.S. and Canadian adults might be advised to exceed 100 mg per day. No wonder the committees charged with publishing recommended intakes for nutrients debate long and hard over vitamin C.[6]

Risks of Overdoses   It is impossible to tell which individuals might have the highest needs for vitamin C just

[6]The long-awaited "1978 RDA" were not completed until 1979 and did not come out until 1980, partly because of the prolonged debate over vitamin C.

by looking at them; they would all have to be tested. At present, the only test that seems reasonable is a test to determine the level of intake at which the tissues are saturated and added vitamin C spills into the urine. But this is an expensive and difficult procedure, and once results have been obtained, their meaning is unclear (what does tissue saturation reflect?). In view of all the uncertainties, some people may decide to exceed the recommended intakes, "just to be on the safe side." Then the question arises, How much is safe?

The risks of overdoses are briefly discussed in Chapter 10, and aside from those mentioned there, no serious harm seems to result in many cases from intakes as high as 4,000 mg (4 g) a day, and possibly higher. In other words, the safe range for vitamin C seems to be very broad, in contrast to such vitamins as A, D, and K and many of the minerals. No one choosing to dose himself at this level has any guarantee, however, that his own body would not react adversely. There is probably as great a variety in different people's tolerance to megadoses as there is in their minimum needs. Later we may find that serious harm is caused by megadoses and that in the 1970s we hadn't discovered it yet because we hadn't known where to look.

One of the chief arguments

Mini-Glossary

placebo (pla-SEE-bo): an inert, harmless medication given to provide comfort and hope.

placebo effect: the healing effect that faith in medicine, even inert medicine, often has.

In any experiment in which a variable (see p. 51) is being tested, one group of subjects must be studied for the effect of that variable while a second group is followed—the **control group,** which is similar in all respects to the first except for that variable.

A **blind** experiment is one in which the subjects do not know whether they are members of the experimental or the control group.

A **double blind** experiment is one in which neither the subjects nor those conducting the experiment know which subjects are members of the experimental group and which are serving as control subjects, until after the experiment is over.

Repeating an experiment and getting the same results is called **replication.** The skeptical scientist, on hearing of a new, exciting finding will ask, "Has it been replicated yet?"

If it hasn't, he will withhold judgment regarding its validity.

indexes: books in which the articles published in journals are indexed by author, title, or topic (see Figure 1).

The white blood cells referred to here are the **leukocytes** (LOO-ka-sites). Their anti-infective activity is phagocytosis.

leukos = white
kytos = cell

phagocytosis (FAG-oh-sigh-TOE-sis): the engulfing of large particles by a cell.

phagein = to eat
osis = intensive

anecdote: story of a single episode; a joke.

testimonial: a statement of appreciation.

A quack may sometimes refer to his anecdotes as "case histories," but a true **case history** is a well-documented study of a single patient's case, reported in a reliable medical or scientific journal. Examples of true case histories are cited in Chapter 10.

---

for taking large doses of vitamin C is that most animals synthesize their own in large quantities. In fact, almost the only animal useful for laboratory studies on this vitamin is the guinea pig, because it is almost the only animal other than humans that needs the vitamin in its diet. We—and guinea pigs—need the vitamin from food because at some time in our evolutionary history we lost (stopped inheriting) the genes that enabled us to produce the enzymes to synthesize the vitamin. Dr. Pauling argues that our ancestors, 25 million years ago, ingested large quantities of vitamin C with their fruit-and-vegetable diet and that they became deficient in it when they shifted to meat. His argument is logical, but it is only logic. It needs testing.

Dr. Pauling seldom mentions the common cold any more but still believes that vitamin C has antiviral and antibacterial activity and enhances the anti-infective activity of the white blood cells. This notion has been tested in several ways, however, and doses of 2 g per day were found to *impair* the activity of white blood cells.[7] Pauling also suggests that vitamin C megadoses protect against and cure cancer and tells of personal experiences to back up this notion. He suggests that vitamin C may cure cancer by stimulating collagen-containing connective tissue to wrap the cancer and keep it from spreading. Again, this idea is plausible—but not yet tested.

In a lecture we heard in late 1979, Dr. Pauling told several stories of extraordinary cancer cures that seemed to result from megadoses of vitamin C.[8] He wasn't lying; he was reporting and attempting to account for what he had seen—some interesting individual cases. His theories about them may all be proved correct in time. The great usefulness of his theories is that they can be tested, and valuable research will emerge from his brilliant ideas. Meanwhile—and this is unfortunate—Dr. Pauling's stories of dramatic cures must be classed with all other such stories as mere anecdotes and testimonials.

One of the easily recognized marks of a quack is that he supports his claims with testimonials and "case histories" rather than with scientifically derived evidence and then tries to sell you something he has "proved" you need. Dr. Pauling has few of the marks of a quack. When he was designing and executing the brilliantly conceived experiments that revealed the structure of proteins, he was one of our most outstanding scientists. His findings have become the foundation of much fruitful research into protein structure and function, and they won him the Nobel Prize in 1954. But his new ideas on vitamin C have not yet been phrased into experimental designs that will yield such solid findings. Until they are, his testimonials and case histories are in the same class with any other story you might hear from your neighbor over the backyard fence.

A FLAG SIGN OF A SPURIOUS CLAIM IS:

The quoting of "evidence" that consists only of testimonials and anecdotes.

The special involvement of vitamin C in dramatic cures—if it exists at all—cannot be explained by a theory until the theory has been proved by testing. Until then, any theory is equally reasonable. Cancer is stressful, and a high dose of vitamin C might relieve a deficiency caused by the stress, facilitating more efficient use of the body's resources in fighting the disease. Anxiety is also stressful, and cancer

[7]Vitamin C and phagocyte function, *Nutrition Reviews* 36 (June 1978):183-185.

[8]L. C. Pauling, lecture at Florida State University, Tallahassee, Florida, October 26, 1979.

causes great anxiety. The placebo effect of vitamin C in relieving anxiety might greatly reduce the stress level, thus affecting recovery very indirectly. Controlled, careful, meticulously designed and executed experiments are urgently needed to reveal the mode of action, if any, of vitamin C in relation to cancer.

Is Dr. Pauling wrong to present his ideas to the world? No one is wrong who presents a theory as a theory only. Even if it is proved wrong, it will have value in stimulating research from which new knowledge comes. Out of the vast research that is taking place in an attempt to discover the modes of action of vitamin C will eventually come better understanding, and we will all be indebted to Pauling for his vigorous expression of his ideas. In the meantime, the best evidence seems to be that vitamin C may have an important impact on many stressful conditions not yet understood but that in doses as great as 2 g and more, there may also be risks as yet unknown.

To Explore Further

Wilson, C. W. M., and Loh, H. S., Common cold and vitamin C, *Lancet* 1 (1973):638-641 is the report of a 1973 study that took place in four boarding schools in Dublin in 1967-1968. The con-

clusion was that vitamin C significantly reduced the severity and total intensity of colds in girls but did not benefit cold symptoms in boys.

For the study reported in Karlowski, T. R., Chalmers, T. C., Frendel, L. D., Kapikian, A. Z., Lewis, T. L., and Lynch, J. M., Ascorbic acid for the common cold: A prophylactic and therapeutic trial, *Journal of the American Medical Association* 231 (1975):1038-1042, the National Institutes of Health supplied 311 employees. The conclusion was that vitamin C had at best only a minor influence on the duration and severity of colds and that the demonstrated effects might be explained equally well by a break in the double blind of the experiments.

The study reported in Coulehan, J. L., Eberhard, S., Kapner, L., Taylor, F., Rogers, K., and Garvy, P., Vitamin C and acute illness in Navajo schoolchildren, *New England Journal of Medicine* 295 (1976):973-977 involved 868 subjects and showed no preventive or curative effect of vitamin C.

This 1979 study involving 674 Marine recruits also showed no effect: Pitt, H. A., and Costrini, A. M., Vitamin C prophylaxis in Marine recruits, *Journal of the American Medical Association* 241 (1979):908-914.

Most of the March/April 1978 issue of *Nutrition Today* was devoted to a lively debate between Dr. Pauling and several prominent nutrition authorities. The debate brings out the major issues surrounding Pauling's new ideas about vitamin C and the differences in attitude among

people attempting to assess the validity of his theories.

The most famous and fascinating story about vitamin C is the story of how Norman Cousins, the *Saturday Review* editor, recovered from a supposedly incurable disease. Cousins researched some of the medical literature, decided that vitamin C would cure him, removed himself from the hospital, and got well with the help of vitamin C megadoses and laughter. His account of the experience is intriguing and thought-provoking, telling how the patient's attitude, relief from stress, and faith affect healing. Highly recommended:

Cousins, N., Anatomy of an illness (as perceived by the patient), *Nutrition Today*, May/June 1977, pp. 22-28; reprinted from the *New England Journal of Medicine*.

The sequel, which explores further the attitudes of doctors and patients and the importance of the patient's involvement in his own cure, is also stimulating reading:

Cousins, N., What I learned from 3,000 doctors, *Saturday Review*, February 18, 1978, pp. 12-16.

Vitamin C

Look up and record your recommended intake of vitamin C (from the RDA tables on the inside front cover or from the Canadian Dietary Standard in Appendix O). Also record your actual intake, from the average derived on Form 2 in the Self-Study at the end of the introduction to Part One (p. 16). What percentage of your recommended intake did you consume? Was this enough? What foods contribute the greatest amount of vitamin C to your diet? If you consumed more than the recommendation, was this too much? Why or why not? In what ways would you change your diet to improve it in this respect?

Optional Extras

● Find a substitute for fruit sources of vitamin C. Suppose a person dislikes fruits but likes vegetables. How much of a serving of greens would she have to consume daily to meet her recommended intake for vitamin C? How many servings of potatoes would meet the recommended intake?

Cabbage is a favorite vegetable of the Chinese. How much cabbage must a person eat to consume the recommended intake of vitamin C?

Mexicans eat citrus fruits infrequently but use chili peppers and tomatoes daily. Can they meet their vitamin C needs this way?

● Return to the health food store and ask about the virtues of vitamin C supplements. Jot down the claims and the evidence cited to substantiate them. Which claims are you inclined to believe? Which seem spurious?

CHAPTER 11

CONTENTS

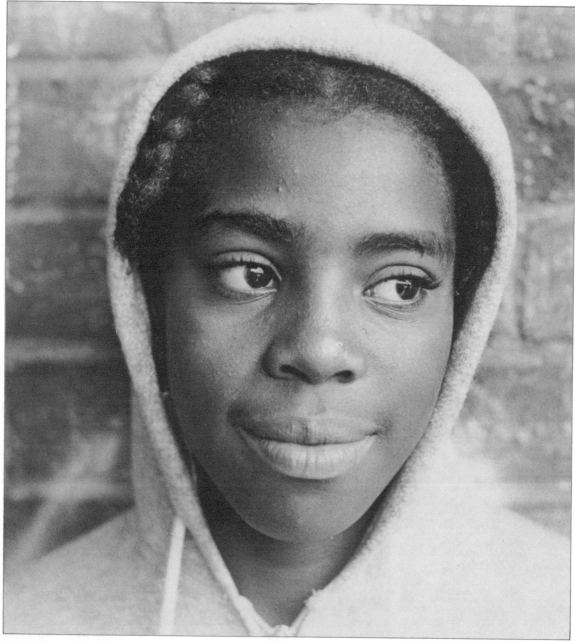

The health of the eyes depends on vitamin A.

THE FAT-SOLUBLE VITAMINS: A, D, E, and K

I remember well the time when the thought of the eye made me cold all over.

CHARLES DARWIN

Has it ever occurred to you how remarkable it is that you can see things? As an infant you were enchanted with the power this gave you. You closed your eyes and the world disappeared. You opened them and made everything come back again. Later you forgot the wonder of this phenomenon, but the fact remains: Your ability to see brings everything into being for you, more so than any of your other senses. Light reaching your eyes puts you in touch with things outside your body, from your friend sitting on the couch near you to stars in other galaxies.

Has it ever occurred to you how extraordinary it is that a child grows? From a mere nothing, a speck so tiny that it is invisible to the naked eye, each person develops into a full-size human being with arms and legs, teeth and fingernails, a beating heart and tingling nerves. Years go into the making of an adult human being, with each day bringing changes so gradual they seem undetectable. Only if you are absent during a part of this process do you notice it on your return and remark to a child, "My, how you've grown!"

And when did you last think about your breathing? In, out, in, out, day and night, year after year, you take in the oxygen you need and release it, disposing of the used-up carbons whose energy moves you and keeps you alive. The nutrients discussed in this chapter—vitamins A, D, E, and K—are vital for these and other processes that you may often take for granted.

The Roles of Vitamin A

Vitamin A has the distinction of being the first fat-soluble vitamin to be recognized. It may also be one of the most versatile, because of its role in several important body processes.

Vision   At the place where light hits the retina of the eye, profoundly informative communication occurs between the environment and the person. The eye receives the signal—light—and transforms it into informational signals that travel to the interior of the brain. There a

retina (RET-in-uh): the layer of light-sensitive cells lining the back of the inside of the eye; consists of rods and cones.

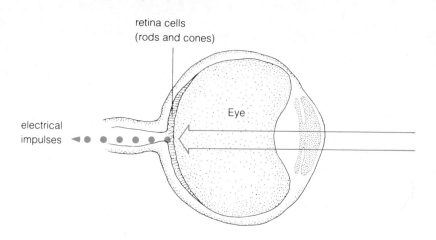

retina cells
(rods and cones)

Eye

electrical
impulses

pigment: a molecule capable of absorbing certain wavelengths of light, so that it reflects only those that we perceive as a certain color.

rhodopsin (ro-DOP-sin): the light-sensitive pigment of the rods in the retina.

iodopsin (eye-o-DOP-sin): the light-sensitive pigment of the cones in the retina. Both rhodopsin and iodopsin contain retinal; the proteins are different.

retinal (RET-in-al): an active form of vitamin A. For the structure of this and other forms, see Appendix C.

cones: the cells of the retina that respond to light by day.

rods: the cells of the retina that respond to light by night.

mental picture forms of what the light conveys. For this to happen, the eye performs a remarkable transformation of light energy into nerve impulses. The transformers are the molecules of pigment (rhodopsin, iodopsin, and others) in the cells of the retina.

Experts have written whole volumes about the eye, but it is not our intent to convey more than the briefest summary of the way its intricate machinery works. (A clear and accurate explanation is given in one of the references suggested at the end of this chapter.) From the standpoint of nutrition, what is important is to know that this extraordinary capability, like so many others already discussed, depends first on the perfect structures and functions of protein and other molecules, which are synthesized following instructions coded in the genes, and depends second on obtaining in the diet pieces of those molecules that the body cannot synthesize—the essential nutrients. The description that follows identifies the cells in the retina, which respond to light by day and by night; the pigments within those cells, which absorb the light; and the way they convert light into nerve impulses, which are interpreted in the brain as a picture. The punchline is that a portion of each pigment molecule is the compound retinal, a compound the body can synthesize only if vitamin A or its relatives are supplied by the diet.

A mechanical genius could not have designed such a system better. Light itself cannot be conducted through the solid material of the brain, so it is changed into signals transmitted by nerves. But light comes in different colors (wavelengths), which reveal a lot about the environment. To keep the colors sorted out, the eye uses different light-sensitive cells (cones) to receive them. Blue light is absorbed by one set of cells, green by another, and yellow-red by a third. By day, combinations of these give the full range of color vision. By night, the light entering the eye is of low intensity, and the set of cells (rods) that can receive this light are of one kind only, so that by night a person can normally discern only the presence of light but not its color.

What absorbs the light is the pigment molecules inside the cells. Each pigment molecule is composed of a protein called opsin bonded to a molecule of retinal. When a particle of light (a photon) enters the eye, it is absorbed into the retinal molecule, which responds by changing shape (it actually changes color too, becoming bleached). In its altered form retinal cannot remain bonded to opsin and so is released. This disturbs the shape of the opsin molecule.

This shape change is used to send a message saying, in effect, "Light has entered here." By a mechanism not completely understood, the cell membrane is disturbed by the pigment's change in shape and permits charged ions to enter and leave the cell. The cell hyperpolarizes (that is, the electrical charge across its membrane changes), and an electrical impulse is generated that travels along the cell's length. At the other end of the cell, the impulse is transmitted to a nerve cell, which conveys it deeper into the brain. Thus the message is sent.

Meanwhile, back in the retina and once again in the dark, the changed molecule of retinal is converted back to its original form and rejoined to opsin to regenerate the pigment rhodopsin. Many molecules of retinal are involved in this process. There are about 6 to 7 million cone cells and 100 million rod cells in the retina, and each cell contains about 30 million molecules of visual pigment. Repeated small losses incurred by visual activity, necessitate the constant replenishment of retinal or its precursors from the blood, which brings a new supply of these compounds from the body stores. Ultimately, vitamin A and its relatives in food are the source of all the retinal in the pigments of the eye.

Bright light seen at night destroys much more retinal than light seen by day, for three reasons. First, the pupil is wide-open at night, to allow as much light as possible to enter the eye. Second, there is an adaptation in the retina itself: A shadowing pigment protects the rods by day (they are not needed in bright light) but withdraws at night, leaving them exposed. Third, there are many more rods than cones. Hence if a bright light suddenly shines at night through the wide-open pupil onto the unprotected rods, much of the pigment in them is bleached and momentarily inactivated. More retinal than usual is freed, and more is lost. A moment passes before the pigments regenerate and sight returns. You no doubt have experienced this phenomenon when you were "blinded" by a flashlight shining directly into your eyes. People who must do a lot of night driving, facing headlights from oncoming cars, thus need an increased amount of vitamin A.

The eye is not designed for night driving or, in general, for accommodating itself to bright light at night. The mechanisms of vision evolved over millions of years, before humankind had harnessed electricity and lit up the night with headlights, beacons, and streetlights. In nature, animals in the wilderness have no need to adapt to sudden flashes of bright light at night, because they occur so seldom.

Vitamin A is undeniably an important nutrient, if for no other reason

opsin (OP-sin): the protein portion of the visual pigment molecule (rhodopsin) in the rods.

photon (FOE-ton): a particle of light energy. Depending on its wavelength, a photon conveys different colors of light.

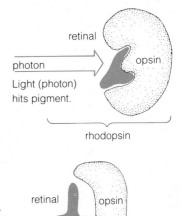

Retinal changes shape and is released from opsin. Opsin changes shape.

than that it plays a vital role in vision. But only one-thousandth of the vitamin A in the body is in the retina. It does other things as well.

mucosa (myoo-COH-suh): the membranes, composed of cells, that line the surfaces of body tissues.

urethra (you-REE-thruh): the tube through which urine from the bladder passes out of the body.

The cells on the surface are known as **epithelial** (ep-i-THEE-lee-ul) **cells.**

mucus (adjective **mucous**): a substance secreted by the epithelial cells of the mucosa; mucopolysaccharide (see also p. 160).

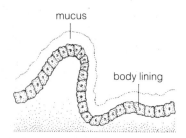

keratin (KAIR-uh-tin): a water-insoluble protein; the normal protein of hair and nails. Keratin may be produced under abnormal conditions by cells that normally produce mucus.

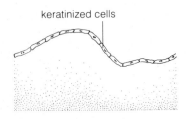

Body lining in vitamin A deficiency.

Maintenance of Linings Fortunately for you, your mucosa are all intact. You may not properly appreciate what these membranes do for you, but consider how important it is that each of these surfaces should be smooth: the linings of the mouth, stomach, and intestines; the linings of the lungs and the passages leading to them; the linings of the urinary bladder and urethra; the linings of the uterus and vagina; the linings of the eyelids and sinus passageways. The cells of all these surfaces—epithelial cells—secrete a smooth and slippery substance (mucus) that coats and protects them from invasive microorganisms and other harmful particles. The mucous lining of the stomach also shields its cells from digestion by the gastric juices. In the upper part of the lungs, these cells also possess little whiplike hairs (cilia), which continuously sweep the coating of mucus up and out, so that any foreign particles that chance to get in are carried up and away by the flow. (When you clear your throat and swallow, you are excreting this waste by way of your digestive tract.) In the vagina, similar cells sweep the mucus down and out. During an infection in any of these locations, these surface cells secrete more mucus and become more active, so that a noticeable discharge occurs; when you cough it up, blow your nose, or wash it away, you help to rid your body of the infective agent.

Vitamin A plays a role in maintaining the integrity of all these membranes. When vitamin A is not present, the cells cannot produce the carbohydrate normally found in mucus and produce a protein called keratin instead. As you might predict, greater losses of vitamin A occur during infection than under normal conditions.

The mucous membranes line an area within the body larger than a quarter of a football field, so this function of vitamin A accounts for most of the body's vitamin A need. And as if this weren't enough, vitamin A is also essential for healthy skin, another one or two square meters of body surface. Thus all surfaces, both inside and out, are maintained with the help of vitamin A.

Besides its roles in vision and in the maintenance of internal and external linings, vitamin A has an important part to play during growth.

Bone Growth "Growth is when everything gets bigger all together" is the definition given by a five-year-old. Certainly that is how it looks from the outside. A baby's hands, feet, arms, legs, and internal organs are all baby-size; an adult's are all relatively larger. Actually, however, the organs and body parts all grow at different rates and experience growth spurts at different times. The brain, for instance, reaches 80 percent of its adult size by the time a child is two, but the testes are still baby-size when a male first enters his teens. Furthermore, they do not just "get bigger"; bones are a case in point.

To enlarge the interior of a brick fireplace, the first thing you have to do is remove some of the old bricks. Similarly, to make a bone larger requires remodeling, as the picture in the margin shows. To convert a small bone into a large bone, the bone-remodeling cells must "undo" some parts of the small bone as they go.

It is in the undoing that vitamin A is involved. Some of the cells involved in bone formation are packed with sacs of degradative enzymes that can take apart the structures of bone. With the help of vitamin A in a carefully controlled process, these cells release their enzymes, which gradually eat away at selected sites in the bone, removing the parts that are not needed as the bone grows longer. (A similar process occurs when a tadpole loses its tail and becomes a frog. As you know, the tail doesn't simply fall off; rather it is resorbed, "growing" shorter and shorter until it disappears. As a fetus you also had a tail and lost it, a process that depended on vitamin A.)

These sacs of degradative enzymes are **lysosomes** (LYE-so-zomes).

lyso = to break
soma = body

The cells are osteoclasts (see p. 399).

Vitamin A's role in promoting good night vision, the health of mucous membranes and skin, and the growth of bone are well known although still not completely understood. Others, less well understood, include roles it plays in reproduction, in maintaining the stability of cell membranes, in helping the adrenal gland to synthesize a hormone (corticosterone), in helping to ensure a normal output of thyroid hormone (thyroxin) from the thyroid gland, in helping to maintain nerve cell sheaths, in assisting in immune reactions, in helping to manufacture red blood cells, and many others. Vitamin A research still in progress is yielding many new answers to the questions of how this nutrient functions in the body

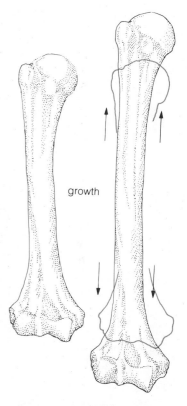

growth

Vitamin A Deficiency

Up to a year's supply of vitamin A may be stored in the body, 90 percent of it in the liver. If you stop eating good food sources of the vitamin, deficiency symptoms will not begin to appear until after your stores are depleted. Then, however, the consequences are profound and severe. Table 1 itemizes some of them. Some have to do with the role of vitamin A in vision, some with its functions in epithelial tissue, some with its part in growth; others are as yet unexplained.

As bone lengthens, vitamin A helps remove old bone.

Impaired Night Vision If sufficient retinal is not available (from the blood bathing the cells of the retina) to rapidly regenerate visual pigments bleached by light, then a flash of bright light at night will be followed by a prolonged spell of night blindness. This is one of the first detectable signs of vitamin A deficiency. Because night blindness is easy to test, it is a symptom that aids in diagnosis of the condition. (Of course it is only a symptom and may indicate some condition other than vitamin A deficiency.)

night blindness: slow recovery of vision after flashes of bright light at night; an early symptom of vitamin A deficiency.

Night blindness.

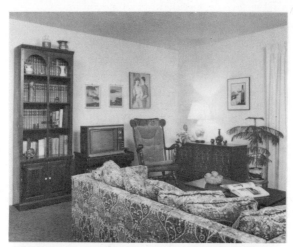

In bright light you can see all the details in this room.

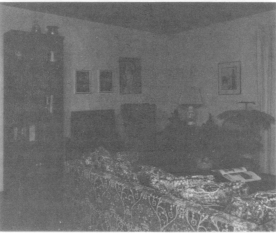

When the lights are turned out, you are momentarily blinded.

normal
night
vision

defective
night
vision

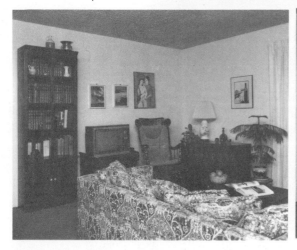

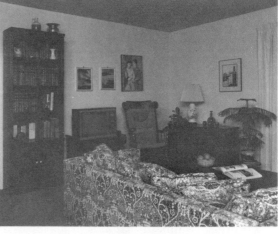

Then you recover your vision and can again see the details in the semidarkness.

A vitamin A deficiency makes this recovery of night vision impossible.

Table 1. Vitamin A Deficiency

Area affected	Main effect	Technical name for symptoms
Eye		
retina	night blindness	
membranes	failure to secrete mucopolysaccharide causes changes in epithelial tissue and hyperkeratinization	
general*	drying (mildest form) irreversible drying and degeneration of the cornea causing blindness (most severe)	**xerosis** **keratomalacia**
Skin	hair follicles plug with keratin forming white lumps	**hyperkeratosis**
GI tract	changes in lining; diarrhea	
Respiratory tract	changes in lining; infections	
Urogenital tract	changes in lining favor calcium deposition resulting in kidney stones, bladder disorders	
Bones	bone growth ceases; shapes of bones change	
Teeth	enamel-forming cells malfunction, teeth develop cracks and tend to decay; dentin-forming cells atrophy	
Nervous system	brain and spinal cord grow too fast for stunted skull and spine; injury to brain and nerves causes paralysis	
Blood	anemia, often masked by dehydration	

*The eye's symptoms of vitamin A deficiency are collectively known as xerophthalmia.

enamel: the hard mineral coating of the outside of the tooth, composed of calcium compounds embedded in a fine network of keratin fibers.

dentin: the softer material underlying the enamel of the tooth, composed of calcium compounds embedded in a network of collagen fibers.

For a picture of tooth structure, see p. 471.

Roughened Surfaces Instead of staying smooth and well-rounded and producing normal mucus, the epithelial cells flatten and harden with vitamin A deficiency, losing their protective mucous coating and filling with keratin instead. In the eye this process leads to drying and hardening of the cornea, which may progress to blindness. In the

The epithelial cells fill with keratin in a process known as **keratinization.** The progression of this condition to the extreme is **hyperkeratosis.**

hyper = too much

In the eye, the symptoms of vitamin A deficiency are collectively known as **xerophthalmia** (zer-off-THAL-mee-uh).

xero = dry
ophthalm = eye

An early sign is **xerosis** (drying of the cornea); the latest and most severe is **keratomalacia** (total blindness).

malacia = softening, weakening

cornea (KOR-nee-uh): the transparent membrane covering the outside of the front of the eye.

The accumulation of this hard material, keratin, around each hair follicle is **follicular hyperkeratosis.**

follicle (FOLL-i-cul): a group of cells in the skin from which a hair grows.

mouth, drying and hardening of the salivary glands makes them susceptible to infection; failure of mucous secretion in the mouth may lead to loss of appetite. Mucous secretion in the stomach and intestines is reduced, hindering normal digestion and absorption of nutrients, causing diarrhea, and so indirectly worsening the deficiency. Infections of the respiratory tract, the urinary tract, and the vagina are also made more likely by vitamin A deficiency. On the outer body surface, the cells also harden and flatten, making the skin dry, rough, scaly, and hard. Around each hair follicle an accumulation of hard material makes a lump.

Abnormal Growth   Because growth and development of the brain and eyes are most rapid in the unborn and in the very young baby, the effects of vitamin A deficiency are most severe in and around the time of birth. For example, in a child of one or two, abnormal growth of the skull may cause crowding of the brain (which is growing rapidly at that age). Tooth growth may also be abnormal. Crooked teeth in a child may reflect a vitamin A deficiency suffered by its mother while its jawbones were forming during her pregnancy. Damage to the eyes is also most pronounced in the young, with blindness the result in thousands of cases of vitamin A deficiency throughout the world. Vitamin A deficiency is second only to protein-kcalorie malnutrition as a nutritional problem afflicting the young of the world.

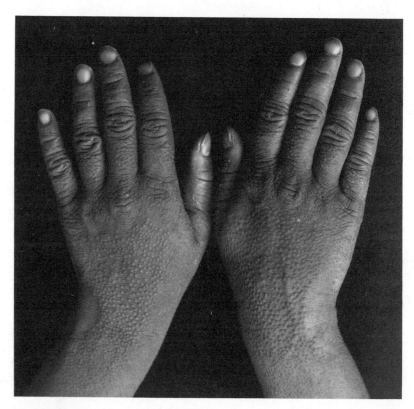

Follicular hyperkeratosis.
Photo courtesy of Parke-Davis & Company.

Naivete on the part of the well-intentioned can cause more harm than good, as is often observed when attempts are made to remedy the problem of malnutrition in the underdeveloped countries. An awareness of the way nutrients function in the body and of their interdependence must precede efforts to correct malnutrition problems as the case of vitamin A illustrates.

Vitamin A depends on proteins for its functions and transport in the body. In protein-kcalorie malnutrition, when vitamin A stores are also low, there is a balance of a kind. But when protein is given without supplemental vitamin A, protein carriers that may be synthesized deplete the liver of the last available stores of vitamin A, thus precipitating a deficiency.[1] Administration of protein has been observed to cause an epidemic of blindness, as when skim milk was offered by UNICEF to children in Brazil (in 1961). Vitamin A capsules were supplied with the milk, but the parents often ate the capsules or sold them, giving only the milk to the children.[2]

The mineral zinc is also needed for the body to use vitamin A properly. An apparent vitamin A deficiency may reflect an underlying zinc deficiency that must first be corrected.

> Knowledge of nutrition must accompany the giving of nutritional help.

In the United States as well, the problem of vitamin A deficiency is all too common. The Ten-State Survey revealed that a third of the children under six who were examined had less than the recommended vitamin A intakes.[3] Spanish-Americans and blacks exhibited the most pronounced evidence of deficiency. Some subgroups of the Canadian population are also deficient, notably Canadian and Eskimo women, especially during their pregnancies.

Results of surveys must be interpreted with caution: See Highlight 15.

A major source of vitamin A is the vegetable group, and a probable reason for widespread deficits of vitamin A in children is their refusal to eat these foods. A section of Chapter 15 emphasizes the importance of encouraging children to like vegetables and suggests practical ways to ease their acceptance.

[1] O. A. Roels and N. S. T. Lui, The vitamins, Section A: Vitamin A and carotene, in *Modern Nutrition in Health and Disease*, 5th ed., eds. R. S. Goodhart and M. E. Shils (Philadelphia: Lea and Febiger, 1973), pp. 142-157.

[2] O. A. Roels, Vitamin A physiology, *Journal of the American Medical Association* 214 (1970):1097-1102.

[3] U.S. Department of Health, Education, and Welfare, *Ten-State Nutrition Survey, 1968-1970*, publication no. (HSM) 72-8130 (Atlanta: Center for Disease Control, 1972).

Recommended Intakes of Vitamin A

Vitamin A terminology is in a period of transition. Vitamin A occurs in a number of different forms, and these convert to the active forms in the body with different efficiencies. Now that the chemistry and conversion rates of most of these compounds are known, it makes sense to state the recommended amounts of vitamin A and the amounts found in foods in terms of the total activity available from the various forms after they have been converted to the active form. The active form used for reference is retinol, and the recommended amounts of vitamin A are stated in terms of retinol equivalents (RE). As of 1980, both U.S. and Canadian authorities were using this terminology and were recommending 1,000 RE per day for adult men and 800 RE for women.

The amounts of vitamin A found in *foods*, however, are reported using an older system of measurement, international units (IU), which are based on some assumptions that are now known to be not completely correct. In the future, tables of food composition will report the vitamin A activity of foods in RE, but until they do, you will have to do some computing. If you wish to use a table like Appendix H or Table 3 in this chapter to compute your vitamin A intake, you will have to remember both terms, RE and IU, and the fact that 1 RE is roughly equivalent to 5 IU. Some additional guidelines for interpreting vitamin A measures given in IU are offered after the next section.

retinol: one of the active forms of vitamin A, similar to retinal. Retinol is an alcohol; retinal is an aldehyde (see pp. 351, 68, and Appendix C).

RE (retinol equivalent): a measure of vitamin A activity; the amount of retinol that a vitamin A compound will yield after conversion.

IU (international unit): a measure of vitamin A activity, determined by such biological methods as feeding a given compound to vitamin A-deprived animals and measuring the number of units of growth produced. IUs were used to measure vitamin A before chemical analysis of the vitamin A compounds and their precursors was possible.

1 RE ~ 5 IU. More accurately, 1 RE = 3.33 IU from animal foods or 10.0 IU from plant foods.

Vitamin A Toxicity

Vitamin A toxicity is not likely if you depend on foods for your nutrients, but if you take pills or supplements containing the vitamin, toxicity is a real possibility. Overdoses have serious effects on many of the same body systems that vitamin A helps when ingested in proper amounts (see Table 2). Children are most likely to be affected, because they need less, they are smaller and more sensitive to overdoses, and it is easy to make the mistake of giving them too much in pill form or in other concentrates. The availability of breakfast cereals, instant meals, fortified milk, and chewable candy-like vitamins each containing 100 percent of the recommended daily intake of vitamin A makes it possible for a well-meaning parent to provide several times the daily allowance of the vitamin to a child in a few hours. Serious toxicity is seen in small infants when they are given more than ten times the recommended amount every day for weeks at a time. A child herself may also overdose: Liking vitamin pills and thinking of them as candy, she may eat several.

There is a wide range of vitamin A intakes in which neither deficiency nor toxicity symptoms appear. Recommended intakes in both the United States and Canada are set at about double the minimum

Table 2.   Vitamin A Toxicity

Disease	Area affected	Main effects
Hypervitaminosis	bones	increased activity of osteoclasts causes decalcification, joint pain, fragility, stunted growth, thickening of long bones; pressure increases inside skull, mimicking brain tumor.
	blood	red blood cells lose hemoglobin and potassium; menstruation ceases; clotting time slows; bleeding is easily induced
	nervous system	loss of appetite, irritability, fatigue, restlessness, headache, nausea, vomiting, muscle weakness, interference with thyroxin
	GI tract	nausea, vomiting, abdominal pain, diarrhea, weight loss
	skin	dryness, itching, peeling, rashes, dry scaling lips, loss of hair, brittle nails
	liver	jaundice, enlargement
	spleen	enlargement
Hypercarotenemia	skin	yellow color

osteoclasts: the cells that destroy bone during its growth. Those that build bone are **osteoblasts.**

osteo = bone
clast = break
blast = build

jaundice: yellowing of the skin; a symptom of liver disease, in which bile and related pigments spill into the bloodstream.

necessary to prevent deficiency. Doubtless, many people need not consume amounts this high. The exact upper limit of safety can't be determined exactly, because people's tolerances to overdoses vary. Probably the amount of added vitamin A that anyone can tolerate depends on the length of time he takes it and on how much of the vitamin has already accumulated in his body stores before he begins to overdose.

In one case, only one month of daily doses of 10 times the recommended intake has been reported as having toxic effects,[4] but in others it may take 40 times the recommended intake for several months to elicit symptoms of toxicity.[5] The National Nutrition Consortium advises that adults should avoid daily intakes of more than 5 to 10 times the recommended amounts to ensure safety.[6] In general, it makes sense to get your vitamin A from natural, mostly plant, sources.

[4]S. J. Yaffe and L. J. Filer, Jr., American Academy of Pediatrics, Joint Committee Statement on Drugs and on Nutrition, The use and abuse of vitamin A, *Pediatrics* 48 (1971):655-656.

[5]D. R. Davis, Using vitamin A safely, *Osteopathic Medicine* 3 (October 1978):31-43.

[6]Committee on Safety, Toxicity, and Misuse of Vitamins and Trace Minerals, National Nutrition Consortium, *Vitamin-Mineral Safety, Toxicity, and Misuse* (Chicago: The American Dietetic Association, 1978).

Acne: see also zinc, pp. 469-470.

Adolescents should be warned that massive doses of vitamin A taken internally will have no beneficial effect on acne but may cause the miseries itemized in Table 2. The belief that vitamin A cures acne arises from the knowledge that it is needed for the health of the skin. As with all nutrients, however, the vitamin promotes health when enough is supplied; more than enough has no further beneficial effects.

However, a relative of vitamin A, vitamin A acid does sometimes help relieve the symptoms of acne when applied directly to the skin surface. The acid helps loosen the plugs that may accumulate in pores, allowing the skin to cleanse itself naturally. Such a treatment should of course be undertaken only on a doctor's recommendation.[7]

preformed vitamin A: vitamin A in its active form. See vitamin A (below).

precursor: a compound that can be converted into active vitamin A (see also p. 67).

beta-carotene: a vitamin A precursor found in plants (see provitamin A carotenoids, below).

vitamin A: the family of compounds found in animal foods, similar to and including retinol and retinal, which have high vitamin A activity.

provitamin A carotenoids: the family of compounds found in plant foods, similar to and including beta-carotene, which have less vitamin A activity and convert relatively inefficiently to vitamin A.

It is possible to suffer toxicity symptoms only when excess amounts of the preformed vitamin from animal foods or supplements are taken. The precursor, beta-carotene, which is available from plant foods, is not converted to vitamin A rapidly enough in the body to cause toxicity but is instead stored in fat depots as carotene. Being yellow in color, it may accumulate under the skin to such an extent that the overdoser actually turns yellow.

Vitamin A in Foods

Most of the vitamin A compounds found in animal foods have activities similar to that of retinol, and these are known as the vitamin A family. There is another family of compounds found in plant foods that have considerably less activity but can convert to active vitamin A with a low efficiency. For example, 6 μg of the plant pigment beta-carotene can convert to 1 μg of retinol in the body. The family of plant pigments similar to beta-carotene is known as the provitamin A carotenoids.[8]

[7]For further information on nutrition and acne, read Controversy 18: Acne, in E. M. N. Hamilton and E. N. Whitney, *Nutrition: Concepts and Controversies* (St. Paul: West, 1979), pp. 445-446.

[8]This terminology was agreed on by several nutrition, biochemistry, and medical societies and published in 1979: American Institute of Nutrition, Committee on Nomenclature, Nomenclature policy: Generic descriptors and trivial names for vitamins and related compounds, *Journal of Nutrition* 109 (1979):8-15.

In earlier years it was thought that the carotenoids had greater activity than we now know they have. (It was thought that about two units of carotene converted to one unit of vitamin A; now the ratio appears to be closer to six to one.[9]) The vitamin A "activity" listed in the food tables we still use today used the older, incorrect assumption. Thus the vitamin A contents of the *plant* foods shown in Appendix H and Table 3 of this chapter look bigger than they really are. If you seek to meet the recommended intake for vitamin A using plant foods, you might well aim high. Since the carotenoids are not toxic, there is probably no harm in daily intakes of about 15,000 IU for adults.

Table 3 shows the vitamin A contents of 50 common foods. If we could show you a color photograph of these foods, you would notice immediately that the top 15 items are all brightly colored—green, yellow, orange, and red. Any food with significant vitamin A activity must have some color, since the vitamin and its plant precursor carotene are colored compounds themselves (vitamin A is a very pale yellow; carotene is a rich, deep yellow, almost orange). The dark-green leafy vegetables contain abundant amounts of the green pigment chlorophyll, which masks the carotene in them. A skilled hostess or restauranteur knows that an attractive meal includes foods of different colors that complement one another but may not be aware that such a meal probably ensures a good supply of vitamin A as well.

On the other hand, food with a yellow or orange color does not invariably have vitamin A or carotene. Many of the compounds that give foods their colors, such as the yellow and red xanthophylls, are unrelated to vitamin A and have no nutritional value.

On the third hand (this chapter has three hands), if a food is white or colorless, it contains little or no vitamin A. Notice that many of the foods at the bottom of Table 3 are in this category.

About half of the vitamin A activity in foods consumed in the United States comes from fruits and vegetables, and half of this comes from the dark leafy greens (not iceberg lettuce or green beans) and the yellow or orange vegetables, such as yellow squash, carrots, and sweet potatotes. The other half comes from milk, cheese, butter and other dairy products, eggs, and meats. Since vitamin A is fat-soluble, it is lost when milk is skimmed. Skim milk is often fortified with 5,000 IU (the intake recommended for men) of vitamin A per quart to compensate.[10] The butter substitute, margerine, is usually fortified with 15,000 IU per pound.[11]

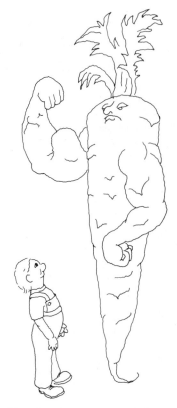

The vitamin A contents of plant foods may look greater than they really are.

chlorophyll: the green pigment of plants, which absorbs photons and transfers their energy to other molecules, initiating photosynthesis.

photosynthesis: the synthesis of carbohydrates by plants from carbon dioxide and water, using the sun's energy.

Fortified: see p. 443.

[9]Other reasons for considering the vitamin A activity of plant foods presently listed in tables to be an overstatement: The carotenoids other than beta-carotene are less than half as active; many are less well absorbed (perhaps only a third as well), and individual variability makes some of them still less well utilized by some individuals.

[10]In Canada, 1,500 IU per liter.

[11]Milks and margarines are also usually fortified with vitamin D.

Table 3. Vitamin A Contents of 50 Common Foods*

Ex-change group[†]	Food	Serving size[‡]	Vita-min A (IU)	Ex-change group[†]	Food	Serving size[‡]	Vita-min A (IU)
5M	Beef liver	3 oz	45,420	1	Yogurt (made with whole milk)	1 c	340
4	Pumpkin	3/4 c	10,943[§]	2	Green beans	1/2 c	340
2	Dandelion greens	1/2 c	10,530	4	Corn on cob	1 small	310
2	Carrots	1/2 c	7,610	3	Orange juice	1/2 c	275
2	Spinach	1/2 c	7,200	3	Orange	1	260
2	Collard greens	1/2 c	5,130°	6	Cream, light	2 tbsp	260
4	Winter squash	1/2 c	4,305	4	Lima beans	1/2 c	240
4	Sweet potatoes	1/4 c	4,250	6	Cream, heavy	1 tbsp	230
2	Mustard greens	1/2 c	4,060	4	Corn	1/3 c	230
3	Cantaloupe	1/4	3,270	1	2% fat fortified milk	1 c	200
2	Broccoli	1/2 c	2,363	5L	Sardines	3 oz	190
3	Dried apricots	4 halves	1,635	6	Soft margarine	1 tsp	156
3	Peach	1	1,320	3	Blackberries	1/2 c	145
2	Cooked tomatoes	1/2 c	1,085	3	Banana	1/2 med	115
2	Tomato juice	1/2 c	970	5M	Creamed cottage cheese	1/4 c	105
2	Asparagus	1/2 c	605	4	Corn muffin	1	100
5M	Egg	1	590	3	Raspberries	1/2 c	80
5L	Oysters	15, 3/4 c	555	5L	Chicken, meat only	3 oz	80
3	Pink grapefruit	1/2	540	4	Yellow grits	1/2 c	75
4	Green peas	1/2 c	430	4	Pancake	1	70
2	Summer squash	1/2 c	410	5L	Canned tuna	3 oz	70
2	Brussels sprouts	1/2 c	405	3	Blueberries	1/2 c	70
1	Canned evaporated milk	1/2 c	405	3	Strawberries	3/4 c	68
3	Tangerine	1	360	5L	Canned salmon	3 oz	60
1	Whole milk	1 c	350	3	Pineapple	1/2 c	50

*These are not necessarily the best food sources but are selected to show a range of vitamin A contents. Note how many 2s and 3s are at the top of the left-hand column and how many 5s are at the bottom.

[†]The numbers refer to the exchange lists: 1 is milk; 2, vegetables; 3, fruit; 4, bread; 5L, lean meat; 5M, medium-fat meat; 6, fats and oils.

[‡]Serving sizes are the sizes listed in the exchange lists, except for meat.

[§]Vitamin A activity reported in plants may be spuriously high. The actual amount of active vitamin A derived from plants depends on the body's conversion of the precursor, carotene, to the active vitamin.

°One serving of any of the first six foods contains the RDA (for an adult male) of 5,000 IU.

The safest and easiest way to meet your vitamin A needs, then, is to consume generous servings of a variety of dark-green, deep-orange, and other richly colored vegetables and fruits. A 1-c serving of carrots, sweet potatoes, or dark greens such as spinach would provide such liberal amounts of carotenoids that, even allowing for inefficient absorption and conversion, intake would be sufficient. Alternatively, a diet including more or larger servings of medium sources would ensure an ample intake. No doubt you can find food sources of the vitamin that appeal to you and can easily calculate the minimum amounts you should eat in order to meet your needs.

The fruit and vegetable family is one of the Four Food Groups. Its importance for meeting vitamin A needs is reflected in the recommendation that adults have at least four servings a day, including "at least one dark-green or deep-orange" item every other day.

Fast foods are notable for their *lack* of vitamin A.[12] Anyone who dines frequently on hamburgers, french fries, shakes, and the like is well advised to emphasize vegetables heavily at other meals.

One animal food notable for its vitamin A content is liver. A moment's reflection should reveal the reason for this: Vitamin A not needed for immediate use is stored in the liver.[13] Some nutritionists recommend that people include a serving of liver in their diets every week or two, partly for this reason. Because the vitamin A in liver is preformed, active vitamin A, an intake of 5,000 IU in this form is probably equivalent to an intake of at least 15,000 IU in plant carotenoids.

People sometimes wonder if vitamin A toxicity can result from using liver too frequently. This problem has never been observed except in the Arctic, where explorers who have eaten large quantities of polar bear liver have become ill with symptoms probably indicating vitamin A toxicity. Liver is an extremely nutritious food, and its periodic use is highly recommended.

Recall that one of the B vitamins—folacin—is found most abundantly in dark-green vegetables.

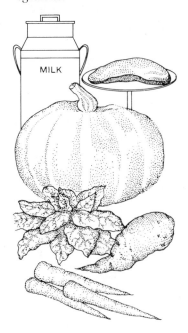

The Bone Vitamin: D

Vitamin A helps to remodel bones; vitamin D helps to grow them. Vitamin A is versatile and important in many body systems; vitamin D seems to play its part only in connection with the minerals of the bone system. That part is considerable, however, and vitamin D is indispensable to keep the system working during periods of bone growth or remodeling. Vitamin D is a member of a large and cooperative bone-making and maintenance team made up of nutrients and other compounds, including vitamins C and A; the hormones parathormone and calcitonin; the protein collagen, which precedes bone; and the minerals calcium, phosphorus, magnesium, fluoride, and others, of which the bone is finally composed.

Blood calcium is very active metabolically. It has been estimated that about a fourth of the calcium in the blood is exchanged with bone calcium every minute. The special function of vitamin D is to help make calcium and phosphorus available in the blood that bathes the bones so that they can be deposited there as the bones grow (harden or mineralize).

Parathormone and calcitonin: see p. 425.

Collagen: see p. 363.

mineralization (calcification): the process in which calcium, phosphorus, and other minerals crystallize on the collagen matrix of a growing bone, hardening the bone.

[12]C. P. Greecher and B. Shannon, Impact of fast food meals on nutrient intake of two groups, *Journal of the American Dietetic Association* 70 (1977):368-372.

[13]Liver is not the only organ that stores Vitamin A. The kidneys, adrenals, and other organs also perform this function, but liver is the only one that is usually eaten.

Vitamin D raises blood concentrations of these minerals in three ways: by stimulating their absorption from the gastrointestinal tract; by helping to withdraw calcium from bones into the blood; and by stimulating calcium retention by the kidneys. The star of this particular show is calcium itself; vitamin D is a supporting actor. A description of how calcium moves from food into the blood and into and out of bone is reserved for Chapter 12, where a closer view of the whole system is provided. The object here is to make you aware of the importance of vitamin D, the risks of deficiency and toxicity, and the ways in which it can be obtained from foods.

A note should be made here of one way this nutrient is unique: The body can synthesize its own vitamin D in the skin with the help of sunlight. In this sense vitamin D is not an essential nutrient. Given enough sun, you need consume no vitamin D at all in the foods you eat. Rather, it is like a hormone—a compound manufactured by one organ of the body that has effects on another.

The precursor of vitamin D made in the liver is 7-dehydro-cholesterol, which is made from cholesterol. This is one of the body's many "good" uses for cholesterol.

The liver manufactures a vitamin D precursor, which is released into the blood and circulates to the skin. When ultraviolet rays from the sun hit this compound, it is converted to previtamin D_3, which works its way back into the interior of the body. Slowly, then, over the next 36 hours, the previtamin is converted with the help of the body's heat to vitamin D_3. Two more steps occur before the vitamin becomes fully active: The liver adds an OH group and then the kidney adds another at specific locations to produce the active vitamin.[14]

The technical name for the final product, active vitamin D, is 1,25-dihydroxycholecalciferol—dihydroxy vitamin D for short.

There are thus two ways to meet your vitamin D needs: self-synthesis and consumption of foods containing the preformed vitamin—chiefly animal foods.[15]

Vitamin D Deficiency and Toxicity

Both inadequate and excessive vitamin D intakes take their toll in the United States, despite the fact that the vitamin has been known for decades to be essential for growth and toxic in excess. The Ten-State Survey revealed that nearly 4 percent of the children under six who were examined showed evidence of vitamin D deficiency, with several cases of overt rickets. The National Nutrition Survey in Canada revealed low intakes of vitamin D in women and children but no overt cases of rickets—although they may exist in persons not tested. Worldwide, rickets still afflicts large numbers of children.

Results of surveys must be interpreted with caution (see Highlight 15).

rickets: the vitamin D-deficiency disease in children.

A rare type of rickets, not caused by vitamin D deficiency is known as **vitamin D-refractory rickets.**

[14]The whole story is told by one of the principal investigators in this area, whose meticulous work has revealed many more details than are presented here. See DeLuca, 1979 in this chapter's To Explore Further.

[15]A plant version of vitamin D (ergosterol) may also yield an active compound, vitamin D_2 (calciferol), on irradiation, but less is known about the body's further use of this compound. Thus animal sources of vitamin D are considered the only reliable ones.

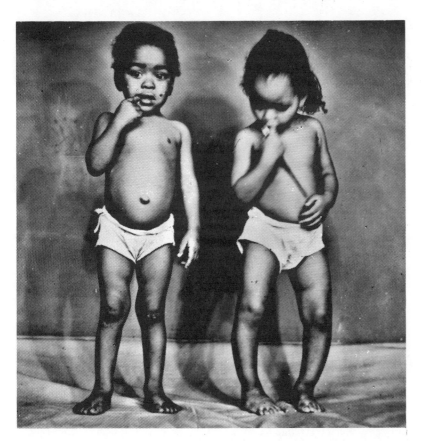

Rickets.

Photo courtesy of Parke-Davis & Company.

The symptoms of an inadequate intake of vitamin D are those of calcium deficiency, as shown in Table 4. The bones fail to calcify normally and may be so weak that they become bent when they have to support the body's weight. A child with rickets who is old enough to walk characteristically develops bowed legs, often the most obvious sign of the disease.

Adult rickets, or osteomalacia, occurs most often in women who have little exposure to sun and who go through repeated pregnancies and periods of lactation. The bones of the legs may soften to such an extent that a woman who was tall and straight before her first pregnancy becomes bent, bowlegged, and stooped after her second or third.

Vitamin D deficiency depresses calcium absorption and results in low blood calcium levels and abnormal mineralization of bone. An excess of the vitamin does the opposite, as shown in Table 5: It increases calcium absorption, causing abnormally high concentrations of the mineral in the blood, and promotes return of bone calcium into the blood as well. The excess calcium in the blood tends to precipitate in the soft tissues, forming stones. This is especially likely to happen in the

osteomalacia (os-tee-o-mal-AY-shuh): the vitamin D-deficiency disease in adults.

osteo = bone
mal = bad (soft)

Osteomalacia may also occur in calcium deficiency; see Chapter 12.

Bowing of the ribs causes the symptom known as **pigeon breast.** The beads that form on the ribs resemble rosary beads; thus this symptom is known as **rachitic** (ra-KIT-ik) **rosary** (the rosary of rickets).

fontanel: the open space in the top of a baby's skull before the skull bones have grown together.

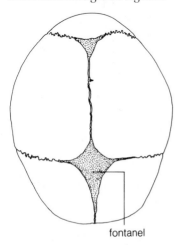

fontanel

thorax: the part of the body between the neck and the abdomen.

alkaline phosphatase: an enzyme in blood.

Table 4.   Vitamin D Deficiency

Disease	Area affected	Main effects
Rickets	bones	faulty calcification resulting in misshapen bones (bowing of legs) and retarded growth
		enlargment of ends of long bones (knock-knees)
		deformities of ribs (bowed, with beads or knobs)
		delayed closing of fontanel results in rapid enlargement of head
	blood	decreased calcium and/or phosphorus
	teeth	slow eruption; teeth not well-formed; tendency to decay
	muscles	lax muscles resulting in protrusion of abdomen
	excretory system	increased calcium in stools, decreased calcium in urine
	glandular system	abnormally high secretion of parathyroid hormone
Osteomalacia	bones	softening effect: deformities of limbs, spine, thorax, and pelvis; demineralization; pain in pelvis, lower back, and legs; bone fractures
	blood	decreased calcium and/or phosphorous, increased alkaline phosphatase
	muscles	involuntary twitching, muscle spasms

kidneys, which concentrate calcium in the effort to excrete it. Calcification or hardening of the blood vessels may also occur. This process is especially dangerous in the major arteries of the heart and lungs, where it can cause death.

The range of safe intakes of vitamin D is narrower than that of vitamin A. Half the recommended intake is too little, but over a few

Table 5.   Vitamin D Toxicity

Disease	Area affected	Main effects
Hypervitaminosis D	bones	increased calcium withdrawal
	blood	increased calcium and phosphorus concentration
	nervous system	loss of appetite, headache, excessive thirst, irritability
	excretory system	increased excretion of calcium in urine; kidney stones; irreversible renal damage
	tissues	calcification of soft tissues (blood vessels, kidneys, lungs), death

times the recommended intake may be too much. Intakes of 4,000 IU per day cause high blood calcium levels in infants, but some are sensitive to lower doses than this. Intakes of 10,000 IU per day for four months or 200,000 IU per day for two weeks cause toxicity in children and, if further prolonged, in adults. The amounts of vitamin D found in foods available in the United States and Canada are well within these limits, but pills containing the vitamin in concentrated form should definitely be kept out of the reach of children.

Vitamin D activity was previously expressed in international units (IU) but as of 1980 is expressed in micrograms of cholecalciferol. To convert, use the factor:

100 IU = 2.5 μg
400 IU = 10 μg.

Vitamin D from Sun and Foods

In rapidly growing children, an intake of close to 400 IU of vitamin D a day is recommended; mature adults need half as much. Only a few animal foods supply significant amounts of the vitamin, notably, eggs, liver, and some fish, and even these vary greatly, depending on the animal's exposure to sun and on its consumption of the vitamin in its foods. The fortification of milk with 400 IU per quart (360 IU per liter in Canada) is the best guarantee that children will meet their vitamin D needs and underscores the importance of milk in children's diets.

The RDA for vitamin D for adults over 22 is 5 μg cholecalciferol (200 IU).

Canadian Dietary Standard: 2.5 μg cholecalciferol.

   Significant amounts of vitamin D can be made with the help of sunlight. No exact measures have been made, but it is generally agreed that most adults, especially in the sunnier climates, need not make special efforts to obtain vitamin D in food. However, people of all ages need vitamin D; if you are not outdoors much or if you live in a northern or predominantly cloudy or smoggy area, you are advised to make sure your milk is fortified with vitamin D, to drink at least 2 c a day, and to make frequent use of eggs and periodic use of liver in menu planning.

Exposure to sun should be reasonable. Excessive exposure to sun may cause skin cancer.

Vitamin E

Antioxidant: see p. 364.

oxidant: a compound (such as oxygen itself) that oxidizes other compounds.

As we stated at the start, this book is intended to give you a sense of what to believe and what not to believe, presenting well-known and documented research in the chapters and reserving recent, speculative, and controversial material for the Highlights. Much of what is presently being said about vitamin E is too uncertain to have won the security of a textual presentation and so is addressed in Highlight 11. However, there is one role vitamin E plays—as an antioxidant—that is quite well understood.

Like vitamin C, vitamin E is readily oxidized. If there is plenty of vitamin E in a mixture of compounds exposed to an oxidant, chances are this vitamin will take the brunt of the oxidative attack, protecting the others. Because it is soluble in fat, vitamin E is found in fat-rich fluids and tissues of the body in association with the lipids of cell membranes and with the other fat-soluble vitamins. Because of this and its relative abundance in the diet, it is especially effective in preventing the oxidation of vitamin A and the polyunsaturated fatty acids. It also helps vitamin A to be absorbed.

Of 12 possible diseases associated with vitamin E deficiency in animals, only one has been demonstrated in human beings. When the blood concentration of vitamin E falls below a certain critical level, the red blood cells tend to break open and spill their contents, probably due to oxidation of the polyunsaturated fatty acids (PUFAs) in their membranes. (Cell membranes are rich in PUFAs, and those of the red blood cells in particular are exposed to high concentrations of oxygen because of their repeated circulation through the lungs.) In animals, this action tends to occur more readily if the diet is high in PUFAs, suggesting that it is indeed vitamin E's role in protecting PUFAs from oxidation that prevents the deficiency disease. A person's need for vitamin E may therefore depend on the amount of PUFAs consumed. Fortunately, vitamin E and the polyunsaturates tend to occur together in the same foods.

erythrocyte hemolysis (eh-REETH-ro-cite he-MOLL-uh-sis): the vitamin E-deficiency disease in human beings.

erythrocyte: red blood cell.

erythro = red
cyte = cell

hemolysis: bursting of red blood cells.

hemo = blood
lysis = breaking

Vitamin E is readily destroyed by heat processing and oxidation, so fresh or lightly processed foods are preferable as sources of this vitamin. The processed and convenience foods often used by the elderly and nursing homes may contribute to a vitamin E deficiency if their use continues over several years.[16]

Vitamin E is the only one of the fat-soluble vitamins for which toxicity symptoms are unknown in humans; even prolonged intakes of many times the recommended intake have few observable effects. Sensitive individuals may complain of nausea and intestinal discomfort, but the general impression seems to be that for most people intakes from pills of up to 300 IU per day are harmless—and useless.[17]

[16]H. H. Koehler, H. C. Lee, and M. Jacobson, Tocopherols in canned entrees and vended sandwiches, *Journal of the American Dietetic Association* 70 (1977):616-620.

[17]For more information on vitamin E myths and realities, read Controversy 20: Vitamin E, in E. M. N. Hamilton and E. N. Whitney, *Nutrition: Concepts and Controversies* (St. Paul: West, 1979), pp. 481-482.

About 60 percent of the vitamin E in the diet comes directly or indirectly from vegetable oils in the form of margarine, salad dressings, and shortenings; another 10 percent comes from fruits and vegetables; smaller percentages come from grains and other products. Soybean oil and wheat germ oil have especially high concentrations of E; cottonseed, corn, and safflower oils rank second, with a tablespoon of any of these supplying more than 15 mg of the vitamin. Other oils contain less (for example, peanut oil supplies about half as much per tablespoon). Animal fats such as butter and milk fat have negligible amounts of vitamin E.

The RDA for vitamin E for adults: 10 mg for men, 8 mg for women. Canadian Dietary Standard: 8-9 mg for men, 6 mg for women.

Vitamin E units: 1 mg = 1 IU.

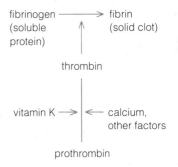

The clotting process

K stands for the Danish word *Koagulation* (coagulation or clotting).

Thrombin: see p. 136.

hemorrhagic (hem-o-RAJ-ik) **disease:** the vitamin K-deficiency disease.

hemophilia: a hereditary disease having no relation to vitamin K but caused by a genetic defect that renders the blood unable to clot because of lack of ability to synthesize certain clotting factors.

The bacterial inhabitants of the digestive tract are known as the **intestinal flora.**

flora = plant inhabitants

Provisional RDA for vitamin K (1980): 70-140 μg.

sterile: free of microorganisms, such as bacteria.

The synthetic substitute usually given for vitamin K is **menadione** (men-uh-DYE-own); see Appendix C.

The Blood-Clotting Vitamin: K

Like vitamin D, vitamin K seems to be limited in its versatility. But like D, its presence can make the difference between life and death. At least 13 different proteins and the mineral calcium are involved in making a blood clot, and vitamin K is essential for the synthesis of at least 4 of these proteins, among them the protein thrombin.

When any of these factors is lacking, blood cannot clot and hemorrhagic disease results; if an artery or vein is cut or broken under these circumstances, bleeding goes unchecked. (As usual, this is not to say that the cause of hemorrhaging is always vitamin K deficiency. Another cause is hemophilia, which is not curable by vitamin K.) Deficiency of vitamin K may occur under abnormal circumstances when absorption of fat is impaired (that is, when bile production is faulty or in diarrhea). The vitamin is sometimes administered preoperatively to reduce bleeding in surgery but is only of value at this time if a vitamin K deficiency exists. Toxicity can result when too much vitamin K is given, especially to an infant or to a pregnant woman.

Again, like vitamin D, vitamin K is made within your body—but not by you. In your intestinal tract there are billions of bacteria, which normally live in perfect harmony with you, doing their thing while you do yours. One of their "things" is synthesizing vitamin K that you can absorb. You are not dependent on bacterial synthesis for your K, however, since many foods also contain ample amounts of the vitamin, notably, green leafy vegetables, members of the cabbage family, and milk.

Brand new babies are commonly susceptible to a K deficiency, for two reasons. First, a baby is born with a sterile digestive tract; he has his first contact with intestinal bacteria as he passes down his mother's birth canal, and it takes the bacteria a day or so to establish themselves in the baby's intestines. Second, a baby may not be fed at the very outset (and breast milk is a poorer source of vitamin K than cow's milk). A dose of vitamin K (usually in a synthetic form similar but not identical to the natural vitamin) may therefore be given at birth to prevent hemorrhagic disease of the newborn; it must be administered carefully to avoid toxic overdosing. People taking sulfa drugs, which destroy intestinal bacteria, may also become deficient in vitamin K.

Putting It All Together

This chapter concludes the treatment of the vitamins. Another look at diet adequacy and balance is in order at this point. For the B vitamins, meat, milk, breads, cereals, and vegetables are good sources; for vitamin C, the fruits are important. With this consideration of the fat-soluble vitamins, the sixth group of foods in the exchange system, namely the fat group, assumes significance. The diagram that follows shows how the selection of foods from all six exchange groups ensures that each nutrient discussed so far will be consumed in the recommended amounts. The individual lines of the web may be of interest, but the main point of the figure is that it is a web: Different foods supply different assortments of nutrients, so that a wide and varied selection is the best guarantee of adequacy for all.

Note: Some vitamins known to be essential in human diets have not been studied sufficiently to permit setting recommended intakes. Food sources of these nutrients are less well known. However, the variety of

Food group

Supplies substantial amounts of

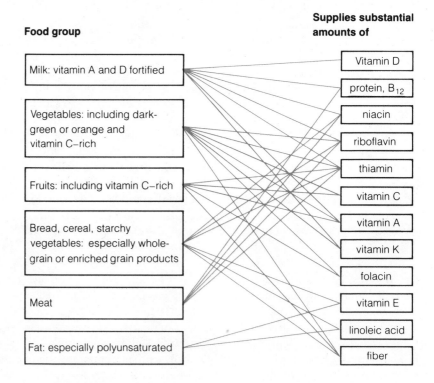

selections suggested above is so great that chances are good they will supply most nutrients in amounts sufficient to meet the needs of virtually all members of a healthy population. This diagram will be repeated at the end of Chapter 13, where it will be shown that some modifications are necessary to ensure adequacy for certain minerals.

Summing Up

Vitamin A as part of the visual pigment rhodopsin is essential for vision, especially in dim light. Vitamin A is involved in maintaining the integrity of mucous membranes throughout the internal linings of the body and thus in promoting resistance to infection. It helps maintain the health of the skin and is essential for the remodeling of bones during their growth or mending; it also plays a part in cell membrane functions, in hormone synthesis, in reproduction, and other functions.

Deficiency of vitamin A causes night blindness due to the failure to regenerate rhodopsin; a failure of mucous secretion, which can lead by way of keratinization of the cornea to blindness; disorders of the respiratory, urogenital, reproductive, and nervous systems; and abnormalities of bones and teeth. Toxicity symptoms are caused by large excesses (10 times the recommended intake or more) taken over a prolonged period and result only from the preformed vitamin (from supplements or animal products such as liver)—not from the precursor carotene and its relatives, the yellow pigments found in plants.

The recommended intake for vitamin A (800 RE for women, 1,000 RE for men) is easily met by periodically consuming the vitamin's richest food sources, such as liver or dark-green leafy vegetables, or by consuming other concentrated sources daily, such as carrots, cantaloupe, yellow squash, or broccoli. All food sources of vitamin A or the carotenoids have some color.

Vitamin D promotes intestinal absorption of calcium, mobilization of calcium from bone stores, and retention by the kidneys and is therefore essential for the calcification of bones and teeth. Given reasonable exposure to sun, humans can synthesize this vitamin in the skin from a precursor manufactured by the liver. Deficiency of vitamin D causes the calcium deficiency diseases (rickets in children and osteomalacia in adults); excesses cause abnormally high blood calcium levels, due to excessive GI absorption and withdrawal from bone, and result in deposition of calcium crystals in soft tissues, such as the kidney and major blood vessels. The recommended intake of 400 IU (2.5 μg cholecalciferol) per day is best met by drinking fortified milk; food sources of vitamin D are unreliable. However, exposure to sunlight probably ensures vitamin D adequacy for the average adult.

The best-substantiated role of vitamin E in humans is as an antioxidant that protects vitamin A and the polyunsaturated fatty acids

(PUFAs) from destruction by oxygen. Although many vitamin E-deficiency symptoms have been observed in animals, only one has been confirmed in humans: hemolysis of red blood cells due to oxidative destruction of the PUFAs in their membranes. The recommended intake of about 6 to 10 mg per day for adults is more than adequate to prevent this. The human requirement for vitamin E is known to vary with PUFA intake; since the vitamin occurs with PUFAs in foods, it is normally supplied in the needed amounts. Deficiences are seldom observed but there is some concern that the overuse of processed foods may make deficiences more likely. Toxicity symptoms are rare.

Vitamin K, the coagulation vitamin, promotes normal blood clotting; deficiency causes hemorrhagic disease. The vitamin is synthesized by intestinal bacteria and is available from foods such as green vegetables and milk. Deficiency is normally seen only in newborns, whose intestinal flora have not become established, in people taking sulfa drugs, or in people whose fat absorption is impaired.

Adequate intakes of all the nutrients discussed so far are ensured by selecting a variety of foods from all six of the food exchange groups, as shown in the diagram on p. 410; inclusion of polyunsaturated oils promotes ample intakes of both linoleic acid and vitamin E.

To Explore Further

This beautifully illustrated biology textbook provides in Chapter 26 a clear, accurate, and detailed explanation of the way the eye works:

Biology Today (Del Mar, Calif.: CRM Books, 1972).

The vast problem of vitamin A deficiency throughout the world is summarized in an 88-page booklet available from the World Health Organization (address in Appendix J):

WHO/USAID Joint Meeting, *Vitamin A Deficiency and Xerophthalmia*, Technical Report Series 590 (Albany, N.Y.: Q Corporation, 1976).

Vitamin A deficiency may be implicated in some kinds of cancer. The story is still far from complete, but you might like to look up these three articles:

Basu, T. K., Vitamin A and cancer of epithelial origin, *Journal of Human Nutrition* 33 (February 1979):24-31.

Sporn, M. B., Dunlop, N. M., Newton, D. L., and Smith, J. M., Prevention of chemical carcinogenesis by vitamin A and its synthetic analogs (retinoids), *Federation Proceedings* 35 (1976):1332-1338.

Vitamin A, tumor initiation and tumor promotion, *Nutrition Reviews* 37 (May 1979):153-156.

Recent research on vitamin D is summarized by one of the major investigators in the area in a featured article in *Nutrition Reviews:* DeLuca, H. F., The vitamin D system in the regulation of calcium and phosphorus metabolism, *Nutrition Reviews* 37 (June 1979):161-193. This would make stiff reading for the general reader, but it is recommended to anyone who wants to gain an appreciation of all the complexities. Of special interest is the new hope this research brings to renal patients, whose bone disease was untreatable until the kidney's role in vitamin D metabolism was understood.

A two-page summary of vitamin E myths and realities, assembled by a committee of experts, is available free from General Mills (address in Appendix J):

Expert Panel on Food Safety and Nutrition, Committee on Public Information, Institute of Food Technologists, Vitamin E, *Contemporary Nutrition* 2 (November 1977).

Other interesting and useful information on the vitamins can be found in the general references listed in Appendix J.

You are watching a movie about the early days in the Old West. A wagon is parked in the woods. A man is mixing a batch of something in a washtub and then ladling it into medicine bottles. The scene shifts to the nearby town. The man is now dressed in a high silk hat and swallow-tailed coat and is hawking the "medicine" from a makeshift stage on the rear of the wagon. The camera shows the faces in the crowd, mesmerized by the man's tale of the wonderful cures this medicine has effected. "Step right up, folks, and buy this time-tested medicine, only a dollar for the giant bottle, and it will cure lumbago, the ague, and rheumatism." The faces in the crowd register concern over some private ailment they wish could be cured by this magical medicine. As you watch the film, you wonder how the people could have been duped by such a show.

HIGHLIGHT 11

Vitamin E: A Cure-All?

Is it likely that the RDA Committee is grossly in error about the amounts of vitamin E needed for optimum health? One "common sense" way of approaching such questions (which might be called a "biological" approach) is to consider that mankind evolved on the food it could readily obtain, and that one should not expect to find large natural barriers blocking access to foods needed for health. Let us see what one would have to eat to get 1,500 IU of vitamin E each day. . . . [It] would require some eight or nine pounds of oil, something over a gallon a day.

RONALD M. DEUTSCH

Today's magical medicine barkers don't wear high silk hats or mix their potions in washtubs. Those props have gone out of style along with the ailments the old barkers sought to cure. Only the faces in the crowd remain the same. They listen avidly now as the authors of a book on vitamin E hawk their wares on a television talk show. The authors sound knowledgeable, sure of the truth of what they are saying.

There must be some reasonable explanation for so many honest people believing the many claims of the curative powers of vitamin E, especially as research shows that human beings are rarely deficient in this vitamin. Let's examine what is known about this vitamin, which has caught the public's fancy as a cure for everything from impotence in males to the healing of burns.

Animal Research Male rats deprived of vitamin E cease to manufacture sperm. Their testes become atrophied, brownish, and flabby. The rabbit, dog, and monkey show similar damage, but the mouse seems remarkably resistant, taking a great deal longer to exhibit these signs.[1]

In pregnant female rats on a diet lacking vitamin E, the

[1]M. K. Horwitt, The vitamins, Section D: Vitamin E, in *Modern Nutrition in Health and Disease*, 5th ed., eds. R. S. Goodhart and M. E. Shils (Philadelphia: Lea and Febiger, 1973), pp. 175-190.

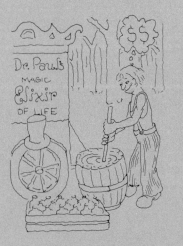

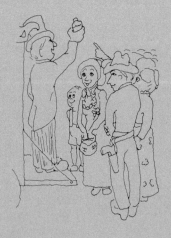

fetus dies during the first week. If vitamin E is restored to the diet during the first week of pregnancy, the fetus can be saved, indicating that a vitamin E deficiency damages the blood supply between the uterus and the placenta.[2]

In animals on a vitamin E-deficient diet, the muscles become weak and a kind of muscular paralysis sets in; this too can be reversed by restoring the vitamin to the diet. The extent of the paralysis seems to be related to the amount of polyunsaturated fat in the tissues. The heart muscles of rabbits, sheep, and cattle (plant-eating animals) seem to be especially vulnerable. Fatal heart attacks are not uncommon, and they take place before overt signs of the deficiency have developed.[3]

These results of studies of vitamin E-deficient animals indicate a possible role for the vitamin in prolonging virility in males, carrying a fetus to full term in females, and keeping muscles healthy, particularly heart muscles. The next logical quest is to see if the vitamin is necessary for maintenance of these functions in human beings.

The search to find such a role for vitamin E in humans has continued for over 30 years, but thus far it has produced only negative results. However, the "faces in the crowd" continue to look to vitamin E as the potion that will prolong virility, abolish miscarriages, and cure muscular weakness like that in muscular dystrophy.

Why is it that laboratory findings on vitamin E deficiencies in animals cannot be applied to humans? To answer this question, we must examine nutrition research on animals.

Animal Research Methods   Two steps are necessary in both animal and human research to show that lack of a nutrient is causing a certain symptom. First, a diet lacking that nutrient and only that nutrient must be fed. The administration of this diet must result consistently in the appearance of the deficiency symptom. Then, when the nutrient is returned to the diet, the deficiency symptom must disappear. Furthermore, in nutrient research using animals, several preparatory steps must be taken.

● An animal must be found that does not synthesize the nutrient. For example, vitamin C-deficiency research cannot be carried out on rats, because rats synthesize vitamin C. Guinea pigs have to be used instead.

● A laboratory feed must be prepared that contains all essential nutrients except the one under study. This is not the simple task of finding a food for the animal; it entails mixing the nutrients in the correct proportion. The result is usually a mixture of synthetic nutrients, since natural foods would very likely contain traces of the nutrient being excluded. Moreover, chemical analysis must show that the mixture is indeed free from the nutrient and that it is not lacking in another essential nutrient. (Alternatively an antinutrient can be used to bind, inactivate, or compete with the nutrient in question, but then the researcher must distinguish between the effects of the nutrient's lack and those of the antinutrient's presence.)

● The animals must have a common heredity and be maintained on similar diets for the same length of time prior to the start of the experiment.

● Other variables may need to be controlled for specific nutrients. For example, if it has been shown in other work that a nutrient's absorption is under seasonal hormone control,[4] that fact will need to be considered in the design of the experiment.

When the deficiency symptom has been produced in the laboratory animal and alleviated with the addition of the missing nutrient, researchers can say that in that

[2]Horwitt, 1973.

[3]Horwitt, 1973.

[4]H. Weindling and J. B. Henry, Laboratory test results altered by "the pill," *Journal of the American Medical Association* 229 (1974):1762-1768.

species they have found the lack of a particular nutrient caused a particular symptom. When other laboratories have replicated these results, they are accepted—for that species. Until laboratory research has shown this relationship to be true for another species of animal, researchers can only theorize that the relationship may be true in both.

Applications to Humans

It is much trickier to apply knowledge gained from research with laboratory animals to humans than to transfer knowledge gained from one species to another in the laboratory. The experimental animal is caged, thus assuring that feed, fluid, temperature, and most of the factors in his environment will be controlled. It is also possible to allow the experiment to continue until death intervenes, after which an autopsy can show the effects of the nutritional deficiency on the internal organs.

In research with humans, the intake of food and fluid cannot be controlled except in very short-term experiments. In addition, there is no way of knowing that each subject is in a similar nutritional state prior to the beginning of the experiment. This fact necessitates the use of large numbers of human subjects so that the results can be averaged. Finding a large enough population hinders the launching of such an

Mini-Glossary

ague (AY-gyoo): a chill; a fit of shivering, an old-fashioned term.

lumbago (lum-BAY-go): rheumatic pain in the joints, an old-fashioned term.

muscular dystrophy (DIS-tro-fee): a hereditary disease in which the muscles gradually weaken; its most debilitating effects arise from weakening of the respiratory muscles.

nutritional muscular dystrophy: a vitamin E-deficiency disease of animals, characterized by gradual paralysis of the muscles.

rheumatism: pain in the joints, an old-fashioned term.

experiment and adds to the cost. Experimentation on human beings must also depend on subjects who are free to break the restrictions of the diet or to drop out of the experiment at any time, even if they are being paid to be subjects.

In the case of vitamin E research on human beings, there have been several unique obstacles in addition to these:[5]

● Vitamin E is widely distributed in foods. It is, therefore, difficult to compose a diet totally devoid of it.

[5]Committee on Nutritional Misinformation, Food and Nutrition Board, NAS/NRC, Who needs vitamin E? *Journal of the American Dietetic Association* 64 (1974):365-366.

● Vitamin E is one of the fat-soluble vitamins and as such is stored in abundance in the tissues of the body, particularly in adipose tissue. Therefore, it takes a long period of deficiency for the body to be depleted.

Another type of study that can be carried out with humans is that in which results from many case studies involving a possible vitamin E deficiency are pooled to see if there is a common thread of truth. For the most part, these efforts have been unproductive. Vitamin E has been shown to be ineffective in the treatment of such diseases as muscular dystrophy, reproductive failure, and heart disease. It seems that these conditions in humans are not the result of vitamin E deficiency.[6]

In summary, when a symptom has been shown to be caused by a deficiency of a nutrient in several species of laboratory animals, this fact can be used as a pointer toward the existence of the same relationship in humans. However, until a deficiency symptom can be produced in human subjects by a diet deficient in the nutrient and then cured by the restoration of that nutrient, it cannot be claimed that the symptom is caused by the lack of that nutrient.

[6]Editorial: Vitamin E in clinical medicine, *Lancet* 1 (1974):18.

The Committee on Nutritional Misinformation of the Food and Nutrition Board of the NAS/NRC prepared a statement that reads in part, "How did these claims [for vitamin E] come about? To some extent, they arose from a misinterpretation of the results of research on experimental animals. . . . The widespread presence of the vitamin in human diets has prevented a deficiency, such as seen in animals under experimental conditions."[7]

The amount of misinformation that has arisen out of the public's failure to understand these distinctions and the profit-making incentive of those who promote misunderstandings of this kind has cost the public millions of dollars every year.

A FLAG SIGN OF A SPURIOUS CLAIM IS THE USE OF:

Animal research findings misapplied to humans.

[7]Committee on Nutritional Misinformation, 1974.

The Appeal of Myths

There would seem to be another factor operating in the public's ready acceptance of claims that cannot be substantiated in human beings. The areas where animal research suggests a possible role for vitamin E in the human body are the same that currently are of the greatest concern to people. Emotional appeals for belief in the efficacy of vitamin E fall on willing ears when it is claimed that supplements of it will cure, for example, muscular dystrophy. *Hereditary muscular dystrophy* is a disease afflicting children, who usually die at an early age when their respiratory muscles cease to function properly. *Nutritional muscular dystrophy,* however, is the muscular weakness produced in many animals by a deficiency of vitamin E. This deficiency leads to an atrophy of the muscles; it can be cured by reintroducing vitamin E into the diet. At no time has there been any evidence in reliable literature that links this condition to hereditary muscular dystrophy.

It is easy to understand how the public might be confused by the use of these similar terms for separate conditions, but a nutritionist should be aware of the difference. Some years ago a popular writer on nutrition published in her book an account of a child with muscular dystrophy being cured

through early administration of vitamin E.[8] Throughout the several pages devoted to vitamin E, it was apparent that she was not aware of the difference between muscular dystrophy and nutritional muscular dystrophy. The cruelty of such a promise to parents of children with the disease is unconscionable.

In this discussion of vitamin E we have focused on the inadequacy of animal research for finding out about human nutrition. If we were to present a more balanced picture of the research on vitamin E, we would include the problems of finding standards for evaluating tissue status in humans, enzyme functions, absorption and turnover, and many other problems unique to vitamin E. J. G. Bieri has examined these in *Nutrition Reviews' Present Knowledge in Nutrition,* which is recommended in the To Explore Further section at the end of this Highlight.

Vitamin E in Foods   We have made the point that vitamin E is widespread in food and stored in the body so that it is quite difficult to deplete the tissues of it. Nutritionists are looking, however, at one area of food consumption that may be a cause for concern: the use of

[8]A. Davis, *Let's Eat Right to Keep Fit* (New York: Harcourt Brace Jovanovich, 1970), chap. 20.

highly processed food, such as frozen dinners and food from vending machines.[9] It is known that these are deficient in vitamin E, and if they are used consistently over a number of years, a vitamin E deficiency could possibly develop. People at risk for such a deficiency might be patients in institutions that make use of highly processed foods or might be older people who use convenience foods such as frozen dinners because it is too much trouble to prepare food "from scratch." The children of busy parents also may be at risk—if the parents repeatedly give them TV dinners or money to buy food from vending machines. We have no data at present to tell us the effect of a vitamin E-deficient diet over a period of five to ten years, which is the period of time some people may rely on frozen dinners.

With all of the uncertainty regarding people's vitamin E status, and with the public's belief in the dire effects of deficiencies, many people are resorting to the use of supplements "as an insurance measure." Luckily, none of the work that has been done on humans indicates that vitamin E toxicity develops at the levels usually taken in supplements.[10] It may be that a person's belief that vitamin E is helping to alleviate a condition—for instance, sexual impotence—may provide a helpful psychological boost that in itself is worth the price of the vitamin. There is one dangerous aspect that should be noted, however: If taking a vitamin lulls a user into avoiding the correct diagnosis and treatment of a serious condition, the vitamin supplement may cost more than anyone can afford to pay. In the meantime, the modern-day hawkers of vitamin E supplements get richer, but as far as we know, no one gets any healthier.

To Explore Further

This article reviews the research on vitamin E and helps to explain why knowledge of it is tentative:

Bieri, J. G., Vitamin E, in *Nutrition Reviews' Present Knowledge in Nutrition*, 4th ed. (New York: The Nutrition Foundation, 1976), chap. 11.

Another helpful reference is *Vitamin E—Miracle or Myth*, U.S. Department of Health, Education, and Welfare, Public Health Service, Publication no. (FDA) 76-2011, available from the U.S. Government Printing Office (address in Appendix J).

A teaching aid, *Vitamin E* by A. L. Tappel, contains 12 slides that explore the cellular function of vitamin E. It can be ordered from the Nutrition Today Society (address in Appendix J).

[9]H. H. Koehler, H. C. Lee, and M. Jacobson, Tocopherols in canned entrees and vended sandwiches, *Journal of the American Dietetic Association* 70 (1977):616-620.

[10]Editorial: Vitamin E, 1974.

The Fat-Soluble Vitamins

Exercises 1 to 3 make use of the information you recorded on Forms 1 to 3 in the Self-Study at the end of the introduction to Part One.

1. Look up and record your recommended intake of vitamin A (from the RDA tables on the inside front cover or from the Canadian Dietary Standard in Appendix O). Note that this recommendation is stated in RE units.

2. Estimate your actual intake of vitamin A by restudying Form 1 (in the Self-Study following the introduction to Part One, p. 14) in light of what you now know from reading Chapter 11. List all the foods you ate during your three-day self-study period that contributed more than 100 IU of vitamin A. Sort the amounts of vitamin A they contributed into two columns: one for animal foods, the other for plant foods. Add up these two columns separately. Now, using the rule of thumb that 10 IU of vitamin A from plant foods or 3.33 IU from animal foods is approximately equivalent to 1 RE, divide the amount in your plant-food column by 10. Divide the amount in your animal-food column by

3.33. Then add the two columns together to express your three-day vitamin A intake in RE. Finally, divide this number by 3 (days) to derive your average estimated intake of vitamin A per day in RE.

3. What percentage of your recommended intake of vitamin A did you consume? Was this enough? What foods contribute the greatest amount of vitamin A to your diet? What percentage of your intake comes from plant foods? If you consumed more than the recommendation, was this too much? Why or why not? In what ways would you change your diet to improve it in this respect?

Optional Extras

Tables of food composition do not show vitamins D, E, and K, but you can guess at the adequacy of your intake.

● For vitamin D, answer the following questions: Did you drink fortified milk (read the label)? Eat eggs? Fortified breakfast cereals? Liver? Are you in the sun frequently? (Remember, though, that excessive exposure to sun can cause skin cancer in susceptible individuals.)

● For vitamin E, consider the foods you ate in 24 hours. Vitamin E often accompanies linoleic acid in foods. Did you consume enough linoleic acid? (The recommendation is 2 percent of total kcalories from linoleic acid, as specified in the Self-Study on Fat, p. 94.)

● For vitamin K, does your diet include 2 c of milk or the equivalent in milk products every day? Does it include leafy vegetables frequently (every other day)? Do you take antibiotics regularly (which inhibit the production of vitamin K by your intestinal bacteria)?

● Return to the health food store and ask some more questions, this time about the fat-soluble vitamins. Does the salesperson try to alert you to the risks of overdosing with these vitamins?

CHAPTER 12

CONTENTS

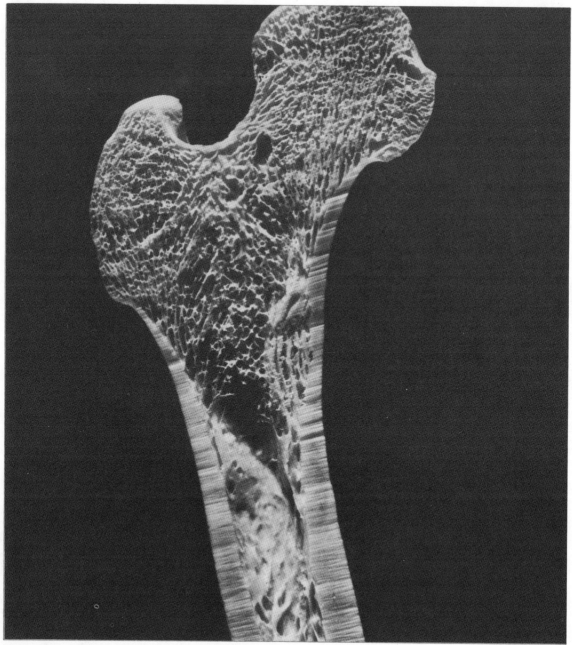

Cross section of bone, showing trabeculae.

THE MAJOR MINERALS

Professor C. Culmann of Zurich was . . . designing a crane, and during a visit to the laboratory of his friend and colleague, Professor Meyer, the anatomist, he saw the trabeculae in the head of a bisected femur. With a sudden flash of insight he exclaimed, "That's my crane!" . . . The cells which deposit the bone [are] sensitive to tensions and compressions . . . . They deposit bone with respect to these lines of force.

JOHN TYLER BONNER

Chapters 1 to 11 have been devoted to the first four of the six classes of nutrients: carbohydrates, fat, protein, and vitamins. Now we move on to the minerals. A few generalizations about minerals that distinguish them from vitamins were presented in the introduction to Part Two. (You may want to review those points before you continue.)

Because the amounts of the minerals found in the body and needed in the diet vary so widely, many authorities have divided them into two categories: the major minerals (sometimes called macrominerals) and the trace minerals (sometimes called microminerals).

Major minerals:	Trace minerals:
calcium	iron
phosphorus	iodine
potassium	zinc
sulfur	selenium
sodium	manganese
chlorine	copper
magnesium	molybdenum
	cobalt
	chromium
	fluorine
	silicon
	vanadium
	nickel
	tin
	arsenic (?)
	cadmium (?)

The major minerals are sometimes called the **macrominerals.** They are needed in amounts on the order of 0.1 g or more each day. They comprise 0.1% of the body weight or more.

The trace minerals are sometimes called the **microminerals.** They are needed in amounts on the order of 0.01 g or less each day and comprise 0.01% of the body weight or less.

Figure 1 shows how much the human body needs of some of these minerals.

Figure 1 The amounts of minerals in a 60-kilogram human body. A line separates the major minerals from the trace minerals. The major minerals are those present in amounts larger than 5 g (a teaspoon). A pound is about 454 g; thus only calcium and phosphorus appear in amounts larger than a pound. There are more than a dozen trace minerals, although only four are shown here; not shown are fluoride, silicon, vanadium, chromium, cobalt, nickel, zinc, selenium, molybdenum, and tin.

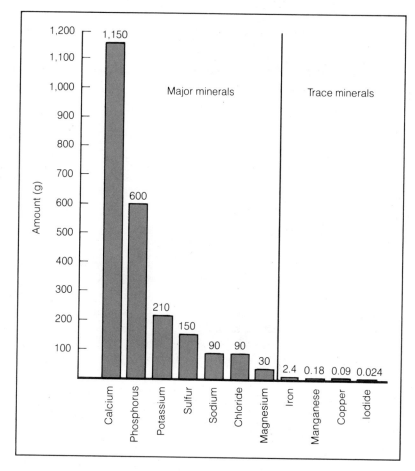

The influence of the minerals on the acid-base balance of the body fluids is proportional to the amounts found in the body. Thus the major minerals have a much greater effect than the trace minerals on this balance. The special roles of minerals in regulating the pH of body fluids depend on their interaction with water, the last nutrient to be discussed in this book. Chapter 14 is reserved for a discussion of these roles, and Table 1 in that chapter shows the major minerals divided into the acid- and base-forming classes.

In addition to the mineral elements listed above, most of which have long been familiar to nutritionists, others that are needed in the daily diet in very tiny amounts have recently come to light. The list of needed mineral elements is still growing longer as research continues. Perhaps 30 or more minerals will eventually prove to be essential in the human diet. This means that the amount of information available on the minerals, like that on the vitamins, is overwhelmingly great and cannot be treated exhaustively in an introductory textbook. What is probably most important is for you to be aware of the minerals that are presently known to be lacking in the diets of significant numbers of people. Those most needing emphasis by this criterion are calcium, iron,

iodine, zinc, and fluorine. Calcium will be emphasized most heavily in this chapter; the others, being trace minerals, will be discussed in Chapter 13.

Calcium

A popular book on nutrition that has enjoyed wide sales over the past 30 years makes extravagant claims for calcium.[1] The writer implies that even a very slight decrease in dietary intake causes these symptoms: air swallowing and indigestion; insomnia and other forms of the inability to relax; irritability of the muscles, including cramps and spasms; menstrual cramps; hypersensitivity to pain; a tendency to hemorrhage; cataracts; tooth decay; and complications in childbirth. Since there is hardly anyone in the world who is free of all of these symptoms, the naive reader might be led to believe that calcium is a virtual cure-all and that people must make special efforts to procure adequate amounts of this extremely important, even miraculous, nutrient.

The claims made for this wonderful nutrient are based on a misunderstanding of the facts about the roles it plays in the body. A deficiency of calcium caused by failure of the *body* to maintain a proper concentration can cause some of these symptoms, but a *dietary* deficiency cannot. In fact, a dietary calcium deficiency has little or no effect on its blood concentration or on the functions mentioned above.

The Roles of Calcium Calcium's most obvious role is as a component of bones and teeth: 99 percent of the calcium in the body is found in these structures. The remaining 1 percent circulates in the watery fluids of the body, where it performs a number of important functions. Some calcium is found in close association with cell membranes; it appears to be essential for their integrity. The calcium found between and among cells is essential for keeping them in association with one another. In some way it helps to support or maintain the intercellular cement—collagen. In association with cell membranes, calcium helps to regulate the transport of other ions into and out of cells. In association with the membranes of muscle cells, calcium is essential for muscle relaxation and so helps maintain the heartbeat. Calcium must be present between nerve and nerve, and between nerve and muscle, for the transmission of nerve impulses.

Collagen: see pp. 136, 363.

The mineral must also be present if blood clotting is to occur, because it is one of the 14 factors directly involved in this process. (The other 13 are proteins; vitamins, such as vitamin K, are also needed for the synthesis of some of these proteins.) Calcium is also needed as a cofactor for several enzymes, acting like a coenzyme.

cofactor: a mineral element that, like a coenzyme, works with an enzyme to facilitate a chemical reaction.

Coenzyme: see p. 326.

[1]A. Davis, *Let's Eat Right to Keep Fit* (New York: Harcourt Brace Jovanovich, 1970), chap. 21. This and other unreliable books are on a list of nutrition books that are not recommended, available on request from the American Medical Association (address in Appendix J).

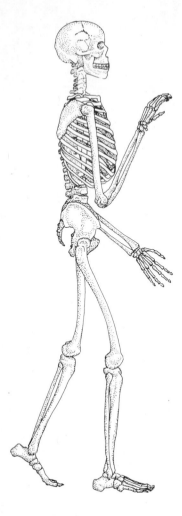

An awareness of all these functions might lead you to believe that a deficiency of calcium in food would cause nerve and muscle irritability and possibly nervous tension, hemorrhaging, and the other symptoms mentioned earlier. Yet in fact none of these things happens with a dietary deficiency of calcium. The reason for this is that the amount of calcium found in the blood remains remarkably constant over a wide range of dietary intakes; a deficiency affects the calcium stores in bones.

Why the Blood Calcium Level Does Not Change   It is an axiom of nature that if a function is vital to life it will be maintained against tremendous odds. Breathing is such a function; there is no way you can stop breathing voluntarily, as you may remember learning when you were a very small child. A child having a tantrum will make furious efforts to hold his breath until he is blue in the face. But even as he starts to lose consciousness, his automatic, instinctive reflexes take over and he begins to breathe again. In the same way, if the beating of the heart is stopped by a heart attack, which affects the node of cells in the heart muscle known as the pacemaker, a second node of cells nearby takes over and keeps the heartbeat going—albeit at a slower pace. Or if the secretion of pancreatic enzymes fails, a second set of enzymes similar to the pancreatic ones, produced by the small intestine, continue to work so that some digestion will still proceed.

These examples could be multiplied many hundreds of times to show that wherever there is a vital function, backup systems provide for it to be carried out in emergencies. You can tell how important a body function is for survival by observing how many different systems serve the backup function. By this criterion it is obvious that maintenance of the blood's calcium concentration is extremely important for overall health and even life, for calcium is the most closely regulated ion in the body.

The bones hold the body upright, but from the blood's point of view, this is not their primary role. The bones serve as a "bank" for calcium and other minerals. The minerals can be readily withdrawn from bone when blood levels begin to fall, and they can be redeposited into bone if blood levels rise too high. The 99 percent of the body's calcium stored in bone constitutes a tremendous "savings account."

The concentration of ionic calcium in the blood is maintained within very narrow limits, around 10 mg/100 ml of blood. If it falls or rises ever so slightly, it is immediately corrected. Four separate systems serve to maintain the blood calcium level. Some calcium in the blood itself is reversibly bound to such blood proteins as the albumins and globulins. The first line of defense against falling blood calcium is the release of this bound calcium from the proteins. The other three systems are regulated with the help of vitamin D and hormones.

One of these systems is the absorption system. A calcium-binding protein is made by the intestinal cells with the help of vitamin D, and

albumins (al-BYOO-mins) and **globulins** (GLOB-yoo-lins): two major classes of blood proteins.

more of this protein is made if more calcium is needed. Thus you will absorb more when you need more. This system is most obviously reflected in the increased absorption by a pregnant woman. She may drink the same amount of milk that she did before she was pregnant but absorbs 50 percent of the calcium from it; formerly she absorbed only 30 percent. Thus her body's calcium supply almost doubles, even if her food intake does not change at all. Similarly, growing children absorb 50 or 60 percent of ingested calcium; when their growth slows or stops (and their bones no longer demand a net increase in calcium content each day), their absorption falls to the adult level of about 30 percent.

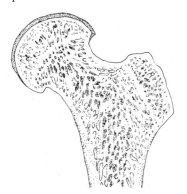

trabeculae (tra-BECK-you-lie), singular **trabecula:** lacy filaments inside bone that serve as a storage site for calcium and phosphorus. They are readily broken down and built up again in response to the body's changing needs for these minerals.

The second system is a storage system. Calcium is reversibly stored in the trabeculae of the bones. When blood calcium concentration rises, more is put away inside these lacy filaments. When calcium is needed in the blood, the trabeculae break down again. The photograph at the opening of this chapter shows the exquisite architecture of bone.

The third system involves the kidneys. The kidneys are sensitive to blood calcium concentrations and excrete more when blood calcium rises above the acceptable level and less when it falls.

These three systems are regulated by two hormones, one secreted by the parathyroid glands and the other secreted by both the thyroid and the parathyroid glands. The first, parathormone, is released whenever blood calcium falls below 7 mg/100 ml. Parathormone affects all three systems, stimulating increased absorption in the intestines, release of calcium from bone trabeculae, and increased retention by the kidneys. The other hormone, calcitonin, is secreted by both the thyroid and parathyroid glands when blood calcium rises above tolerance. Calcitonin inhibits the release of calcium from bone. For these reasons, blood calcium concentrations are very little affected by varying dietary intakes.

To say that food calcium never affects blood calcium is not to say that blood calcium never changes. In fact, sometimes blood calcium does rise above normal, causing a condition known as calcium rigor. When this happens, the muscle fibers contract and cannot relax. Similarly, calcium levels may fall below normal in the blood, causing calcium

parathyroid (para-THIGH-royd) **glands:** 4 small glands situated on the surface of the thyroid gland, 2 on each side; they produce the hormones parathormone and calcitonin.

thyroid glands: 2 glands in the neck, one on each side; they produce the hormones thyroxin (see p. 245) and thyrocalcitonin (see below).

parathormone (para-THOR-mone): hormone secreted by the parathyroid glands in response to low blood calcium concentrations; causes increased intestinal absorption, release from bones, and increased renal resorption of calcium.

calcitonin (cal-si-TONE-in): one form, **thyrocalcitonin,** is secreted by the thyroid glands in response to high blood calcium concentration, inhibiting release of calcium from bone; the other is secreted by the parathyroid.

calcium rigor: hardness or stiffness of the muscles.

calcium tetany: intermittent spasms of the extremities due to nervous and muscular excitability.

tetany—also a situation characterized by uncontrolled contraction of muscle tissue, due to a change in the stimulation of nerve cells. These conditions do not reflect a dietary lack or excess of calcium but are due to a lack of vitamin D or to glandular malfunctions resulting in abnormal amounts of the hormones that regulate blood calcium concentration.

On the other hand, a chronic dietary deficiency of calcium or a chronic deficiency due to poor absorption can, over the course of years, diminish the savings account in the bones. It is the bones, not the blood, that are depleted by calcium deficiency.

rickets: the calcium- (or vitamin D-) deficiency disease in children.

Calcium Deficiency   The disease rickets has been mentioned in connection with vitamin D deficiency. Often in rickets the amount of calcium in the diet is adequate, but it passes through the intestinal tract without being absorbed into the body, leaving the bones undersupplied. Vitamin D deficiency, by depressing the production of the calcium-binding protein, is the most common cause of rickets. (The symptoms have been described in Table 4 of Chapter 11.) In children, the failure to deposit sufficient calcium in bone causes growth retardation, bowed legs, and other skeletal abnormalities. In adults, the disease may set in after a normal childhood, during which calcium intake and absorption were adequate, and after the skeleton has become fully calcified. Prolonged inadequate calcium uptake during adulthood, often due to vitamin D deficiency, may cause the gradual and insidious removal of calcium from the bones, resulting in altered composition or reduced density of the bones in old age, which makes them fragile.

Altered composition of the bones is reflected in **osteomalacia**, the condition in which the bones become soft (see p. 405).

Reduced density of the bones results in **osteoporosis** (oss-tee-oh-pore-OH-sis), literally porous bones.

The fragility of the bones is most severe in the pelvic bone, which may become so brittle that it breaks when the person is walking. You may have heard of an old person who fell and broke her hip. What often actually happens is that her hip breaks while she is walking, and then she falls. The pelvic bone may shatter into countless fragments, so that it can never be repaired but has to be replaced with an artificial hip.

Many older people are severely afflicted with osteoporosis. The causes seem to be multiple, but a calcium deficiency during the growing years is a factor always present. This fact underscores the importance of prevention: Drink plenty of milk while you are young to have strong bones in later life.

A net calcium loss occurs in many adults, especially in women after menopause or hysterectomy, suggesting that hormonal changes are responsible. Many minerals and vitamins are required to form and stabilize the structure of bones, including magnesium, fluoride, vitamin A, and others. Any of these may be essential for preventing osteoporosis. One obvious line of defense, however, is to maintain a lifelong adequate intake of calcium.

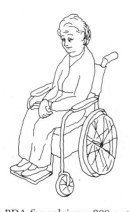

The RDA for calcium: 800 mg.

Canadian Dietary Standard: 800 mg for men, 700 mg for women.

Food Sources of Calcium   The recommended intake of calcium, arrived at by way of balance studies, is 700 to 800 mg (0.7 to 0.8 g) per day for adults in both the United States and Canada. Adults can stay in balance on intakes lower than this if they adapt over a long period of time to lower intakes, and the World Health Organization recommends only 400 to 500 mg per day for adults. However, high phosphorus intakes increase calcium excretion, and in the United States and Canada, where the diets are rich in phosphorus-laden protein, 700 to 800 mg seems to be a protective recommendation.

Calcium is found almost exclusively in a single class of foods—milk and milk products—as shown in Table 1. For this reason, if for no other, members of this group must be included in the diet daily. Because a cup of milk contains almost 300 mg calcium, an intake of 2 c milk provides an amount nearly adequate for most people. The other dairy food that contains comparable amounts of calcium is cheese. One

Table 1.   Calcium Contents of 50 Common Foods*

Exchange group[†]	Food	Serving size[‡]	Calcium (mg)	Exchange group[†]	Food	Serving size[‡]	Calcium (mg)
5L	Sardines with bones	3 oz	372	6	Cream, light	2 tbsp	30
1	2% fat fortified milk	1 c	352	4	Winter squash	1/2 c	29
1	Canned evaporated milk	1/2 c	318	2	Turnips	1/2 c	27
1	Skim milk	1 c	296	5M	Egg	1	27
1	Dry skim milk	1/3 c	293	2	Summer squash	1/2 c	26
1	Whole milk	1 c	288	3	Dried fig	1	26
1	Yogurt	1 c	272	2	Onions	1/2 c	25
5L	Oysters	3/4 c	170	4	Whole wheat bread	1 slice	25
5L	Canned salmon with bones	3 oz	167	2	Brussels sprouts	1/2 c	25
2	Collard greens	1/2 c	145	4	Mashed potato	1/2 c	24
2	Dandelion greens	1/2 c	126	2	Carrots	1/2 c	24
2	Spinach	1/2 c	106	3	Blackberries	1/2 c	23
2	Mustard greens	1/2 c	97	4	White bread	1 slice	21
4	Corn muffin	1	96§	3	Pink grapefruit	1/2	20
5M	Creamed cottage cheese	1/4 c	58	3	White grapefruit	1/2	19
4	Pancake	1	58	4	Rye bread	1 slice	19
3	Orange	1	54	4	Green peas	1/2 c	19
2	Broccoli	1/2 c	49	5M	Peanut butter	2 tbsp	18
4	Dried beans	1/2 c	45	3	Strawberries	3/4 c	17
4	Pumpkin	3/4 c	43	5L	Chipped beef	3 oz	17
4	Muffin	1	42	2	Asparagus	1/2 c	15
4	Lima beans	1/2 c	40	4	Hamburger bun	1/2	15
3	Tangerine	1	34	3	Raspberries	1/2 c	14
2	Cabbage	1/2 c	32	3	Cantaloupe	1/4	14
2	Green beans	1/2 c	32	4	Sweet potatoes	1/4 c	14

*These are not necessarily the best food sources but are selected to show a range of calcium contents. Study of the left-hand column will help you to generalize about which foods contain the most calcium.

†The numbers refer to the exchange lists: 1 is milk; 2, vegetables; 3, fruit; 4, bread; 5L, lean meat; 5M, medium-fat meat; 6, fats and oils.

‡Serving sizes are the sizes listed in the exchange lists, except for meat.

§To this point, all foods supply at least 10 percent of the recommended intake (for a man) of 800 mg.

slice of cheese (1 oz) contains about two-thirds as much calcium as a cup of milk. For people who don't drink milk, greens are an important food; a 1-c serving provides as much calcium (and riboflavin) as a cup of milk.

The absurdity of attempting to meet calcium needs in any way other than by consuming two servings a day of these foods can be demonstrated by listing the amounts of other foods you would have to consume instead: 6 heads of iceberg lettuce, 10 c of cooked green beans, 12 oranges or eggs, or 20 c of strawberries!

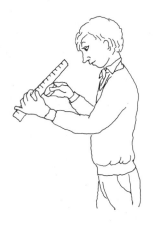

The amount of calcium recommended for the daily diet is so great that it cannot be packaged in a single pill that could be swallowed. To be absorbed, calcium is combined into an organic salt such as calcium gluconate or calcium lactate—a process that makes the pill extremely bulky. To get 600 mg of calcium in this salt you would have to take six pills the diameter of a quarter and the thickness of four quarters. You therefore never find significant amounts of calcium in vitamin-mineral supplements of the type that are to be taken once a day. Many vitamin-mineral supplements do contain some calcium, however.

There are two ways to read a label: One is to read what it contains, and the other is to read how much. A list of the ingredients in a pill that contains calcium might mislead unaware consumers into believing that their calcium needs would be met by the pill. However, often the label lists the calcium content of each pill as 10 mg. Only when you compare this amount with the recommended intake (800 mg) do you realize that you would have to take 80 of these pills to meet your calcium needs. This discussion should remind you of a point made once before (p. 122): Use a yardstick.

It is important to remember, too, that pills do not supply the relative amounts of nutrients that are in the best balance for your overall health. A typical calcium supplement, for example, is labeled with the instructions to take six a day. Yet six pills a day supply less than 50 percent of the recommended intake of calcium and 500 percent of the vitamin D. (Vitamin D is added to the pill to enhance the absorption of calcium.)

On the other hand, 2 c of vitamin A & D-fortified skim milk would supply the following percentages of the nutrients an adult man needs: calcium, 60 percent; vitamin D, 50 percent; protein, 40 percent; vitamin A, 50 percent; thiamin, 12 percent; riboflavin, 50 percent; plus 24 g carbohydrate in the form of lactose. You will recall from Chapter 6 that calcium absorption is enhanced by some of these other nutrients. Once again, a point made previously (p. 6) is relevant: There are fringe benefits to eating a nutrient in a natural food as opposed to a purified nutrient preparation.

For most people, the obvious way to meet calcium needs is to include milk and milk products in the diet daily. This is especially important for pregnant or lactating women and for children in the growing years (their calcium balance must be positive to permit good skeletal growth). Adults concerned with feeding children who dislike milk may find it helpful to learn how to conceal milk in foods. Ice cream, ice milk, and yogurt are acceptable substitutes for regular milk, and puddings, custards, and baked goods can be prepared in such a way that they also contain appreciable amounts of milk. Powdered skim milk, which is an excellent and inexpensive source of protein, calcium, and other nutrients, can be added to many foods (such as cookies and meatloaf) in preparation. For children with a milk allergy, a calcium-rich substitute such as fortified soy milk must be found. Butter and cream contain negligible calcium, because calcium is not soluble in fat.

The word *daily* should be stressed with respect to food sources of calcium. Because of its limited ability to absorb calcium, the body cannot handle massive doses periodically but instead needs frequent opportunities to take in small amounts.

Calcium must be soluble if it is to be absorbed. The hydrochloric acid in the stomach increases solubility, as do vitamin C and some of the amino acids. But a high-fat diet may inhibit the absorption of calcium by forming insoluble soapy scums with calcium, which are then excreted in the feces. This may be the case in any of the diseases that affect the absorption of fat, leaving a high fat content in the intestine to combine with calcium.

The lactose in milk forms a soluble compound with calcium. This enhances the value of milk as one of the best food sources of calcium. (Remember, too, that milk is chosen as the vehicle for fortification with vitamin D.) Calcium levels are lower in breast milk than in cow's milk, but babies absorb it better from breast milk, probably because of the higher lactose content of breast milk.

An important relationship exists between calcium and phosphorus. Each is better absorbed if they are ingested together. Authorities differ on the ratio that might best favor health, but it seems probable that most would agree on a 1:1 ratio; perhaps any ratio from 3:1 to 1:3 is all right.

Some foods contain certain compounds, called binders, that combine chemically with calcium (and other minerals such as iron and zinc) to prevent their absorption, carrying them out of the body with other wastes. For example, phytic acid and oxalic acid render the calcium, iron, and zinc in certain foods "unavailable." Phytic acid is found in oatmeal and other whole-grain cereals, and oxalic acid in peanuts, rhubarb, and spinach, among other foods.[2] The calcium-binding properties of these binders in no way affect the overall value of the foods. Whole grains and greens are nutritious for so many reasons that no one should hesitate to include them in menu planning.

[2]Oxalate content of common foods, *Nutrition and the MD*, September 1979.

The Four Food Group Plan recommends daily milk servings:

Children under 9	2-3 c
Children 9-12	3+ c
Teenagers	4+ c
Adults	2 c
Pregnant women	3+ c
Lactating women	4+ c
Older women	3 c

milk allergy: the most common food allergy; caused by the protein in raw milk. Milk allergy is sometimes overcome by cooking the milk to denature the protein, sometimes "cured" by abstinence from and gradual reintroduction to milk. See also the discussion of lactose intolerance, p. 32.

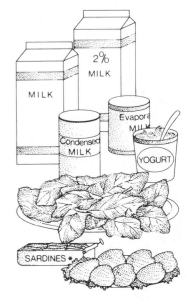

binders: chemical compounds occurring in foods that can combine with nutrients (especially minerals) to form complexes that the body cannot absorb. **Phytic** (FIGHT-ic) and **oxalic** (ox-AL-ic) **acids** are examples of such binders.

A generalization that has been gaining strength throughout this book is supported by the information given here about calcium: A balanced diet that supplies a variety of foods is the best guarantee of adequacy for all essential nutrients. All food groups should be included, and none should be overused. Calcium is found lacking wherever milk is underemphasized in the diet—whether through ignorance, simple dislike, lactose intolerance, or allergy. By contrast, iron is found lacking whenever milk is overemphasized, as Chapter 13 shows.

Phosphorus

Phosphorus is the mineral in second largest quantity in the body. About 85 percent of it is found combined with calcium in the crystals of the bones. Its concentration in blood plasma is less than half that of calcium: 3.5 mg/100 ml plasma. But as part of one of the body's major acids (phosphoric acid), it is a part of the structure of all body cells.

The average person hears very little about phosphorus, even though it plays a critical part in all cell functions. This lack of publicity in popular nutrition writing is probably due to the fact that deficiencies are unknown. Phosphorus is widespread in foods in association with calcium and protein; if these nutrients are adequate in the diet, then phosphorus is too.

Phosphorus is intimately associated with the calcium in bones and teeth as calcium phosphate, one of the compounds in the crystals that give strength and rigidity to these structures.[3] It is also a part of DNA and RNA, the genetic code material present in every cell. Thus phosphorus is necessary for all growth, because DNA and RNA provide the instructions for new cells to be formed.

Phosphorus plays many key roles in the cells' transfers of energy. Many enzymes and the B vitamins become active only when a phosphate group is attached. The B vitamins, you will recall, play major roles in energy metabolism. Again, phosphorus is critical in energy exchange. ATP itself, the energy carrier of the cells, contains three phosphate groups and uses these groups to do its work.

Some lipids contain phosphorus as part of their structure. These phospholipids help to transport other lipids in the blood; they also form a part of the structure of cell membranes, where they affect transport of nutrients into and out of the cells.

Phosphorus in the plasma is one of the most important buffers. A diagram in Chapter 14 shows how a buffer works in a solution such as blood to maintain the required acid-base balance.

Animal protein is the best source of phosphorus, because phosphorus is so abundant in the energetic cells of animals. People in the developed countries eat large quantities of animal protein and so

[3]The suffix *ate* in *calcium phosphate* indicates that oxygen is bound to the phosphorus.

excrete more phosphorus than people who consume a protein-poor diet. The extra phosphorus they excrete carries some calcium with it. This is why the recommended intakes for calcium in the United States and Canada are higher than they are for other countries. The recommended intakes for phosphorus are the same as those for calcium: 700 to 800 mg per day for adults.

The RDA for phosphorus: 800 mg.

Canadian Dietary Standard: 800 mg for men, 700 mg for women.

Sodium

Sodium is the positive ion in the compound sodium chloride, ordinary table salt. Salt has been known throughout recorded history. The Bible's saying, "You are the salt of the earth," means that a person is valuable. If, on the other hand, "you are not worth your salt," you are worthless. Even the word *salary* comes from the word *salt*. Carnivores generally do not travel to find salt, because they get it from eating other animals, but a grazing animal will travel many miles to a salt lick, driven by its body's need for sodium.

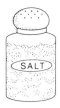

There is seldom a sodium shortage in the diet. Foods usually include more salt than is needed, and it enters the body fluids freely. The kidneys filter the surplus out of the blood into the urine. They can also sensitively conserve salt and return it to the blood in the event of a deficiency, which might occur during heavy sweating or starvation. Intakes vary widely, especially because of cultural differences in diets. Orientals, who use a great deal of soy sauce and monosodium glutamate (MSG or Accent) for flavoring, consume about 30 to 40 g of salt per day; most people in the United States average about 6 to 18 g of salt per day. Vegetarians probably consume much less than this.

The total amount of fluid in the body depends primarily on the sodium and potassium ions present. Cells can move these ions across their membranes, and they work constantly to keep sodium on the outside and potassium on the inside. Nerve transmission and muscle contraction depend on the cells' permitting a temporary exchange of sodium and potassium ions across their membranes. About 30 to 45 percent of the body's sodium is thought to be stored on the surface of the bone crystals, where it is easy to recover if the blood level drops.

The activity of the kidney in regulating the body content of sodium is remarkable. Sodium is absorbed easily from the intestinal tract, then travels in the blood, where it ultimately passes through the kidney. The kidney filters all the sodium out, then with great precision returns to the bloodstream the exact amount needed. Normally, the amount excreted equals the amount ingested that day.

If the blood level of sodium rises, as it will after a person eats heavily salted foods, the thirst receptors in the brain will be stimulated. The fluid intake will increase to make the sodium-to-water ratio constant. Then the extra fluid will be excreted by the kidneys along with the extra sodium.

Dieters sometimes think that eating too much salt or drinking too much water will make them gain weight, but this is not the case. Excess water is excreted immediately. Excess salt is excreted as soon as enough water is drunk to carry the salt out of the body. From this perspective, then, the way to keep body salt (and "water weight") under control is to drink more, not less, water.

If the blood level of sodium drops, as it does during vomiting, diarrhea, or heavy sweating, both water and sodium must be replenished. If only water is replaced, the blood concentration of sodium drops and water migrates into the cells. This results in symptoms of water intoxication: muscle weakness, apathy, nausea, and loss of appetite. Times when such a condition might exist are during athletic contests or heavy physical work in the heat, after extensive burns, or following accidents or surgery that involve loss of blood. Overly strict use of low-sodium diets in the treatment of kidney or heart disease may also deplete the body of needed sodium. The symptoms quickly vanish with the return of both sodium and water.

No recommendation needs to be made for daily sodium intake, because of the sensitive controls operating in the body. Furthermore, cooks add salt generously in food preparation, and diners add more from the salt shaker on the table. The highest concentrations in foods are in cured ham, bacon, pickles, potato chips, and cold cuts, where the salt acts as a preservative. Pregnant women should normally not restrict their salt intake (see Chapter 15).

The use of highly salted foods may contribute to high blood pressure. This may be true only for those who have a genetic tendency to develop high blood pressure. Black Americans are especially at risk in this respect. With a high sodium level in the blood, the volume of the blood increases. As this greater volume courses through the arteries, it expands them and puts their walls under tension. The heart then must work harder to pump the extra fluid throughout the system. It is presently recommended that we reduce our sodium intake by cutting our salt intake to not more than 5 g added salt a day (that is, salt added by manufacturers and consumers above and beyond that already in the food as grown). In practice, this would mean avoiding highly salted foods and removing the salt shaker from the table. (Appendix I shows the sodium contents of foods.)

Public water can contribute significant sodium to people's intakes. In some areas, where the water supply contains more than 100 mg of sodium per liter, some people's blood pressure is affected. Where highways are salted in winter to melt the snow, the runoff may contribute to this problem by adding more salt to the underground

Estimated safe and adequate daily dietary intake of sodium (Committee on RDA): 1.1-3.3 g.

High blood pressure is often called **hypertension.** People sometimes confuse hypertension with stress, but hypertension is an internal and stress an external condition. Stress may cause hypertension in sensitive people, however.

5 g of salt would be about 2 g of sodium.

1 g salt = 1/5 tsp

water. A sodium standard for public water of perhaps 20 mg per liter might need to be adopted in these areas.[4]

Chlorine

The element chlorine occurs naturally as a poisonous gas, but when it combines with sodium in salt, it is not poisonous but is part of a life-giving compound. It occurs in salt as the negative chloride ion.

The chloride ion is the major negative ion of the fluids outside the cells, where it is found mostly in association with sodium. Chloride can move freely across membranes and so is also found inside the cells in combination with potassium.

In the stomach, the chloride ion is part of hydrochloric acid. This is what maintains the strong acidity of the stomach. The cells that line the stomach continuously expend energy to push chloride into the stomach fluid. One of the most serious consequences of vomiting is the loss of chloride ions from the stomach, which upsets the acid-base balance of the body.

A chlorine compound is added to public water to sterilize it before it flows through pipes into people's homes. Turning to the deadly poisonous gas chlorine, it kills dangerous microorganisms that might otherwise spread disease, and then evaporates, leaving the water safe for human consumption. The addition of chlorine to public water is one of the most important public health measures ever introduced in the developed countries and has eliminated such water-borne diseases as typhoid fever, which once ravaged vast areas, killing thousands of people.

Estimated safe and adequate daily dietary intake of chloride (Committee on RDA): 1,700-5,100 mg.

Potassium

Potassium is critical to maintaining the heartbeat. The sudden deaths that occur in severe diarrhea, and in children with kwashiorkor may often be due to heart failure caused by potassium loss. As the principal positively charged ion inside body cells, it plays a major role in maintaining water balance and cell integrity. In water loss from the body in which sodium is lost, the ultimate damage comes when potassium is pulled out of the cells and excreted. Dehydration is especially scary, because potassium deficiency affects the brain cells early, making the victim unable to decide that she needs water.

[4]E. J. Calabrese and R. W. Tuthill, A review of literature to support a sodium drinking water standard, *Journal of Environmental Health* 40 (September/October 1977):80-83.

During nerve transmission and muscle contraction, potassium and sodium briefly exchange places. Nerve and muscle cells, then, are especially rich in potassium, but all cells must contain some. Potassium is also known to play a catalytic role in carbohydrate and protein metabolism, but the exact nature of this role is not known.

A deficiency of potassium from getting too little in the diet is unlikely. Abnormal conditions like diabetic acidosis or loss of large volumes of water can cause potassium deficiency, however. One of the earliest symptoms is muscle weakness.

Estimated safe and adequate daily dietary intake of potassium (Committee on RDA): 1,875-5,625 mg (1.9-5.6 g).

The warning implied by this information is that water loss from the body can be a grave danger. Adults are warned not to take diuretics (water pills) except under the direction of a physician; if another physician is consulted for a different health problem, he should be alerted to the fact that a diuretic is in use.

Gradual potassium depletion can occur when a person sweats profusely day after day and fails to replenish his potassium stores. A study of this effect shows that up to about 3 g of potassium can be lost in a day. The average diet in this country supplies about 1.5 to 2.5 g. If a person sweats heavily and often, the authors of this study recommend that he eat about five to eight servings of potassium-rich food each day.[5]

Potassium-rich foods include bananas, orange juice and many other fruit juices, and potatoes, tomatoes, and many other vegetables. For details, see Appendix I.

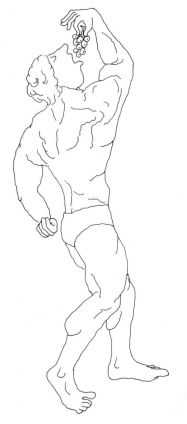

It has been pointed out several times previously that there are advantages to eating food instead of taking supplements. Salt tablets contain sodium and chloride, but foods contain a multitude of minerals. The body evolved in dependence on foods, not supplements. Men who think fruit is only for dainty ladies might take note that because of the potassium it contains, fruit may do more for their muscles than meat.

A borderline food is the liquid "sweat replacer," such as Gatorade, designed especially for athletes like football players. In choosing one of these, the buyer should look for potassium on the label.

The principal sources of potassium among foods commonly eaten are orange juice, bananas, dried fruits, and potatoes. Potassium supplements are not advisable except when prescribed, because too much potassium is as dangerous as too little. Even salt substitutes containing potassium should be avoided, especially by heart patients, except as recommended by a physician.

[5]H. W. Lane and J. J. Cerda, Potassium requirements and exercise, *Journal of the American Dietetic Association* 73 (1978):64-65.

Sulfur

Sulfur is present in all proteins and plays its most important role in determining the contour of protein molecules. Sulfur helps the strands of protein to assume a particular shape and hold it—and so to do their specific jobs, such as enzyme work. Some of the amino acids contain sulfur in their side chains, and once built into a protein strand, these amino acids can link to each other by way of sulfur-sulfur bridges. The bridges stabilize the protein structure. Skin, hair, and nails contain some of the body's more rigid proteins, and these have a high sulfur content.

There is no recommended intake for sulfur, and no deficiencies are known. Only if a person lacks protein to the point of severe deficiency will he lack the sulfur-containing amino acids.

Magnesium

Magnesium barely qualifies as a major mineral. Only about 1 3/4 oz are present in the body of a 130-pound person. Most of this is in the bones. Bone magnesium seems to be a storage reservoir to ensure that some will be on hand for vital reactions regardless of recent dietary intake.

Magnesium also acts in all the cells of the soft tissues, where it forms part of the protein-making machinery and where it is necessary for the release of energy. Its major role seems to be as a catalyst in the reaction that adds the last high-energy phosphate bond to ATP. Magnesium also helps relax muscles after contraction and promotes resistance to tooth decay by holding calcium in tooth enamel.

A dietary deficiency of magnesium does not seem likely, but deficiency may occur as a result of vomiting, diarrhea, alcoholism, or protein malnutrition; in postsurgical patients who have been fed incomplete fluids into a vein for too long; or in people using diuretics.

It is interesting to note that in areas with a high magnesium content in the water supply, there is a lower incidence of sudden death from heart failure.[6] A severe deficiency causes tetany, an extreme and prolonged contraction of the muscles very much like the reaction of the muscles when calcium levels fall. Magnesium deficit is also thought to cause the hallucinations experienced by alcoholics during withdrawal from alcohol.

Recommended intakes of magnesium are 300 to 350 mg a day for adult males, 250 to 300 mg for females. The amounts in foods have not been thoroughly studied as yet, but good food sources include nuts, legumes, cereal grains, dark-green vegetables, seafoods, chocolate, and cocoa. The kidney acts to conserve magnesium; that not absorbed is excreted in the feces.

The RDA for magnesium: 350 mg for men, 300 mg for women.

Canadian Dietary Standard: 300 mg for men, 250 mg for women.

[6]M. S. Seelig and H. A. Heggtreit, Magnesium interrelationships in ischemic heart disease: A review, *American Journal of Clinical Nutrition* 27 (1974):59-79.

Summing Up

Of the major minerals—calcium, phosphorus, potassium, sulfur, sodium, chlorine, and magnesium—calcium was selected for emphasis in this chapter because the risks of deficiency are the greatest. About 99 percent of the body's calcium is a structural component of the bones and teeth; these structures, in addition to their obvious roles, serve as a reserve to help maintain blood calcium at a constant concentration. The 1 percent of body calcium found in body fluids helps maintain cell membrane integrity, intercellular cohesion, transport of substances into and out of cells, and transmission of nerve impulses. It is also an essential factor for blood clotting and acts as a cofactor in some enzyme systems.

Ionic calcium concentration in the blood is held constant by equilibrium between free and bound calcium and by the hormones parathormone and calcitonin (with the help of vitamin D). Abnormal calcium concentrations in blood reflect abnormal amounts of these hormones or of vitamin D in the system; a lack of dietary calcium has its impact on bone, not blood.

Calcium deficiency in the body may be caused directly by inadequate calcium intakes over a prolonged period of time or indirectly by vitamin D deficiency, which suppresses calcium absorption. The diseases that result are rickets, osteomalacia, and osteoporosis, which are described in Chapter 11.

The recommended calcium intake is easily met by consuming 2 c or more of milk or equivalent dairy products such as cheese; fortified soy milk is an alternative in the case of milk allergy or lactose intolerance. The only other rich food source of calcium is dark-green leafy vegetables, 1 c cooked greens being equivalent to 1 c milk in calcium content. Daily consumption of calcium-containing foods is preferable to infrequent large amounts.

Phosphorus, another major mineral, is abundant in foods, and therefore deficiencies are highly unlikely. It participates with calcium in forming the crystals of bone and therefore composes a large proportion of the minerals found in the body.

Sodium is also abundant in the diet, as part of salt, and is efficiently handled by the body. Deficiencies are rare except in dehydration. Genetically sensitive people may develop high blood pressure in response to too-high sodium intakes; control of dietary salt is recommended for these people. Chlorine, also part of salt, contributes to the formation of the stomach's hydrochloric acid. Both sodium and potassium are important in body fluids (see Chapter 14).

Potassium, which can also form salts, is primarily involved in the working of nerve and muscle cells. A deficiency caused by protein deprivation or dehydration can stop the heart; excess potassium is also dangerous.

Sulfur, like phosphorus, is a major mineral constituent of body tissues. It is abundant in the diet, and deficiencies are unknown.

Magnesium plays a role in the synthesis of body proteins and so is in a key position with respect to all body functions. It is seldom found lacking in human beings, except in conditions that aggravate dietary protein deficiency, such as kwashiorkor and alcoholism. A deficiency of magnesium causes severe neuromuscular and cardiovascular disorders.

To Explore Further

The general references listed in Appendix J contain additional information on all the minerals covered in this chapter, and they also lead to further reading.

Nutrition Labeling

[If a] shopper is thoughtful, . . . [he] scratches his head. How much thiamin, he asks himself, is .09 mg?

RONALD M. DEUTSCH

Would you buy an article of clothing if the merchant would not let you see its size, color, or fabric? Not likely. If it was attractively packaged, with a picture of the garment on the outside, and it assured you that "one size fits all" would you buy it? Maybe. However, if you became disenchanted with this type of packaging, you would demand to see inside the package before you paid your money.

This is the situation that consumers of food products found themselves in some years ago. They were buying new products on the basis of advertising claims and continuing to use them if the taste, quality, convenience, or price were right. But as consumers became more knowledgeable about nutrition, they realized that qualities such as taste and price were not satisfactory guidelines and that they needed knowledge about the nutrients contained in the food products before they paid their money. Advertising claims

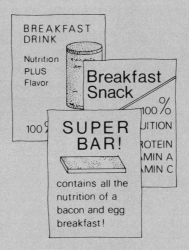

that a product was a substitute for breakfast (see Highlight 1) were not satisfactory to the new breed of consumer. The smart consumer read the fine print that listed the ingredients and understood that they were listed in descending order of predominance—but then wanted to know more. If sugar was listed in first place, the buyer wanted to know, "How much sugar?"

As the new consumer evolved, advertisers of food products responded quickly. They touted the nutritional superiority of their products: high in protein, low in kcalories, more polyunsaturates, builds bones and teeth, provides energy for active children, a substitute for dairy products, and many other such claims. The advertisers knew that good nutrition had become a salable item. Many new products came on the market—convenience foods and imitations of traditional foods—that were not familiar to the consumer, who was forced to

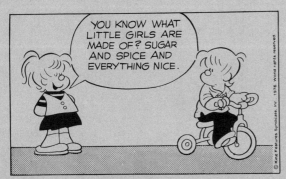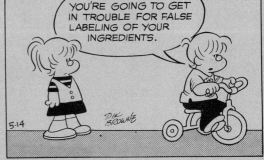

rely solely on advertising blurbs or label statements about these foods because there was no other source of information. Nutrition educators became concerned over the misinformation that was being promulgated in pseudo-scientific advertisements.

These developments and others led to the recognition that today's buyers need to "see inside the package" before they pay their money. In other words, consumers should be protected by their government from fraudulent advertising and label claims, especially in an area as vital to good health as food purchases. However, the objections of manufacturers and processors, that the revelation of their recipes would be an unfair trade practice, also needed to be resolved.

Thus it came about that the White House Conference on Food, Nutrition, and Health of 1969 recommended that the FDA develop nutrition labeling. Several studies by government, industry, university research departments, and consumer groups followed to determine the type of information that would be most meaningful to the consumer. One of these studies found that not many people would make direct use of nutrition information on labels. But of 4,400 people interviewed during the study, 88 percent thought such labeling was desirable and 98

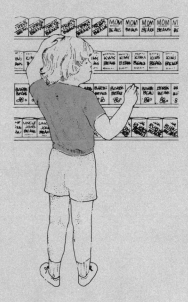

percent thought that consumers had a right to have the nutritional information available, whether or not they used it to make wiser choices.[1]

The combined efforts of manufacturers, educators, consumers, and the FDA resulted in the publication of new food labeling regulations in 1972, to which the public was asked to respond. In 1973, the final regulations were published with full compliance required by 1976.[2] Three sections dealt with nutrition, an area that was relatively new to FDA regulations. The three were nutrition labeling, nutritional

quality guidelines, and imitation foods.[3]

Nutrition Labeling

Authority for the government to move into the field of nutrition labeling comes from the Food, Drug, and Cosmetic Act of 1938. Regulations under this act require that labels state:[4]

● The common name of the product.

● The name and address of the manufacturer, packer, or distributor.

● The net contents in terms of weight, measure, or count.

● The ingredients listed in order of descending predominance.

However, in conforming to these regulations, manufacturers often printed the information in type too small to be read and placed it in an inconspicuous part of the label.

In 1966 Congress passed the Fair Packaging Labeling Act which required, in part, that information for the consumer's use be put in a prominent place on the label and that words used to convey this information be those ordinarily used. For instance, adjectives such as *economy* or

[1]M. L. Ross, What's happening to food labeling? *Journal of the American Dietetic Association* 64 (1974):262-267.
[2]*Federal Register* 38 (January 19, 1973):2131.

[3]O.C. Johnson, The Food and Drug Administration and labeling, *Journal of the American Dietetic Association* 64 (1974):471-475.
[4]Ross, 1974.

giant could not be used to describe the size of the package, because they do not ordinarily have a size connotation.[5] With these new regulations, labels began to be much more informative than in the past.

As the various interested groups were designing the new nutrition labels, they discovered that "percentage of RDA" was the most meaningful way to express amounts to consumers. But which value of the RDA tables should be used? Obviously, to include values for all the ages and both sexes would make the label unwieldy. This led to the introduction of a new term: U.S. RDA. The U.S. RDA is "the highest value for each nutrient given in the RDA tables for males and nonpregnant, nonlactating females, 4 or more years of age, except for calcium, phosphorus, biotin, pantothenic acid, copper, and zinc."[6] Thus the U.S. RDA for iron is 18 mg, because this is the RDA for adult females who have the highest need. The U.S. RDA for riboflavin is 1.7 mg, because this is the RDA for adult males who have the highest need.

The U.S. RDAs for calcium and phosphorus are not quite as high as the highest values in the RDA tables but were set at 1 g each because of their bulk and solubility and the wide variability in age-

[5]Ross, 1974.

[6]*Federal Register*, January 19, 1973.

Mini-Glossary

FDA: Food and Drug Administration.

imitation food: a substitute for a food that is nutritionally inferior, as defined by law, to the food imitated.

nutrient density: a characteristic of a food such that it provides a high quantity (relative to need) of one or more nutrients with a small quantity (relative to need) of kcalories. Among measures of nutrient density are the NCBR (nutrient-kcalorie benefit ratio) and the INQ (index of nutritional quality).

RDA tables: tables of the Recommended Dietary Allowances for 17 distinct age-sex groups (inside front cover).

Standard of Identity: a published standard stating what ingredients must be in a product and in what amounts, if the product is to bear a certain name; the name alone may then be listed on the label without a listing of ingredients.

U.S. RDA: a table of the maximum values from the RDA tables, used as a standard for statements of the nutrient content of foods on labels (see Table 1).

---

based requirements. Biotin, pantothenic acid, copper, and zinc had not been included in the RDA tables but were generally recognized as essential for human nutrition. The FDA believed that setting amounts for these nutrients would allow manufacturers

to list them if they wished to do so. It was expected that the values would be amended as more information on human nutrition became available.[7] In fact, these nutrients were included in the revised RDA tables of 1980; however, the values for the U.S. RDA remained the same (see Table 1).

The FDA's Bureau of Foods, Nutrition and Food Sciences, which has the responsibility for publishing the U.S. RDA, did not revise the U.S. RDA for several reasons. From a regulatory standpoint the current values are satisfactory. Since the higher 1968 RDAs are safe to consume and since there is always the possibility that the public might think of the RDAs as maximums (which would result in poor diets) the FDA felt it was wise to stay with the 1968 values.

Also, it would cost the industry a lot of money to relabel all the food packages now ready for distribution. A third reason was the confusion which would result for foods labeled as either "enriched" or "fortified." Nutrients inserted at levels higher than 50 percent in a food now must be labeled as "supplement." By lowering the U.S. RDA to agree with the 1980 RDAs some "enriched" and "fortified" foods might end up as "supplements" and so be subject to further regulations and defi-

[7]*Federal Register*, January 19, 1973.

Table 1.   U.S. Recommended Daily Allowances (U.S. RDA's) for Essential Nutrients[*]

Nutrients which MUST be declared on the label:[†]	Infants Birth to 12 months (Tentative)	Children Under 4 Years of Age	Adults and Children 4 or More Years of Age	Pregnant or Lactating Women
Protein (g), PER ≥ casein	20	45	45	45
Protein (g), PER < casein	28	65	65	65
Vitamin A (IU)	1,500	2,500	5,000	8,000
Vitamin C (ascorbic acid) (mg)	35	45	60	60
Thiamin (vitamin B_1) (mg)	0.5	0.7	1.5	1.7
Riboflavin (vitamin B_2) (mg)	0.6	0.8	1.7	2.0
Niacin (mg)	8	9	20	20
Calcium (g)	0.6	0.8	1.0	1.3
Iron (mg)	15	10	18	18
Nutrients which MAY be declared on the label:				
Vitamin D (IU)	400	400	400	400
Vitamin E (IU)	5	10	30	30
Vitamin B_6 (mg)	0.4	0.7	2.0	2.5
Folic acid (folacin) (mg)	0.1	0.2	0.4	0.8
Vitamin B_{12} (μg)	2	3	6	8
Phosphorus (g)	0.5	0.8	1.0	1.3
Iodine (μg)	45	70	150	150
Magnesium (mg)	70	200	400	450
Zinc (mg)	5	8	15	15
Copper (mg)	0.6	1	2	2
Biotin (mg)	0.05	0.15	0.3	0.3
Pantothenic acid (mg)	3	5	10	10

[*]Adapted from *Food Technology* 28(7):5, 1974
[†]Whenever nutrition labeling is required

nitions. Whenever new regulations are costly to industry, the cost is borne ultimately by the consumer. The FDA did not believe that changing the U.S. RDA would result in a benefit that was worth the rise in price.

You will notice that the U.S. RDA for protein in Table 1 gives two values. The manufacturer may use the lower value as a standard if the protein in the product is of high quality (PER equal to or greater than the PER of casein, the protein of milk). If the protein is of lower quality (PER less than that of casein), the higher U.S. RDA has to be used. This rule is an advantage to the consumer who should not be expected to understand these distinctions.

Table 1 shows that there are four different U.S RDAs. The set of figures in the third column is the one seen on most labels. This set is intended to express the nutrient contents of foods in terms of the allowances for adults and children four years of age and older. The other three are for products intended for special categories of people: infants under one year of age, children under four years of age, and pregnant or lactating women.

The four sets of U.S. RDAs have survived much court litigation in which many other labeling proposals have fallen by the wayside. The U.S. RDA for adults promises to be the standard on nutrition labels for years to come and is the single set of figures most understandable by the public. The more varied and specific RDA figures will continue to be used for research.

Several types of claims on labels are forbidden: (1) that a food is effective as a treatment for a disease; (2) that a balanced diet of ordinary foods cannot supply adequate amounts of nutrients (excepting the iron requirements of infants, children, and pregnant or lactating women); (3) that the soil on which food is grown may be responsible for deficiencies in quality; (4) that storage, transportation, processing, or cooking of a food may be responsible for deficiencies in its quality; (5) that a food has particular dietary qualities when such qualities have not been shown to be significant in human nutrition; and (6) that a natural vitamin is superior to a synthetic vitamin.[8]

Manufacturers of food products have the freedom to add or not add nutrients to their products and to advertise or not advertise the nutritional superiority of such products. However, if they decide to add the nutrient (for example, adding vitamin C to a breakfast drink) or to

[8]M. Stephenson, Making food labels more informative, *FDA Consumer* 9(8) (1975):13-17.

advertise its nutritional qualities (for example, advertising orange juice as a source of vitamin C) then they must comply *fully* with the nutrition labeling regulations. Without this complete information panel, nutrition claims could deceive the consumer about the true nutritional value of a food.

If any nutrition information or claim is made on the label of a food package, it must conform to the following format under the heading "Nutrition Information":

● Serving or portion size

● Servings or portions per container

● Calorie content per serving

● Protein grams per serving

● Carbohydrate grams per serving

● Fat grams per serving

(When fatty acid composition is declared, the information must be placed on the label immediately adjacent to the statement on fat content; when cholesterol content is declared, the information must immediately follow the

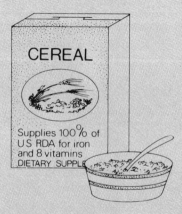

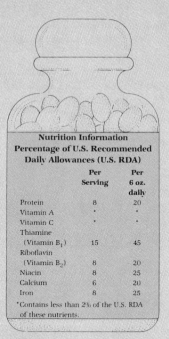

Nutrition Information
Percentage of U.S. Recommended
Daily Allowances (U.S. RDA)

	Per Serving	Per 6 oz. daily
Protein	8	20
Vitamin A	*	*
Vitamin C	*	*
Thiamine (Vitamin B$_1$)	15	45
Riboflavin (Vitamin B$_2$)	8	20
Niacin	8	25
Calcium	6	20
Iron	8	25

*Contains less than 2% of the U.S. RDA of these nutrients.

statement on fat content— and fatty acid content, if stated.)

● Protein, vitamins, and minerals as percentages of the U.S. RDAs (No claim may be made that a food is a significant source of a nutrient unless it provides at least 10 percent of the U.S. RDA of that nutrient in a serving. No claim may be made that a food is nutritionally superior to another food unless it contains at least 10 percent more of the U.S. RDA of the claimed nutrient per serving.)[9]

Nutritional Quality Guidelines Guidelines for the regulation of nutritional quality have been proposed by the FDA for such highly processed foods as frozen

[9]*Federal Register* 38 (March 14, 1973):6950.

CEREAL

Supplies 100% of U.S RDA for iron and 8 vitamins DIETARY SUPPLE

Table 2. Required Nutrient Content of Highly Processed Foods Such as Frozen Dinners*

Nutrient	For Each 100 Calories Required Components	For the Combined Required Components Regardless of Calories
Protein, grams	4.60	16.0
Vitamin A, IU	150.00	520.0
Thiamin, mg	0.05	0.2
Riboflavin, mg	0.06	0.2
Niacin, mg	0.99	3.4
Pantothenic acid, mg	0.32	1.1
Vitamin B_6, mg	0.15	0.5
Vitamin B_{12}, μg	0.33	1.1
Iron, mg	0.62	2.2

*Stephenson, M.: Making food labels more informative. *FDA Consumer* 9(8):13-17, 1975.

dinners; breakfast cereals; meal replacements; noncarbonated, vitamin C-fortified fruit or vegetable beverages; and main dishes such as pizza or macaroni and cheese.

For frozen dinners, there must be at least three components: one or more sources of protein from meat, poultry, fish, cheese, or eggs and these must make up at least 70 percent of the total protein; potatoes, rice or a cereal-based product; one or more vegetables or vegetable mixtures other than potatoes, rice, or cereal-based products; and the dinner must have a minimum nutrient level of several nutrients for each 100 kcal, according to Table 2.

Under the Food, Drug and Cosmetic Act, foods given Standards of Identity are exempt from listing the mandatory ingredients, although many manufacturers do so voluntarily. Standards of Identity have been issued for such foods as bread and mayonnaise—common foods which at one time were usually prepared at home and for which the basic recipe was understood by almost everyone. Certain ingredients must be present in a specified percentage in order for the food to use the standard name. For example, any product called mayonnaise must contain 65 percent by weight vegetable oil, either vinegar or lemon juice, and egg yolk.[10] The FDA does not now have the authority to require that the mandatory ingredients be listed in standardized foods. However, it is urging manufacturers to provide more detailed information.

[10]Stephenson, 1975.

The terms *enriched* and *fortified* are used in the titles of some Standards of Identity, like those for enriched bread. Separate definitions for enriched and fortified were deleted in 1980 but the titles still must be used for specific standards. In the Standards, enriched has generally meant the addition of specific nutrients so that the final product will have the levels of the nutrients that the original food had before processing. Fortified generally has meant the addition of nutrients that were not necessarily found in the food originally, or the addition of nutrients in amounts well in excess of those normally found. Sometimes the food selected for fortification is a food which contains other nutrients and its value is enhanced by the added nutrient—as when milk is fortified with vitamin D to aid in the absorption of its calcium. At other times—as in the case of vitamin C-fortified beverages—there may be few nutrients present except for those added. The alert consumer should realize that the word *fortified* refers only to the specific nutrient added. Thus orange juice contains more nutrients than most vitamin C-fortified fruit drinks, even though the drinks may be higher in vitamin C content.

Imitation Foods A section of the original Food, Drug and Cosmetic Act of 1938 re-

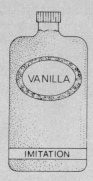

quired that a food that was an imitation of a traditional food must state this fact on its label. With new food technology, many food products on the market may not be nutritionally inferior to traditional foods. It is misleading to the consumer for these to be called imitation because the word implies that the product is inferior. For this reason, recent FDA regulations require that the word *imitation* be used on the label only if the product is "a substitute for and resembles another food but is nutritionally inferior to the food imitated." Nutritional inferiority is defined as any reduction in the content of an essential vitamin or mineral or of protein that is present in a measureable amount where there is no reduction in the caloric or fat content.[11]

Thus if you read *imitation* on a label, you should consider the product carefully. This may be of no consequence in a food that usually would not be depended on for nutrients like the flavoring, vanilla. But if it is a fruit

[11]*Federal Register*, January 19, 1973.

drink which you consume daily, and if you usually include no other fruits or vegetables in your diet, then the label may alert you to a needed change.

Nutrition Labels of the Future The labeling regulations are revised and added to as consumers express new labeling needs, and as new technologies create problems unmet by the old regulations. While this book is in print, new regulations will doubtless come into being that change or add to what is being said here. But it seems important, nevertheless, to clarify the current regulations which affect the issues that knowledgeable consumers and nutritionists are most concerned about at the present time.

Nutrition Today carried a debate about labeling in which D. M. Hegsted, a well-recognized authority in nutrition, stated that the average consumer might be led to feel, erroneously, that a product claiming to give him 100 percent of the U.S. RDA would allow him to then forget about nutrition.[12] That impression, of course, could be misleading to the consumer. However, even with that possibility, no nutritionist proposes that labeling be abandoned. The crux of

[12]D. M. Hegsted and L. M. Ausman versus R. J. Williams, Nutrition contretemps (a debate), *Nutrition Today*, March/April 1974, pp. 9-10, 29-30.

the matter is for the ordinary person to be able to interpret the labels and use them for his benefit.

Some claims now made in advertising and on labels are true and are within the law but may not reveal all of the facts of interest to consumers and may then be misleading. For example, the label on a fabricated food may claim that the amounts of protein, fat, carbohydrate, and certain vitamins and minerals are the same as those found in a meal of traditional foods. The label would not usually mention other differences such as: the carbohydrate may be mostly sugar (in comparison to the complex carbohydrates in the original, imitated food), or there may be more salt in the fabricated food, or the traditional foods contain nutrients other than those required on a nutrition label. An example of this kind of food— breakfast bars—was described in Highlight 1.

Nutritionists know of the existence of many nutrients that are needed in the diet. The ones listed on labels are only indicator nutrients; if they are present you can generally assume that others are also. However, in fabricated foods these other important nutrients may not be present in the same amounts as in the traditional foods and some may be totally absent.

A desirable solution might be to relieve the consumer altogether of the burden of reading labels by allowing certain foods to state that they are nutritious. If the word *nutritious* were given a legal meaning and prohibited from being used except within the confines of that meaning, then judging the nutritional value of a food might be easier for consumers. As you might expect, a number of proposals for this definition have already been made. All such proposals make use of the concept of nutrient density.

The object is to distinguish between nourishing foods— those that provide some nutrients besides kcalories— and *nutritious foods*, a term which requires a very precise definition. One version shows the definition as having two parts:

● Each nutrient in the food is scored against the kcalories in the food. If a serving of the food provides 10 percent of the RDA for kcalories but 30 percent of the RDA for vitamin C, then it gets a 30/10 score—or a 3—for vitamin C.

● If the food has a score of 1 for at least four nutrients or a score of 2 for at least two nutrients, it can be defined as a nutritious food.

Obviously, the manufacturer could add a few nutrients to almost any food to achieve good scores, so that possibility has to be ruled out:

● Such a term can be applied "only to food derived directly or indirectly from animal or vegetable products which can be expected to supply small but important amounts of many other naturally occurring essential nutrients and which have not been fortified to levels more than 15 percent above those of their unprocessed forms."[13]

This proposal illustrates the kind of guidelines by which labels of the future may be simplified, or by which you may measure the nutritional value of the foods you select for yourself. The scores given to foods have been called the NCBR (nutrient-calorie benefit ratio) or INQ (index of nutritional quality), and the details of how they are calculated are still being worked out. But they all have the same objective: to help you distinguish between truly nutritious foods and those whose stated value is inflated. Recognizing nutrient density, you will be able to choose foods with greater sophistication than if you were simply to reject all processed foods and embrace all natural, unprocessed foods. An exercise in the use of this concept is presented at the end of this Highlight.

Supplements   The labeling of vitamin and mineral supplements also comes under the jurisdiction of the FDA. The idea that there need be no concern about high or excessive consumption of vitamin and mineral supplements because excesses are excreted is misleading.[14] The great majority of the research of the past 30 years has been directed toward defining the requirements and the biochemical mechanisms of their functioning and almost no work has concerned the effects of either acute or chronic consumption of elevated levels of supplemental nutrients.

It is well known that the fat-soluble vitamins A and D, when excess amounts are consumed for prolonged periods, have adverse effects. The consumption of the water-soluble vitamins at elevated levels appears to be less dangerous; but the relative rarity of reported adverse effects must be balanced by the relative rarity of research directed toward study of the hazard/benefit of regular consumption of therapeutic (or higher) dosages of these nutrients. Mineral toxicities are reasonably well known and combination supplements (vitamins and minerals) rarely exceed 150-200 percent of the recommended daily allowances; but multiple consumption from a variety of products, each containing the recommended allowance, should be viewed with concern and hesitancy.

[13]H. A. Guthrie, Concept of a nutritious food, *Journal of the American Dietetic Association* 71 (1977):14-19.

[14]Vitamins, minerals and FDA, *FDA Consumer*, reprinted by the Department of Health, Education, and Welfare, publication no. (FDA) 74-2001 (Washington, D.C.: Government Printing Office, 1973).

Back in the early 1960s there appeared to be a real nutrient-power race underway, both in the proliferation of supplements and the addition to foods. In an attempt to maintain rationality in this trend, the FDA proposed a standard for vitamin/mineral supplement products. Considering the state of knowledge then (and now) the proposal was quite conservative, requiring the presence of most essential nutrients in a balanced potency range between 50 and 150 percent of the daily recommendations. Potencies or combinations beyond those of the standard would not be available as over-the-counter (nonprescription) drugs in the same manner as aspirin, mouth washes, or laxatives. There were many objections to the proposal, so after more than 10 years, including 2 years of hearings, a tentative final regulation was published but it was still viewed as too conservative and restrictive.

Legal appeals and Congressional action resulted in very substantial changes in the restrictiveness of the standard. The essence of those actions was to define the supplements as food and, for adults (12 years and older, not pregnant or lactating), removed the potency and combination limits unless the FDA could prove toxicity.[15]

During this interval, vita-

mins A and D were placed in a prescription category if the potency exceeded 10,000 IU and 400 IU, respectively. Court action also brought about the removal of that requirement. As of 1980, the standard and its associated labeling requirements, such as changing to U.S. RDA from the old MDR (minimum daily requirements), and dating are still not final regulations.

The arguments for and against such regulation by the FDA center around an evolving concept of what constitutes a drug. When a person takes a vitamin capsule in amounts that would be the equivalent of, say, a gallon of food, is that person taking a vitamin supplement or a drug? Of course, the second issue, personal freedom (and its counterpart, personal responsibility), is an emotionally charged one, and it is difficult to decide at what point a government agency should step in to protect a private citizen against the consequences of his own actions.

Highlight 13 examines other substances that come under the surveillance of the FDA. There, too, you will see the conflict between principles of government protection and the exercise of personal freedom.

To Explore Further

A good discussion of how food is improved by enrichment, resto-

ration, and fortification appears in Improvement of the nutritive quality of foods, *Journal of the American Medical Association* 225 (1973):1116-1118. Reprint requests should be made to the American Medical Association (address in Appendix J).

Dr. Harper is recognized as an authority on nutrition labeling:

Harper, A. E., Nutritional regulations and legislation: Past developments, future implications, *Journal of the American Dietetic Association* 71 (1977):601-609.

The final policy statement on Nutritional Quality of Food by the Food and Drug Administration was published in:

Federal Register 45 (January 25, 1980):6314-6324.

Advertising must also concern nutrition educators:

Schwartzberg, L., George, C., and Phillips, M. C., Issues in food advertising: The nutrition educator's viewpoint, *Journal of Nutrition Education* 9 (1977):60-63.

To size up the new foods and for help in designing a healthful diet, the interested reader will find these two paperbacks useful:

Fremes, R., and Sabry, Z., *Nutriscore: The Rate-Yourself Plan for Better Nutrition* (New York: Methuen/Two Continents, 1976).

Jacobson, M. F., *Nutrition Scoreboard* (New York: Avon Books, 1974).

For a comprehensive scoring of many foods on the basis of their nutrient density, *Nutrition and the MD* recommends:

Hanse, R. G., *Index of Nutritional Quality Food Profiles*.

[15]*Federal Register* 43 (March 14, 1978):10,552.

This 184-page book is available for $10.80 from the Utah State University Bookstore, Utah State University, UMC 01, Logan, UT 84322.

A miniversion of the same kind of effort is Gifft, H., *Guide to Nutritive Value.* This is a 2-page chart, showing nutrients as a percentage of the U.S. RDA in common foods, that uses shading to indicate a significant source of a nutrient. It is available for $.25 from Mailing Room 7, Research Park, Cornell University, Ithaca, NY 14853.

For help in reading labels, many booklets are available. One we like is *Inside Information about the Outside of the Package*, available free from Pillsbury Company, 1177 Pillsbury Building, 608 Second Avenue South, Minneapolis, MN 55402.

A helpful cassette is *A Practical Nutrient Density-Nutritional Quality Index for Food*, by B. Wyse, R. G. Hansen, and A. W. Sorenson, available from the American Dietetic Association (address in Appendix J). The Association also makes available a cassette, *Food Labeling*, prepared by M. Robinson.

Look up and record your recommended intake of calcium (from the RDA tables on the inside front cover or from the Canadian Dietary Standard in Appendix O). Also record your actual intake, from the average derived on Form 2 (p. 16). What percentage of your recommended intake did you consume? Was this enough? What foods contribute the greatest amount of calcium to your diet? If you consumed more than the recommendation, was this too much? Why or why not? In what ways would you change your diet to improve it in this respect?

Optional Extras

● Compute your sodium intake, using Appendix I. A dietary goal quoted in Chapter 12 is to restrict added salt intake to 5 g a day or less. This means 2 g (2,000 mg) sodium in the added salt. (By

SELF-STUDY

Major Minerals

"added salt," we mean salt added in processing or by you in cooking or at the table. It is assumed that foods you eat already contain about 3 g naturally occuring salt. So in calculating, count only the sodium you find in processed foods and in the salt shaker.)

Is your salt intake ample? Excessive? Should you consider making any changes, and if so, what kind?

Some authorities feel that the dietary goal for sodium should not apply to everyone but only to those who have a hereditary tendency toward heart disease, especially hypertension. Are these conditions characteristic of your family? The quiz in Highlight

6 (p. 209) gives you a means of estimating your risk of heart disease. The higher your score on that quiz, the more critical your sodium intake probably is.

● Find alternative calcium sources for someone who doesn't drink milk. Plan a day's menus around this person's favorite foods.

● Consider nature's arrangement of nutrients in foods: Phosphorus is critical in the transfer of energy, the structure of genetic material, the transport of substances across cell membranes, the structure of the skeleton, and the maintenance of the acid-base balance. It is so widespread in foods that we need not worry about suffering a deficiency. Why is this? Can you see any evolutionary reason why this vital nutrient should happen to be so abundant in the animal and plant tissues that we use as food?

Nutrient Density

Highlight 12 describes food labels and the need for consumers to know how nutritious the foods are that they buy. The concept of nutrient density helps people estimate the nutritional value of foods. Using this concept, you can decide which of your favorite foods are the most nutritious.

Pick a food, any food you are curious about, and follow this procedure using Form 1 to record the information:

1. Record your recommended kcalorie intake and your recommended intakes for protein, vitamins, and minerals from the inside front cover or from Appendix O. (The Self-Study at the end of Highlight 7 directed you to calculate how much energy you need for a typical day. You could use this personalized calculation in place of your recommended kcalorie intake if you feel it is more accurate.)

2. Look up in Appendix H the number of kcalories

Form 1. Nutrient Density of a Food

Food chosen for analysis: _____

		Energy (kcal)	Protein (g)	Calcium (mg)	Iron (mg)	Vitamin A (IU)	Thiamin (mg)	Riboflavin* (mg)	Vitamin C (mg)
1	Your recommended intake								
2	Amount provided by one serving of the food								
	Percentage of recommended intake provided by 1 serving	(3) Comparison number	4						4
5	Nutrition score								

6. Is the food nutritious? _____

*A complete calculation would include niacin, but we have omitted it because of the difficulty in estimating niacin derived from tryptophan (see Chapter 9).

and the amounts of protein, vitamins, and minerals provided by a serving of the food you are interested in, and list these numbers under your recommended intakes.

3) Determine what percentage of your recommended intake for kcalories a serving of the food provides. This will be your comparison number.

4) Determine what percentage of your recommended intake a serving of the food provides for each nutrient.

5) Divide each percentage derived for the nutrients by the comparison number to give each nutrient a score.

6) By the standard suggested in Highlight 12, the food is nutritious if it receives a score greater than 1 for each of four nutrients or greater than 2 for each of two. By this standard, how nutritious is the food you selected?

Repeat this procedure several times to study a variety of the foods in your diet that you are curious about.

Finally, review your food records (p. 14) and list from them the foods that made the major contributions to your kcalorie intakes on the days you studied. Jot down by each food your reason for choosing it:

● Personal preference (I like it)

● Social pressure (it was offered; I couldn't refuse)

● Familiarity (I often eat it)

● Availability (I was hungry and it was the only food offered)

● Economy (it was the only food I could afford)

● Convenience (I was too rushed to prepare anything else)

● Nutritional value (I thought it was good for me)

● Other (explain)

From what you know now, you can make a good guess about the nutritive value of each of these foods. In some cases you will find that a food chosen primarily because it tastes good to you is also nutritious—a happy surprise. In others, you may find that a food you thought was nutritious is not especially noteworthy in this sense. Such insights can help guide you toward food selections that meet your needs for pleasure as well as for good nutrition.

Optional Extra

You may want to know if the U.S. RDA used on labels is similar to your own RDA, so that the label information applies to you. Jot down your RDA for each nutrient from the inside front cover, and the U.S. RDA from Table 1 in Highlight 12 and compare them. Which of your RDAs are out of line with the U.S. RDA? (For example, a food that contains only 50 percent of the U.S. RDA for iron would contain almost 100 percent of a man's iron RDA.)

CHAPTER 13

CONTENTS

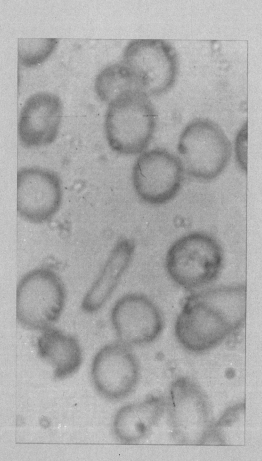

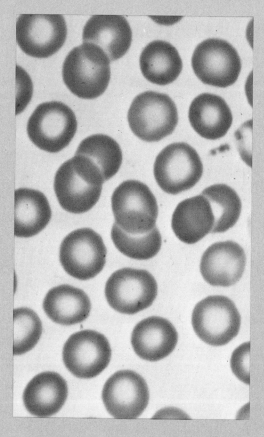

Blood cells in iron-deficiency anemia.

Normal blood cells.

THE TRACE MINERALS

If you could remove all of the trace minerals from your body, you would have only a bit of dust, hardly enough to fill a teaspoon. You would also die instantly. Although present in tiny quantities, each of the trace minerals performs some vital role for which no substitute will do. A deficiency of any of them may be fatal, and an excess of many is equally deadly. Remarkably, the way you eat and the way your body handles these minerals enables you to maintain a supply that is just sufficient for health and within the limits of toxicity.

Laboratory techniques developed in the past two decades have enabled scientists to detect the minute quantities of trace minerals in living cells for the first time. Study of the "new" trace elements, using animals, is one of the most active areas of research in nutrition today. An obstacle to determining the precise role of a trace element lies in the nearly impossible task of providing an experimental diet devoid of that element. Even the dust in the air or the residue left on laboratory equipment by the rinsing water may contaminate the feed enough to prevent a deficiency. Thus research in this area is limited to the study of small laboratory animals, which can be fed highly refined, purified diets in an atmosphere free of all contamination.

The best-known trace elements—iron, iodine, and zinc—have been so thoroughly studied that we can describe many of their roles with certainty. Government authorities have established recommended daily intakes for these three. For six others, the Committee on RDA published tentative ranges for safe and adequate daily intakes for the first time in 1980. Five others are known to be essential nutrients, but the amounts needed are so tiny that they have not yet been measured. Many others are presently under study to determine whether they too perform indispensable roles in the body.

Whole books have been published just on the trace minerals.[1] In selecting the information to present in this chapter we have chosen to give most attention to those that are likely to have the greatest impact on your health. Iron, for example, is often deficient in the diets of

---

[1]For example, E. J. Underwood, *Trace Elements in Human and Animal Nutrition*, 4th ed. (New York: Academic Press, 1977).

people the world over, and an iron deficiency profoundly hurts the quality of life. Iodine is easy to obtain in adequate amounts, but simple ignorance can precipitate a deficiency, with tragic and irreversible consequences. Until recently, zinc and chromium deficiencies were unheard of, but now that we know of their existence and their effects, we see the need to help people protect themselves from these conditions too. No doubt the years to come will bring new knowledge of equal importance about some of the other trace elements, but an acquaintance with these few can enable you to take action — to select a diet composed of protective foods that will ensure adequacy for all the essential nutrients.

Iron

Of all the trace minerals, iron deserves the most attention. It is a problem nutrient for millions of people. If you want to plan and consume a diet adequate in iron, you must be well informed.

Iron in the Body   Iron is found in every cell, not only of the human body but of all living things, both plant and animal. It occurs in many vital proteins, including those involved in cell respiration and DNA synthesis. It is part of many major enzymes.

hemoglobin: the oxygen-carrying protein of the red blood cells.

hemo = blood
globin = globular protein

myoglobin: the oxygen-carrying protein of the muscle cells.

myo = muscle

The **ferrous** ion has a +2 charge; **ferric** iron has a +3 charge.

Most of the iron in the human body is a component of the proteins hemoglobin and myoglobin. Both these proteins carry oxygen and release it. As the cells' environments change, ionized iron can change from a +2 charge to +3 and back again, thereby releasing or holding on to oxygen, which has a −2 charge.

Hemoglobin is the oxygen carrier in the red blood cells, and its iron can have either charge. Myoglobin is in the muscle cells, and its iron can have only a +2 charge. Myoglobin therefore has a greater holding capacity for oxygen and so serves as a reservoir for oxygen; its presence in the muscle cells seems to draw oxygen into them. The muscle cells use this oxygen as the receiver for used-up carbon and hydrogen atoms flowing down the glucose-to-energy pathway. These atoms combine to make carbon dioxide and water, the final waste products of metabolism. Thus oxygen keeps the energy-yielding pathway open so that the muscles can remain active. As the muscles use up and excrete their oxygen (combined with carbons and hydrogens), the red blood cells shuttle between muscles and lungs to maintain fresh supplies.

The average red blood cell lives about four months. When it has aged and is no longer useful, it is removed from the blood by liver cells, which take it apart and prepare many of the degradation products for excretion. Its iron, however, is attached to a protein carrier. The iron is returned to the bone marrow, where new red blood cells are constantly being produced. Thus although red blood cells are born, live, and die within a four-month cycle, the iron in the body is recycled through each new generation. Only tiny amounts of iron are lost, principally in urine, sweat, and shed skin.

About 75 percent of the iron in the body is in the red blood cells, so iron losses are greatest whenever blood is lost. For this reason, "women need more iron," as a well-known television commercial proclaims: Menstruation incurs losses that make a woman's iron needs up to twice as great as a man's.

To replace the lost iron, the body provides special proteins to absorb it from food and carry it to the liver, bone marrow, and other blood-manufacturing sites. Iron absorbed into the intestinal cells from food is captured by a blood protein, transferrin, that carries it to tissues throughout the body. Each tissue takes up the amount of iron that it needs: The bone marrow and liver take large quantities, other tissues take less. In a pregnant woman, the placenta is avid for iron, devouring large quantities for delivery to the fetus even if this means depriving the mother's tissues of iron. Should there be a surplus, special storage proteins in the bone marrow and other organs store it.

transferrin (trans-FURR-in): the body's iron-carrying protein.

The storage proteins are **ferritin** (FAIR-i-tin) and **hemosiderin** (heem-oh-SID-er-in).

Iron routes in the body.

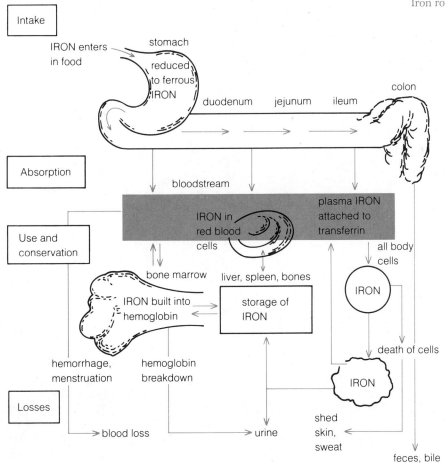

Iron clearly is the body's gold, a precious mineral to be hoarded and closely guarded. The number of special provisions for its handling show that it is as vital as calcium. At the receiving end, in the intestines, another provision shows this even more clearly. Normally only about 10 percent of dietary iron is absorbed. But if the body's supply is diminished or if the need increases for any reason, absorption increases. More transferrin (the carrier that picks up iron from the intestines) is produced so that more than the usual amount of iron can be absorbed. Only if this measure fails and the stores are used up do the red cells become depleted. Then anemia sets in.

Iron absorption responds to the body's need. (This figure does not show how the intestinal cells also help to regulate iron absorption.)

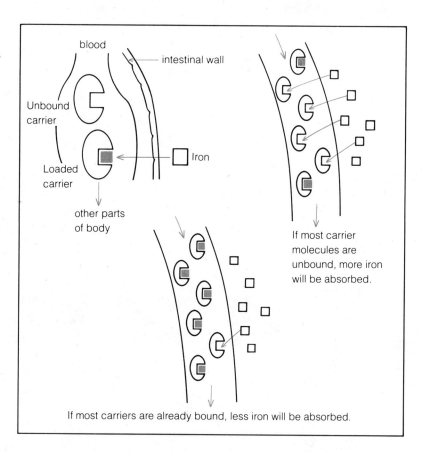

The most common tests for iron deficiency are measures of the number and size of the red blood cells and of their hemoglobin concentration. But before these levels fall, at the very beginning of an iron deficiency, the transferrin concentration *rises*. There is a sensitive test that will detect a developing iron deficiency before it is full-blown; it tests the amount of transferrin in the blood and the amount of iron that it is carrying.

Technically, this technique is known as measuring the total iron-binding capacity (TIBC) and the transferrin saturation.

For women only: You are often told that you need more iron, yet you may often have had your blood cell count or hemoglobin level pronounced normal. Does this mean that you don't need more iron? Not necessarily. The difference between you and the men you know is a difference in your body stores of iron, which doesn't show up in these tests. Most men eat more food than women do, because they are bigger, and so their iron intakes are higher. Besides, women menstruate, and so their iron losses are greater. These two factors—lower intakes and higher losses—put you much closer to the borderline of deficiency. Even though you may never have been diagnosed as iron-deficient, you are likely to be deficiency-prone. Should you lose blood for any reason (even by giving a blood donation) or become pregnant (so that your blood volume would need to increase), you would need to pay special attention to your diet in an effort to maintain your iron stores. The information about iron in foods, which appears later in this chapter, is especially important for you.

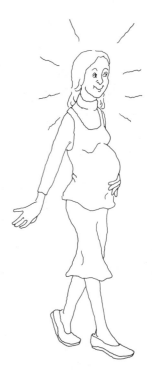

Iron-Deficiency Anemia If iron stores are exhausted, the body cannot make enough hemoglobin to fill its new red blood cells. Without enough hemoglobin, the cells are small. Since hemoglobin is the bright red pigment of the blood, the skin of a fair person who is anemic may become noticeably pale. A sample of iron-deficient blood examined under the microscope shows smaller cells that are a lighter red than normal (see the photograph at the start of this chapter). The undersized cells can't carry enough oxygen from the lungs to the tissues, so energy release in the cells is hindered. Every cell of the body feels this effect; the result is fatigue, weakness, headaches, and apathy.

Long before the mass of the red blood cells is affected, however, a developing iron deficiency may affect other body tissues, including the brain. As researchers have become better acquainted with iron, they have learned that it plays roles in the body, including brain functions, not earlier appreciated. For example, iron works with an enzyme that helps to make neurotransmitters, the substances that carry messages from one nerve cell to another. Children deprived of iron show some psychological disturbances, such as hyperactivity, decreased attentiveness, and even reduced IQ. These symptoms are among the first to appear when the body's iron level begins to fall and among the first to disappear when iron intake is increased again.[2]

In a dark-skinned person, this symptom can be observed by looking in the corner of the eye. The eye lining, normally pink, will be very pale, even white.

Iron-deficiency anemia is a **microcytic** (my-cro-SIT-ic) **hypochromic** (high-po-KROME-ic) **anemia.**

micro = small
cytic = cells
hypo = too little
chrom = color

[2] R. L. Leibel, Behavioral and biochemical correlates of iron deficiency: A review, *Journal of the American Dietetic Association* 71 (1977):399-404; and E. Pollitt and R. L. Leibel, Iron deficiency and behavior, *Journal of Pediatrics* 88 (1976):372-381.

Maximum treadmill work time in women with different hemoglobin levels. The numbers within the bars show how many women were tested at each level. The chart shows that the lower a woman's hemoglobin level, the less muscular work she can perform.

Adapted from G. W. Gardner, V. R. Edgerton, B. Senewiratne, R. J. Barnard, and Y. Ohira, Physical work capacity and metabolic stress in subjects with iron deficiency anemia, *American Journal of Clinical Nutrition* 30 (1977):910-917. Courtesy of the authors and publisher.

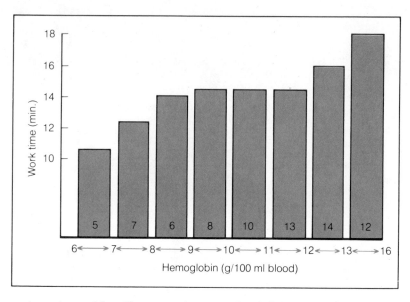

pica (PIE-ka): a craving for unnatural substances.

picus = woodpecker or magpie

A curious side effect seen in some iron-deficient subjects is an appetite for ice, clay, starch, and other nonnutritious substances. People have been known to eat as many as eight trays of ice in a day, for example. This behavior has been observed for years, especially in women and children of low-income groups, and has been given the name pica. Pica clears up dramatically within days after iron is given, long before the red blood cells respond.[3]

Muscle tissue, too, is sensitive to depletion of iron stores. By the time the stores are exhausted, work capacity begins to be profoundly affected. One study has shown this especially clearly: As women's hemoglobin levels fell from normal to half of normal, their work capacity declined in proportion. At the lowest level they were unable to do much work at all.

Many of the symptoms described here are easily mistaken for "mental" symptoms. A restless child who fails to pay attention in class might be thought contrary. An apathetic homemaker who has let her housework pile up unattended-to might be thought lazy. But the possibility is real that both these persons' problems are nutritional.

No responsible nutritionist would ever claim that all mental problems are caused by nutritional deficiencies. But nutrition is always a possible cause or contributor to problems like these. When you are seeking the solution to a behavioral problem it makes sense to check the adequacy of the diet and to have a routine physical examination before going the more expensive and involved route of consulting a mental health professional.

[3]Leibel, 1977.

It is conventional to measure the body's iron status by measuring the amount of hemoglobin (in grams per 100 milliliters of blood). The normal level is considered 14 to 15 g/100 ml for adult men, 13 to 14 g/100 ml for women. Yet many people who have values lower than this have no obvious symptoms. American blacks have average values about half a gram lower than these; it is not known whether this is a racial characteristic or is due to insufficient iron intakes. Some women have no symptoms of anemia—at least as measured by the performance of mental tasks—at levels as low as 10 g or even 8 g.[4] Doubtless people vary: One man may feel miserable with a hemoglobin of 12 g, another may feel no effects at a drastically low level of, say, 6 g: "Who, me? Anemic?"[5] Still, such symptoms as fatigue, weakness, and the like are often seen at levels not much below the standards.

When hemoglobin begins to fall, it is a sign that a long period of depletion of body stores has already occurred. In view of this fact and in light of the behavioral effects of iron deficiency in children, it seems reasonable to aim at "normal" hemoglobin levels for the general population: 14 to 15 for men, 13 to 14 for women. Values much below these represent a real hazard to health and to the quality of life.

Norms for children:

Ages 2-5	11 g/100 ml
Ages 6-12	11.5 g/100 ml

Note that hemoglobin is measured in grams per 100 ml, but we often just use the number alone in speaking of it: "Hemoglobin, 14."

A low hemoglobin level may represent a dietary iron deficiency, and if it does, the doctor may prescribe iron supplements. But the cause of an iron deficiency may be something else. For example, a vitamin B_6 deficiency can indirectly cause anemia, because B_6 is required to make the iron-containing portion of the hemoglobin molecule. A vitamin E deficiency can cause anemia by making the red blood cell membranes so fragile that the cells lose their hemoglobin. A vitamin B_{12} or folacin deficiency can cause it, because these vitamins are used in making new red blood cells to replace the old ones as they die. A vitamin C deficiency can cause it by reducing the absorption of iron.[6] Recently it has been learned that vitamin A, too, is involved in the making of red blood cells and that some people's low hemoglobin levels can be corrected only by administering vitamin A.[7]

Feeling fatigued, weak, and apathetic is a sign that something is wrong but does not indicate that you should take iron supplements. It indicates that (you guessed it!) you should consult your doctor. The doctor herself must use all her knowledge to diagnose correctly

[4]P. C. Elwood and D. Hughes, Clinical trial of iron therapy on psychomotor function in anaemic women, *British Medical Journal* 3 (1970):254-255.

[5]W. H. Crosby, Current concepts in nutrition: Who needs iron? *New England Journal of Medicine* 297 (1977):543-545.

[6]R. H. Matthews and M. Y. Workman, Nutrient content of selected baby foods, *Journal of the American Dietetic Association* 72 (1978):27-30.

[7]R. E. Hodges, H. E. Sauberlich, J. E. Canham, D. L. Wallace, R. B. Rucker, L. A. Mejia, and M. Mohanram, Hematopoietic studies in vitamin A deficiency, *American Journal of Clinical Nutrition* 31 (1978):876-885.

secondary nutrient deficiency:
one caused indirectly—not by
inadequate intake but by the
deficiency of another nutrient,
interference with absorption,
disease, or other causes.

the primary cause of a secondary anemia; you don't have a chance at
making this kind of diagnosis. In fact, taking iron supplements may
be the worst possible thing you could do, because they may mask a
serious medical condition, such as hidden bleeding from cancer or
an ulcer. Once again, this caution deserves repeating:

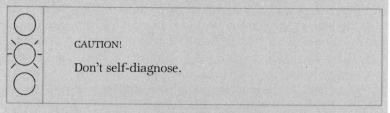

CAUTION!

Don't self-diagnose.

However, the role of all these nutrients in making and maintaining red blood cells dictates a preventive measure: Eat right! A study
of over 200 older adults in Boston provides evidence to support this
recommendation. These people all had moderately low hemoglobin
levels (below 13 g/100 ml) to begin with. Two-thirds were given
iron-fortified foods; the other third received foods without added
iron. At the end of the study, *all* had higher hemoglobin levels. Food
made a difference, iron supplements did not.[8] The appropriate
risk-free "supplements," then, are nutritious foods.

By these criteria, iron-deficiency anemia is a major health problem in
both the United States and Canada and even more so in the rest of the
world. It is especially common in older infants, children, women of
childbearing age, and people in low-income and minority groups. The
incidence of iron deficiency in these groups ranges from 10 to over 50
percent.[9] It tends to cluster with other indicators of low socioeconomic
status, such as family instability, little money spent on food, little
attention given to children.[10] But no segment of society is free of
iron-deficiency anemia, and these groups are not the only ones affected.
For example, 1 out of every 20 Canadian men is at moderate risk
(hemoglobin 12 to 14), and 1 out of every 100 is at high risk
(hemoglobin below 12).[11]

[8]S. N. Gershoff, O. A. Brusis, H. V. Nino, and A. M. Huber, Studies of the elderly in Boston:
I. The effects of iron fortification on moderately anemic people, *American Journal of
Clinical Nutrition* 30 (1977):226-234.

[9]M. Winick, Nutritional disorders of American women, *Nutrition Today*,
September/October-November/December 1975, pp. 26-28.

[10]D. M. Czajka-Narins, T. B. Haddy, and D. J. Kallen, Nutrition and social correlates in
iron deficiency anemia, *American Journal of Clinical Nutrition* 31 (1978):955-960.

[11]Z. I. Sabry, J. A. Campbell, M. E. Campbell, and A. L. Forbes, Nutrition Canada,
Nutrition Today, January/February 1974, pp. 5-13.

Iron Overload   Iron toxicity is rare but not unknown. The body protects itself against absorbing too much iron by setting up a "block" in the intestinal cells. A protein traps extra absorbed iron and holds it until it can be shed from the body when the mucosal cells are shed. The average life of an intestinal cell is only three days, so this method efficiently removes excess iron from the system. Still, the mucosal block can be overwhelmed, and iron overload is the result.

Two kinds of iron overload are known. One is caused by a hereditary defect, the other by ingesting too much iron. Tissue damage, especially to the liver, occurs in both, but it is most severe in those who also drink large quantities of alcohol.[12] Alcohol increases the absorption of ferric iron, and wines contain substantial amounts of iron, so the overconsumption of wine is particularly risky.

Iron overload is more common in men than in women. An argument against the fortification of foods with iron to protect women is that it might put more men at risk of overload. Indeed, there is some evidence from Sweden, where foods are generously fortified with iron, that this measure has increased the incidence of iron overload in men. It is too bad that a measure meant to promote the health of one sex might put the other sex at risk.

The ingestion of massive amounts of iron can cause sudden death. The second most common cause of accidental poisoning in small children is ingestion of iron supplements or vitamins with iron (the first is aspirin).[13] As few as 6 to 12 tablets have caused death in a child.[14] A child suspected of iron poisoning should be rushed to the hospital to have his stomach pumped; 30 minutes may make a crucial difference.

Iron in Foods   The usual Western mixed diet provides only about 5 to 6 mg of iron in every 1,000 kcal. The recommended daily intake for an adult man is 10 mg and most men require more than 2,000 kcal, so a man can easily meet his iron needs without special effort. The recommendation for a woman, however, is 14 to 18 mg per day. Because women typically consume fewer than 2,000 kcal per day, they understandably have trouble achieving this intake. A woman who wants to meet her iron needs from foods must increase the iron-to-kcalorie ratio of her diet so that she will receive about double the

mucosal block to iron absorption: the provision of a binding protein (ferritin) in the mucosal cells which captures and holds unneeded iron until it is shed with the cells.

iron overload: toxicity from iron overdose.

hemochromatosis (heem-oh-crome-a-TOCE-iss): iron overload characterized by deposits of iron-containing pigment in many tissues, with tissue damage; an inborn error (see p. 537).

hemosiderosis (heem-oh-sider-OH-sis): iron overload characterized by excessive iron deposits in hemosiderin, the normal iron-storage protein.

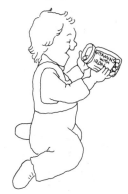

[12]The detection of early hemochromatosis, *Nutrition Reviews* 36 (March 1978):76-79; and C. V. Moore, Major minerals, Section C: Iron, in *Modern Nutrition in Health and Disease*, 5th ed., eds. R. S. Goodhart and M. E. Shils (Philadelphia: Lea and Febiger, 1973), pp. 297-323.

[13]W. H. Crosby, Prescribing iron? Think safety, *Archives of Internal Medicine* 138 (1978):766; abstract in *Journal of the American Dietetic Association* 73 (1978):344.

[14]Committee on Safety, Toxicity, and Misuse of Vitamins and Trace Minerals, National Nutrition Consortium, *Vitamin-Mineral Safety, Toxicity, and Misuse* (Chicago: The American Dietetic Association, 1978).

Recommended intakes of iron:

Men	10 mg/day
Women	14 mg/day (Canada)
	18 mg/day (U.S.)

How recommended daily intake for iron is calculated (for example, for an adolescent girl):

Losses from urine and shed skin: 1/2-1 mg

Losses through menstruation (about 15 mg total averaged over 30 days):   1/2 mg

Net for growth: 1/2 mg

Average daily need (total):
                    1-1/2-2 mg

Only 10 percent of ingested iron is absorbed, so this girl must ingest 15-20 mg per day.

Meeting iron needs from food (example):

Food choice	Iron (mg)	Energy (kcal)
1 egg	1.1	80
3 oz beef	2.9	245
3 slices bread	1.5	165
1/2 c tomatoes	0.6	25
1/2 c broccoli	0.6	40
1 small apple	0.4	70
1/2 small banana	0.4	50
1 sweet potato	1.0	155
2 c milk	0.4	320
Total	8.9	1,150

This example shows that selection of a variety of nutritious foods according to the Four Food Group Plan rule—without any added butter, margarine, or sugar—uses up 1,150 of a woman's 2,000 kcal and supplies fewer then 10 mg of iron.

average amount of iron—at least 10 mg per 1,000 kcal. This means she must emphasize the most iron-rich foods in every food group.

In considering which foods are the best sources of iron it is important to know that iron is absorbed differently from various foods. The average amount of iron absorbed is 10 percent, but up to 40 percent of the iron in meat-fish-poultry, and soybeans may be absorbed. Less than 10 percent of the iron in eggs, whole grains, nuts, and dried beans is absorbed. At the bottom of the list is spinach: Only 2 percent of its iron is absorbed. The listing of common foods in Table 1 does not take iron's varying absorbability into account, but even so, meat-fish-poultry are at the top. Obviously, then, a woman who includes some meat in everyday meal planning will get a head start toward meeting her iron needs, especially if she makes periodic use of liver and other organ meats.

Foods in the milk group do not appear in Table 1 at all. Milk and cheese are notoriously poor iron sources, as poor in iron as they are rich in calcium. Although these foods are an indispensable part of the diet, they should not be overemphasized. In considering the grain foods,

Meat-fish-poultry contain about half their iron bound into molecules of **heme** (HEEM), the nonprotein part of the hemoglobin and myoglobin proteins. Heme iron is much more absorbable than nonheme iron. Meat-fish-poultry also contain a factor other than heme that promotes the absorption of iron, even of the iron from other foods eaten at the same time as the meat.

Overconsumption of milk is a common cause of iron deficiency in children; the resulting anemia is known as **milk anemia**.

Table 1. Iron Contents of 50 Common Foods*

Ex-change group[†]	Food	Serving size[‡]	Iron (mg)	Ex-change group[†]	Food	Serving size[‡]	Iron (mg)
5L	Oysters	3/4 c	10	3	Dried apricots	4 halves	.8
5M	Beef liver	3 oz	8	4	Winter squash	1/2 c	.8
4	Bran flakes, enriched	1/2 c	6.2	4	Whole-wheat bread	1 slice	.8
5M	Beef heart	3 oz	5	3	Blackberries	1/2 c	.7
5L	Chipped beef	3 oz	4	4	Pumpkin	3/4 c	.7
5L	Lean beef roast	3 oz	2.9	5L	Canned salmon	3 oz	.7
5L	Veal roast	3 oz	3	4	Cooked cereal	1/2 c	.7
5M	Hamburger	3 oz	2.7	3	Blueberries	1/2 c	.7
3	Prune juice	1/4 c	2.6	4	Spaghetti, enriched	1/2 c	.7
5L	Sardines	3 oz	2.5	4	Macaroni, enriched	1/2 c	.7
4	Dried beans	1/2 c	2.5	2	Broccoli	1/2 c	.7
2	Spinach	1/2 c	2.4	4	Potato chips	15	.6
4	Lima beans	1/2 c	2.2	3	Raspberries	1/2 c	.6
5L	Ham	3 oz	2.2	5M	Peanut butter	2 tbsp	.6
5L	Canned tuna	3 oz	1.6	4	White bread	1 slice	.6
2	Dandelion greens	1/2 c	1.6	3	Dried fig	1	.6
4	Green peas	1/2 c	1.5	4	Muffin	1	.6
5L	Leg of lamb	3 oz	1.4	4	Corn muffin	1	.6
5L	Chicken, meat only	3 oz	1.4	3	Applesauce	1/2 c	.6
2	Mustard greens	1/2 c	1.3	2	Cooked tomatoes	1/2 c	.6
3	Strawberries	3/4 c	1.1	4	French-fried potatoes	8	.6
5M	Egg	1	1.1	4	Popcorn, no fat	3 c	.6
2	Tomato juice	1/2 c	1.1[§]	3	Pear	1	.5
4	Rice, enriched	1/2 c	.9	4	Potato	1 small	.5
2	Brussels sprouts	1/2 c	.9	4	Corn on cob	1 small	.5

*These are not necessarily the best food sources but are selected to show a range of iron contents. Note the preponderance of 5s at the top of the left-hand column and the total absence of 1s in this table. Remember, too: Iron is better absorbed from meat-fish-poultry and soybeans than from other foods.

[†]The numbers refer to the exchange lists: 1 is milk; 2, vegetables; 3, fruit; 4, bread; 5L, lean meat; 5M, medium-fat meat. Note that milk exchanges (1) are missing.

[‡]Serving sizes are those in the exchange lists, except for meat.

[§]To this point, all foods supply at least 10 percent of the recommended intake (for a man) of 10 mg.

remember that iron is one of the enrichment nutrients. Whole-grain or enriched breads and cereals—not refined, unenriched pastry products—are the best choices. Finally, among the vegetables, the legume family and the dark greens are the most iron-rich; among the fruits, dried fruits are the best. A set of guidelines, then, for planning an iron-rich diet:

enrichment: the addition of iron, thiamin, riboflavin, and niacin to refined grain products to restore approximately their original contents (see p. 337).

- *Milk and cheese.* Don't overdo these foods (but don't omit them either; you need them for calcium). Drink skim milk to free up kcalories to be invested in iron-rich foods.

- *Meat.* Use liver and other organ meats frequently, perhaps every week or two. Meats, fish, and poultry are excellent iron sources.

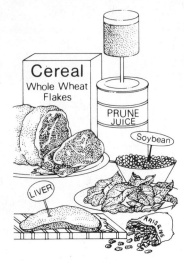

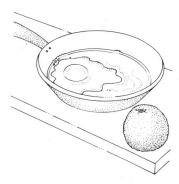

fortification: the addition of nutrients to a food—but not necessarily the nutrients that were originally found there.

- *Meat substitutes.* Don't forget legumes: A cup of peas or beans can supply up to 5 mg iron.
- *Breads and cereals.* Use only whole-grain, enriched, and fortified products.
- *Vegetables.* The dark-green leafy vegetables are rich in iron.
- *Fruits.* Dried fruits like raisins, apricots, peaches, and prunes are high in iron.

Knowledgeable cooking and menu planning can enhance the amount of iron delivered by your diet. The iron content of 100 g of spaghetti sauce simmered in a glass dish is 3 mg, but it's 87 mg when the sauce is cooked in an unenameled iron skillet. Even in the short time it takes to scramble eggs, their iron content can be tripled by cooking them in an iron pan. Foods containing 25 mg or more of vitamin C can more than double the amount of iron absorbed from iron sources eaten at the same meal.[15] Therefore, two additional suggestions are:

- Cook with iron skillets whenever possible.
- Serve vitamin C-containing foods at every meal.

Even after taking all of these precautions, a woman may not accumulate enough storage iron to prepare her for the increased demands of pregnancy and childbirth. In 1974 the Committee on RDA acknowledged for the first time that pregnant women might need supplemental iron. The Canadian Dietary Standard also includes this statement. However, the iron from supplements is far less well absorbed than that from food, and the doses have to be as high as 50 mg per day. Absorption of iron from supplements can be improved by taking them with meat or with vitamin C-rich foods or juices.

The use of fortified foods is another option. Some breakfast cereals boast that they contain 100 percent of the recommended daily intake of iron. The use of these may indeed boost the day's iron intakes, even though absorption of the iron used in them is poor. A number of proposals have been made for further fortification. Canada is considering adding iron to milk;[16] other ideas are to add it to coffee, to junk foods, even to salt. At present, 25 percent of all the iron consumed in the United States derives from fortified foods. A proposal to increase further the iron level in enriched bread has been defeated.[17] Ultimately, it is up to the consumer herself to see that she gets enough iron.

[15]M. Balsley, Soon to come: 1978 Recommended Dietary Allowances, *Journal of the American Dietetic Association* 71(1977):149-151; and J. D. Cook and E. R. Monsen, Vitamin C, the common cold, and iron absorption, *American Journal of Clinical Nutrition* 30 (1977):235-241.

[16]D. Rosenfield, Nutritional optimization of new foods (commentary), *Journal of the American Dietetic Association* 72 (1978):475-477.

[17]For a full description of the disagreements surrounding this decision, see Controversy 13: Iron Superenrichment, in E. M. N. Hamilton and E. N. Whitney, *Nutrition: Concepts and Controversies* (St. Paul: West, 1979), pp. 292-294.

Iodine

Iodine occurs in the body in an infinitesimally small quantity, but its principal role in human nutrition is well known and the amount needed is well established. Iodine is a part of thyroxin, a hormone secreted by the thyroid gland. Thyroxin is responsible for the basal metabolic rate. The hormone enters every cell of the body to control the rate at which the cell uses oxygen. This is the same as saying that thyroxin controls the rate at which energy is released.

Thyroxin: see also p. 245.

Iodine must be available for thyroxin to be synthesized. The amount in the diet is variable and generally reflects the amount present in the soil in which plants are grown or on which animals graze. Iodine is plentiful in the ocean, so seafood is a completely dependable source. In the United States, in areas where the soil is iodine-poor (most notably the Plains states), the use of iodized salt has largely wiped out the iodine deficiency that once was widespread.

> People sometimes wonder whether sea salt, made by drying ocean water, is preferable to purified sodium chloride for use in the salt shaker. Sea salt does contain trace minerals, but it loses its iodine during the drying process. Thus in a region where goiter is a risk, iodized sodium chloride is the salt to choose.

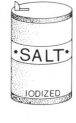

When the iodine level of the blood is low, the cells of the thyroid gland enlarge in an attempt to trap as many particles of iodine as possible. If the gland enlarges until it is visible, it is called a simple goiter. Goiter is estimated to affect 200 million people the world over. In all but 4 percent of these cases the cause is iodine deficiency. Furthermore, 8 million people have goiter because they overconsume plants of the cabbage family and others that contain an antithyroid substance whose effect is not counteracted by dietary iodine.[18] The goitrogens present in plants serve as a reminder that food additives may not be such great offenders as some natural components of foods (see Highlight 13).

goiter (GOY-ter): an iodine-deficiency disease. Goiter caused by iodine deficiency is **simple goiter**.

goitrogen: a thyroid antagonist found in food; causes **toxic goiter**.

In addition to causing sluggishness and weight gain, an iodine deficiency may have serious effects on the development of an infant in the uterus. Severe thyroid undersecretion during pregnancy causes the extreme and irreversible mental and physical retardation known as cretinism. A cretin has an IQ as low as 20 and a face and body with

cretinism (CREE-tin-ism): an iodine-deficiency disease characterized by mental and physical retardation.

[18]F. M. Strong, Toxicants occurring naturally in foods, in *Nutrition Reviews' Present Knowledge in Nutrition*, 4th ed. (Washington, D.C.: Nutrition Foundation, 1976), pp. 516-527.

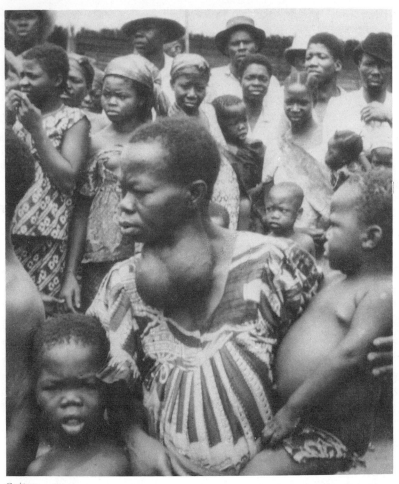

Goiter.

Courtesy of FAO.

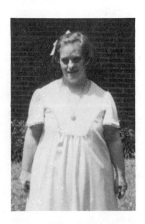

Laura Drake, age 38, a cretin.

abnormalities like those shown in the margin. Much of the mental retardation associated with cretinism can be averted by early diagnosis and treatment.

The iodization of salt in the Plains states eliminated the widespread misery caused by goiter and cretinism in the local people during the 1930s. Once these scourges had disappeared, a new generation of children grew up who never saw the problem and so had no appreciation of its importance. Rejecting iodized salt out of ignorance, they allowed iodine deficiences to creep back into their lives. Hopefully, now, education is keeping them informed of the need to continue using iodized salt.

The recommended intake of iodine for adults is 100 to 150 μg a day, a miniscule amount. Like chlorine, iodine is a deadly poison in large amounts, but traces of it are indispensable to life. The need for iodine is easily met by consuming seafood, vegetables grown in iodine-rich soil, and (in iodine-poor areas) iodized salt. In the United States, you have to read the label to find out whether salt is iodized; in Canada all table salt is iodized.

The RDA for iodine: 150 μg.

Canadian Dietary Standard: 140-150 μg for men, 100-110 μg for women.

Many of the minerals share with the fat-soluble vitamins the characteristics of being toxic in excess. Iodine, in particular, is notorious in this respect. The skull and crossbones on the iodine bottle warns the user that this substance is a deadly poison and that it must be kept out of the reach of children.

Much of the prejudice against iodized salt and fluoridated water arises from the conclusion that these minerals must be avoided altogether because they are dangerous when used in excess. This misconception raises an important point about all the nutrients and many other substances: They may work one way at a high concentration and another at a low concentration. There is not a simple linear relationship between the dose level and its effects.

Let's take three examples—a hormone, a vitamin, and a drug. The hormone insulin, at physiological doses, lowers blood glucose concentrations by facilitating the transport of glucose into cells. At a much higher dose (100 or 1,000 times more than is normally found in the body), insulin seems to *raise* blood glucose concentrations. When the insulin dose exceeds a threshold level, the body responds by secreting an antagonistic hormone (glucagon) in such large amounts that a backlash occurs; the normal effects are reversed.

The distinction being made here is that between normal doses and massive doses of the same compound; that is, the distinction between a pharmacological dose and a physiological dose. At the high level used in some experiments the vitamin acts as a drug, overwhelming body systems that at normal concentrations are impervious to it. It is as if a different compound altogether were acting in the body.

Drugs are similar. The antibiotic streptomycin works by interfering with protein synthesis in growing cells. Since protein synthesis must occur for growth to occur and since bacterial cells grow rapidly, the drug rapidly kills these cells without affecting the more slowly growing cells of the human digestive tract. At a higher dose level, the drug would also kill the cells of the human body.

Thus if you read or hear one report of a certain substance having a certain effect on people, you cannot necessarily conclude that the substance is "good" or "bad." You must ask what dose was used and whether the same effect would have been observed if the substance had been used at a higher or lower concentration. Two corollaries to this observation might be the following:

linear relationship: a relationship between two variables in which one increases in direct proportion to the other.

nonlinear relationships:

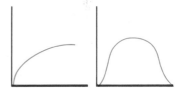

Variable: see p. 51.

physiological dose: a dose equivalent to the amount of a nutrient (or hormone) normally found in the body.

pharmacological dose: a much higher dose, at which unexpected, druglike effects are often observed.

CAUTION WHEN YOU READ!

What is a poison at a high concentration may be an essential nutrient at a low concentration. (What is "bad" high may be "good" low.)

What is a needed nutrient at a low concentration may be toxic at a high concentration. (More is not necessarily better.)

Additives proven to cause cancer at any dose are prohibited. See discussion of the Delaney Clause in Highlight 13.

Laboratory scientists responsible for investigating the effects of additives in foods have discovered these facts over the years. They have realized that it is necessary to demonstrate that an additive causes harm *at the dose level we can realistically expect to find in our foods* before concluding that it is dangerous. If the general public understood this, many of the scares that appear from time to time in the media would lose their impact. For many reasons, massive doses of many substances have undesirable effects, but in the real world of real people, effects like these are not so often felt.

In the interest of selling a product or an idea, promoters sometimes appeal to emotions; a most powerful emotion is fear. "This additive causes cancer, and they are using it in bread." When you feel physically threatened you may not stop to reason and seek out the evidence; you may just do what you are told—in this case avoid the grocery store product and buy the promoter's product instead because it makes you feel safe. Yet the additives in foods are extensively tested before they are approved for general use, and the laws that regulate their use are well enforced. Each additive is there for a reason.

The situation is complex and requires an understanding of many subtleties. To be fair, no simple statement can be made about the effects of all the additives. Each must be investigated individually. Still, it should be clear from this Digression that you need not feel fear each time someone claims that our foods are being contaminated with poisons.

A FLAG SIGN OF A SPURIOUS CLAIM IS:

Scare tactics

To balance this discussion, remember that sometimes you are right to be scared. An occasional outbreak of food poisoning does occur, for example, showing that the inspection system failed to catch a hazard in time. Occasionally a food product is removed from the market when a previously unsuspected side effect of one of its constituents becomes evident. The rarity of these occurrences, however, testifies to the overall effectiveness of the consumer protection agencies. Highlight 13 is devoted to some further aspects of consumer protection and additives.

Zinc

Zinc occurs in a small quantity in the body (about 2 g) but is a helper for some 20 enzymes and forms part of the structure of bone. High concentrations of zinc appear in the eye, liver, muscles, and male reproductive organs. It is involved in DNA and protein synthesis, the action of insulin, the immune reactions, and the utilization of vitamin A. With all of these vital roles, it is not surprising that zinc is necessary for the healing of wounds; a deficiency of zinc can seriously retard this process. Zinc is also required for a normal sense of taste. The impressive accumulation of new information about zinc in recent years has led to the conclusion that this mineral is as important as protein in the normal processes of growth and maintenance of body tissues.

A deficiency of zinc was first observed in humans in the 1960s in the Middle East, where a diet high in cereal and low in animal protein was common. Cereal grains, although rich in zinc, contain fibers and phytic acid, which hinder the absorption of zinc. The zinc deficiency was marked by growth retardation, especially of sexual organs, and loss of taste; these symptoms responded to the administration of zinc. Since then, zinc deficiencies have also been identified in schoolchildren in at least one U.S. city (Denver), and are suspected to exist among preschoolers, older people, hospital patients, and other populations whose protein intakes may be limited.

Animal foods are good sources of zinc, with the richest being oysters, herring, milk, and egg yolks. Among plant foods, whole grains are richest in zinc, but it is not so well absorbed from them as from meat. The recommended intake of 9 to 15 mg a day for adults is probably easily met by the diet of the average middle-class person, but deficiency is likely if animal protein is underemphasized. As a rule of thumb, two small servings of animal protein a day will provide sufficient zinc.

Teenagers and young college students who are concerned about acne may learn that zinc has been effective in its treatment in cases where vitamin A has not been.[19] However, self-dosing with zinc can cause

The Egyptian boy in this picture is seventeen years old but is only four feet tall, like a seven-year-old in the United States. His genitalia are like those of a six-year-old. The retardation is ascribed to zinc deficiency.

Reproduced with permission of *Nutrition Today* magazine, P.O. Box 1829, Annapolis, Maryland, 21404, March 1968.

Phytic acid: see p. 429.

The RDA for zinc: 15 mg.

Canadian Dietary Standard: 10 mg for men, 9 mg for women.

[19] G. Michaëlsson, L. Juhlin, and A. Vahlquist, Effects of oral zinc and vitamin A on acne, *Archives of Dermatology* 113 (1977):31-36.

toxicity with severe consequences: muscle incoordination, dizziness, drowsiness, lethargy, renal failure, anemia, and others.[20] As with all the nutrients, and especially the trace minerals, overdoses of zinc are dangerous. The appropriate strategy would be to consult a physician about using zinc for acne.

The "Newer" Trace Elements

Iron, iodine, and zinc are the best known of the trace elements, but six others have recently become better recognized through inclusion in the RDA tables. They deserve a bit of individual attention.

Copper   The body contains about 75 to 100 mg of copper, which performs several vital roles. As a catalyst in the formation of hemoglobin, it helps to make red blood cells. It is involved in the manufacture of collagen and helps to maintain the sheath around nerve fibers. Most of what is known about copper is from animal research, which has provided clues about its possible roles in humans. Copper's critical roles seem to have to do with helping iron shift back and forth between its +2 and +3 states. This means that copper is needed in many of the reactions related to respiration and the release of energy.

A copper deficiency is rare but not unknown. It has been seen in children with kwashiorkor and with iron-deficiency anemia and can severely disturb growth and metabolism.

The best food sources of copper include grains, shellfish, organ meats, legumes, dried fruits, fresh fruits, and vegetables—a long list showing that copper is available from almost all foods. About a third of the copper taken in food is absorbed, and the rest is eliminated in the feces.

Manganese   The human body contains a tiny 20 mg of manganese, mostly in the bones and glands. Still, this represents billions on billions of molecules. Animal studies suggest that manganese cooperates with many enzymes, helping to facilitate dozens of different metabolic processes. Manganese deficiency in animals deranges many systems, including the bones, reproduction, the nervous system, and fat metabolism.

Deficiencies of manganese have not been seen in humans, but toxicity may be severe. Miners who inhale large quantities of manganese dust on the job over prolonged periods show many of the symptoms of a brain disease, with frightening abnormalities of appearance and behavior: "Facial expression is mask-like, the voice

Estimated safe and adequate daily dietary intake of copper (adults): 2-3 mg.

Estimated safe and adequate daily dietary intake of manganese (adults): 2.5-5.0 mg.

---

[20]Questions doctors ask . . . , *Nutrition and the MD,* October 1978.

monotonous; and intention-tremor, muscle rigidity and spastic gait appear."[21]

The example of manganese underlines again the fact that toxicity of the trace elements occurs at a level not far above the estimated requirement. Thus it is as important not to overdose as it is to have an adequate intake. The Committee on RDA underscores this point by adding the special warning to its trace-mineral table, not to exceed the upper end of the range of recommended intakes. The National Nutrition Consortium, too, worries that now more trace minerals are known, they will be added to vitamin-mineral pills, making toxic overdoses more likely. The FDA is not permitted to enforce limits on the amounts of trace minerals added to supplements, so this is an area in which the consumer himself has to be careful and aware.[22]

CAUTION:

Beware of supplements containing trace minerals.

It is safer to consume a diet that provides foods from a variety of sources than to try to put together, without causing toxicity, a combination of pills that will meet all your needs.

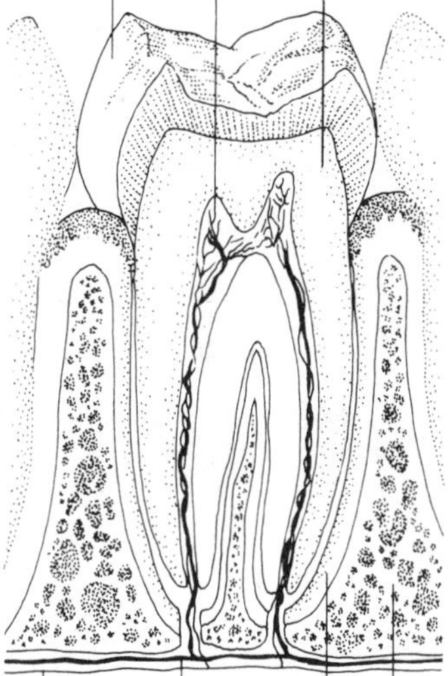

The outer two layers of the teeth, enamel and dentin, are composed largely of calcium compounds, including hydroxyapatite and fluorapatite.

Fluoride   Only a trace of fluoride occurs in the human body, but studies have demonstrated that where diets are high in fluoride, the crystalline deposits in bones and teeth are larger and more perfectly formed. When bones and teeth become calcified, first a crystal called hydroxyapatite is formed from calcium and phosphorus. Then fluoride replaces the hydroxy (OH) portions of the crystal, rendering it insoluble in water and resistant to decay.

Drinking water is the usual source of fluoride, although fish and tea may supply substantial amounts. Where fluoride is lacking in the water supply, the incidence of dental decay is very high. Dental problems can

hydroxyapatite (high-droxy-APP-uh-tite): the major calcium-containing crystal of bones and teeth.

fluorapatite (fleur-APP-uh-tite): the stabilized form of bone and tooth crystal, in which fluoride has replaced the hydroxy groups of hydroxyapatite.

[Diagram labels: pulp (blood vessels, nerves); enamel; dentin; nerve; gum; blood vessel; bone]

[21]T. K. Li and B. L. Vallee, Trace elements, Section B: The biochemical and nutritional role of trace elements, in *Modern Nutrition in Health and Disease*, 5th ed., eds. R. S. Goodhart and M. E. Shils (Philadelphia: Lea and Febiger, 1973), pp. 372-399.

[22]Annual report from the National Nutrition Consortium (update), *Journal of the American Dietetic Association* 70 (1977):538-540.

Unprotected teeth decay extensively. This child's teeth were frequently bathed with apple juice.

Courtesy of H. Kaplan and V. P. Rabbach.

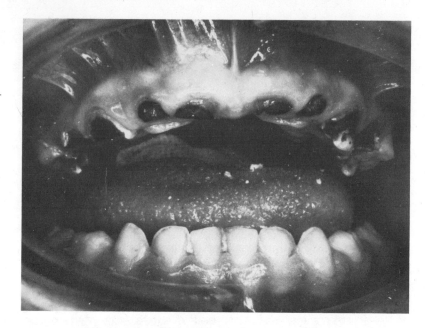

fluorosis (fleur-OH-sis): mottling of the tooth enamel; due to ingestion of too much fluoride during tooth development.

osis = too much

cause a multitude of other health problems, affecting the whole body. Fluoridation of community water where needed, to raise its fluoride concentration to one part per million (1 ppm), is thus an important public health measure. Fluoridation of community water is presently practiced in more than 5,000 communities across the United States, and about 100 million people are drinking it (see Figure 1).

In some communities the natural fluoride concentration in water is high, 2 to 8 ppm, and children's teeth develop with mottled enamel. This condition, called fluorosis, is not harmful (in fact, these children's

Figure 1 Fluoridation in the United States.

From D. P. DePaola and M. C. Alfano, Diet and oral health, *Nutrition Today*, May/June 1977, pp. 6-11, 29-32. Courtesy of the authors and of *Nutrition Today* magazine, 703 Giddings Avenue, Suite 6, Annapolis MD 21401, © May/June 1977.

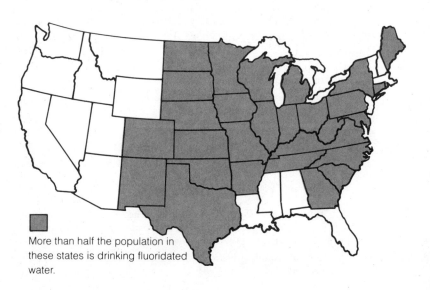

More than half the population in these states is drinking fluoridated water.

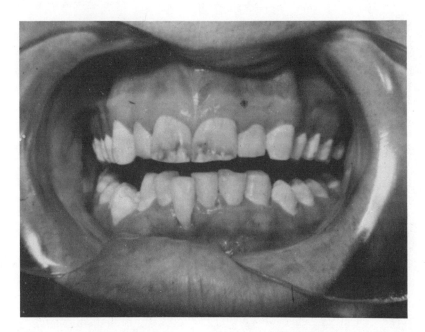

Fluorosis.

Courtesy of H. Kaplan and V. P. Rabbach.

teeth are extraordinarily decay-resistant), but violates the prejudice that teeth "should" be white. Fluorosis does not occur in communities where fluoride is added to the water supply.

Not only does fluoride protect children's teeth from decay, but it makes the bones of older people resistant to the degeneration of osteoporosis. Fluoride is also required for growth in animals and is an essential nutrient for humans; in fact, the continuous presence of fluoride in body fluids is desirable. Luckily, all normal diets include fluoride. It is toxic in excess, but toxicity symptoms appear only after chronic intakes of 20 to 80 mg a day over many years. The amount consumed from fluoridated water is typically about 1 mg a day. Despite its value and the limited possibility of receiving excessive fluoride in the water supply, violent disagreement often surrounds the introduction of fluoride to a community.

People in unfluoridated communities need to find alternative means of protecting their children's teeth. The best temporary solution seems to be to use fluoride toothpastes and/or to have children obtain a topical fluoride application yearly. Fluoride tablets are also available. For infants there are vitamin drops with fluoride in them, but their effectiveness is limited.

Osteoporosis: see p. 426.

Estimated safe and adequate daily dietary intake of fluoride (adults): 1.5-4.0 mg.

topical: a surface application.

Chromium The element chromium has been shown to remedy impaired carbohydrate metabolism in several groups of older people in the United States.[23] Experiments on animals have shown that

[23]K. M. Hambidge, Chromium nutrition in man, *American Journal of Clinical Nutrition* 27 (1974):505-514.

chromium works closely with the hormone insulin, facilitating the uptake of glucose into cells and then the breakdown of that glucose with the release of energy. When chromium is lacking, the effectiveness of insulin is severely impaired, and a diabetes-like condition results.

Like iron, chromium can have two different charges: The +3 ion seems to be the most effective in living systems. It also occurs in association with several different complexes in foods. The one that is best absorbed and most active is a small organic compound named the glucose tolerance factor (GTF). This compound has been purified from brewer's yeast and pork kidney and is believed to be present in many other foods. It may be that when more is known the GTF, rather than chromium, will be dubbed an essential nutrient and classed among the vitamins.

GTF (glucose tolerance factor): a small organic compound containing chromium.

Depleted tissue concentrations of chromium in human beings have been linked to adult-onset diabetes and growth failure in children with protein-kcalorie malnutrition.

Estimated safe and adequate daily dietary intake of chromium (adults): 0.05-0.2 mg.

selenium (se-LEEN-ee-um)

Estimated safe and adequate daily dietary intake of selenium (adults): 0.05-0.2 mg.

Selenium   Selenium, too, is a trace element that functions as part of large molecules, especially certain enzymes. It also acts alone as an antioxidant and can substitute for vitamin E in some of that vitamin's antioxidant activities. Deficiencies are unknown, and food sources are abundant.

molybdenum (mo-LIB-duh-num)

Estimated safe and adequate daily dietary intake of molybdenum (adults): 0.15-0.5 mg.

Molybdenum   Finally, molybdenum has also been recognized as an important mineral in human and animal physiology. It functions as a working part of several enzymes, some of which are giant proteins. One, for example, contains two atoms of molybdenum and eight of iron. Deficiencies of molybdenum are unknown in animals and humans, because the amounts needed are miniscule—as little as 0.1 part per million parts of body tissue. Excess molybdenum causes toxicity in animals, but this effect has not been seen in humans.

These six "newer" trace minerals have not been known for long. Others are even more recent newcomers. Nickel is now recognized as important for the health of many body tissues, and deficiencies cause harm to the liver and other organs. Silicon is known to be involved in bone calcification, at least in animals. Tin is necessary for growth in animals and probably in humans. Vanadium, too, is necessary for growth and bone development and also for normal reproduction; human intakes of vanadium may be close to the minimum needed for health. Cobalt is recognized as the mineral in the large vitamin B_{12} molecule; the alternative name for B_{12}, cobalamin, reflects the presence of cobalt. In the future we may discover that many other trace minerals also play key roles: silver, mercury, lead, barium, cadmium. Even arsenic—famous as the poisonous instrument of death in many

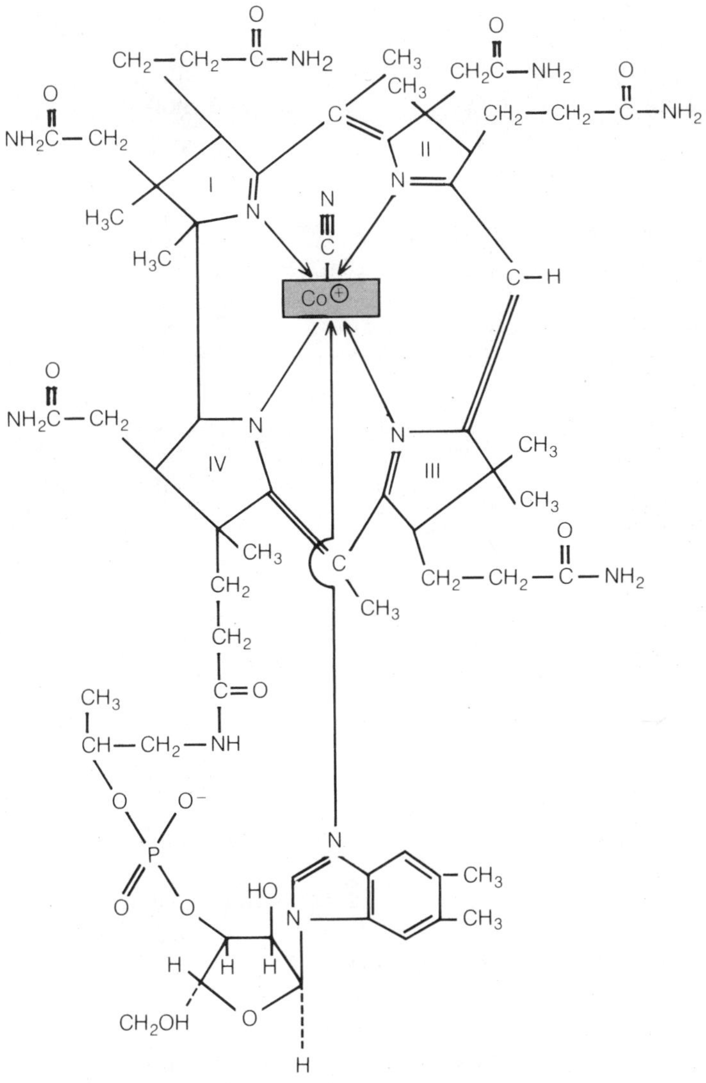

The intricate vitamin B_{12} molecule contains one atom of cobalt.

murder mysteries—may turn out to be an essential nutrient in tiny quantities.[24]

As research on the trace minerals continues, many interactions between them are also coming to light. An excess of one may cause a deficiency of another. A slight manganese overload, for example, may aggravate an iron deficiency. And a deficiency of one may open the way for another to cause a toxic reaction. Iron deficiency, for example, makes the body much more susceptible than normal to lead poisoning. The continuous outpouring of new information about the trace minerals is a sign that we have much more to learn.

[24]The "newer" trace elements, *Nutrition and the MD*, November 1975.

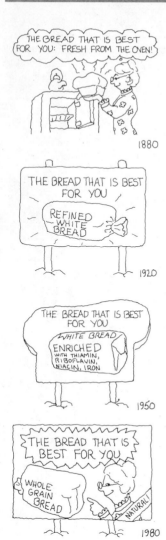

Putting It All Together

One reason the trace minerals are receiving increased attention today is that the food supply has increasingly been refined. As more people turn to refined, processed, and prepared foods and away from the crude products of the farm, they enjoy a saving in convenience and time but suffer a loss of the richness and variety of nutrients that occur in less-pure foods. As a result, deficiencies crop up where the existence of a needed nutrient might never before have been suspected. A case in point is chromium, which is lost when sugar and whole grains are refined. Humans need unbelievably small amounts of chromium, but when it is lacking, severe disorders in body physiology occur. Another case is zinc, which is lost when cereal grains are refined. Deficiencies of zinc are no longer unknown in the United States, and their effects can be devastating. The increasing use by the wealthy nations of highly refined, processed foods concerns nutritionists; they fear that the advice to consume "a balanced diet" no longer is enough to protect people against serious nutritional deficiencies and imbalances.

A "balanced diet," as recommended by the Four Food Group Plan (see Appendix M), consists of (for an adult):

- Milk or milk products, 2 cups
- Meat or meat substitutes, 2 servings
- Fruits and vegetables (1 C-rich, 1 A-rich), 4 servings
- Breads and cereals (whole-grain or enriched), 4 servings

But the optimum diet may need to be more carefully defined than this. Meat substitutes, for example, may lack the iron sorely needed by groups at risk for iron deficiency. Legumes, being rich in iron, and especially soybeans, whose iron is well absorbed, may be acceptable meat substitutes—but other meat substitutes made from other vegetable proteins may be iron-poor. Breads and cereals that have been refined and then enriched may be good sources only of the nutrients on the label; overusing enriched breads may mean risking deficiencies of chromium, zinc, and other minerals. In the case of two other nutrients—iodine and fluorine—food sources are so unreliable in some geographical locations that the definition of an adequate diet must be expanded to include iodized salt and fluoridated water or fluoride supplements.

A diagram at the end of Chapter 11 demonstrated that foods from all six exchange groups are necessary for an adequate diet. With the qualifications made here, that diagram has to be modified. If you are curious about the adequacy of your diet, you might ask yourself if you have all your nutrient bases covered by using the following diagram as a checklist:

Does your diet include this food group?

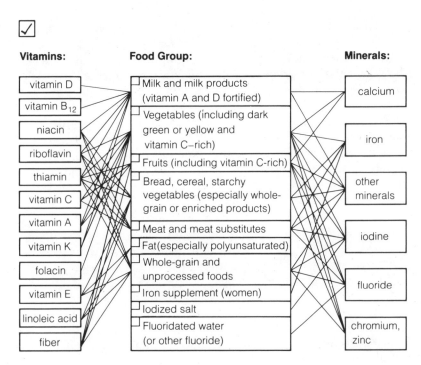

Vitamins:

- vitamin D
- vitamin B$_{12}$
- niacin
- riboflavin
- thiamin
- vitamin C
- vitamin A
- vitamin K
- folacin
- vitamin E
- linoleic acid
- fiber

Food Group:

- Milk and milk products (vitamin A and D fortified)
- Vegetables (including dark green or yellow and vitamin C–rich)
- Fruits (including vitamin C-rich)
- Bread, cereal, starchy vegetables (especially whole-grain or enriched products)
- Meat and meat substitutes
- Fat(especially polyunsaturated)
- Whole-grain and unprocessed foods
- Iron supplement (women)
- Iodized salt
- Fluoridated water (or other fluoride)

Minerals:

- calcium
- iron
- other minerals
- iodine
- fluoride
- chromium, zinc

Summing Up

Iron is found principally in the red blood cells, where it comprises part of the oxygen-carrier protein hemoglobin. When red blood cells die and are dismantled in the liver, the iron is retrieved and transported by iron-carrier proteins back to bone marrow, where new red blood cells are synthesized. There is no route of excretion for iron; losses are small except when blood is lost, as in menstruation or hemorrhage. Thus women's needs for iron are greater than men's (14 to 18 mg a day for women, 10 mg for men).

Iron-deficiency anemia, one of the world's most widespread malnutrition problems, is most common in women and children; it causes weakness, fatigue, headaches, and pallor. Food sources of iron for women must be chosen carefully if even two-thirds of the recommended intake is to be met within a kcalorie allowance that is not excessive. The enrichment of breads and cereals somewhat improves women's iron intakes, but iron enrichment or fortification of other foods may produce iron overload in men. Addition of an iron supplement to the diet may be advisable for some women.

Foods relatively rich in iron include (in roughly descending order) liver and other organ meats, soybeans, dried beans and legumes, red meats, and dark-green vegetables. Other significant contributors are enriched breads and cereals, eggs, and dried fruits such as raisins and prunes. Iron is better absorbed from meats and soybeans than from other foods, and its absorption is enhanced by eating vitamin C at the same meal. Milk and milk products are notable for their lack of iron.

Zinc is necessary for normal development, including sexual development, and for wound healing and the sense of taste. Deficiencies of zinc have been observed in some children in the United States as well as in children in the Middle East. Diets in the Middle East are high in whole-grain cereals, which contain absorption-inhibiting fiber and phytic acid.

Iodine forms part of the thyroid hormone; deficiency causes goiter (enlargement of the thyroid gland), slowed metabolism, and stunted growth and mental retardation in children. Addition of iodine to salt in minute quantities protects against deficiency, provided the iodized salt is used. Education must accompany this measure to make it effective.

Copper is important for red blood cell formation, collagen synthesis, and central nervous system function. Manganese aids many body enzymes, but its safe range is narrow, with toxicity causing a severe brain-disease syndrome in humans.

The fluoride ion combines with calcium and phosphorus to stabilize the crystalline structure of bones and teeth against resorption or decay. In communities where the water contains fluoride, dental caries and osteoporosis are less prevalent than in communities where the water supply is low in fluoride.

Chromium, as part of the glucose tolerance factor, works with insulin in promoting glucose uptake into cells and normal carbohydrate metabolism. Chromium deficiency is now believed to have a significant incidence among older people and to be responsible for some cases of maturity-onset diabetes; it may cause growth failure in children as well.

Other trace minerals include selenium, important as an antioxidant and in fat metabolism, and molybdenum, a part of several enzyme systems. Many other trace minerals are under investigation.

In light of the increased use of refined, highly processed foods by the wealthy nations, a balanced diet (as outlined by the Four Food Group Plan) may not provide adequacy for all the trace minerals. Some women may need iron supplements, and it may be desirable as well to use whole-grain rather than refined (even enriched) products for their chromium and zinc, to use iodized salt in iodine-poor areas, and to use fluoride supplements in unfluoridated communities.

To Explore Further

A teaching aid with slides, *Iron* by C. A. Finch, can be ordered from the Nutrition Today Society (address in Appendix J).

A cassette tape, *Trace Elements in Nutrition* (CAM 2-75), can be ordered from the American Dietetic Association (address in Appendix J).

Additional information on all the trace elements is presented in the general references recommended in Appendix J.

HIGHLIGHT 13

Additives in the Food Supply

Give me neither poverty nor riches; feed me with the food that is needful for me.

PROVERBS 30:8

To many people, the word *additive* is frightening. Every day, it seems, news reports carry the story of one more chemical in our food supply that is now suspected of causing a health risk. These additives are a common topic of conversation—mothers discuss the improvement in their children's behavior now that they are eating an "additive-free" diet, and young people declare that they eat only fresh fruits and vegetables and buy only flour that doesn't have bleaches or preservatives in it.

Most of these people are not "health freaks" or just following the crowd in a new fad. They are seriously concerned about what is going into their bodies and are accepting personal responsibility for it. But they have a problem: They don't know where to find valid information on additives or how to make judgments about whom to believe. Thus they fall prey to a common human frailty: They follow the person who speaks with the most confidence. When they themselves are wavering on the issue of radically changing their diet, they become uncomfortable with remarks like "there is conflicting evidence" or "further experimentation is needed."

If you go to the public library for answers to your questions about additives, you will find books and articles that support the scare stories as well as ones that tell you there is nothing to worry about. A better source of balanced, reliable information is the scientific reports in journals, but you may be overwhelmed by the amount of reading involved. Each of the reports is about just one additive—and thousands of chemicals must be tested, interactions between chemicals and nutrients studied, and the application of results from animal research to humans debated. The flow of reports is never-ending. Small wonder that many people give up trying to obtain a total picture and instead follow one writer who commands them to a certain course of action.

The tremendous amount of literature on the subject of additives posed a special problem for us. The subject could be handled more properly in a food science text-book, but nutrition students have questions, serious ones, about their food supply. The best that we can do under these circumstances is to explain the regulatory laws and provide a perspective that we have gained from our own reading.

The term food additive means any substance that becomes part of a food supply when added either directly or indirectly. Intentional (or direct) food additives are added to produce a desired effect. Other unintentional (or indirect) food additives find their way into various foods during processing, packaging, or storage, such as chemical substances that may migrate from plastic packaging. Substances which can get into food by accident, such as pollutants, are incidental food additives. Intentional additives are listed on food labels—so you can decide if you wish to consume them. On the other hand, you must depend on the Federal government to regulate safe levels of indirect food additives and to inspect foods to keep out harmful incidental additives.

The term color additive is defined under a separate amendment of the law while new animal drugs are covered under still other provisions of the law. There are special provisions for the use of these substances. All of the substances mentioned are the responsibility of the Food and Drug Administration (FDA).

There are also provisions for the use of pesticides that are covered separately under the law administered by the Environmental Protection Agency.

Many writers have pointed out that the highly complex food industry could not have developed without the advent of intentional additives to ensure stability of products. Without additives, for instance, it would be impossible for some foods to survive processing, packaging, long-distance transportation, and storage on the store shelf before being consumed. If intentional food additives were sweepingly eliminated, many foods would disappear from grocery shelves and chaos and widespread starvation would result before another system evolved. The alternative to eliminating additives, it seems, is to find ways of ensuring that the additives are safe in the amounts and under the conditions they are used in. The agency charged with this responsibility in the United States is the Food and Drug Administration.

Mini-Glossary

carcinogen (car-SIN-oh-gen): a substance that causes cancer either directly or indirectly (after metabolism in the body).

Delaney Clause: a clause in the 1958 Food Additives Amendment that prohibits use of any chemical in foods that has been shown to cause cancer in man or animal.

GRAS (pronounced GRASS) **list:** a list of additives whose food uses are not restricted because they are generally recognized as safe.

hazard: the capacity of a chemical to harm living organisms under conditions of normal use.

incidental food additive: a chemical that has gotten into a food through an accident in processing or from pollution.

intentional (direct) food additive: a chemical added to a food to achieve a particular quality. Some of these are:

   coloring agents: to increase acceptability and attractiveness.

emulsifiers, stabilizers, thickeners: to give texture, smoothness, or other desired consistencies.

flavoring agents: to add or enhance flavor.

nutrients: to improve nutritive value.

preservatives, antioxidants, sequestrants, antimyotics: to prevent spoilage, rancidity of fats, and microbial growth.

margin of safety: as used when speaking of food additives, a zone between the concentration normally used and that at which a hazard exists.

toxicant: a poison.

toxicity: the ability of a substance to be toxic. All substances are toxic if high enough concentrations are used.

unintentional (indirect) food additive: a chemical that migrates into food during processing, packaging, or storage.

FDA Regulation of Food Additives   In Highlight 12 we discussed the role of the FDA in the labeling of foods; another job assigned to the FDA is regulation of what substances can be put into food products and in what amounts. The 1958 Food Additives Amendment and the 1960 Color Additives Amendment to the Food, Drug, and Cosmetic Act regulate food additives. The amendments authorize FDA to regulate additives only on the basis of safety. The Food Additives Amendment requires that food processors who wish to add a substance to a food must first "submit a petition to FDA, accompanied by extensive information on chemistry, use, function, and safety."[1]

After careful review of the data in the petition and other relevant material the agency will conclude on the safe use of the food additive and issue a regulation, if warranted,

[1]Consumer forum, *FDA Consumer* 9:7 (1975):3.

prescribing conditions under which it may be safely used. The published order will provide for any person who will be adversely affected by the regulation to submit written objections and request a public hearing on the stated objections. In the few instances thus far where evidence has been developed that seriously questions the essential safety of a food additive, the additive has been banned or its use restricted.

FDA in recent years has done much to improve its ability to listen to the public. These openings of the channels of communications have gone far beyond the letter of the law. "It [FDA] has stated how to petition the FDA . . . . It has begun publishing a weekly 'public calendar' so everyone may know with whom key FDA officials are meeting, and why . . . . And, it has taken a number of steps to create greater public understanding of the protections it offers, the limitations of these protections, and the public's own responsibilities for self-protection."[2]

When the Food Additives Amendment was passed, many substances which were in common use were exempted from the definition of "food additive." They were put on what is known as the GRAS (generally recognized as safe) list. Anytime there is substantial scientific evidence

or public outcry that questions the safety of any of the substances on the GRAS list, a special reevaluation of the substance is made. The FDA is now reevaluating all the items on the GRAS list; this investigation will obviously take a number of years to complete.[3]

One of the safety standards an additive must meet is that it must not have been found to cause cancer in any test on animals or humans. The Delaney Clause of the Food Additives Amendment of 1958 is very straightforward in speaking to the problem of carcinogens in foods. It states that "no additive shall be deemed to be safe if it is found to induce cancer when ingested by man or animal."[4]

In recent years, the Delaney Clause has come under fire because of the amount of a food a human would have to consume to obtain the amount of a carcinogen given to test animals. When the artificial sweetener cyclamate was banned in 1969, it was estimated that a human would have to drink at least 138 12-oz bottles of diet soft drinks a day in order to ingest an amount of cyclamates comparable to the

quantity given animals in the tests that caused the ban.[5] The FDA was criticized for banning cyclamates, but under the law it had no alternative.

In the early twentieth century when the food laws were being enacted, today's problems could not have been foreseen. The problem now and in the future, in view of our more complex food supply and our new skills in chemical analysis, will be to quantify risk. It is now possible to detect an almost infinitesimal amount of a chemical, even lower than the amount that may be present naturally in foods.[6] There will need to be input from scientists in developing a risk-benefit equation. "The Delaney Clause is only a partial answer and not necessarily the best one even for its limited coverage."[7]

FDA Monitors Chemical Residues in Foods
Through its Total Diet Study, the FDA keeps tabs on the kinds and amounts of residues of pesticides, heavy metals, and industrial chemicals consumed in food and drink. To make sure there's

[2]T. Larkin, Ten fallacies about FDA, *FDA Consumer* 9:9 (1975):21.

[3]P. Lehman, More than you ever thought you would know about food additives, *FDA Consumer*, April 1979.

[4]FDA clears some food items, bans others, *Chemical and Engineering News* 52:40 (1974):12.

[5]R. D. Middlekauf, Legalities concerning food additives, *Food Technology* 28:5 (1974):42-49.

[6]J. M. Coon, Natural food toxicants: A perspective, *Nutrition Reviews* 32:11 (1974):321-332.

[7]V. O. Wodicke, Risk and responsibility, *Nutrition Reviews* 38 (1980):45-52.

no chance of underestimating the average person's intake, the study is based on the awesome appetite of a teenage boy. These foods are bought in the public market, are then divided into categories, and the categories are chemically analyzed for the presence and level of these residues. This method, commonly called the Market Basket Survey, has shown that the level of DDT has declined dramatically since it has been banned from agricultural use.[8]

People concerned about substances which find their way into the food supply should remember that those found in foods are not the only ones that enter the body. Public water can be a carrier of accidental chemicals, also. Chapter 14 discusses some of the undesirable compounds found in the water supply.

Perspective on Additives
Since it would be a mammoth job to educate yourself about each of the more than 3,000 additives, it would be well to look at the additives in total and at the news accounts about additives and develop a kind of perspective that would be a guiding principle in your food selection.

There are now in use about 3,890 substances

which are added to foods. Of these, about 2,080 are regulated food additives and about 950 are on the GRAS list. It may be surprising that sugar (sucrose) is in the largest amount of any of the additives; in fact, 102 pounds per year per person of sugar is used and this is more than the weight of all the other additives combined. Salt is the second most common legal additive and United States citizens use about 15 lb per person per year in this way, not including the salt from the salt shaker at home. Corn syrup is consumed at 8.4 lb per person per year, dextrose at about 4.2 lb per person per year, and the remaining legal food additives are used at a total of slightly more than 9 lb per year.[9]

Of the 9 lb per year of other additives, 7.8 lb are accounted for by 32 commonly used additives such as leavening agents, agents to control acidity and alkalinity, flavoring agents, propellents, and nutrient supplements. The remaining 1900 direct additives account for only 1.8 lb per person per year which is about 1 part per billion of the daily diet for each additive.[10]

It seems then that we ought not to worry about our food supply. However, accidents have happened and news stories occasionally reflect inadequacies in con-

sumer protection, but the dangers associated with the additives in our food supply have been exaggerated. In fact, profits are sometimes made by means of scare tactics. As one of hundreds of possible examples: *Nutrition Today* reported in 1975 that a "Sioux City, Iowa, firm is frightening shoppers into buying a product called 'Homaganized Bakon'— exact composition unrevealed except that it contains no nitrites or nitrates," implying that regular bacon would cause cancer.[11] The editorial in that issue of *Nutrition Today* is recommended reading for anyone attempting to get a sense of perspective. It concludes, "No one has the right to stand up in our perturbed and restless society and cry, without adequate cause, 'Cancer! Alarm! Cancer!' " The analogy is to the tragic deaths that occur when the audience in a crowded theater panics at someone's crying "Fire!"— and in that case, a public law has made such an outcry illegal. Perhaps we need a law against the shouting of false alarms about the dangers of our food supply.

One reason for the public's sometimes unreasonable fear of additives is a generalized fear of anything "chemical" or "synthetic." Many deadly poisons are "natural" substances found in foods or

[8]H. Hopkins, Finding out what else you eat, *FDA Consumer* 9 (6) (1975):8-15.

[9]Middlekauf, 1974.

[10]Middlekauf, 1974.

[11]F. J. Ingelfinger, A matter of opinion, *Nutrition Today* 10:4 (1975):11, 28.

produced by living organisms (consider mushrooms). Many plant products can make people sick, not because they contain additives but because they contain substances to which people are allergic. In a letter to the editor of the *Journal of the American Medical Association*, a physician expressed concern over illness caused by herbal teas. Camomile tea, for example, provokes a violent allergic reaction in people who get hay fever from ragweed pollen.[12]

Another reason for exaggerated alarm about additives is the public's failure to understand the difference between *toxicity* and *hazard*. "Toxicity—the capacity of a chemical substance to harm living organisms—is a general property of matter; hazard is the capacity of a chemical to produce injury under conditions of use. All substances are potentially toxic, but are hazardous only if consumed in sufficiently large quantities."[13]

If there is a hazard associated with additives, it is very small compared with many other food-associated

hazards that get less attention from the public. In 1975, the former Commissioner of Food and Drugs put additives sixth and last among the "broad areas of hazard" that people are concerned about. In order of concern, hazards associated with foods are:

1. Food-borne infection, which is increasing because of large-scale operations and multiple transfers involving handling
2. Nutrition, which requires close attention as more artificially constituted foods appear on the market
3. Environmental contaminants, which are increasing yearly in number and in concentration and whose consequences are difficult to foresee and forestall
4. Naturally occurring toxicants in foods, which occur randomly at arbitrary levels and constitute a hazard whenever people turn to consuming single foods either by choice (fad diets) or by necessity (famine)
5. Pesticide residues
6. Food additives, listed last "because so much is known about them, and all are now, and surely will continue to be, well regulated."[14]

One of the reasons additives are used, of course, is to protect against the development and growth of microorganisms in food. Serious

illness and even death from food-borne infections can occur whenever batches of contaminated foods escape detection and are distributed. Batch numbering makes it possible to recall all food items from a contaminated batch through public announcements on TV, radio, and through other public media. Close monitoring of commercial processing, preparation, and distribution of food is extraordinarily effective, but individual consumers must be vigilant and knowledgeable in order to protect themselves against occasional hazards resulting from their care of the food after purchase.

Prevention of food poisoning is another concern that justifies the use of some additives. For example, nitrates and nitrites have been opposed because of their possible link to cancer. Nitrates can be converted to nitrites which then can combine with amines in the stomach to form nitrosamines, and these in turn can cause cancer.[15] However, nitrates and nitrites occur naturally in some vegetables, and even in the body, in much higher levels than those added to bacon, ham, and hot dogs. They are added to these meats to prevent the botulism organism from

[12]W. H. Lewis, Reporting adverse reactions to herbal ingestants (letter to the editor), *Journal of the American Medical Association* 240 (1978):109-110.

[13]W. H. Strong, Toxicants occuring naturally in foods, in *Nutrition Reviews' Present Knowledge in Nutrition*, 4th ed. (Washington, D.C.: Nutrition Foundation, 1976), pp. 516-527.

[14]A. M. Schmidt, Food and drug law: A two-hundred-year perspective, *Nutrition Today* 10:4 (1975):29-32.

[15]N. P. Sen, Nitrosamines, in *Toxic Constituents in Animal Foodstuffs*, ed. I. E. Liener (New York: Academic Press, 1971), pp. 131-195.

producing its toxin. Botulism is the most potent biological poison known and a more immediate hazard than cancer. Therefore, viewed in terms of risk versus benefit, the use of nitrates and nitrites appears to be justified. At present, we seem to have no better alternative.

On the other hand, when a chemical finds its way into the food supply and constitutes a risk, no matter how small, that is not outweighed by the benefits, we can afford to do without it. An example is provided by DES (diethylstilbestrol), a hormone added to cattle feed to promote growth. DES can cause cancer. At first it could not be detected in meats from cattle whose feed had contained it, but when tests became sensitive enough to detect its presence at extraordinarily low levels, its use was banned.[16]

When an additive is used for esthetic reasons only, restrictions can be stringent. In line with this principle, the FDA is clearing the GRAS list of all color additives and adding back only those which are thoroughly tested.[17] Attractive colors add more appeal to food than their opponents may give them credit for, but their use is still "only" esthetic. "Today the abundance of our food supply permits the luxury of trying to avoid any and all risk. We can afford to seek the ideal of absolute safety."[18]

At present, in the minds of many consumers, the ideas about what constitutes safety are rather hazy. In the laws as they are stated, the concept of safety seems to be based on a *margin of safety.* Most chemicals that involve risk are allowed in foods only at levels 100 times below those at which there is no adverse effect at all when the chemical is ingested by animals.[19] This margin of safety is said to be 100. Experiments for this purpose involve feeding test animals the substance at different concentrations throughout their lifetimes. In many foods, naturally occurring substances appear at levels such that the margin of safety is closer to 10. Even some nutrients, as you have seen, involve risks at high dosage levels. The margin of safety for vitamins A and D is 25 to 40; it may be less than 10 in infants (see Chapter 11). For some trace elements it is about 5. Many people consume common table salt every day in amounts only three to five times less than those that cause serious toxicity.[20]

Not only are the allowable concentrations of any potentially toxic substances extremely low, but the toxicities also do not add to each other. For example, if you dosed yourself with 100 different compounds, each at a hundredth of what would cause toxicity, you would still have one-hundredth the chance of experiencing a toxic reaction. Often there are antagonisms as well: "The toxicity of one element is offset by the presence of an adequate amount of another."[21]

Food itself also protects against toxicity: fat mammals, birds, and fish are more resistant to the insecticide DDT than their thinner counterparts; DDT depletes the liver of vitamin A, so that a vitamin A deficient diet increases the risk from DDT; cadmium is a toxic substance present in some soils and thus in foods, but its toxicity seems to be reduced by adequate zinc in the diet; and dietary calcium can alter the effect of too much zinc since calcium increases the zinc requirements, especially when there is an abundance of phytic acid.[22] (If you find all these interactions confusing, welcome to the club.

[16]A. M. Schmidt, The benefit-risk equation, *FDA Consumer* 8:4 (1974):27-31.

[17]H. Hopkins, Countdown on color additives, *FDA Consumer* 10:9 (1976):5-7.

[18]Schmidt, 1975.

[19]J. M. Coon, Natural food toxicants: A perspective, in *Nutrition Reviews' Present Knowledge in Nutrition*, 4th ed. (Washington, D.C.: Nutrition Foundation, 1976), pp. 528-546.

[20]Strong, 1976.

[21]Coon, 1976.

[22]R. A. Shakman, Nutritional influences on the toxicity of environmental pollutants, *Archives of Environmental Health* 28 (1974):105-113.

The experts are confused. It is only the people who are not trying to see the total picture who are making blanket indictments of additives.)

There is much yet to learn about additives and their interactions with body substances, but some surprising results have come already. BHA (butylated hydroxyanisole) and BHT (butylated hydroxytoluene) are antioxidants widely used to control rancidity of oils, but they have been the target of campaigns to get them out of the food supply. Now, however, research indicates that maybe, just maybe, BHA and BHT protect against carcinogens in some way. It would be ironic if these reputed demons should turn out to be beneficial after all.[23]

This attempt to put in perspective the chemicals that find their way into our food supply has shown that there are many reasons why we need not be alarmed at the presence of intentional additives in our foods: They are needed; they are not hazardous; they are thoroughly tested; they are permitted in foods only with a wide margin of safety; and they are listed on the food labels. When an additive fails to meet our stringent requirements, action follows promptly. A familiar instance is that of saccharin; we will take a closer look at this one substance in order to illustrate some principles that operate to protect our food supply.

Saccharin, a Case Study
After the ban on cyclamates, saccharin became the major artificial sweetener used in diet foods and beverages and as a sugar substitute. Then reports were made public that saccharin, too, was a carcinogen. Rats fed large quantities of saccharin in their feed showed a higher incidence of bladder cancer than did control rats. Some evidence followed from human studies suggesting that saccharin caused bladder cancer in humans as well.[24] As a result, the FDA removed saccharin from the GRAS list in 1971 and banned it from use in 1977.

Ironically, the public responded without gratitude for the vigilance of the FDA. Within 8 weeks of the proposed ban, 25,000 people responded—the greatest response the FDA had ever received—and most of them were opposed to banning saccharin. Opposition to the ban became so strong that Congress decided to allow its continued use but to require food manufacturers to label all foods containing it:

Use of this product may be hazardous to your health. This product contains saccharin, which has been determined to cause cancer in laboratory animals.

The intention was to reduce the use of saccharin by 90 percent and to eliminate the risk to children altogether. Thus an additive that has been seen to cause cancer in animals remains on the market, and it is left to the consumer to decide whether to use it or not.

An important issue to understand before deciding is whether, and how far, animal test results can be extended to apply to human beings. Laboratory animals are much smaller than human beings, their metabolism is faster, and their life spans are shorter. To test the toxicity of a substance for human beings, animal experiments must be designed so that the total dose received by a small number of animals during the testing period will provide enough information so that the experimenters can draw conclusions about the probable effects of the substance on the people in the entire U.S. population throughout their life times. This entails giving the animals much larger doses than a person would take, balancing this effect by using a much shorter testing period, and making several assumptions that may or may not be valid.

One of the major assump-

[23]A. B. Lowenfels and M. E. Anderson, Diet and cancer, *Cancer* 39 (1977):1809-1814.

[24]G. R. Howe, J. D. Burch, and A. B. Miller, Artificial sweeteners and human bladder cancer, *Lancet*, 17 September 1977, pp. 578-581.

tions is that the relationship of the dose level to its effects is linear (see p. 467). That is, if 10 units cause 10 episodes of illness, then 100 units will cause 100. This assumption is not valid for some substances, where sublethal doses may show no effect (and if metabolized, no cumulative effect), but where, above a certain threshold, a dose will kill all the animals exposed to it. An example is that of a nutrient such as iodine: If large doses of iodine were given to test animals to determine its safety for humans, the animals would die, and the erroneous conclusion might be drawn that iodine at any dose was unsafe for human use.

However, with carcinogens, the assumption seems to be more valid. A carcinogen does not work by reaching a certain threshold level and then overwhelming the host, like a poison. Rather, a single molecule of the carcinogen can cause an event in a single cell of the host, so that the cell becomes cancerous and begins to multiply out of control. The more molecules of the carcinogen there are, and the longer the exposure time, the more likely this event becomes, so there is no dose level at which a carcinogen can be guaranteed safe. It is on this reasoning that the Delaney Clause is based: Even a very low dose of a carcinogen can initiate cancer.

On the other hand, the effect of low doses of a carcinogen may be canceled by the body's defense mechanisms. Even after the initiating event has occurred, cancer is not inevitable, because many steps must still ensue. (Highlight 2 discussed these steps.) The body is protected at many of these steps by a nutritious diet rich in vegetables and fiber.[25] Thus, although any dose of a carcinogen can theoretically cause cancer, the chance with low doses is small, and may even be negligible.

Another question about the relevance of animal findings is whether the animals and humans are equally susceptible to the carcinogen. Sometimes the metabolism of a test animal will differ from that of human beings. Experiments using rabbits to get information about cholesterol metabolism in human beings have had to be discarded, because rabbits' metabolism of cholesterol happens to differ significantly from that of humans. But with cancer, the National Re-

search Council reports, "Virtually every form of human cancer has an experimental counterpart, and every form of multicellular organism is subject to cancer."[26] It seems, from what we know, that it is legitimate to apply rat results to humans in the case of the bladder cancers caused by saccharin.

Animal experiments are of great value in predicting the consequences of human intake of certain substances where the direct study of humans would be unethical or would take too long to be of value for the present generation. Each must be scrutinized on its own merits, however. Not treated here have been several questions:[27]

● The route of administration. If humans take the substance by mouth, then it should be given by mouth to the animals.

● The determination of excretion. Does the substance actually get into the body?

● The study of metabolism. If the substance is metabolized in the human to some other substance (for example, nitrates to nitrosamines), then the metabolite should be tested in animals.

[25]J. Arehart-Treichel, Chemical carcinogens: Part of the problem, *Science News* 115 (1979):411-412. Sauerkraut, coleslaw, brussels sprouts, and broccoli have especially been noted as being negatively correlated with cancer of the colon: S. Graham, H. Dayal, M. Swanson, A. Mittleman, and G. Wilkinson, Diet in the epidemiology of cancer of the colon and rectum, *Journal of the National Cancer Institute* 61 (1978):709-713.

[26]National Research Council, as quoted in *Science News* 112 (2 July 1977):12-13.

[27]T. H. Jukes, Fact and fancy in nutrition and food science, *Journal of the American Dietetic Association* 59 (1971):203-211.

To make a long story short, these problems would seem to have been satisfactorily dealt with by the rat-saccharin investigators.

The rat-saccharin experiments have been questioned from another angle, too. Critics have said that the cancers seen in the experimental animals were caused not by the saccharin itself but by impurities in the commercial preparations used in the tests or by derivatives of these impurities produced in the animal's body.[28] Saccharin for human use does not contain these impurities, so if this is true, the rat results have no relevance to humans. In one experiment, when highly purified saccharin was used in a very sensitive test, it appeared to cause no mutations down to a very low frequency. However, in another very sensitive kind of test, purified saccharin did cause mutations, proving to be a true carcinogen, although a "weak" one.[29] Frustrating as it may be for the public to wait, it seems that further testing may be needed to completely resolve the issue. Meanwhile, the likelihood is that saccharin is a weak carcinogen.

The most-discussed result with human beings is from a Canadian study in which the investigators reported that males with bladder cancer had used more saccharin than those without cancer—but the females who developed cancer had used less saccharin. If the results for the two sexes were averaged, a critic says, the difference between the saccharin users and the nonusers would be insignificant.[30] This review again suggests that the risks with normal use are very small.

The consumer faced with deciding whether or not to use saccharin might want to compare its risks with the benefits in his own individual case. For example, people with diabetes may have an irresistible craving for sweets, which saccharin can satisfy. If the use of saccharin helps to curb their weight-gaining tendencies, then the benefits may well outweigh the risks. The president of the American Cancer Society is quoted as saying that saccharin has "great value" in this respect.[31] On the other hand, a pregnant woman who uses saccharin exposes not only herself but also her unborn baby to it, and might decide that the risks in her case outweigh the benefits.

Perhaps moderation in the use of saccharin is the choice for some. A guideline as to what constitutes moderation is provided by the Canadian Dietetic Association, which says that an intake of 50 mg a day can be considered moderate.[32] (Over-the-counter sale of saccharin is now prohibited in Canada, and it is recommended that pregnant and lactating women not use it at all.) This is conservative. A 12-oz drink containing 10 mg per oz provides a total of 120 mg of saccharin, and a tablet equivalent to the sweetness of a teaspoon of sugar provides about 8 mg. Thus we might limit ourselves to two or three diet drinks a week, or use only a few tablets a day.

Personal Strategies   It seems that on the whole you can have confidence in the food supply. Thanks to our regulatory agencies, it is one of the safest in the world. If there is any area in which a little healthy fear may be justified, it is probably in your own kitchen. When a normally healthy person eats a normal amount of food and gets sick from it, it is seldom if ever because the food-as-purchased was bad; it is

[28]R. P. Batzinger, S.-Y. L. Ou and E. Bueding, Saccharin and other sweeteners: Mutagenic properties, *Science* 198 (1977):944-946.

[29]S. Wolff and B. Rodin, Saccharin-induced sister chromatid exchanges in Chinese hamster and human cells, *Science* 200 (1978):543-545.

[30]Bladder cancer and saccharin, *Lancet,* 17 September 1977, pp. 592-593.

[31]*Nutrition Today,* July/August 1977, p. 4.

[32]M. Hollands and J. Goeller, A guideline to the use of saccharin, *Journal of the Canadian Dietetic Association* 38 (July 1977):198, abstract cited in *Journal of the American Dietetic Association* 71 (1977):572.

almost always because of careless food handling. Our regulatory agencies can't enforce the washing of home kitchen utensils in hot, soapy water with each use, nor can they require the refrigeration of egg-milk dishes. Food poisoning is a real possibility for the careless handler of food.

Otherwise, harm from food almost always results from consumption of abnormally large quantities of a single food, as when someone eats tuna three times a day for a year, or from an abnormality of the individual, such as allergy, inborn error, or disease.[33]

To protect yourself against possible harm from additives, you can apply the principle of dilution: Eat a wide variety of foods. Suppose, for example, that you are concerned about the nitrates used in the preservation of meats. How can you dilute these? Of course, you could abstain from eating any processed meat, but when you do that you may unknowingly be increasing some other harmful substance. A smarter way, perhaps, is to eat a variety of fresh meats and only occasionally to have cold cuts or ham. Sometimes children will use cold cuts for between-meal snacks. A wise parent will offer cheese and fruits instead, and reserve the nitrates for a time when the

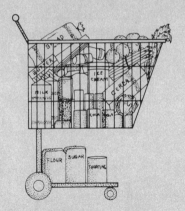

entire family wants to enjoy ham. In other words, don't eliminate a class of foods altogether lest you overburden your body with another. Just introduce more variety. As J. M. Coon wrote in *Nutrition Reviews*, "The wider the variety of food intake, the greater is the number of different chemical substances consumed and the less is the chance that any one chemical will reach a hazardous level in the diet."[34]

Finally, if you are still concerned about the presence of an additive in the food supply, it seems to us inappropriate to cry, "Fire!" Rather, it behooves the consumer to inform himself diligently, to exercise his right to choose in the market place those foods he considers safe, and, if he is very concerned about the food supply, to campaign actively in the political arena for whatever changes he believes are needed.

To Explore Further

The two sides of the question of additives can be reviewed in these two books:

Hunter, B. T., *The Mirage of Safety* (New York: Scribner's, 1975).

Whelan, E., and Stare, F. J., *Panic in the Pantry* (New York: Atheneum, 1975).

A symposium presented at the Massachusetts Institute of Technology in September 1979 explored the risk versus benefits of chemicals found in our food supply:

Risk versus benefits: The future of food safety, *Nutrition Reviews* 38 (1980):35-64.

Three reprints on food additives can be ordered from U. S. Government Printing Office (address in Appendix J):

P. Lehman, More than you ever thought you would know about food additives, FDA Consumer (1979) April, May, and June, HEW Publication No. 5 (FDA) 79-2115, 79-2118, and 79-2119.

Shakman, R. A., Nutritional influences on the toxicity of environmental pollutants, *Archives of Environmental Health* 28 (1974):105-113 includes an interesting discussion of how the diet influences the toxicity of trace minerals and oxidant air pollutants.

Two other books on additives that present thought-provoking views are:

Jacobson, M., *Eater's Digest: The Consumer's Factbook of Food Additives* (New York: Doubleday, 1972).

Benarde, M., *The Chemicals We*

[33]Coon, 1976.

[34]Coon, 1976.

Eat (New York: McGraw-Hill, 1975).

Short articles on additives that make interesting reading:

Hall, R. L., Food additives, *Nutrition Today,* July/August 1973, pp. 20-28.

Hall, R. L., Safe at the plate, *Nutrition Today,* November/December 1977, pp. 6-9, 28-31. This one pokes fun at all the scare stories.

Kermode, G. O., Food additives, *Scientific American* 226 (1972):15-21. This, although older, remains one of the sanest and most balanced views available in short form.

Helpful pamphlets, free from General Foods (address in Appendix J) are:

Today's Food and Additives, 1976.

Focus on Food Additives, 1976.

A poster that lists about 50 common additives and classifies them as safe, unsafe, or questionable is available for $1.75 from the Center for Science in the Public Interest, Box 3099, Washington, DC 20010. This might stimulate good discussion, in light of the perspectives offered in this book.

A general review of all color additives and how the FDA regulates them:

Damon, G. E., and Jannsen, W. F., Additives for eye appeal, *FDA Consumer,* July/August 1973, pp. 15-18.

A teaching aid, *Additives* by R. L. Hall, can be ordered from the Nutrition Today Society (address in Appendix J).

We wish to thank Emil Corwin, Public Information Officer, Food and Drug Administration, and Dr. Katherine Clancy, Nutritionist, Federal Trade Commission, for their help with the details of the law relating to consumer issues.

Trace Minerals

Look up and record your recommended intake of iron (from the RDA tables on the inside front cover or from the Canadian Dietary Standard in Appendix O). Also record your actual intake, from the average derived on Form 2 in the Self-Study at the end of the introduction to Part One (p. 16). What percentage of your recommended intake did you consume? Was this enough?

Which of the foods you eat supply the most iron? Rank your top five iron contributors: How many were meats? Legumes? Greens? Did any of them fall outside these classes? If so, what were they? How much of a contribution does enriched or whole-grain bread or cereal make to your iron intake? Are there refined bread/cereal products in your diet, such as pastries, that you could replace with enriched or whole-grain products to increase your iron intake?

Optional Extras

● If you have a need to learn more about individual foods and their contributions of iron to the diet, look up some of the following in Appendix H: different kinds of liver; different green, leafy vegetables; various breads and cereals (do enriched breads have more or less iron than whole-grain breads, or are they about the same?); nuts and legumes; dried fruits; molasses and other sugar sources. Pay particular attention to the foods you eat. Then plan several days' menus you would enjoy that provide your recommended intake.

● Are you in an area of the country where the soil is iodine-poor? If so, do you use iodized salt?

● Is the water in your county fluoridated? If not, how do you and your family ensure that your intakes of fluoride are optimal?

● Review your three-day food record (p. 14) and separate the foods you ate into two categories: predominantly natural, unprocessed foods like those on the exchange lists (Appendix L) and highly processed foods, such as TV dinners, pastries, and potato chips. By each food, record its kcaloric value. How many total kcalories did you consume in three days? Of these, what percentage came from highly processed foods? In light of the discussion of trace elements in Chapter 13, what implications do you suppose this estimate has for the nutritional adequacy of your diet?

Scoring Your Diet against the Four Food Group Plan

With all the possible food choices that people can make, many different patterns of food intake can add up to an adequate diet. It is obvious that the best guidelines for a nutritious diet are those a well-informed individual chooses for herself. There is no one right way. However, if you seek a single guide, the most serviceable and long-lived one is the Four Food Group Plan. Representatives of all four food groups appear in the diets of almost all the world's people. Wherever all four groups are fairly represented, there is likely to be adequate nutrition.

To help people discover how well-planned their own diets are, nutrition educators sometimes employ a scorecard like that shown in Form 1. Such a scorecard can be most helpful, especially when your diet planning is based on the Four Food Group system. If you have completed the Self-Studies up to this point, you can now compare the usefulness of this quick scoring system with that of the detailed analysis you have already done. Some people find that they can rely entirely on a nutrition scorecard like this. Others find it too simple to be satisfactory.

The scorecard can be off in two ways. A high score can be belied by poor nutrient intakes if the particular selections from the food groups are poor. This may mean you should reexamine the food groups to find better sources of the nutrients you lack. Conversely, your diet can meet 100 percent of the recommended intakes for all of the indicator nutrients without scoring well on the scorecard. If this is the case, you may want to note and remember what special foods are meeting your nutrient needs.

The scorecard illustrates a point that is important in diet planning. Notice that it allows points for foods from each of the four food groups to a maximum of 25. The only way you can score a perfect 100 is to choose from all four groups. The message is to diversify your investment. Don't overdo any one food or food group; and don't leave one out without compensating carefully. This way you will reap the benefits not only of the nutrients you know are in the foods you

choose but also of those that are unlisted—vitamin D, zinc, vitamin B_6, iodine, folic acid, and some 30 others. A diet that provides an abundance of all the familiar nutrients is virtually guaranteed to supply the others equally generously.

To use the scorecard, list the foods you ate in one day on Form 1 and score as directed. Repeat for each additional day. How does your daily diet score by this method? Are these scores fair? Why or why not?

This is the last of the exercises we will suggest to help you study your own diet. Review the work you have done and summarize your most important findings. What changes, if any, have you made in your diet as a result of these Self-Studies? What effect have these changes had on you so far? (Do you feel better? Have you had to change your lifestyle at all? Are you spending more or less money for food? Has your weight changed?) What changes do you still intend to make?

Form 1. Food Selection Scorecard

Food group and recommended intake	Your score	Your intake from group (specify food and amount)
Fruits & vegetables—4 or more servings (1/2 c cooked edible portion or 3-4 oz, 100 g, raw); at least one raw daily		
One serving vitamin A-rich dark green or deep orange fruit or vegetable (any food with more than your RDA) = 10 points (no more than 10 points allowed)		
One serving vitamin C-rich fruit or vegetable (any food with more than your RDA) = 10 points (no more than 10 points allowed)		
Other fruits and vegetables, including potatoes = 2.5 each		
Subtotal (no more than 25 points allowed)		
Breads & cereals—4 or more servings of whole-grain or "enriched" (1 oz dry-weight cereal or 1-oz slice bread or equivalent grain product)		
One serving cereal or 2 bread equivalents = 10 points (no more than 10 points allowed)		
Other bread equivalents = 5 points each		
Subtotal (no more than 25 points allowed)		
Milk & milk products—2 or more servings (8 oz fluid milk; calcium equivalents are 1 1/3 oz hard cheese, 1 1/3 c cottage cheese, 1 pint ice milk or ice cream)		
One serving = 12.5 points		
Subtotal (no more than 25 points allowed)		
Meat & meat substitutes—2 or more servings (2-3 oz cooked lean meat, fish, poultry; protein equivalents are 2 eggs, 2 oz hard cheese, 1/2 c hard cheese, 1/2 c cottage cheese, 1 c cooked legumes, 4 tbsp peanut butter, 1 oz nuts or sunflower seeds); count cheese either in milk group or in meat group, not both		
One serving = 12.5 points		
Subtotal (no more than 25 points allowed)		
GRAND TOTAL (no more than 100 points)		

The above are FOUNDATION FOODS. ADDITIONAL FOODS are those that do not fit into the above groupings but add flavor, interest, variety, and (often) kcalories. List those eaten:

_____   _____   _____

_____   _____   _____

_____   _____   _____

CHAPTER 14

CONTENTS

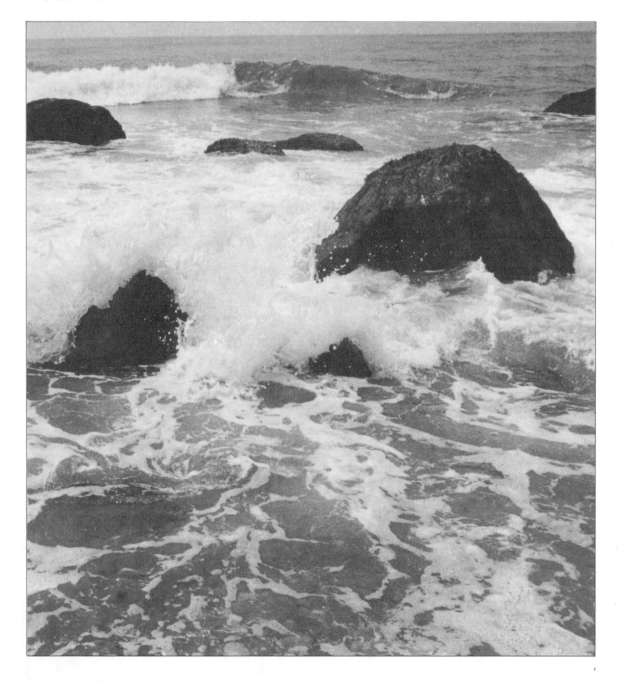

WATER AND SALTS

It was assuredly not chance that led Thales to found philosophy and science with the assertion that water is the origin of all things.

LAWRENCE J. HENDERSON

Water and salts provide the medium in which nearly all of the body's reactions take place, participate in many of them, and supply the means for transporting vital materials to cells and waste products away from them. Every cell in the body is bathed in water of the exact composition that is best for it. The fluid found in the eye contains the dissolved materials necessary for the health of the rod and cone cells; the fluid inside the spinal column is perfectly constituted for nerve cell function; the fluid at each point along the GI tract is ideal for the activities of the cells in that part of the tract—and so on.

Each of these fluids is constantly undergoing loss and replacement of its constituent parts as cells withdraw nutrients and oxygen from them and excrete carbon dioxide and other waste materials into them. Yet the composition of the body fluids in each compartment remains remarkably constant at all times. We have provided details about two examples of this constancy: the regulation of blood glucose concentration (Chapter 1) and that of blood calcium (Chapter 12). On closer examination, it becomes apparent that every important constituent of body fluids is similarly regulated. The interstitial fluid, for example, always has a high concentration of sodium and chloride ions and lower concentrations of about eight other major ions. The intracellular fluid always has high potassium and phosphate concentrations and lower concentrations of other ions. These special fluids regulate the functioning of cells; the cells in turn regulate the composition and amount of the fluids. The entire system of cells and fluids remains in a delicate but firmly maintained state of dynamic equilibrium.

The maintenance of this balance is so important that it is credited with our ability and that of other animals to live on land. Our single-celled ancestors depended totally on the sea water they lived in to provide nutrients and oxygen and to carry away their waste. We have managed over the course of our 2-billion-year evolutionary history to internalize the ocean—to continue bathing our cells in a warm nutritive fluid that keeps them alive. It is interesting to note that the amounts of salts in our body fluids, and their temperature, are believed to be the same as in the ocean—not as it is now, but as it was at the

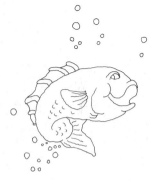

We, too, live in water.

Ionic compounds: see Appendix B.

dynamic equilibrium: a state of balance in which rapid exchange is taking place. For example, body fluids, bones, and fat maintain a constant composition but exchange materials continuously with their surroundings. As opposed to a condition of **static equilibrium**, dynamic equilibrium is a condition of **homeostasis** (see p. 179).

Salt does not refer only to sodium chloride but also to ionic compounds, as defined in Appendix B.

495

time when our ancestors emerged onto land. The ocean has since become more salty, but we still carry the ancient ocean within us.

The Uniqueness of Water

Water in the body is not simply a river coursing through the arteries, capillaries, and veins, carrying the heavy traffic of nutrients and waste products. Some of the water is a part of the chemical structure of compounds that form the cells, tissues, and organs of the body. For example, protein holds water molecules within its structure. This water is locked in and is not readily available for any other use.

> The water held in protein molecules often discourages the very obese person who has starved himself and lost lean body mass. When he first eats a small amount of food, restoring even a pound of his protein tissue brings with it the retention of 4 lb water. Small wonder that the obese person thinks that any tiny amount of food causes him to gain enormous amounts of weight. As a result, he concludes that dieting is futile for him.

Water also participates actively in many chemical reactions, instead of being merely the medium in which they take place. A good example of this is the splitting of two glucose units (a disaccharide). Water participates by being split, with a hydrogen going to one glucose and an oxygen and hydrogen going to the other. By this action, the bond that held the two glucose units together is broken.

As the medium for the body's chemical traffic, water is very nearly a universal solvent. Luckily for our body integrity, this is not quite the case, but water does dissolve amino acids, glucose, minerals, and many other substances needed by the cells. Fatty substances are specially wrapped in water-soluble protein so that they too can travel freely in the blood and lymph. Water thus makes an ideal transportation medium.

Another important characteristic of water is its incompressibility: Its molecules resist being crowded together. Thanks to this characteristic, water acts as a lubricant around joints. For the same reason, it can protect a sensitive tissue, such as the spinal cord, from shock. The fluid that fills the eye serves in a similar way to keep optimal pressure on the retina and lens. The unborn infant is cushioned against blows by the bag of water it develops in. Water also lubricates the digestive tract and all tissues moistened with mucus.

Still another of water's special features is its heat-holding capacity. This characteristic of water is well known to coastal dwellers, who know that land surrounded by water is protected from rapid and wide variations in temperature from day to night. Water itself changes temperature slowly; at night, when the land cools, the water holds its heat and gives it up gradually to the air, moderating the coolness of the night. In contrast, the desert has a wide variation in temperature from day to night because of the lack of water on the land and in the air. In our bodies, water helps to maintain our temperature at a constant 98.6° F (37° C) by resisting fluctuations in temperature.

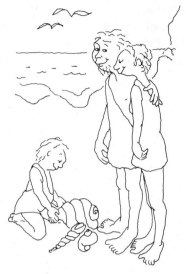

Related to this characteristic is the fact that a great deal of heat is required to change water from a liquid to a gas. This serves the body when cooling is needed. In a very hot environment, we sweat: Water is brought to the body surface through the sweat glands. When the sweat evaporates, it carries off all the absorbed heat and so cools the body.

Another fascinating characteristic of water that makes life possible on earth is the fact that it contracts as it gets colder but that, unlike other substances, it expands as it freezes. (It is most dense at 4° C.) Ice is thus lighter than cold water and so floats instead of sinking. This protects the water beneath from the coldness of the air. Thus pond water below a protective sheet of ice can remain unfrozen, and living things in a pond can survive through hard winters, even when the temperature of the air falls many degrees below freezing.

The expansion of water during freezing explains why packages of frozen food tell you "Do not refreeze." As it freezes, the water disrupts the structure of the food and so changes its texture. People sometimes wonder if there is any danger in eating a twice-frozen food. Provided that they haven't let it spoil while it was thawed, the only problem is that the food may be less appealing. Its nutrient content is not affected by refreezing.

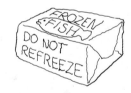

The Constancy of Body Water

Water constitutes 55 to 60 percent of your body weight, and it is fortunate that the total amount of water remains constant. That it does so is a consequence of two delicate balancing systems that regulate both its intake and its excretion.

Water Intake: Thirst   When you need water, you drink. Everybody knows that, but it takes a thinking physiologist to ask why. The evidence from experiments with thirst points to the possibility that several mechanisms operate in its regulation. One is in the mouth itself: When the blood is too salty (having lost water but not salts), water is withdrawn from the salivary glands into the blood. The mouth becomes dry as a result, and you drink to wet your mouth. Another thirst mechanism is in a brain center, where cells sample and monitor

Water follows salt, moving in the direction of higher osmotic pressure (see p. 500).

The brain center described here is the **hypothalamus** (hy-po-THAL-a-mus).

the salt concentration in the blood. When they find it too high, they initiate impulses that travel to brain centers that in turn stimulate drinking behavior. The stomach may also play a role. Thirsty animals drink until nerves in their stomachs, known as stretch receptors, are stimulated enough to turn off the drinking. More must be learned about these mechanisms, but it is clear from what we know already that thirst is finely adjusted to provide a water intake that exactly meets the need.

Water Excretion   This mechanism is better understood. The cells of the hypothalamus, which monitor salt concentration in the blood, stimulate the pituitary gland to release a hormone, ADH, whenever the body's salt concentration is too high. ADH stimulates the kidneys to hold back (actually reabsorb) water, so that it recirculates in the body rather than being excreted. Thus the more water you need, the less you excrete. There are also cells in the kidney itself that are responsive to the salt concentration in the blood passing through them. When they sense a too-high salt concentration, they too release a substance. By a

---

Two mechanisms control the way the kidney retains water: the ADH mechanism and the aldosterone mechanism.

The ADH mechanism directly causes water retention by the kidneys.

ADH (antidiuretic hormone): a hormone released by the pituitary gland in response to high osmotic pressure of the blood. Target organ: the kidney, which responds by reabsorbing water.

Hormone: see p. 165.

The aldosterone mechanism indirectly causes water retention by the kidney:

1. The kidney releases renin in response to high osmotic pressure of the blood.
2. The renin converts angiotensinogen (an-gee-o-ten-SIN-o-gen) in the blood to angiotensin (an-gee-o-TEN-sin).
3. Angiotensin stimulates the adrenal gland to release aldosterone.
4. Aldosterone stimulates the kidney to reabsorb sodium.
5. Water follows sodium and is reabsorbed.

aldosterone (al-DOSS-ter-OWN): a hormone released by the adrenal gland in response to the presence of angiotensin. Target organ: the kidney, which responds by reabsorbing sodium.

roundabout route, this substance causes the adrenal gland to release a hormone—aldosterone—that in turn causes the kidneys to retain more water. Again, the effect is that when more water is needed, less is excreted.

These renal excretion mechanisms cannot work by themselves to maintain water balance unless you drink enough. This is because the body must excrete a minimum amount of water each day—the amount necessary to carry out of the body the waste products generated by the day's metabolic activities. Above this minimum (about 900 ml a day), the amounts of water you excrete can be adjusted to balance your intake. The urine merely becomes more dilute. Hence drinking plenty of water is never a bad idea.

Metabolic wastes: ketones and urea (see pp. 234, 228).

Water Imbalance   Water deficiency, or dehydration, occurs whenever there is a massive loss of body water (as in kidney malfunction, blood loss, vomiting, or diarrhea) or when water becomes unavailable. Since the consequences are related to losses of the salts that accompany the water, this phenomenon is discussed below. Excess water in the body is reflected in the symptoms of edema, hypertension, or both; these too are related to the body's salt retention.

But consider sweating (see p. 507).

Massive loss of body water through the kidneys is **diuresis** (dye-yoo-REE-sis).

Losses from lungs and skin are called **insensible water losses.**

The Constancy of Total Body Water   In addition to the obvious dietary source, water itself, all foods contain water (as a look back at the figures on p. 5 will remind you). In addition, water is generated from the energy nutrients in foods (recall that the Cs and Hs in these nutrients combine with oxygen during metabolism to yield CO_2 and H_2O). Daily water intake from these three sources totals about 2 1/2 liters.

In addition to the water excreted via the kidneys, some water is lost from the lungs as vapor, some in feces, and some from the skin. The losses of all of these also total about 2 1/2 liters a day.

2 1/2 l is about 2 1/2 qt.

How Salts Behave

The regulation of body water distribution and transportation is intimately associated with the regulation of salt distribution. A closer look at the way the body handles this problem will pave the way for an understanding of the causes and consequences of imbalances.

Interestingly enough, the very minerals that are most important in regulation of the water balance—sodium, chlorine, phosphorus, and potassium—are those that are most abundant in the diet and thus are very rarely deficient in humans. This is no coincidence. The regulation of water balance is so vital that our bodies have evolved to use these abundant elements for this purpose. Any other course would have brought the process of evolution to a dead halt.

Water intake:

Liquids	950—1,500 ml
Food	700—1,000 ml
Metabolic water	200— 300 ml
	1,850—2,800 ml

Water output:

Kidneys	900—1,400 ml
Lungs	350 ml
Feces	150 ml
Skin	450— 900 ml
	1,850—2,800 ml

Na = sodium

Cl = chlorine

salt: a compound composed of charged particles (ions). However, a compound in which the cations are H^+ is an acid; a compound in which the anions are OH^- is a base.

cation (CAT-eye-un): a positively charged ion.

anion (AN-eye-un): a negatively charged ion.

For a closer look at ions, see Appendix B.

chloride: the ionic form of chlorine.

dissociation: physical separation of the ions in an ionic compound. A salt that partly dissociates in water is an **electrolyte**.

electrolyte solution: a solution that can conduct electricity.

milliequivalent: a number of ions equal to the number of H^+ ions in a milligram of hydrogen. This is a useful measure, because when we are considering ions we are usually interested in the number of positive or negative charges present in a solution rather than in their weight.

This force is known as the **osmotic pressure** of a solution. Water flows in the direction of the higher osmotic pressure. Whatever is dissolved in the water, that creates this pressure, is the **solute** (SOLL-yute).

To understand how cells regulate the amount of water they contain, it is necessary to take a closer look at the minerals as ions, the form in which cells use minerals for water regulation. Cell membranes are freely permeable to water, which flows back and forth across them all the time. Yet they neither lose all their water, shrinking down and collapsing, nor do they overfill with water, swelling up and bursting like balloons. Along the evolutionary path they have contrived a method of keeping their water constant; they do this beautifully by employing the salts to assist them. They make use of the principle that water follows salt.

Chemists use the term *salt* to include many inorganic substances, not just the ordinary table salt most of us are familiar with. To denote table salt, the chemist refers to table salt as sodium chloride, NaCl. Sodium chloride is a good example to use in a discussion of salts. In the white crystalline substance the sodium and chlorine atoms are bound together by strong electrostatic forces in a rigid crystalline structure. Outwardly, the crystals exhibit no electrical charge. However, when dissolved in water, the rigid structure relaxes. Some of the sodium moves about freely as positively charged ions, and some of the chloride also dissociates and moves about as negatively charged ions. The salt thus reveals itself as a compound composed of charged particles. The positive ions are cations; the negative, anions.

A salt that partly dissociates in water, as sodium chloride does, is known as an electrolyte. Since the fluids of the body are composed of water and partly dissociated salts, they are electrolyte solutions.

Electrolyte solutions are always electrostatically balanced. There is no such thing as a test tube filled with sodium ions. Sodium ions are always positvely charged, and so they cannot exist apart from negatively charged ions. Therefore, in any fluid with dissolved electrolytes there will always be the same number of positive and negative ions. For instance, in the extracellular fluid, the numbers of cations and anions both equal 155 milliequivalents per liter (mEq/l). Of the cations, sodium ions make up 142 mEq/l, and potassium, calcium, and magnesium ions make up the remainder. Of the anions, chloride ions number 104 mEq/l, bicarbonate ions number 27 mEq/l, and the remainder is provided by phosphate ions, sulfate ions, organic acids, and protein. If an anion enters a cell, a cation must accompany it or another anion must leave so that electroneutrality will be maintained.

We stated above that water follows salt. More precisely, there is a force that moves water into a place where a solute, such as sodium chloride, is concentrated. This force can operate only if the divider separating the two fluid solutions is permeable to water but not permeable (or less freely permeable) to the solute. The following figure shows this force in operation. In the top part, equal amounts of solute on both sides of the divider cause the amounts of water to be equal also. In the bottom part, the presence of more solute on side B has drawn water across the divider so that the *concentration* of solute on both sides becomes equal.

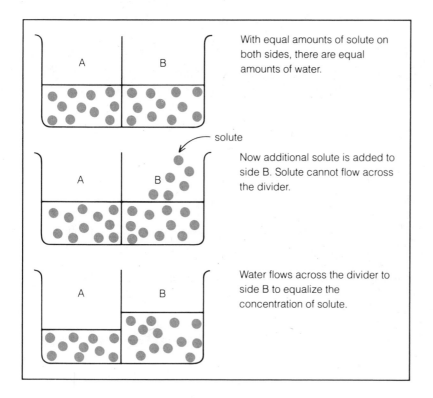

With equal amounts of solute on both sides, there are equal amounts of water.

— solute

Now additional solute is added to side B. Solute cannot flow across the divider.

Water flows across the divider to side B to equalize the concentration of solute.

You have seen this force at work if you have ever salted a lettuce salad an hour before eating it. When you came back to the salad, the lettuce was wilted and there was water in the salad bowl. The high concentration of salt (and therefore low concentration of water) on the outside of the lettuce cells caused water to leave the inside of the cells. They collapsed (the lettuce wilted), and the water puddled in the salad dish. Sugar would have caused the same reaction as the salt. There is one way you could have prevented this (here's a cooking lesson for the novice): You could have coated the lettuce lightly with oil, then salted it or put salad dressing containing salt on it; the oil would have acted as a barrier against the salt, keeping the lettuce crisp.

The Body's Use of Salts

With the previous diagram in mind, you can see how the living cell manages to move water in and out as it needs to. It is obvious how vital salts are to the body's well-being.

Water Balance   The divider between the water inside and outside of a cell is the cell membrane. The cell cannot pump water directly across its membrane, but it does have proteins in its membrane that can

Other terms used to describe electrolyte solutions:

isotonic: having the same osmotic pressure as a reference solution. For example, a saline solution may be made isotonic to human blood.

hypertonic: having a higher osmotic pressure than a reference solution.

hypotonic: having a lower osmotic pressure than a reference solution.

The salty water on the outside of the lettuce cells is hypertonic to the water inside the cells, so it attracts water out of the cells.

The cell membrane is **semipermeable:** more permeable to some substances (such as water) than to others. This is the condition necessary for osmotic pressure to operate.

For more about the cell-membrane pumps, see p. 196.

attach to sodium ions and move them from one side of the membrane to the other. When these sodium pumps are active, they pump out sodium faster than it can diffuse into the cell. Water follows the sodium. When potassium pumps are active, they pump in potassium, and water follows this ion. By maintaining a certain concentration of sodium outside and potassium inside, the cell can exactly regulate the amount of water it contains.

Acid-Base Balance   In addition to regulating the amount of water found in each body compartment, the body uses its ions to regulate the acidity (pH) of its fluids. The major minerals are most important in this regard, since they are present in the highest concentrations. The chloride ion, for example, shifts back and forth across the membranes of the red blood cells, helping the blood fluid to maintain the proper degree of acidity as the blood travels to and from the lungs. As the blood leaves the lungs bearing red blood cells loaded with oxygen, the chloride ion travels in the plasma. When the cells deliver their oxygen, the plasma picks up carbon dioxide from the tissues and carries it as bicarbonate ions. Thus the plasma's bicarbonate concentration rises. The chloride ions then shift into the red blood cells to keep the total acidity constant. After the blood has passed through the lungs and the bicarbonate level has been lowered, the chloride ions shift back into the blood fluid to maintain the acid-base balance.

The chloride ion, Cl^-, is a negatively charged, acid-forming ion.

The bicarbonate ion, HCO_3^-, is also a negatively charged, acid ion.

The electrolyte mixtures in the body fluids, as well as the proteins, also protect the body against changes in acidity by acting as buffers—substances that can accommodate excess plus or minus charges. The action of a buffer is shown in Figure 1.

buffer: a substance or mixture capable in solution of neutralizing both acids and bases and thereby capable of maintaining the original concentration of hydrogen ions (pH) in the solution.

Acid- and Base-Formers   Some of the major minerals are acid-formers; others are base-formers. Table 1 divides these minerals into the acid- and base-forming classes. Foods, too, can be classified as acid- or base-formers, depending on which of these minerals predominate in them. Grains contain the acid-forming minerals; fruits and vegetables contain base-formers.

The base-forming nature of fruits may come as a surprise to people who think of fruits as being acid. You may have heard someone say, for example, "I can't eat oranges; they're too acid for me." In truth, although fruits may taste sour or acid in the mouth, their ash is composed of base-forming minerals. After the *organic* acids have been digested, metabolized, and excreted, only the base-forming minerals are left. Therefore fruits and vegetables are ultimately alkaline to the body as a whole.

A buffer is a large molecule, usually protein, that can accommodate excess plus or minus charges (ions).

Figure 1   Action of a buffer.

A buffer can be neutral (an equal number of plus and minus charges).

A buffer can be acidic (an excess of plus charges).

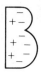

A buffer can be alkaline, or basic (an excess of minus charges).

In a solution, a buffer helps the solution keep its acid-base balance by soaking up excess plus or minus charges or by giving them up to the solution.

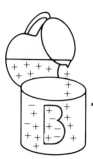

If the solution receives excess plus charges, tending to make it acidic,

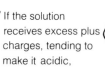

If the solution loses plus charges, tending to make it alkaline (basic),

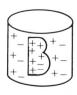

the buffer will pick these up. The solution keeps its acid-base balance.

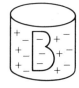

the buffer will give up its plus charges. The solution keeps its acid-base balance.

Table 1   The Major Minerals*

Acid-formers	Base-formers
Chlorine	Calcium
Sulfur	Magnesium
Phosphorus	Sodium
	Potassium

*The task of remembering each of these seven elements as either an acid-former or a base-former is somewhat simplified if you are aware that each of these elements forms a common compound whose name reveals its role. For example, a compound of calcium is calcium hydroxide. Hydroxides are bases—and thus calcium is a base-former. With phosphorus, a common compound is phosphoric acid; thus phosphorus is an acid-former. The compound of sulfur, sulfuric acid, tells you that sulfur is an acid-former. The rule is consistent: For chlorine, remember hydrochloric acid; for magnesium, sodium, and potassium, the hydroxides.

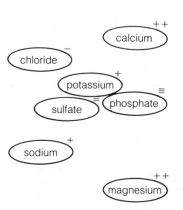

Major mineral ions.

Table 2 Acid- and Base-Forming Foods

Acid-forming foods	Base-forming foods
Meat, fish, poultry 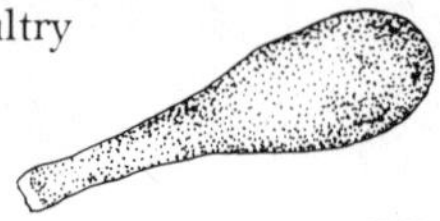	Milk 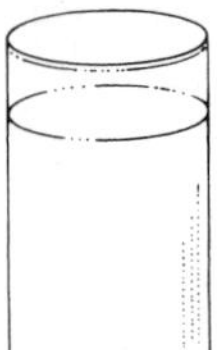
Eggs 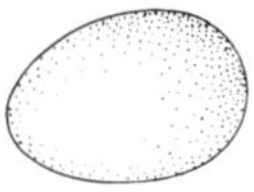	
Cheese 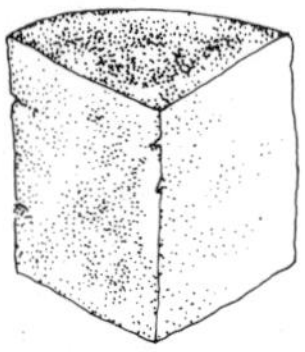	Vegetables 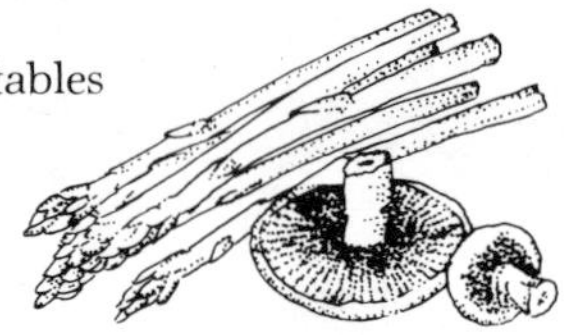
Grains (breads and cereals) 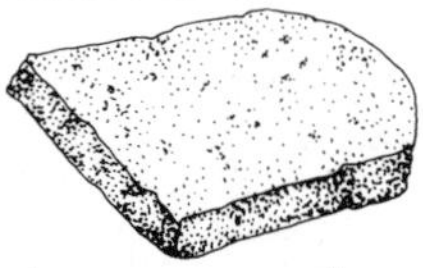	Fruits (except cranberries, prunes, and plums) 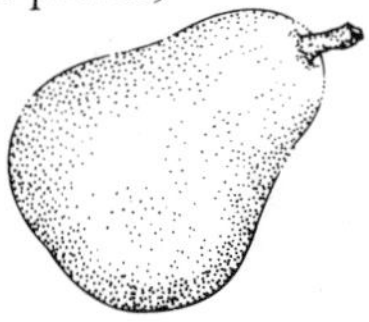
Fruits (cranberries, prunes, and plums only)	

Meat, eggs, poultry, and fish contain the acid-forming minerals. Milk and milk products contain both acid- and base-formers. The breakdown of the protein in milk does produce some acid temporarily, but the large amounts of calcium cause milk to be classified as a base-former in the body. Table 2 shows the acid- and base-forming foods.

The Constancy of Total Body Salts

Surprisingly, although one person may eat more base-forming foods and another more acid-forming foods, the body's total content of electrolytes remains constant. The job of regulating the body's salt population is largely delegated to the kidneys, under the supervision of several monitoring systems, notably the adrenal and pituitary glands. The net effect of all the homeostatic balancing systems is to ensure that output balances intake. A person who eats a lot of table salt, for example, excretes more sodium and chloride in his urine than one who eats only a little. Thus the *body's* total electrolytes remain constant, and it is the composition of the *urine* that is affected by what you eat.

If the kidneys are asked to excrete very high concentrations of minerals, or if some part of their intricate machinery is damaged by poison or a mistake in heredity, they may develop stones—deposits of

adrenal glands: the two small glands nestled into the tops of the kidneys. Among the hormones secreted by these glands are the stress hormones (catecholamines: see p. 180) and aldosterone (p. 498).

ad = on top
renal = of the kidney

pituitary gland: the master gland in the brain; secretes many hormones, including ADH (see p. 498).

Kidney stones are deposits of minerals that have crystallized within the kidney. Technically, they are termed **renal calculi** (REE-nul CAL-kyoo-lie).

renal = of the kidney
calculus = a small stone

minerals that they were unable to dissolve in water and excrete. A person who has alkaline stones (for example, calcium stones) in her kidneys may be told to eat an "acid ash diet" so that her urine will be acidic, to prevent the further precipitation of such stones. She would be told, then, to cut down on her fruit and vegetable intake and to eat more grains and protein-rich foods (except milk). A person with acid stones (for example, uric acid) would be put on an alkaline ash diet.

Kidney disorders impair the body's ability to regulate its fluid and electrolyte balances. To keep a renal patient alive, the physician may have to resort to the use of a kidney machine, a large apparatus connected directly to the patient's blood supply that filters it and adjusts the concentrations of its dissolved materials. Between sessions with the machine, the burden falls on the dietitian to regulate the renal patient's intakes of electrolytes. The dietitian may have to calculate a diet that precisely specifies the sodium, potassium, calcium, water, and many other constituents. (A dietitian in this very sophisticated medical specialty requires several years of schooling.)

It is not known whether any regulating system other than the kidneys governs the body's salt contents. We have thirst, to govern our intake of water, but do we have a salt hunger to govern our intake of sodium? Salt hunger is well known in plant-eating animals like cattle, which will travel long distances to a salt lick when they have been depleted of sodium. The tongue, in both animals and humans, is equipped with taste receptors that respond only to salt, hence the ability to distinguish a salty taste. Animals know instinctively when to seek this stimulus, but humans may seek it when they have no need. Future research may determine whether a true salt hunger operates in humans.

Water and Salt Imbalances

You are well protected from imbalances of water and electrolytes. Through intake and excretion, your whole body can achieve the optimal levels of fluid and electrolytes over a wide range of different conditions. By these mechanisms your body's cells are supplied with the total amounts of sodium, potassium, and other ions that they need in order to maintain their own local balances. However, you may be thrown into situations that your kidneys, thirst instinct, and cell membranes cannot compensate for. This is the case when large amounts of fluid and electrolytes are lost in an emergency. The most familiar conditions in which this happens are discussed below. As you read, remember that sodium and chloride are the principal cation and anion outside the cell and that potassium and phosphate are the principal cation and anion inside the cell.

Losses of Water and Salt   When you vomit, you lose large amounts of water and hydrochloric acid from your stomach. This leaves you

acid ash diet: a diet of acid-forming foods (foods that, if burned to ash, would be found to contain acid-forming minerals). Such a diet contributes to acidity of the urine, because the kidney collects the excess acid-forming minerals into the urine for excretion.

alkaline ash diet: a diet of base-forming foods.

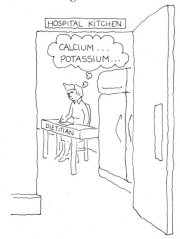

There are 4 kinds of taste receptors on the tongue: those sensitive to salt, sweet, sour, and bitter flavors.

Technically, these kinds of imbalances are known as **fluid-and-electrolyte imbalances**.

Alkalosis, acidosis: see p. 133.

dehydrated and, because of the loss of acid, may initially throw you into alkalosis. If you have a prolonged attack of diarrhea, you lose a more alkaline fluid from the lower portion of the GI tract, consisting largely of sodium ions. This too can leave you dehydrated but will throw you into acidosis. Both vomiting and diarrhea reflect losses of fluid from one body compartment—the gastrointestinal tract.

When either vomiting or diarrhea occurs, an astonishing amount of fluid is involved. One cannot help but wonder where it all comes from. Normally we are not conscious of the large amount of fluid involved in the digestive process, because our bodies are so wonderfully made that we don't have to drink the fluid necessary for digestion. You may recall from Chapter 5 that water is added to the GI tract contents at each step along the way—via saliva, via gastric, intestinal, and pancreatic juices, and via bile—but then is normally reabsorbed in the colon and recycled. The amount of digestive secretions put forth in the average adult has been estimated at over 9 liters/day, or more than three times as much as the water taken in with food and drink and produced during metabolism. It is obvious that replacement of this fluid is of prime importance in the medical and nutritional management of diarrhea and vomiting. Over half of the deaths in children under four are due to diarrhea.

Normally the ratio of mineral particles to water particles (the concentration) is the same on both sides of cell membranes:

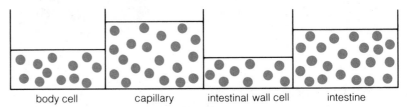

body cell   capillary   intestinal wall cell   intestine

If diarrhea occurs, water flows from the intestinal wall to replace the water lost from the intestine:

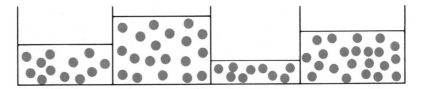

Eventually water flows out of every cell. This is dehydration:

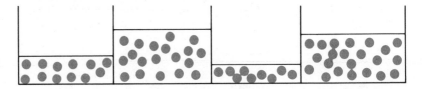

A domino effect operates when the body attempts to maintain water balance: Each fluid compartment is affected in turn by a change in the concentration of the fluids of adjacent compartments. For instance, in prolonged diarrhea, when a large amount of sodium has been lost from the GI tract, sodium and water move into the tract from the nearby interstitial and intravascular spaces. These spaces are continuous throughout the body, and their loss of sodium causes cells all over the body to compensate by shifting potassium out into the interstitial space. Meanwhile, since the whole fluid volume of the blood has decreased, the kidneys are experiencing dehydration and are attempting to retrieve needed water. Their principal means of doing this is to retain sodium, because water travels with sodium. The kidneys thus return sodium from the urine filtrate back to the blood. As the sodium enters, potassium must be exchanged; thus, potassium is lost in the urine. The end result, then, is excretion of potassium that came from cells far removed from the site of the original disturbance. The loss of potassium ions severely affects intracellular functions and, if great enough, can lead to cardiac arrest, since potassium ions are needed for the contractions of the heart muscle.

The examples of vomiting and diarrhea illustrate the body's responses to major fluid losses. If you understand the principles, you can predict what will happen in other fluid-loss situations. For example, when you sweat excessively, you are losing fluid largely from the interstitial space. The dehydration that results affects not only this space but also the vascular and intracellular spaces and other imbalances follow. If you replace the lost water without replacing the salt, you may suffer a severe depletion of your body sodium and chloride. Since these are the major electrolytes lost in sweat, the Food and Nutrition Board offers a rule of thumb: If you have drunk more than about 3 liters of water in a day to replace water lost in heavy sweating, you should take two or more grams of sodium chloride with each additional liter.

One additional example will illustrate another class of fluid loss: loss from the intracellular space, as when a person is severely burned. In this instance, the electrolytes potassium and phosphate and others are lost. Since the salts lost in this case are the chemist's salts, and not the single compound sodium chloride, their replacement must be managed by a physician. The physician's first and most important concern in treating a burn patient is to assess the fluid and electrolyte balance and to plan a careful replacement that will not upset the balance further.

Excess Salt   As you have probably anticipated, there is a risk of overcompensating. Excessive salt intake can be as serious as insufficient intake. (As you know, people lost at sea will die sooner if they drink the salt water.) To excrete excess sodium, the kidneys must excrete a certain amount of water along with it. Thus too much salt can as readily cause dehydration as too little water. When the kidneys are diseased, a moderate salt intake is especially critical. Unexcreted salt accumulates

A liter is roughly the same size as a quart. A U.S. quart is a little smaller and a Canadian (imperial) quart a little bigger than a liter.

1 g of sodium chloride = 1/5 tsp salt

Salt tablets are often 1 g each.

Edema: see also p. 132.

High blood pressure is the same as hypertension.

Still another fluid-loss situation has been described: the taking of diuretics (p. 287). This discussion shows why self-prescribed diuretics are dangerous.

in extracellular fluids and so may cause either edema or high blood pressure or both.

The details of electrolyte balance are among the most important ones that medical students must learn. Mastery of the details is appropriately left to them and to their medical associates. For the general reader and the student of nutrition, it is necessary only to appreciate the importance of this balance and the principles by which it is maintained and to be aware of the situations that threaten it. When any of these gets out of control, a red-hot medical emergency may exist. The most appropriate action is to call the doctor. The water and salts, which we take for granted and usually ignore, are more vital to life than any of the other nutrients considered in this book.

The Water Supply

When you draw water from the tap into a glass and drink it, it is not only water that you are drinking. Chlorine may have been added to it, to kill microorganisms that might otherwise convey disease. Fluoride may have been added to it, if your community has adopted fluoridation (see p. 472). In addition, it contains naturally occurring minerals, toxic heavy metals, live microorganisms, and a miscellany of organic compounds. Most people in the more developed countries take their water supply for granted and assume that it is pure water, and is safe. At the same time, they may be very much concerned over the presence of incidental additives in food. Actually water, too, may contain "incidental additives" of considerable significance to nutrition.

The quality of water varies, depending on its source. It may carry large quantities of dissolved minerals or very few. It may be hard or soft (see below), pure or contaminated. To learn about the water in your particular area, you may want to consult your local health department. The information given here may help you decide what questions to ask. The variables affecting water fall into four groups: minerals, heavy metals, microorganisms, and organic compounds.

Minerals in Water   All of the 20 major and trace minerals discussed in the last two chapters are present in various ground waters in different concentrations. Often they make significant contributions as nutrients to the health of the people who drink the water. A case in point is fluoride, which in some areas occurs naturally at the same concentration as in the ocean where our ancestors evolved. Thus it precisely meets the human nutritional need for fluoride.[1] Few communities have yet analyzed their water supplies completely enough to state which mineral needs they may be helping to meet, but most at least have information about the major minerals.

The distinction between hard and soft water, which has some

[1]W. D. Keller, Drinking water: A geochemical factor in human health, *Geological Society of America Bulletin* 89 (March 1978):334-336.

important health implications, is based on three of these minerals. Hard water usually comes from shallow ground, and it contains high concentrations of the cations calcium and magnesium. Soft water usually comes from deep in the earth, and its principal cation is sodium. Well water is hard or soft, depending on the area. Most people distinguish between these two types of water in terms of their practical experience: Soft water dissolves soap better and leaves less of a ring on the tub; hard water leaves a residue of rocklike crystals in the teakettle after a while, and it turns clothes gray in the wash. Hence consumers often consider soft water to be the more desirable and may even purchase water-softening equipment, which removes magnesium and calcium and replaces them with sodium. However, as far as we know today, hard water seems to have a more favorable impact on health.

Soft water can contribute a lot of sodium to people's diets, and thus it appears to contribute to a higher incidence of high blood pressure and heart disease in areas where it is used. The National Academy of Sciences has suggested a standard for public water allowing no more than 100 mg sodium per liter. This limit would ensure that the water supply would add not more than 10 percent to the average person's total sodium intake. The American Heart Association has recommended a more conservative standard of 20 mg per liter, to protect heart and kidney patients whose sodium intakes must be restricted. At present, about half of the U.S. population drinks water containing more than 20 mg per liter. Where snowy roads are salted, the salt running off into the water supply may raise its sodium content considerably higher than this.[2]

Soft water also dissolves certain metals, such as cadmium and lead, from pipes. Cadmium is not an essential nutrient. In fact, it can harm the body, affecting at least some enzymes by displacing zinc from its normal sites of action. Cadmium has been found in high concentrations in the kidneys and urine of patients with high blood pressure and is suspected of having some causal connection with the condition. A normal intake of zinc may protect against cadmium-induced high blood pressure. Lead is another toxic metal, and the body seems to absorb it more readily from soft than from hard water—possibly because the calcium in hard water protects against its absorption.[3]

The examples just given show that the choice to install a water softener in your home may be unwise, especially if your family may be heart-disease prone. (One family we know solves the problem by connecting the water softener only to the hot-water line, then using only hot water for washing and bathing, and only cold water for cooking and drinking.) These examples also show that the minerals in water interact in unpredictable ways. Someday we may be able to fortify our water with the ideal amounts of trace minerals for human

hard water: water containing high concentrations of calcium and magnesium.

soft water: water containing a high sodium concentration.

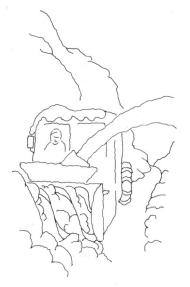

[2] E. J. Calabrese and R. W. Tuthill, Sources of elevated sodium levels in drinking water . . . and recommendations for reduction, *Journal of Environmental Health* 41 (1978):151-155.

[3] Soft water and heart disease, *Nutrition and the MD*, November 1975.

consumption.[4] But before that time arrives, we have much to learn about what is in the water already and what is ideal for humans.

Toxic Metals in the Water Supply   In the wilderness, water cycles rapidly through living systems, undergoing a natural purifying process in every cycle. Animal waste excreted onto the earth is filtered out by the soil before the water arrives underground. Pollutants entering rivers quickly disappear back into the earth as the river flows along, leaving the water pure. But neither the earth nor its rivers can purify completely the heavily polluted water expelled as city sewage or industrial waste. Water leaving a factory may contain concentrations of toxic metals so high that some are still present when it is recycled to become drinking water. And if the water is cycled through the same factory again, it will contain still higher concentrations the next time around.

Human technology bears the burden of purifying water contaminated by human technology. The Public Health Service sets drinking water standards, upper limits for the amounts of toxic metals permitted in water, and public law distributes the responsibility for adhering to these standards among the industries and the water-processing plants.

The metals of greatest concern are mercury, cadmium, and lead. These metals may be absorbed into the body, where they change cell membrane structure, alter enzyme or coenzyme functions, or even change the structure of the genetic material, DNA, causing cancer or birth defects. If they happen to affect the DNA in the germ cells (eggs or sperm), the changes (mutations) will become hereditary. When combined into complexes with organic compounds, these metals may be especially rapidly absorbed and may become even more effective against body tissues.[5]

Mercury is one of the rarer elements in the earth's crust but has been mined extensively for industrial use, and so it is present in our environment in unnaturally high concentrations. Much of it ends up in the water supply as mercury compounds. By far the most toxic of these is methyl mercury, which is efficiently (90 percent) absorbed in the GI tract and accumulates in red blood cells, the brain, and the nerves. In a pregnant woman, methyl mercury becomes concentrated in the growing fetus. Thus it can cause mental and physical defects in the newborn even though the mother has shown no symptoms.

Nerve damage occurs with mercury intakes as low as 300 μg per day, so the Food and Drug Administration has set a limit of one-tenth that amount on the permissible mercury levels in foods and drugs. The acceptable mercury content of water is 0.5 μg per liter.[6] (Monitoring mercury concentrations in water is a task of the public health agencies, such as the Environmental Protection Agency.) Two serious outbreaks

[4]Keller, 1978.

[5]M. M. Varma, S. G. Serdahely, and H. M. Katz, Physiological effects of trace elements and chemicals in water, *Journal of Environmental Health* 39 (1976):90-100.

[6]U.S. Public Health Service standard, in Varma, Serdahely, and Katz, 1976.

of mercury poisoning have occurred in Japan, where people have eaten fish that grew near industrial plants that discharged mercury wastes into the water. Rising levels of environmental mercury have been observed in other industrial countries, including the United States.

Cadmium has already been mentioned in connection with heart disease but has its most toxic effects in the kidney, causing chronic renal disease; in the lungs, causing emphysema; and in the bones, causing osteoporosis and osteomalacia. It has been in commercial use since 1910 and has caused severe outbreaks of disease in Japan. Cadmium in contaminated water can be absorbed into vegetables and grains and so can find its way into human consumers of these foods.[7]

Lead, another highly toxic metal, enters the water supply mostly by being captured in rain falling from atmospheres polluted with automobile exhaust. It is a metabolic poison that prevents hemoglobin formation and the action of several enzymes. Symptoms of mild lead poisoning include lowered hemoglobin, intestinal cramps, fatigue, and kidney abnormalities. These may be reversible if exposure stops. More severe exposure causes irreversible nerve damage, paralysis, mental retardation in children, abortions, and death.[8]

These are only three examples of metal pollutants, but they are enough to illustrate how the purity of the water supply can be threatened by industrial use. Both government and consumer environmental protection groups have to be vigilant in detecting, reporting, and preventing dangerous levels of contamination, because our water is a vital resource.

Microorganisms   Many harmless, even beneficial, bacteria dwell in the human digestive tract and are excreted into sewage. If these were the only inhabitants of sewage, there would be no concern about their presence in drinking water. But disease organisms are also excreted into sewage, and others are introduced into it by flies and other carriers. Before a sewage treatment plant releases its effluent into the water supply, it must reduce the bacterial count enough so that further dilution will make recycled water safe for human use.

An efficient secondary sewage plant may remove 99 percent of the bacteria in the water, which sounds pretty good for a start. But there are typically 10 million bacteria in a milliliter (1/5 tsp) of sewage. After 99 percent removal there will still be 100,000 left. Chlorination then kills another 99 percent, leaving 1,000 bacteria per milliliter. Most of these are harmless, and the few that are harmful can be diluted below the danger point if the water leaving the plant enters a large river.[9] Alternatively, the treatment plant may give the water tertiary treatment, sprinkling it over a large land area so that it will be filtered before re-entering the general water supply.

High standards for sewage treatment in the developed countries

The first step in sewage treatment allows the solids to settle out. This is **primary treatment**.

secondary treatment: removes the suspended matter, including bacteria and some viruses.

tertiary treatment: removes dissolved compounds, both organic and inorganic.

[7]Varma, Serdahely, and Katz, 1976.

[8]Varma, Serdahely, and Katz, 1976.

[9]K. Kawata, Water and other environmental interventions: The minimum investment concept, *American Journal of Clinical Nutrition* 31 (1978):2114-2123.

potable (POTE-uh-bul): suitable for drinking.

potare = to drink

An example of an organic pollutant from insecticide is DDT. A very toxic pollutant is PCB, polychlorobenzene (from the plastics industry). Another potent byproduct of industrial processes is chloroform.

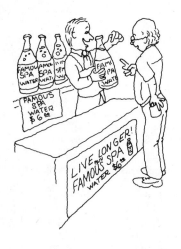

ensure that most people have potable water, but for the rest of the world, microbial contamination remains the primary cause of human diseases and epidemics. Two of the most basic needs of the world's people are safe drinking water and an acceptable standard of waste disposal.[10]

Organics   The fourth class of substances that may occur in water are the organic compounds from sewage, insecticides, petroleum-based and other industries, and other sources. Research on these is less than 20 years old, and few of them have been identified, but many are known to be toxic. Some cause birth defects, some are carcinogenic, some cause permanent alterations of the inherited genetic material.[11] Many contain chlorine, and some may be formed during the chlorination of water. No information is available on the risks now presented by water containing these compounds; standards are only now being established, and new filtering systems may be called for if public water exceeds these standards.[12] The study of organics in the water supply is an increasingly important research area.

Bottled Water   In some regions, consumers have become sufficiently alarmed about their local water supplies to turn to buying bottled water for their own personal consumption. The choice is an individual matter, and we take no position regarding its appropriateness. However, in buying water, as in buying any other product, the consumer needs to be alert to fraudulent claims. Mineral waters sold from "famous spas" offer no known health advantages and may be undesirably high in sodium.[13] On the other hand, bottled water sold in the United States must be tested by the producers once a year for safety and must meet standards set by the Food and Drug Administration for its contents of many chemical substances.[14]

The matter of water quantity still must be discussed. Is there enough to meet our needs? Water is an abundant, natural resource, and until recently its availability has been unquestioned. But the use of water in the industrial countries may put a strain on the supply. Used by agriculture for irrigating and by industry for transporting, dissolving, washing, rinsing, cooling, flushing away waste, and many other purposes, water in huge quantities is diverted from its original, ordinary uses. In the future the water supply may limit human progress. It has been estimated, for example, that if the U.S. population increases by another 20 percent or so, the water supply will be unable to continue meeting all the demands placed on it. We will therefore have to compromise our living standards in order to meet the

[10]Kawata, 1978.

[11]Varma, Serdahely, and Katz, 1976.

[12]N. Wade, Drinking water: Health hazards still not resolved (news and comment), *Science* 196 (1977):1421-1422.

[13]Keller, 1978.

[14]D. C. Fletcher, Safety standards for bottled drinking water (answer to a reader's question), *Journal of the American Medical Association* 238 (1977):2072.

top-priority need for safe, pure water for individual human use.[15]

This book is about individual nutrition and has dealt little with the economic and ecological problems of worldwide supply and demand. This discussion of water brings those problems into the foreground. To continue surviving and to maintain a desirable quality of life in an increasingly crowded and complicated world may mean making some hard choices in the near future.

Summing Up

Water in the body forms part of such chemical compounds as protein, participates in many chemical reactions, and serves as a solvent, transportation medium, and lubricant. Its heat-holding character helps regulate body temperature. Water makes up 55 to 60 percent of the body's weight.

Fluids and electrolytes provide the environment that supports the life of all the body's cells. Their concentration and composition are regulated to remain as constant as possible. Total body water is kept constant by regulating intake and excretion. Intake occurs when the osmotic pressure (solute concentration) of the blood is high, causing withdrawal of water from the salivary glands. The resultant dryness of the mouth stimulates thirst. High osmotic pressure of the blood also stimulates the kidneys to retain water through two hormonal mechanisms, one regulated by the antidiuretic hormone, the other by aldosterone. Excretion occurs whenever body water exceeds needs.

The principal electrolytes in body fluids are sodium, chloride, phosphorus, and potassium; each of these is maintained at a constant concentration by means of renal excretion. Sodium and chloride are the major extracellular electrolytes, and potassium and phosphorus are the major intracellular electrolytes. The electrolytes are involved in moving body water from place to place (by being moved themselves across cell membranes), thus maintaining the water balance. They also determine the pH of body fluids, maintaining the acid-base balance. The total concentrations of electrolytes in all the body compartments are maintained in a vital equilibrium, the electrolyte balance.

In maintaining pH, some major minerals act as base-formers, others as acid-formers. The presence of minerals in foods determines whether the food is an acid-forming or a base-forming food. Thanks to the specialized filtering work of the kidneys, changes in the relative proportions of these foods in the diet alter the acidity of urine but not of the body fluids. In renal disease, dietary concentrations of the major minerals must be strictly controlled.

Fluid and electrolyte imbalances occur when large amounts of fluid

---

[15] R. W. Phillips, Future programs for increasing food production with reference to the pre-school child, in *Pre-School Child Malnutrition: Primary Deterrent to Human Progress*, an international conference on prevention of malnutrition in the pre-school child, Washington, D.C., December 1964, publication 1282 (Washington, D.C.: National Academy of Sciences, National Research Council, 1966).

are lost, as in vomiting, diarrhea, or sweating. Loss of extracellular fluid occurs in these conditions; intracellular fluid then shifts out of cells to compensate, causing abnormal distribution of electrolytes across cell membranes and consequent cellular malfunction. In the case of sweating, the principal electrolytes that are lost are sodium and chloride. Replacement is achieved by increasing water and salt intake. The imbalances caused by vomiting and diarrhea, burns, and hemorrhages are medical emergencies; replacement should be managed by a physician.

Public water may contain significant quantities of minerals, depending on the source and locale. Hard water is rich in calcium and magnesium; soft water is rich in sodium. The relationship of soft water to heart disease has led to the suggestion that an upper limit be established for the amount of sodium permissible in drinking water.

Discharging industrial waste into the environment may add toxic heavy metals like mercury, cadmium, and lead to the water supply, creating a health hazard. A second threat to water is microbial contamination, which can be controlled by sewage treatment that includes chlorination. Nevertheless, contamination of water remains the primary cause of disease in the underdeveloped countries. A third concern is that highly toxic organic compounds may enter the water supply from agricultural and industrial use; little is known about these. As more and more water is diverted to industrial purposes, there is a need for stringent regulation of its use. There may be a need in the future to limit technological uses of water in order to continue providing a sufficient and safe supply to sustain human life.

To Explore Further

Both of the following are classics in the literature of the history of life on earth, revealing facets of the intimate relationship between environmental water and the life of cells. The book is available in paperback.

Oparin, A. I., *Origin of Life* (New York: Dover, 1938).

Wald, G., The origin of life, *Scientific American* 190 (August 1956):44-53 (also Offprint No. 47).

A teaching aid, *Nutrient Metabolism: Water, the Essential Nutrient* by J. Robinson, can be ordered from the Nutrition Today Society (address in Appendix J).

The following references are also recommended:

Calabrese, E. J., and Tuthill, R. W., Sources of elevated sodium levels in drinking water . . . and recommendations for reduction, *Journal of Environmental Health* 41 (1978):151-155.

Keller, W. D., Drinking water: A geochemical factor in human health, *Geological Society of America Bulletin* 89 (March 1978):334-336.

Varma, M. M., Serdahely, S. G., and Katz, H. M., Physiological effects of trace elements and chemicals in water, *Journal of Environmental Health* 39 (1976):90-100.

Applied Nutrition: Food

Knowledge of nutrition is worthless if it is not applied. Although we have stressed an understanding of what nutrients do in our bodies, almost to the exclusion of food, we must recognize that nutrients get into the body only through foods. In addition, we should acknowledge that getting food from source to body takes labor, efficient management of time, fuel, money, and cooking skills. This effort involves a larger segment of the population than just the wife or mother in each family.

So far, the Highlights have been reserved mostly for controversial topics—sugar as poison, vitamin C and colds, vitamin E megadoses. The only thing controversial about this Highlight is whether trained nutritionists are qualified to write about food purchasing and preparation. Traditionally, those who study the science of nutrition do not also study the food sciences, except for those preparing to be dietitians. Even dietitians learn only how to organize large kitchens and prepare food in institutions—not how, say, a college student can eat well on a limited income. However, our experience has been that nutrition students of all ages and both sexes are vitally interested in food-getting problems, and they have pushed us to gather information in this field. In this Highlight we are presenting ideas garnered from all kinds of

Dear Mother,
I was homesick all day yesterday so I cooked some fresh, creamed corn and ate it on vanilla ice cream. For a moment, I was a child and home again. Love,

LI'L NANCY

people living in varied situations on how they managed their time and money while obtaining balanced and varied diets.

The following suggestions are divided into categories according to the kinds of situations people find themselves in at various times in their lives: going on a strict therapeutic diet, living alone, eating in restaurants, or cutting food costs drastically. Naturally we can't include every individual situation, but perhaps you can glean what you need from the following.

I am on a strict therapeutic diet. It is not uncommon for people to be put on a diet which they will have to stay on for a long while, perhaps for life. Some of the diseases that may require dietary con-

trol are diabetes, ulcerative colitis, hypertension, and heart disease. To be told that you have to change your diet permanently can be very traumatic, and it calls upon a person's full adaptive ability to meet the challenge.

If you are one of these people, the one thing that may surprise you is the enormity of the effort that must be expended to follow the diet. Generally speaking, health professionals (doctors, dietitians, and the like) do not appreciate the fact that when they give a dietary order, someone has to do a lot of work to carry it out.

If they order three fruit servings a day, for example, someone must travel to the market—select fruit from the fresh, canned, frozen, or dried fruits—pay for it—carry it home—store it in the refrigerator or freezer or on the shelf—decide which fruit will be served next—wash, pare, and serve the fresh—unwrap, thaw, and serve the frozen—open the canned and serve the contents. If any is to be cooked, he must find a pan, have a stove to cook on, and know how to prepare the fruit. After the food is eaten, he must wash, dry, and put away the dishes, utensils, and pans; wrap and store the leftovers; wipe the kitchen counters and sink; and carry out of the house the wrappings, cans, parings, and table scraps. (Whew! Just for three pieces of fruit!)

All this activity must be

performed by each person for himself or by a parent or caretaker. If you have someone who can take care of these chores for you, it is well that you ponder them anyway, so that you will not make excessive demands of that person. If you must carry out these chores for yourself, we recommend that you read the section for single persons.

Your first task is to completely understand the dietary directions given you. This means asking questions. If you are given a printed booklet to study, read it and then ask questions on your next visit to the doctor. Your second task is to face head-on whatever negative feelings you have about going on this diet. Are you feeling sorry for yourself? Do you feel hostile about having to give up some of your favorite foods? Do you feel someone is punishing you, as if you are a naughty child who is being put to bed without supper? These are normal ways to react to a change in diet, but if you don't wrestle with them, you will fail in the dietary part of your treatment. You may question advice about your feelings coming from a nutrition text. The only reason we include it here is because in the long run they will have an effect on your staying with the diet. And in some diseases, diet can make the difference between life and death.

When you have learned to manage your diet, your next problem will be how to eat away from home. This is a tremendous obstacle for some people. Here are some tricks that help:

● If you can eat nothing your hostess is serving, take small servings and then stir them around on your plate. With practice you can fool the most hovering kind of hostess. Eat when you get home.

● Plan ahead. If it is imperative for you to eat at a particular time or to eat a particular food, take care of this yourself. Do not expect a busy host to do this for you. Eat at home and arrive late, or carry a thermos of whatever it is you must have.

● Manage with as little publicity as possible. Keep the table conversation on world affairs or juicy gossip—anything to keep the spotlight off you and your eating problem.

● One person interviewed for this series said that she was surprised how well it works to say "No, thank you," simply and kindly, and nothing else.

There are textbooks on the market on diet therapy, but these are meant for professionals. Your best sources of information for the details of your diet are the booklets you can get at your doctor's office. In addition, there are some good cookbooks for special problems. We have listed these at the end of the Highlight.

I must live alone now. The preliminary surveys for the 1980 Census showed that there has been an enormous increase in the number of single-person households. Many of these are older people who are choosing the independent life rather than institutional life, and many are young people who are postponing marriage and a family. People who live alone have special marketing and cooking problems. (There seems to be a conspiracy in the grocery store that says everybody is living in a family of four. Bags of potatoes and packages of other vegetables are so large that they rot before a single person can use them.)

Here is a collection of ideas gathered from single people who are doing a good job of getting nourishing food:

● Buy only three pieces of each kind of fresh fruit: a ripe one, a medium one, and a green one. Eat the first right away and the second soon, and let the last one ripen on your windowsill.

● Buy the small cans of vegetables even though they are more expensive. Remember, it is also expensive to buy a regular-size can and let the unused portion spoil in the refrigerator.

● Buy only what you will use.

Don't be timid about asking the grocer to break open a package of wrapped meat or fresh vegetables.

● Think up a variety of ways to use a vegetable when you must buy it in a quantity larger than you can use. For example, you can divide a head of cauliflower into thirds. Cook one third and eat it as a hot vegetable. Put the other two thirds into a vinegar and oil marinade for use as an appetizer or in a salad. You can keep half a package of frozen vegetables with other vegetables to be used in soup or stew.

● Make mixtures, using what you have on hand. A thick stew prepared from leftover green beans, carrots, cauliflower, broccoli, and any meat, with some added onion, pepper, celery, and potatoes, makes a complete and balanced meal—except for milk. But see the uses of powdered milk that follow: You could add some to your stew.

● Buy fresh milk in the size best suited for you. If your grocer doesn't carry pints or half-pints, try a nearby service station or convenience store.

● Buy a half dozen eggs at a time. The carton of a dozen can usually be broken in half. However, eggs keep for long periods in the refrigerator and are such a good source of high-quality protein that you will probably use a dozen before they lose their freshness.

● Set aside a place in your kitchen for rows of glass jars containing shelf staple items that you can't buy in single-serving quantities. These could contain rice, tapioca, lentils or other dry beans, flour, cornmeal, dry skim milk, macaroni, cereal, or coconut, to name only a few possibilities. This will keep the bugs out of the foods indefinitely. They make an attractive display and will remind you of possibilities for variety in your menus. Cut the directions-for-use label from the package and store it in the jar.

● Learn to use dry skim milk. This is the greatest convenience food there is. Dry milk can be stored on the shelf for several months at room temperature. It is fortified with vitamins A and D. It can be mixed with water to make fluid milk in as small a quantity as you like—but once it is mixed, it will sour just like fresh milk. One person says he keeps a jar of dry skim milk next to his stove and "dumps it into everything": hamburgers, gravies, soups, casseroles, sauces, even beverages like iced coffee. The taste is negligible, but five "dumpings" of a heaping tablespoon each would be the equivalent of a cup of fresh milk. Ask a friend who is a member of Weight Watchers to give you some recipes for delicious milkshakes and ice cream using dry skim milk. Their recipes are for single servings.

● Cook for several meals at a time. For example, boil three potatoes with skins. Eat one hot with margarine and chives. When the others have cooled, use one to make a potato-cheese casserole ready to be put into the oven for the next evening's meal. Slice the third one into a covered bowl and pour over it the juice from pickles. The pickled potato will keep several days in the refrigerator and can be used in a salad.

● Experiment with stir-fried foods. Use a frying pan if you don't have a wok. Ask your Chinese friends for some recipes. A variety of vegetables and meat can be enjoyed this way; inexpensive vegetables such as cabbage and celery are delicious when crisp-cooked in a little oil with soy or lemon added. Cooked, leftover vegetables can be dropped in at the last minute. There are also frozen mixtures of Chinese or Polynesian vegetables available in the larger grocery stores. Bonus: only one pan to wash.

● Depending on your freezer space, make double or even six times as much as you need of a dish that takes time to prepare: a casserole, vegetable pie, or meatloaf. Save the little aluminum trays from frozen foods and store the extra servings, labeled, in the trays in the freezer. Be sure to date these so you will use the oldest first. Somehow the work seems worthwhile when you prepare several meals at once.

● Learn to think in terms of socialization and food. Cook for yourself with the idea that you are also preparing for guests you might want to invite. Or turn this suggestion around: Invite guests and make enough food so that you will have some left for yourself at a later meal. These suggestions came from a young widow and an 86-year-old widow. The young widow, after her husband's death, purposely cooked generous amounts so she could make her own frozen dinners from the leftovers. With a wide variety of these on hand, she felt free to invite one or another of her single friends on the spur of the moment to "Come over and share my frozen dinners with me tonight." She says she devised this method of managing her food out of the need to manage her "five o'clock loneliness." The 86-year-old widow invites guests for dinner every Sunday, because "it is no fun to cook for one," and she too loves having the leftovers.

● Buy a loaf of bread and immediately store half, well wrapped, in the freezer. The freezer keeps it fresher than the refrigerator.

● If you have space in your freezing compartment, buy frozen vegetables in the very large bags rather than in the small cartons. You can take out the exact amount you need and close the bag tightly with a rubber band. If you return the package quickly to the freezer each time, the vegetables will stay fresh for a long time.

● If you have ample freezing space, you can buy large packages of such meat as pork chops, ground meat, or chicken when they are on special sale. Immediately divide the package into individual servings. Wrap in aluminum foil, not freezer paper: The foil can become the liner for the pan in which you bake or broil the meat, thus saving work over the sink. Don't label these individually, but put them all in a brown bag marked "hamburger" or "chicken thighs" or whatever the meat is, along with the date. The bag is easy to locate in the freezer, and you'll know when your supply is running low.

● If you have a food processor, prepare your vegetables when you bring them from the market. Then they are ready to use, and you won't have to wash the processor bowls for small quantities each day. A head of cabbage can be shredded, put into freezer bags, and stored in the vegetable bin. A small amount mixed with mayonnaise serves as a salad. Grate half a bag of carrots for carrot salad, and slice the other half for use in stews and soups. These thinly sliced carrots are delicious stir-fried in a little butter. Other vegetables can be treated this way, and you have a ready supply of vegetables every day.

● Look around your office or neighborhood for other singles who would like to eat together. You could take turns being host. When it was your turn, you would have leftovers. And if there were three participants, you would have dishes to wash only twice a week.

You can probably think of many more ideas, but these should give you a start.

I must eat in restaurants. Many people must eat in restaurants, because they are pushed for time or because their jobs take them away from home. A single parent may choose to feed the children with a fast-food meal because he is too tired to prepare supper; a traveling salesperson may have no alternative. In any case, restaurant eating is flourishing in the United States. The main problems with eating at restaurants are cost, lack of variety, and excessive kcalories. Here are some ideas for managing these problems:

● When feeding the children at a fast-food restaurant, pick up fruit at a nearby market and give it to them for dessert or a snack during the evening.

• Look for soup-and-salad restaurants.

• Order fruits, juices, vegetables, or salads whenever they are available. Ask for a vegetable plate even if it isn't on the menu.

• Order from the appetizer or salad sections of the menu; skip the main dishes.

• Ask for a "people" bag as soon as you get your food. Cut portions in half, eat half, and take home the rest for a later time.

• Order fish rather than steak, and ask that it be broiled, not fried.

• Request whole-wheat or other whole-grain bread if given a choice, or refuse the bread basket right away when you sit down, to avoid the temptation.

• Choose baked potatoes rather than french fries.

• Request margarine rather than butter or sour cream for your bread and potatoes. Or don't use the butter. Or cut the amounts they bring you in half.

• Request your salad dressing on the side, or request the salad dry with lemon juice. Ask for dishes without gravy or other sauces.

• Leave food on the plate.

• Frequent a cafeteria where extra servings of french fries or bread and butter are not part of the price.

I must cut my food costs drastically. There are several points to be considered when discussing the cost of food. First of all, many nonfood items are included in your grocery purchases and should be seen for what they are: Cleaning supplies, cosmetics, and the like are not food. Second, there are energy costs associated with food—refrigeration, freezing, cooking, and travel to the market, to name a few. Sometimes, too, you are not purchasing nourishment only for the body but also for the soul: Love, fun, fellowship, and relaxation have a valid claim on your food dollar.

Suppose, however, you do need to economize on food. How can you do it safely? The answers you give to the following questions will alert you to ways you can save money and at the same time improve your nutrition.

• Do you eat more animal protein than you need?

• Do you eat more of any nutrient than you need?

• Do you eat the more expensive meats and seafood?

• Do you eat the more expensive cuts of meat?

• Do you ever substitute cheese, eggs, or legumes and cereal for animal protein?

• Have you tried creative ways of incorporating dry skim milk into your diet?

• Have you served your family's favorite stew or casserole to guests instead of expensive ham or steak?

• Have you investigated the food cooperatives in your town for the purchase of fresh farm vegetables and other groceries at wholesale prices?

• Have you compared different varieties of canned goods—for example, bought three different brands of tomatoes and compared their water content?

• Have you tried the meat analogues (textured vegetable protein—TVP—products that taste like meat) and calculated their cost per ounce of protein?

• Have you done a cost analysis of snack items? Have you ever substituted fruit for potato chips?

• When you eat in a restaurant, do you comparison shop? Do you buy prestige and think you are buying food?

• Have you made master mixes (flour, baking powder, salt, and fat mixed in large quantities for use in making biscuits, pancakes, cakes, and so on) and compared the cost with well-known brands of mixes?

• Do you buy hamburger in bulk at lower prices, then freeze in packages of the right size for your needs?

• Do you keep a jar in your refrigerator for the surplus liquid from cooking vegetables and juice from cooking meats, then use this liquid for gravies or soups?

- Do you boil leftover bones to make soup stock?
- How much of your food cost is for convenience foods? Is there enough convenience to justify that cost?

Some nutrients that you have already paid for are lost—

- When you buy old vegetables and fruits
- When you buy more meat than you can use in leftovers
- When you buy packages of fruits and vegetables that contain more than you need, so that some of them rot
- When you fail to read the nutrition labels, so you buy sugar when you wanted to buy cereal
- When you compare canned goods by looking only at the price, then end up buying water and sugar when you wanted fruit
- When you cook too much food
- When you cook at too high a temperature
- When you leave orange juice exposed to air
- When you pour "pot liquor" down the drain
- When the way you cook food is not appetizing
- When a food is left on the plate
- And so on

Inherent in these suggestions for lowering food costs is the idea that it is nutrients, not foods, you are purchasing. The body cannot distinguish between a nutrient from an expensive food and a nutrient from a cheap food, nor can the body gain any benefits from a nutrient that was thrown away, no matter how expensive it was.

And for the Rest of Us We would have liked to include advice for some other groups of people who need help, such as the young wife and mother or the working mother or the single parent. But even though each situation is different, we felt that many of the ideas in the other categories applied to them too. In addition, the homemaker who does not work outside the home has many avenues open to her for self-education. We assume that since she has chosen her role, she is motivated enough to find the help she needs. Another group we omitted was the very poor. They are hampered in so many ways that their best help may come from social service agencies.

We would like to close by describing a way of cooking that we think is very appropriate in a world where energy must be saved—the Chinese way. The Chinese diet does not follow the pattern of separate meat/fish, vegetable, and starch courses so prevalent in the West. Instead, the Chinese serve a number of dishes in which all three constituents are usually present. Rice is served in separate dishes to each diner at almost every meal except breakfast. Meat, fish, and egg are used sparingly, but the Chinese cuisine still supplies enough protein to meet the recommended intake.

In Chinese cooking, all food is cut into bite-size pieces. Meat seldom dominates a dish and is used to add zest and variety. Vegetables, too, are cut into assorted shapes and then blanched or seared (stir-fried) in hot peanut oil or corn oil to seal in their flavor and maintain crispness and color. Among the favorites are cabbages, greens, squashes, cucumbers, eggplants, mushrooms, sweet potatoes, and red radishes. Soybeans are very abundant, and more than 30 products are manufactured from them.

One disadvantage of Chinese cooking that Westerners need not emulate is the high salt content of their soy sauces. Anyone with hypertension should avoid Chinese restaurants.

Cooking foods the Chinese way tends to preserve nutrients and to conserve energy and land. The small pieces cook quickly with little fuel. Since 80 percent of their diet is from plant food, the Chinese do not use the large amount of land for raising animals that Westerners use. (A million kcalories in wheat can be produced on less than an acre of land; a million kcalories in beef require 17 acres.) The wide variety of foods eaten at every meal supplies a complete complement of vitamins and minerals. In a world in which fuel is becoming increasingly costly and land increasingly scarce, the Chinese way of eating offers a model that industrialized nations might do well to examine closely.

To Explore Further

People who have to change their diets because of heart problems would do well to read:

Bennett, I., *The Prudent Diet* (New York: David White, 1973).

The following cookbooks are recommended for heart patients. The Eshelman and Winston, Mayer, and Rosenthal books are available in paperback.

Eshelman, R., and Winston, M., *The American Heart Association Cookbook* (New York: McKay, 1973).

Heiss, K. B., and Heiss, G., *Eat to Your Heart's Content* (San Francisco: Chronicle Books, 1972).

Keys, A., and Keys, M., *How to Eat Well and Stay Well the Mediterranean Way* (Garden City, N.Y.: Doubleday, 1974).

Mayer, J., *Diet & Your Heart* (Norwood, N. J: Newspaperbooks, 1976).

Rosenthal, S., *Live High on Low Fat* (Philadelphia: Lippincott, 1962).

The following cookbooks are for diabetics:

Jones, J., *The Calculating Cook: A Gourmet Cookbook for Diabetics and Dieters* (San Francisco: 101 Productions, 1977).

Kaplan, D. J., *The Comprehensive Diabetic Cookbook* (New York: Frederick Fell, 1972).

For the person concerned about the shrinking land area available for food production and the rising cost of fuel, a relevant paperback is:

Ewald, E. B., *Recipes for a Small Planet* (New York: Ballantine Books, 1973).

PART THREE

NUTRITION THROUGHOUT LIFE

INTRODUCTION

CHANGING NUTRITIONAL NEEDS

Nutrition undergirds the quality of life throughout the human life cycle: it supports the right to be well born; it ensures optimum growth and development; it maintains productive adulthood; it cushions and enriches old age.

SUE RODWELL WILLIAMS

Part One and Part Two introduced the nutrients and offered guidelines for putting foods together into healthful, balanced, and adequate diets. Part Three views diet from the perspective of the whole person. At different stages in the life cycle, different considerations become important.

During pregnancy, infancy, and childhood, a major factor influencing nutritional needs is growth. Chapter 15 presents the special nutritional problems related to growth and asks what preventive measures can be adopted during these years to promote good health in later life. A major influence on children's eating habits is school, and another is television. To provide good nutrition, these influences have to be taken into account, and they are given attention in Chapter 15.

During the adult years, nutrition becomes the individual's own responsibility. Such factors as drugs, alcohol, and caffeine may complicate the nutritional picture. In the later years, the processes of aging become manifest, further altering nutritional needs. Chapters 16 and 17 ask what nutritional and food-related measures enhance the quality of life during these years.

CHAPTER 15

CONTENTS

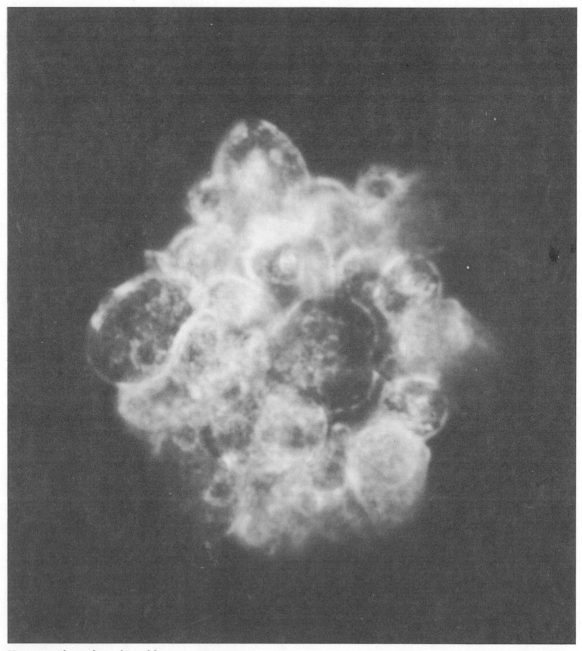

Human embryo three days old.

MOTHER, INFANT, AND CHILD

"I wish you wouldn't squeeze so," said the Dormouse, who was sitting next to her.
"I can hardly breathe."
"I can't help it," said Alice very meekly: "I'm growing."

LEWIS CARROLL

Alice's Adventures in Wonderland

The preceding chapters have been addressed to the adult. Wherever nutrition information has been relevant to your needs and concerns, examples and illustrations involving adults have been given, with only occasional references to infants, children, and older people. The principles of nutrition apply throughout the life span, but some changes in emphasis are appropriate to these other age groups.

Young people, from infancy through the teen years, are growing—a characteristic not shared by adults. In addition to nutritional needs for maintenance, then, young people have special needs related to the growth process. Furthermore, they are growing psychologically. In considering the nutritional needs and the feeding of infants, children, and teenagers, it is important to keep both kinds of growth in mind.

The Processes of Growth

Growth is not a matter of everything simply getting bigger all at once. From conception to adulthood, different organs differentiate, grow, and mature at different rates and times, each with its own characteristic pattern. A few generalizations hold for all growth processes, however, and an understanding of these generalizations underlies knowledge of the special nutritional needs imposed by growth. It is helpful to distinguish three growth levels: that of the whole body, that of the organs and tissues, and that of the cells of each organ or tissue. At each level, different considerations become important.

Whole Body Growth   Between conception and birth, a human being's weight increases from a fraction of a gram to 3,500 grams. The greatest rate of growth is in the fetal period—between 8 weeks and term—when the weight increases over 500 times. After birth, a baby doubles its weight from 7 to 14 pounds in four months, then slows down somewhat and adds another 7 pounds in the next eight months, reaching about 21 pounds at one year. Thereafter, the growth rate slows

The 3 intensive growth periods:

Prenatal period
First year
Adolescence

to 5 pounds a year or less until adolescence, when it again increases dramatically.

A similar pattern holds for height. From a fifth of a millimeter at 3 weeks of gestation, the embryo reaches 3 centimeters at 8 weeks, then 50 centimeters at birth. Thereafter, the increase in height is greatest during the first year (25 centimeters), half that much the second year (12 to 13 centimeters), and then slower still (6 to 7 centimeters a year) until the adolescent growth spurt. At that time, a sudden increase of some 16 to 20 centimeters is achieved in a 2- to 2 1/2-year period.

What is important to notice about all this is that growth does not proceed at a steady pace, that the maximal rate of growth is in the prenatal period, and that the two postnatal periods during which growth is fastest are the first year and the teen years.

Growth of Organs and Tissues The growth of each organ and tissue type has its own characteristic pattern and timing. In the fetus, for example, the heart and brain are well developed at 16 weeks, even though the lungs are still nonfunctional ten weeks later. During the first year after birth, the brain doubles in weight, but it increases only about 20 percent thereafter. In contrast, the muscles will be more than 30 times heavier at maturity than they are at birth.

> The brain and the central nervous system are first to reach maturity.

Each organ and tissue, then, has its own unique periods of intensive growth. Each organ needs the nutrients important for growth during its own intensive growth period. Thus a nutrient deficiency during one stage of development might affect the heart, and at another it might affect the developing limbs.

Cell Growth and Critical Periods At the level of the cells of a single developing organ, a further point becomes apparent: Each organ has its own specific time for cell division, which may not coincide with its time of growth in size. The brain is an interesting case in point. During development of the fetal brain, there is a period when very little increase in overall size is observed but when the cells are increasing dramatically in *number*. Each time a cell divides, it produces two that are half its size. These two do not grow but divide again, producing four cells that are still smaller. At a later time, the cells begin to grow and also continue dividing, so that their *size and number* increase simultaneously. It is during these first two periods that the total number of cells to be found in the brain is determined for life. Later still, cell division ceases, and thereafter the total number of cells is fixed, but they continue to increase in *size*. The development of almost every organ in the body follows a similar three-stage pattern, but each has different timing.

> Stages in organ growth:
>
> **1. hyperplasia** (high-per-PLAY-zee-uh), an increase in cell number
> **2.** simultaneous hyperplasia and **hypertrophy** (high-PER-tro-fee), an increase in cell size
> **3.** hypertrophy (except for the liver)

The third period, during which an increase in cell size is taking place, is the time when the organ is most obviously growing. But the most important events are already over. This fact has important implications for nutrition. The period of cell division is a critical period, critical in the sense that the cell division taking place during that time can occur at only that time and at no other. Whatever nutrients and other environmental conditions are needed for this period must be supplied on time if the organ is to reach its full potential. If cell division and the final cell number is limited at this time, later recovery is impossible. Thus malnutrition at an early period can have irreversible effects that may become fully manifest only when the person reaches maturity.

The effect of malnutrition during critical periods is seen in the shorter height of people who were undernourished in their early years; in the delayed sexual development of those undernourished during early adolescence; in the poor dental health of children whose mothers were malnourished during pregnancy;[1] and in the smaller brain size and brain cell number of children who have suffered from episodes of marasmus or kwashiorkor. Recent research points strongly to the probability that malnutrition in the prenatal and early postnatal periods also affects learning ability and behavior. Clearly, then, it is crucial to provide the best nutrition at early stages of life.

Growth of the Person   The concept of critical periods can also be applied, loosely, to personality growth. From the moment of birth (and perhaps even earlier), the human child is learning what to expect from life and how to cope with life's problems. These learning experiences follow one another in a characteristic sequence, and each must reach some degree of completion before the next can proceed. An infant's earliest impressions mold attitudes that in maturity may still affect behavior. A person who nurtures children must understand what is going on psychologically as well as physically. He must supply the nutrients that children need, and, equally important, he must encourage learning and behavior that will help them to develop fully as human beings.

There are many ways of understanding and interpreting psychological growth and development. The one we have selected to follow is that of Erik Erikson, whose insightful description of the stages of human growth provides a framework for viewing the whole person.[2] Erikson sees human life as a sequence of eight periods, in each of which the individual has a new learning task. To the extent that individuals master each successfully, they develop a strong foundation from which to proceed to the next. To the extent that they fail, they are handicapped in mastering the task at the next level. The stages in life and their respective learning tasks, as identified by Erikson, are:

critical period: a finite period during development in which certain events may occur (but not later) that will have irreversible, determining effects on later developmental stages. A critical period is usually a period of cell division in a body organ.

[1] D. P. DePaola and M. C. Alfano, Diet and oral health, *Nutrition Today,* May/June 1977, pp. 6-11, 29-32.
[2] We are indebted to S. R. Williams, who showed how Erikson's scheme could be integrated with nutrition principles in her book *Nutrition and Diet Therapy* (St. Louis: Mosby, 1973).

- *Infant.* Trust versus distrust
- *Toddler.* Autonomy versus shame and doubt
- *Preschooler.* Initiative versus guilt
- *School-age child.* Industry versus inferiority
- *Adolescent.* Identity versus role confusion
- *Young adult.* Intimacy versus isolation
- *Adult.* Generativity versus stagnation
- *Older adult.* Ego integrity versus despair

Whether you agree with Erikson's view or see human development in some other light, we hope you agree with the principle that understanding the whole person is important, even in the providing of food.

Each section that follows is devoted to a special stage in life, its physical growth and development, the related nutrient needs, and a feeding pattern that will supply the needed nutrients. Each section concludes with an attempt to put these nutrient needs in perspective in relation to the needs of the whole person.

Pregnancy: The Impact of Nutrition on the Future

We normally think of the effects of nutrition as being here-and-now: You feel good this afternoon because you ate a good breakfast this morning, and your friend feels sleepy because she had a sweet dessert after lunch. But the effects of nutrition also extend over years. It has been said that the best way to ensure being healthy when you are old is to be thin while you are young. Your eating habits of today, as part of your lifestyle, may help to determine whether you become a victim of cardiovascular disease (perhaps by eating too much salt), of diabetes (if you allow yourself to become obese), even of cancer (if your diet is rich in kcalories from fat).

At no time is the effect of nutrition on future health more dramatically in evidence than during the early development of an infant in its mother's womb. It is even probable that the nutrition of the infant's *grandmother* during her pregnancy will have permanent effects on the infant when it has become an adult.[3]

Such effects are impossible to demonstrate directly in people, nor would researchers want to experiment on pregnant mothers to see what causes stunting of the body or the brain in their children. But because the questions are important, many of them have been pursued using animals. We have every reason to believe that most findings from

[3]D. B. Coursin, Maternal nutrition and the offspring's development, *Nutrition Today,* March/April 1973, pp. 12-18.

the animal experiments are applicable to human beings. Some have been inadvertently confirmed. Hospital records maintained during the sieges of Holland and Leningrad in World War II gave abundant evidence that the state of the mother's nutrition *prior* to pregnancy was important for the *future* health of her infant.

Growth   Conditions in the uterus at the time of conception determine whether the fertilized egg will successfully implant itself in the uterine wall and begin development as it should. During the two weeks following fertilization, in the implantation stage, the egg cell divides into many cells, and these sort themselves into three layers. Very little growth in size takes place at this time; this is a critical period that precedes growth. Adverse influences at this time lead to failure to implant or other disturbances so severe as to cause loss of the fertilized egg, possibly even before the woman knows she is pregnant. Many drugs affect the earliest intrauterine events and later cross the placenta freely. Most health professionals agree that if possible, a potential

implantation: stage of development (first 2 weeks after conception) in which the fertilized egg embeds itself in the wall of the uterus and begins to develop.

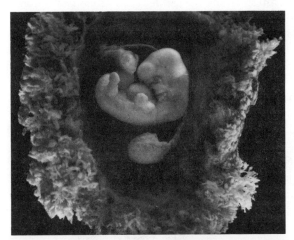

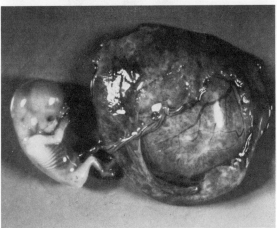

Six-week-old fetus attached to the placenta. At this time the fetus is less than half an inch long.

Courtesy of Dr. Roberts Ruch.

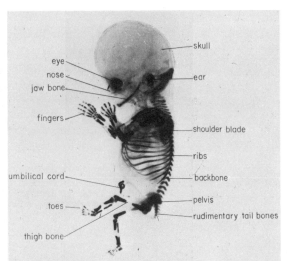

Eight-week-old fetus, showing development of the skeleton. The other tissues were treated so as to be transparent.

Courtesy of Dr. Roberts Rugh.

Ten-week-old fetus attached to the placenta. The blood vessels in the umbilical cord are clearly visible.

Courtesy of Dr. Roberts Rugh.

The 3 layers:

ectoderm (EK-to-derm): the outer layer (presumptive nervous system and skin).

mesoderm (MEZZ-o-derm): the middle layer (presumptive muscles and internal organs).

endoderm (EN-do-derm): the inner layer (presumptive glands and linings).

ecto = outside
meso = middle
endo = inside
derm = skin

embryo (EM-bree-oh): the developing infant during its second to eighth week after conception. Before the second week it is called an **ovum** (OH-vum) or **zygote** (ZYE-goat).

fetus (FEET-us): the developing infant from the eighth week after conception until its birth.

placenta (pla-SEN-tuh): organ inside the uterus in which the mother's and fetus's circulatory systems intertwine and in which maternal and fetal blood exchange materials.

uterus (YOO-ter-us): the womb, the muscular organ within which the infant develops before birth.

amniotic (am-nee-OTT-ic) **sac:** the "bag of waters" in the uterus, in which the fetus floats.

mother should be taking no drugs at all, not even aspirin. Nutrition should be, and should have been, continuously optimal.

The next five weeks, the period of embryonic development, register astonishing physical changes. From the outermost layer of cells, the nervous system and skin begin to develop; from the middle layer, the muscles and internal organ systems; and from the innermost layer, the glands and linings of the digestive, respiratory, and excretory systems. At eight weeks, the 3-centimeter-long embryo has a complete central nervous system, a beating heart, a fully formed digestive system, and the beginnings of facial features. Already the "tail" has formed and almost completely disappeared again, and the fingers and toes are well defined.

The last seven months of pregnancy, the fetal period, bring about a tremendous increase in size. Intensive periods of cell division and growth occur in organ after organ of the fetus.

Meanwhile, the mother's body is undergoing changes. She grows a whole new organ—the placenta—a kind of pillow inside her uterus (womb). In the placenta, the mother's and infant's blood vessels spread out and intertwine. Nutrients and oxygen leave her bloodstream and cross the vessel walls into the infant's bloodstream. Waste materials (carbon dioxide and urea) leave the infant and are carried away by the mother's blood to be excreted through her lungs and kidneys. The amniotic sac fills with fluid to cushion the infant. The mother's uterus and its supporting muscles increase greatly in size, her breasts change and grow in preparation for lactation, and her blood volume almost doubles. Thus the overall gain in weight of mother and child during pregnancy amounts to about 24 pounds (see Table 1).

Nutrient Needs   Nutrient needs during periods of intensive growth are greater than at any other time and are greater for certain nutrients than for others, as shown in Figure 1. Whenever intensive growth is going on, the nutrients protein, calcium, phosphorus, and magnesium

Table 1   Overall Weight Gain during Pregnancy

Development	Weight gain (lb)
Infant at birth	$7 1/2$
Placenta	1
Increase in mother's blood volume to supply placenta	4
Increase in size of mother's uterus and muscles to support it	$2 1/2$
Increase in size of mother's breasts	3
Fluid to surround infant in amniotic sac	2
Mother's fat stores	4
Total	24

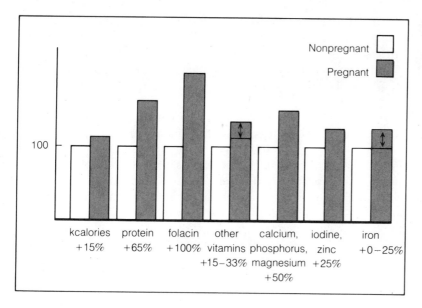

Figure 1 Comparison of the nutrient needs of nonpregnant and pregnant women (over 23 years old). The nonpregnant woman's needs are set at 100 percent, the pregnant woman's needs shown as increases over 100 percent. The pregnant woman's iron needs cannot be met by ordinary diets, and she might need to take an iron supplement. (Calculated from the RDA tables, inside front cover.)

are of greatest importance, because they play major roles in the structure and functions of rapidly dividing or growing cells and growing bones. The extraordinary need for folacin in the pregnant woman is due to the doubling of her blood volume. The frequency of folacin-deficiency anemia in pregnant women often makes it advisable for the physician to prescribe it as a supplement.[4] As you might expect, the vitamin needed in the next highest amount is the other B vitamin associated with the manufacture of red blood cells—B_{12}.

The major route of excretion of iron is menstruation, which ceases during pregnancy. Some of the iron a woman needs to increase her blood stores is saved by having no menstrual losses. As her blood volume increases, so do all its constituents, including the protein that increases absorption of iron from the intestine. An additional adjustment is accomplished by the hormones of pregnancy, which raise the concentration of iron in the blood, either by increasing absorption still further or by mobilizing iron from its storage places in the bone marrow and internal organs or both. Thus a woman *theoretically* needs no more iron during pregnancy than she has needed all along. However, because many women enter pregnancy with inadequate stores, physicians often recommend the use of an iron supplement during this time as a kind of insurance.

How transferrin increases iron absorption: see pp. 455-456.

[4]M. Balsley, Soon to come: 1978 Recommended Dietary Allowances, *Journal of the American Dietetic Association* 71 (1977):149-151.

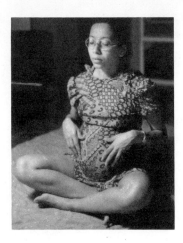

Eating Patterns   If the pregnant woman's dietary pattern is adequate, it can be adjusted to meet changing nutrient needs. The nutrients needing the greatest increase are protein, calcium, phosphorus, magnesium, and folacin, so the foods selected for emphasis should normally be those on the milk, meat, and vegetable exchange lists.

kCalorie needs increase less than nutrient needs. To achieve a slight increase in kcalorie intake with a great increase in nutrient intake, the woman must select foods of high nutrient density. For most women, appropriate choices would be foods like skim milk, cottage cheese, lean meats, eggs, liver, and dark-green vegetables. For vitamin C, a woman should either increase the size of her one serving of a C-rich food, such as citrus fruit or broccoli, or add a second fair C source, such as tomatoes. A suggested food pattern is shown in Table 2.

The pregnant woman must gain weight. Ideally she will have begun her pregnancy at the appropriate weight for her height and will gain about 20 to 24 pounds, most of it in the second half of pregnancy. This sounds like a lot, but a look back at the components of the pregnant woman's weight gain will show that all these pounds—from nutritious kcalories—are needed to provide for healthy placental, uterine, blood, and breast growth of the mother, as well as for a strong 7 1/2-pound baby. There is little place in her diet for the empty kcalories of sugar, fat, and alcohol, whch provide no nutrients to support the growth of these tissues and only contribute to excessive fat accumulation. Much of the weight she gains is lost at delivery; the remainder is generally lost within a few weeks, as her blood volume returns to normal and she loses the fluids she has accumulated.

Table 2   Daily Food Guide for the Pregnant or Lactating Women[5]

	Number of servings		
Food	**Nonpregnant woman**	**Pregnant woman**	**Lactating woman**
Protein foods			
animal (2-oz serving)	2	2	2
vegetable (at least one serving of legumes)	2	2	2
Milk and milk products	2	4	5
Enriched or whole-grain breads and cereals	4	4	4
Vitamin C-rich fruits and vegetables	1	1	1
Dark-green vegetables	1	1	1
Other fruits and vegetables	1	1	1

[5]California Department of Health, as cited in Nutrition and the pregnant obese woman, *Nutrition and the MD*, January 1978.

If the pregnant woman is obese at the time of conception, she should not attempt to lose weight during her pregnancy. Even though excess weight is a disadvantage, it is best lost before the beginning of pregnancy. Authorities recommend not only no dieting but also a weight gain in the obese pregnant woman. A report from the Maternal and Child Health Branch of the California Department of Health, based on the available research, clinical data, and combined judgments of various experts, recommends "a smooth and progressive weight gain of at least 24 pounds—just as would be expected in a non-obese woman."[6]

If the mother does not gain the full amount of weight recommended, she may give birth to an underweight baby. To the uninitiated, this may seem like no catastrophe, and in some instances it is not. A small mother may give birth to a small normal baby, and there is nothing wrong in this. However, on the average, the baby's birthweight reflects the nutritional environment to which it has been exposed, and in general babies of normal weight can be expected to be more healthy. Nutritionists seeking to find a measure by which they can evaluate the outcome of pregnancy have found no better one than birthweight: It is the most potent single indicator of what is to come. A low-birthweight baby, defined as one that weighs less than 5 1/2 pounds (2,500 grams), has a statistically greater chance of contracting diseases and of dying early in life. Its birth is more likely to be complicated by problems during delivery than that of a normal baby (defined as weighing a minimum of 6 1/2 pounds, or 3,000 grams). Low-birthweight infants are sickly, a characteristic often called by health professionals "failure to thrive." Surprisingly, one of the problems some of these infants may later encounter is excessive weight gain and obesity.[7] About 1 in every 15 infants born in the United States is a low-birthweight baby, and about a quarter of these die within the first month of life (see Table 3).

low birthweight: a birthweight of 5 1/2 pounds (2,500 grams) or less, used as a predictor of poor health in the newborn and as an indicator of probable poor nutritional status of the mother during or before pregnancy. Normal birthweight is 6 1/2 pounds (3,500 grams) or more.

Table 3   Infant Death* and Disability in the United States[8]

Category	Number
Total births (1974)	3,159,958
Total low-birthweight infants	233,750
Low-birthweight infants who died in first month of life (1960)	56,865
Low-birthweight infants at risk for lifetime disability	about 60,000

*The United States ranks fourteenth among developed nations in infant mortality rate.

[6]California Department of Health, 1978.

[7]R. L. Huenemann, Environmental factors associated with preschool obesity, part 1: Obesity in six-month-old children, *Journal of the American Dietetic Association* 64 (1974):480-487.

[8]National Institute of Child Health and Human Development, Little babies: Born too soon—born too small, DHEW publication no. (NIH) 77-1079 (Washington, D.C.: Government Printing Office, 1977).

This is **fetal alcohol syndrome**, the cluster of symptoms seen in an infant or child whose mother consumed excess alcohol during her pregnancy. It includes mental and physical retardation with facial and other body deformities.

Prevention of Future Health Problems   The potential impact of harmful influences during pregnancy cannot be overestimated. Excessive alcohol consumption can deprive developing nervous tissue of needed glucose and B vitamins and so cause irreversible brain damage and mental retardation in the fetus.[9] The damage can occur with as little as 2 oz alcohol a day, and its most severe impact is likely to occur in the first month, before the woman even is sure she is pregnant.[10] Smoking restricts the blood supply to the growing fetus and so limits the delivery of nutrients and removal of wastes. It stunts growth, thus increasing the risk of complications at birth and retarded development.[11] Drugs taken during pregnancy can cause grotesque malformations.

Dieting, even for short periods, is hazardous. Low-carbohydrate diets or fasts that cause ketosis deprive the growing brain of needed glucose and cause congenital deformity. Most serious may be the invisible effects. For example, carbohydrate metabolism may be rendered permanently defective.[12] The consequences of protein deprivation may be still more severe. They have been observed most frequently in the underdeveloped countries, but are also seen in this country among vegetarians' children whose height and head circumference are markedly and irreversibly diminished.[13] Iron deficiency during pregnancy in animals has given rise to offspring whose brain cells could never store the needed iron thereafter.[14]

Excessive caffeine ingestion (more than 8 c a day) causes complications in delivery.[15] Saccharin, too, should be avoided; its cancer-causing effects on the offspring of animals have been amply demonstrated. Even sugar consumption during pregnancy has been accused of predisposing the infant to obesity.

It is also important not to gain too much weight. Just as brain cell number can be limited by undernutrition, fat cell number may be increased undesirably by overnutrition, predisposing the newborn to obesity. This effect is even more pronounced later on, when the child is about one to three years old.

[9]J. Martin, The fetal alcohol syndrome: Recent findings, *Alcohol Health and Research World*, Spring 1977, pp. 8-12.

[10]Fetal alcohol syndrome, *Nutrition and the MD*, July 1978.

[11]S. R. Williams, Nutritional guidance in prenatal care, in B. S. Worthington, J. Vermeersch, and S. R. Williams, *Nutrition in Pregnancy and Lactation* (St. Louis: Mosby, 1977), pp. 55-92.

[12]R. M. Pitkin, ed., Nutrition in pregnancy, *Dietetic Currents, Ross Timesaver* 4 (January/February 1977).

[13]D. Erhard, The new vegetarians, part 1: Vegetarianism and its consequences, *Nutrition Today*, November/December 1973, pp. 4-12.

[14]R. L. Liebel, Behavioral and biochemical correlates of iron deficiency: A review, *Journal of the American Dietetic Association* 71 (1977):399-404.

[15]Coffee: Downs and ups, *Nutrition and the MD*, April 1978. "Excessive" means more than 8 c of coffee a day.

An important consideration for the health of subsequent children is the spacing of offspring to allow the mother's body to regain its nutritional balance. A delay of two to three years between births allows the mother's body to replenish any lost nutrient stores. This is of great benefit to the development of the next child. In the developing countries, where food shortages are common, it should be recognized that a nonpregnant woman could live three to six months longer than a pregnant woman on the same amount of food.

The profound effects on human life of nutritional and nutrition-related factors during pregnancy are recognized by policy makers in the United States and across the world. Recognition of the importance of nutrition in this earliest period of life has given rise to programs serving pregnant women with education and nutrient supplements where needed. In the United States, the WIC Program (Women's, Infants' and Children's Supplemental Food Program) was first funded in 1970; by 1977 it was investing $142 million a year in help to low-income pregnant women. Among the most active nongovernmental agencies is the March of Dimes, which promotes nutrition education for pregnant women and measures to prevent birth defects. Worldwide, many countries have similar programs.

Not all birth defects are caused by such factors in the newborn's environment as poor maternal nutrition. Some are inborn errors: inherited disorders caused by genes received from the parents. Diabetes is a possible member of this group; sickle-cell anemia is another. Another well-known and widespread example is lactose intolerance, in which the gene for the intestinal enzyme lactase becomes inactive at about four years of age, so that the child cannot digest the milk sugar, lactose. Many inborn errors involve failure to handle specific nutrients, like lactose, and special diets have to be designed to deal with each of them. Any diet therapy book can show you how this is done.

Troubleshooting To avoid the most common problems encountered during pregnancy, some additional pointers are helpful. Edema is not uncommon. In a poorly nourished woman, it is often part of a larger cluster of symptoms known as toxemia, a condition that requires medical attention. Research has shown that toxemia is preventable by good nutrition prior to and in the early stages of pregnancy, because it seems most often to be due to a lack of protein and/or salt. When the blood concentration of these water-attracting constituents becomes too low, the water balance is disturbed. Fluid leaves the bloodstream to accumulate in the tissues. The ankles and feet may swell, and the face and hands may become puffy. To avert this condition, a pregnant woman should obtain ample protein in her diet, and her salt intake should be about 25 g (5 tsp) a day, about 7 g above the usual intake.[16]

inborn error (of metabolism): an inherited disorder caused by a defective gene, usually the gene for a specific enzyme.

lactose intolerance: an inborn error of metabolism that becomes apparent at about the age of 4; involves failure of the intestinal enzyme, lactase, to digest milk sugar. Symptoms include abdominal pain, nausea, and/or diarrhea after drinking milk.

toxemia (tox-EEM-ee-uh): A cluster of symptoms seen in pregnancy, including edema and often hypertension and kidney complications

tox = poison
emia = in the blood

---

[16]R. M. Pitkin, H. A. Kaminetzky, M. Newton, and J. A. Pritchard, Maternal nutrition: A selective review of clinical topics, *Journal of Obstetrics and Gynecology* 40 (1972):773-785.

This means that there is rarely justification for restricting salt in the diet during pregnancy. However, this increased need is normally met by the increased food intake, and no special efforts to add salt are necessary.

Another common problem in pregnant women is iron-deficiency anemia. Attention should be paid to getting enough iron during this important time. At birth, a baby is supposed to have enough stored iron to last three to six months; this iron must come from the mother's iron stores, which therefore need to have been adequate even before pregnancy began.

A problem often encountered by the pregnant woman is nausea, a symptom that can be caused by folic acid deficiency. The hormonal changes taking place early in pregnancy may cause transient morning sickness, and a hint some expectant mothers have found helpful is to start the day with a few sips of water and a few nibbles of a soda cracker or other bland carbohydrate food, to get something in her stomach before she even gets out of bed. Another problem sometimes seen in pregnancy is vitamin B_6 deficiency which may in some cases cause depression, although depression can have other causes of course.

For causes and remedies of constipation, see Chapter 5.

Later in pregnancy, as the thriving infant crowds her intestinal organs, a woman may complain of constipation; a high-fiber diet and a plentiful water intake will help to alleviate this condition. Calcification of the baby teeth begins in the fifth month after conception; for this and for the bones, fluoride is needed. The woman in a county without fluoridated water may need a prescription from her physician for a supplement that includes fluoride.

What a lot for a woman to remember! And this is only the briefest summary of the nutrient needs in pregnancy. With all of this to worry about, can a woman relax and enjoy expecting her baby?

Psychological Needs of the Pregnant Woman The developing fetus cannot be said to have many psychological needs (although this can be debated), but pregnancy for many women is a time of adjustment to major changes. The woman who is expecting to bear a baby is a growing person in more ways than one. Not only physically, but also emotionally, her needs are changing. If it is her first baby, she knows her lifestyle will have to change as she takes on the new responsibility of caring for a child. Ideally, she will be encouraged to develop this sense of responsibility by caring for herself during pregnancy. According to Erikson, the psychological events of adolescence culminate in the formation of an identity. Experts from many schools of thought agree that one's self-image begins to form early and ideally is strongly positive: "I'm OK!" The expectant mother needs encouragement in thinking of herself as a thoroughly worthwhile and important person with a new and challenging task that she can and will perform well. She is also, as a young adult, still working out her relationship with her mate, and he and she both know that the coming of a first baby will affect that relationship profoundly. There is a need for sensitive communication and understanding on both parts in this time of transition.

A question commonly asked is whether the so-called cravings of the pregnant woman reflect physiological needs. They do in only one known instance—in the behavior called pica. Pica is the habit of poorly nourished women and children of eating clay, cornstarch, ice, paint, or other substances. This craving has been linked to iron deficiency in some instances. Other than pica, the only specific messages the body can send to the brain regarding its needs are for water, possibly salt, and food. In general, most of the cravings of a pregnant woman seem to be psychological, not physiological. If a woman wakes her husband at 2 a.m. and begs him to go to the nearest all-night grocery to buy her some pickles and chocolate sauce, this is probably not because she lacks a combination of nutrients uniquely supplied by these foods. She is expressing a need, however, as real and as important as her need for nutrients—for support, understanding, and love.

Pica: see p. 458.

Nutrition during Breastfeeding

A nursing mother's needs for some nutrients increase even further, because she is feeding a larger infant.

Growth and Nutrient Needs A comparison between a woman's recommended intakes during pregnancy (second half) and during lactation is shown in Figure 2. Inspection of the chart reveals that the nursing mother's needs for several nutrients are down, whereas others

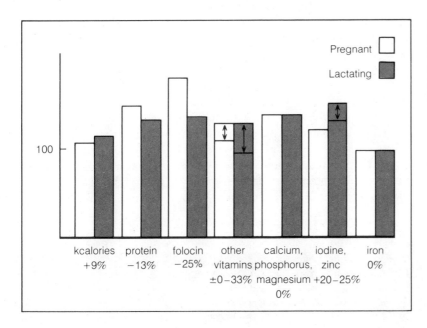

Figure 2 Comparison of the nutrient needs of pregnant and lactating women. The nonpregnant woman's needs are set at 100 percent (calculated from the RDA tables, inside front cover).

increase only slightly. A significant increase is needed for kcalories, both for those that go into her milk and for the energy needed to make the milk. Calcium, phosphorus, magnesium, and protein needs continue to be high. They were going into the baby in the womb; now they are flowing into the baby through the mother's milk. Little iron is secreted in milk, so no increase in iron intake is needed, provided, of course, that the mother's iron nutrition has been good all along. The folacin requirement falls as the mother's blood volume declines.

The secretion of milk by a nursing mother is a beautiful illustration of the ways nature provides for its own. To give but a few examples: The mother's milk supply responds to the infant's needs. If the baby sucks until the breast is empty, a hormone is released that stimulates the mammary glands to produce more milk the next time around; if the baby leaves milk in the breast, the amount secreted is reduced. If a mother is nursing twins, reserving one breast for each, the breasts can even adjust separately to each infant's demands. This same hormone causes the uterus to contract, helping it return to normal size. The infant's crying stimulates a conditioned mother to "let down" her milk. In anticipation of feeding, the milk moves to the front of the breast and, as the infant begins to suck, flows so freely that the infant may have to gulp fast to keep up with the flow. Like many other designs of living systems, the lactation system is a marvel.

> The hormone that controls the breast milk supply is **oxytocin** (oxy-TOCE-in).

> **letdown reflex:** the reflex that forces milk to the front of the breast when the infant begins to nurse.

Eating Patterns   Logically, because the mother is making milk, she needs to consume something that resembles it in composition. The obvious choice is cow's milk. The nursing mother who can't drink milk needs to find nutritionally similar substitutes, like cheese or soy milk and greens. As before, nutritious foods should make up the remainder of the needed kcalorie increase. Because breast milk is a fluid, the mother's fluid intake should be liberal; a busy new mother often forgets this.

The question is often raised whether a mother's milk may lack a nutrient if she is not getting enough in her diet. The answer differs from one nutrient to the next, but in general the effect of nutritional deprivation of the mother is to reduce the quantity, not the quality, of her milk. For the energy nutrients, the milk has a constant composition; if one nutrient is in short supply, correspondingly less milk—but still of the proper composition—will be produced.[17] For the vitamins and minerals, the composition is more variable. But to repeat: Water is the major ingredient of milk, and a nursing mother's fluid intake should be ample.

The period of lactation is the natural time for a woman to lose the extra body fat she accumulated during pregnancy. If her choice of

---

[17]B. Lönnerdal, E. Forsum, M. Gebre-Medhin, and L. Hambraeus, Breast milk composition in Ethiopian and Swedish mothers, part II: Lactose, nitrogen, and protein contents, *American Journal of Clinical Nutrition* 29 (1976):1134-1141; and M. Winick, Nutritional disorders of American women, *Nutrition Today,* September/October-November/December 1975, pp. 26-28.

foods is judicious, a kcalorie deficit and a gradual loss of weight can easily be supported without any effect on her milk output. Fat can only be mobilized slowly, however, and too large a kcalorie deficit will inhibit lactation.[18]

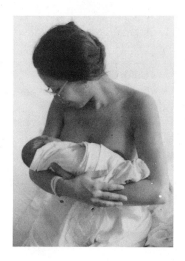

Although there need be no concern about the nutrients in breast milk, a warning is in order for the nursing mother. Chemicals other than nutrients readily enter the milk; in fact, breast milk has been called a "route of excretion" for some compounds. The list of drugs, medical and otherwise, known to be secreted in significant amounts in human milk now numbers over 100 items. Notable among them are nicotine, caffeine, marihuana, morphine, oral contraceptive hormones, and alcohol. A woman who is nursing her baby should abstain from these and all other drugs.

Psychological Needs of the Nursing Mother   To nurse successfully, a woman needs rest and freedom from stress and anxiety. The supportive care of her husband, family, and friends can provide this for her. Many resources are also available to provide her with the information and advice she needs; some are listed in To Explore Further at the end of this chapter.

Nutrition of the Infant

The first year of life is of great importance to the infant's development. What the infant eats, as well as the experience of eating, will affect her for the rest of her life.

Growth and Development   A baby grows faster during the first year than ever again, as Figure 3 shows. As mentioned before, the birthweight doubles in four months, from 7 to 14 pounds, and another 7 pounds is added in the next eight months. (If a ten-year-old girl were to do this, her weight would increase from 70 to 210 pounds in a single year.) By the end of the first year, the growth rate has slowed down, and the weight gained between the first and second birthdays amounts to only about 5 pounds. This tremendous growth is a composite of the differing growth patterns of all the internal organs. The generalization that many critical periods occur early still holds.

Changes in body organs during the first year affect the baby's readiness to accept solid foods. At first, all he can do is suck (and he can do that powerfully), then (at six weeks) he can smile, later (at two months or so) he can move his tongue against his palate to swallow semisolid food. Still later the first teeth erupt, but it is not until sometime during the second year that a baby can begin to handle

[18]M. J. Whichelow, Success and failure of breast-feeding in relation to energy intake, *Proceedings of the Nutrition Society* 35 (September 1976):62A-63A.

Figure 3 Weight gain of human infants (boys) in the first five years.

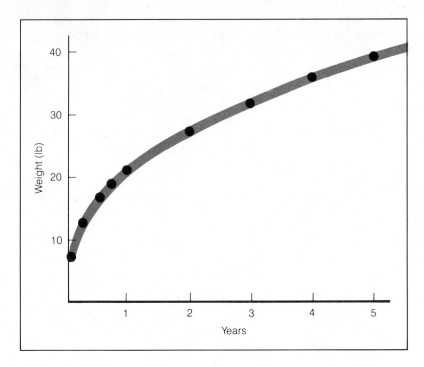

chewy food. The stomach and intestines are immature at first; they can digest milk sugar (lactose) but can't manufacture significant quantities of the starch-digesting enzyme, amylase, until somewhat later and so cannot digest starch until perhaps three months.

The baby's kidneys are unable to concentrate waste efficiently, so a baby must excrete relatively more water than an adult to carry off a comparable amount of waste. This means that dehydration, which can be dangerous, can occur more easily in an infant than in an adult. Because an infant can communicate his needs only by crying, it is important to remember that he may be crying for fluid. A baby's metabolism is fast (the infant heart beats 120 to 140 times a minute, and the respiration rate is 20 times a minute, as compared with an adult's 70 to 80 and 12 to 14, respectively), so its energy needs are high.

Nutrient Needs   The rapid growth and metabolism of the infant demand ample supplies of the growth and energy nutrients—protein, carbohydrate, fat, calcium, phosphorus, and magnesium—and, for their use, the B vitamins and vitamins A, C, and D. Babies, because they are small, need smaller total amounts of these nutrients than adults do. But as a percentage of body weight, babies need over twice as much of most nutrients. Figure 4 compares a three-month-old baby's needs with those of an adult man; as you can see, some of the differences are extraordinary.

Milk for the Infant: Breast versus Bottle   The obvious food to supply the nutrients most needed by the young infant is milk, and if all

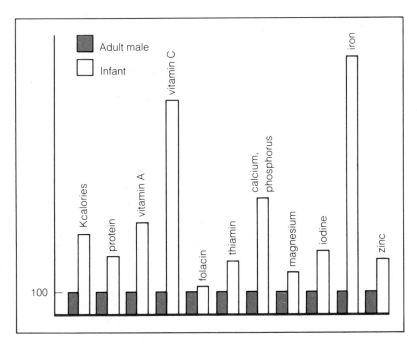

Figure 4 Comparison of the nutrient needs of three-month-old infants with those of adult males (23 years old and up) per pound of body weight. The adult male's needs are set at 100 percent (calculated from the RDA tables, inside front cover).

other things are equal, breast milk is the milk of choice. Tailor-made to meet the nutritional needs of the human infant during the first year, breast milk offers its carbohydrate as lactose, its fat as a mixture with a generous proportion of polyunsaturated fatty acids, and its protein largely as lactalbumin, a protein that the human infant can easily digest. Its vitamin contents are ample. Even vitamin C, for which milk is not normally a good source, is supplied generously by breast milk.

As for minerals, the calcium-to-phosphorus ratio (2:1) is ideal for the absorption of calcium, and both of these minerals and magnesium are present in amounts appropriate for the rate of growth expected in a human infant. Breast milk is also low in sodium.[19] In addition, breast milk contains many factors that favor absorption of the iron it contains. On the average, 49 percent of the iron is absorbed from breast milk, as compared with only 4 percent from fortified formula.[20]

Powerful agents against bacterial infection also occur in breast milk. Among them is lactoferrin, an iron-grabbing compound, which keeps bacteria from getting the iron they need for growth and also works directly to kill some bacteria.[21]

Breast milk also contains antibodies against the intestinal diseases most likely to threaten the infant's young life. Entering the infant's body

lactalbumin (lact-AL-byoo-min): the chief protein in human breast milk, as opposed to **casein** (CAY-seen), the chief protein of cow's milk.

lactoferrin (lak-toe-FERR-in): a factor in breast milk that binds iron and keeps it from supporting the growth of the infant's intestinal bacteria.

[19]J. Mayer, A new look at old formulas, *Family Health / Today's Health,* October 1976, pp. 38, 40, 78.

[20]J. A. McMillan, S. A. Landaw, and F. A. Oski, Iron sufficiency in breast-fed infants and the availability of iron from human milk, *Pediatrics* 58 (1976):686-691.

[21]R. R. Arnold, M. F. Cole, and J. R. McGhee, A bactericidal effect for human lactoferrin, *Science* 197 (1977):263-265.

bifidus (BIFF-id-us, by-FEED-us) **factor:** a factor in breast milk that favors the growth, in the infant's intestinal tract, of the "friendly" bacteria *Lactobacillus* (lack-toh-ba-SILL-us) *bifidus*, so that other less desirable intestinal inhabitants will not flourish.

colostrum (co-LAHS-trum): a milklike secretion from the breast that precedes milk during the first day or so after delivery.

with the milk, these antibodies inactivate bacteria within the digestive tract, where they would otherwise cause harm. Some of the antibodies also "leak" into the bloodstream, because the infant's immature digestive tract cannot completely exclude whole proteins. These antibodies provide additional protection against such diseases as polio.[22] Breast milk also contains a factor that favors the growth of the "friendly" bacteria, *Lactobacillus bifidus*, in the infant's digestive tract, so that other, harmful bacteria cannot grow there.

During the first two to three days of lactation, the breasts produce colostrum, a premilk substance whose antibody content is even higher than that of the milk that comes later. Both colostrum and breast milk are sterile as they leave the breast, and the baby cannot contract a bacterial infection from them even if his mother has one. Both contain active white blood cells in the same concentration as in the mother's blood, to devour enemy agents such as bacteria and viruses. Thus from the start, breast milk protects the infant in many ways that modern medicine (vaccinations) and technology (sanitary water supplies) attempt to do.

In the underdeveloped countries, breastfeeding is indispensable in protecting infants against the ravages of disease caused by unsanitary conditions, poverty, and ignorance. When artificial feeding is substituted, as when an infant is brought into a clinic for treatment of diarrhea, it succeeds only as long as the infant is receiving competent medical care in a sanitary hospital setting. When she takes her baby home, the mother will often have nothing but contaminated well water with which to prepare formula and no equipment for sterilizing bottles and nipples. For a mother to switch to the bottle under such conditions is to pronounce a death sentence on her baby.[23]

Even in a wealthy nation, breastfeeding is preferable whenever possible, because it is less likely than formula to cause allergy. (For the bottle-fed baby who is allergic to cow's milk, a substitute such as goat's milk or soy milk must be provided.) Breastfeeding also seems to produce fewer fat babies than formula feeding does, perhaps partly because the mother does not force her baby to "finish the breast"; she can't see the milk that's left, as she can in a bottle.

A comparison of the nutrient composition of human and cow's milk shows that they do indeed differ. Cow's milk is significantly higher in protein, calcium, and phosphorus, for example, to support the calf's faster growth rate. But a formula can be prepared from cow's milk that does not differ significantly from human milk in these respects. The antibodies in cow's milk do not protect the human baby from disease (they protect the calf), but the high level of preventive medical care (vaccinations) and public health measures achieved in the developed

[22]S. J. Fomon and S. J. Filer, Milks and formulas, in *Infant Nutrition*, 2nd ed., ed. S. J. Fomon (Philadelphia: Saunders, 1974), pp. 359-407.

[23]R. E. Brown, Breast feeding in modern times, *American Journal of Clinical Nutrition* 26 (1973):556-562.

countries, and especially in the United States and Canada, make these considerations less important than they were in the past. Safety and sanitation can be achieved with either mode of feeding by the educated mother whose water supply is reliable.

Even the argument that breastfeeding costs less is not entirely valid. It is true that there is no waste in breastfeeding, but extra money must be spent to feed a baby—whether directly for formula or indirectly for the added food needed by the nursing mother, although the formula costs somewhat more.

As for closeness, clearly that is important. An infant's first impressions of the world relate to the way she is handled during feeding, but holding her with love and a bottle will do more for her psychological development than holding her with resentment at the breast. Moreover, bottle feeding gives the father and other family members a chance to develop a warm, affectionate relationship with the baby, and it may free the mother to work or play more.

Women sometimes hesitate to breastfeed because they have heard that environmental contaminants such as DDT may enter their milk and harm the baby. DDT has been reported in the milk of mothers at higher concentrations than are allowed in cow's milk.[24] The significance of these findings is hard to evaluate, and the decision not to breastfeed on this basis might best be made after consultation with a physician or dietitian familiar with the local circumstances.

Whichever mode of feeding is chosen, the mother should be supported in her choice. Especially with her first infant, she may be experiencing some problems with adjusting. Heavy pressure against either decision constitutes an avoidable stress.

First Foods   The addition of foods to a baby's diet should be governed by three considerations: first, to supply the needed nutrients; second, to supply them in a form the baby is physically ready to handle; and third, to introduce them singly so that allergies can easily be detected.[25] If the baby is breastfed, additions can probably wait until about six months; if formula-fed, a reasonable pattern for adding foods to a baby's diet is shown in Table 4. As for the choice of foods, commercial baby foods in the United States and Canada are generally safe, nutritious, and of high quality. In response to consumer demand, the baby food companies have removed much of the added salt and sugar their products contained in the past,[26] and they also contain few or no additives. They generally have high nutrient density, except for the mixed dinners (which contain little meat) and desserts (which are heavily sweetened). An alternative for the parent who wants the baby to have family foods

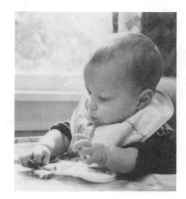

[24]Fomon and Filer, 1974.

[25]Questions doctors ask . . . , *Nutrition and the MD*, October 1977.

[26]Gerber Products Company, Why we put what we put in Gerber baby foods (advertisement), *Nutrition Today*, September/October 1973, p. 24; and J. C. Suerth (chairman of the board, Gerber Products Company), Letter to the editor, *Nutrition Today*, May/June 1977, pp. 34-35.

Meal plan for a one-year-old:

Breakfast
  1 c milk
  2-3 tbsp cereal
  2-3 tbsp strained fruit
  teething crackers

Lunch
  1 c milk
  2-3 tbsp vegetables
  chopped meat
  2-3 tbsp pudding

Snack
  1/2 c milk
  teething crackers

Supper
  1 c milk
  1 egg
  2 tbsp cereal or potato
  2-3 tbsp cooked fruit
  teething crackers

milk anemia: iron-deficiency anemia; caused by drinking so much milk that iron-rich foods are displaced in the diet.

For the special characteristics of juvenile-onset obesity, see Chapter 8.

Table 4   Baby's First Foods*

Age (months)	Addition
0-1	ADC (+ fluoride) supplement (A and D not needed if formula is fortified)
1-2	Diluted orange juice (for vitamin C)
4-6	Enriched rice cereal (for iron; baby can swallow and digest starch now)
7-8	Strained cooked vegetables and strained fruits
9	Finely chopped meat (baby can chew)
Later	Cottage cheese, toast, teething crackers

*For the formula-fed baby. The breastfed baby can wait until 6 months or later before starting foods other than breast milk.

is to "blenderize" a small portion of the table food at each meal. If this choice is made, it is important to take precautions against food poisoning.

At a year of age, the obvious food to supply most of the nutrients the baby needs is still milk; 2 to 3 1/2 c a day are now sufficient. More milk than this would displace foods necessary to provide iron and would cause the iron-deficiency anemia known as milk anemia. The other foods—meat, cereal, bread, fruit, and vegetables—should be supplied in variety and in amounts sufficient to round out total kcalorie needs. A meal plan that meets these requirements for the one-year-old is shown in the margin.

Prevention of Future Health Problems   The first year of a baby's life is the time to lay the foundation for future health. In part, this means taking appropriate measures to avert the likelihood of problems developing later. From the nutrition standpoint, the relevant problems most common in later years are obesity and dental disease. Prevention of obesity should also inhibit the development of the obesity-related diseases—atherosclerosis, diabetes, and cancer.

Infant obesity should at all costs be avoided. Aside from breastfeeding, the most important single measure to undertake during the first year is to encourage eating habits that will support continued normal weight as the child grows. Primarily, this means introducing nutritious foods in an inviting way; avoiding concentrated sweets and empty-kcalorie foods; and encouraging plenty of vigorous physical activity. It has been suggested that the early introduction of sweet fruits to a baby's diet might favor his developing a preference for sweets and lessen his liking for vegetables introduced later. To prevent this, the order should perhaps be changed: vegetables first, fruits later. This practice now has a wide following.

The introduction of solid foods should probably wait until the baby has reached the age of about four to six months, when experience with them is first needed to help the normal swallowing reflex develop.

Earlier, they might have several undesirable effects: displacing breast milk or formula, which is the most perfectly balanced diet for a young baby; increasing or decreasing overall kcalorie intake and so upsetting the physiological course toward normal weight in childhood; or establishing the habit of overeating. It is at six months or later that the transition from breast milk or formula to fluid milk may be made, and at this time, vitamin C and iron need to be supplied from food.

Some parents want to feed solids at an earlier age, on the theory that "stuffing the baby" at bedtime will make him more likely to sleep through the night. There is no proof for this theory. Babies start to sleep through the night at the average age of about nine weeks, regardless of when solid foods are introduced.[27]

To discourage development of the behaviors and attitudes that plague the obese, babies should not learn to seek food as a reward, to expect food as comfort for unhappiness, or to associate food deprivation with punishment. If they cry from thirst, they should be given water, not milk or juice. A baby has no internal "kcalorie counter" and stops eating when his stomach is full, so low-kcalorie foods will satisfy him as long as they provide bulk.

Beyond these recommendations, there is some thought being given to the idea that infants should be started on a "prudent diet"—designed along the lines recommended for heart patients. This means restricting fat in the diet, increasing the ratio of polyunsaturated to saturated fat, and reducing the cholesterol intake. Such a diet has been tried with infants up to three years of age. It seems to have done them no harm while lowering their serum cholesterol.[28] However, this kind of program is only experimental. Babies need the kcalories and fat of normal milk, and most experts agree that they should be fed whole or at least low-fat—not skim—milk until after they are a year old. Tampering with the amount of protein in a baby's diet could be especially undesirable, because altered amounts of protein affect the baby's body composition with unpredictable consequences.[29]

Normal dental development is promoted by the same strategies as those outlined above: supplying nutritious foods, avoiding sweets, and discouraging association of food with reward or comfort. In addition, the practice of giving a baby a bottle as a pacifier is strongly discouraged by dentists on the grounds that sucking for long periods of time pushes the normal jawline out of shape and causes the bucktooth profile: protruding upper and receding lower teeth. In addition, once a baby has some of his teeth, prolonged sucking on a bottle of milk or juice bathes the upper teeth with a continuous flow of carbohydrate-

[27]E. Grunwaldt, T. Bates, and D. Guthrie, Jr., The onset of sleeping through the night in infancy, *Pediatrics* 26 (1960):667-668.

[28]G. Friedman and S. J. Goldberg, An evaluation of the safety of a low-saturated-fat, low-cholesterol diet beginning in infancy, *Pediatrics* 58 (1976):655-657.

[29]L. E. Holt, Jr., Protein economy in the growing child, *Postgraduate Medicine* 27 (1960):783-798.

rich fluid that favors the growth of decay-producing bacteria. Babies permitted to do this are sometimes seen with their upper teeth decayed all the way to the gum line.

Psychological Needs   At birth, a baby's needs are simple—warmth, affection, relief when he feels pain, and constant, consistent feeding when he is hungry. A mother may feel, quite rightly, that her major task at the start is to "keep putting it in one end and keep removing it from the other." However, by the time a baby has reached the age of one, his mother often realizes with consternation that he is no longer the malleable, accepting little creature that he used to be. He is becoming an individual, and the ways he expresses this new development can be exasperating. In recent months he has been "getting into everything"; now that he is learning to walk, his range is broader, and nothing in the house below adult waist level is safe. A toddler explores and experiments endlessly, twisting the knobs on the television set, poking his fingers into the wall sockets, tugging on lamp cords and curtains, pulling all the toilet paper off the roll, stirring the soil in potted plants, and scattering the contents of mother's purse.

He used to be receptive and eager to please; now he is contrary and willful. Whatever mother suggests, he refuses, even if it is something he normally likes to do. When mother tells him to stop hitting the cat with the car keys, he casts an appraising eye at her, hesitates only a moment—and continues hitting the cat.

The wise mother is aware that this is a period in her child's life when these behaviors are normal, natural, and even desirable. The child is developing a sense of *autonomy* that, if allowed to flower, will provide the foundation for later confidence and effectiveness as an individual. A wise mother uses her toddler's short attention span to distract him away from the television set. She absolutely forbids—by force, if necessary—her baby to poke into wall sockets or to eat matches, but also avoids coming down on him too hard. A child's urge to explore and experiment, if consistently denied, can turn to shame and self-doubt.

A one-year-old behaves the same way at the table as in other settings. She displays her urge to experiment by dipping her bananas into the spaghetti, by fingerpainting with the chocolate pudding, or by pouring her milk over the tabletop and watching, fascinated, as it drips onto the floor. Her sense of autonomy is strengthened when she refuses to eat her cereal and insists on having applesauce instead. The dilemma a mother faces, knowing how important it is for her child to eat a balanced diet, can be resolved if she is prepared for these developments and knows how to handle them to best advantage. Although a mother attempts to feed her baby all the necessary nutrients in good balance and in amounts sufficient to promote optimal growth and health, she at the same time wants to encourage the baby to feel secure, confident, and independent and to avoid the techniques of shaming, blaming, and inhibiting the growing child.

In light of these developmental and nutritional needs, and in the face

of the often contrary and willful behavior of the one-year-old, a mother
might find a few feeding guidelines helpful.

Setting the Eating Pattern for Life   If a baby spends 2 1/2 hours a
day eating, the total will be over 1,000 hours a year—as much time as a
college student spends in classes in two years of fulltime study. A baby
is open to new impressions of the world, and the amount of learning
that takes place during the feeding hours is astronomical. Not only does
she obtain needed nutrients for her growth and development, she is
also learning about the world—especially about food, about herself,
and about the behaviors that win approval and those that don't.
Properly handled, eating times can make a tremendous contribution to
a child's future well-being, both physical and psychological. Following
are a few typical problem situations with suggestions for handling
them.

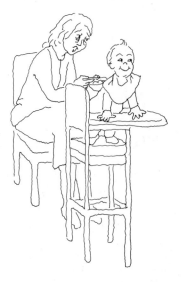

- He stands and plays at the table instead of eating. Don't let him. This
  is unacceptable behavior and should be firmly discouraged. Put him
  down and let him wait until the next feeding to eat again. Be
  consistent and firm, not punitive. If he is really hungry, he will soon
  learn to sit still while eating. Be aware that a baby's appetite is less
  keen at a year than at eight months and that his kcalorie needs are
  relatively lower. A one-year-old will get enough to eat if he lets his
  own hunger be his guide.

- She wants to poke her fingers into her food. Let her. She has much to
  learn from feeling the texture of her food. When she knows all about
  it, she'll naturally graduate to the use of a spoon.

- He wants to manage the spoon himself but can't handle it. Let him
  try. As he masters it, withdraw gradually until he is feeding himself
  competently. This is the age at which a baby can and does learn to
  feed himself and is most strongly motivated to do so. He will spill, of
  course. Mother's best attitude probably is that "one-year-olds don't
  last forever"; he'll grow out of it soon enough.

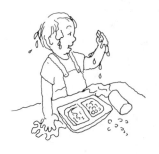

- She refuses food that mother knows is good for her. This way of
  demonstrating autonomy, one of the few available to the one-year-
  old, is most satisfying. Don't force. It is in the one- to two-year-old
  stage that most of the feeding problems develop that can last
  throughout life. As long as she is getting enough milk and is offered a
  variety of nutritious foods to choose from, she can and will gradually
  acquire a taste for different foods—provided that she feels she is
  making the choice. This year is the most important year of a child's
  life in establishing future food preferences. If a baby refuses milk, an
  alternative source of the bone- and muscle-building nutrients it
  supplies must be provided. Milk-based puddings, custards, and
  cheese are often successful substitutes. For the baby who is allergic
  to milk, soy milk and other formulas are available.

- He prefers sweets—candy and sugary confections—to foods

containing more nutrients. Human beings of all races and cultures have a natural inborn preference for sweet-tasting foods. Limit them strictly. There is no room in a baby's daily 1,000 kcal for the kcalories from sweets, except occasionally. The meal plan on p. 546 provides more than 500 kcal from milk; one or two servings of each of the other types of food provide the other 500. If a candy bar were substituted for any of these foods, the baby would lose out on valuable nutrients; if it were added daily, he would gradually become obese.

Nutrition for Children

After the age of one, a child's growth rate slows. But during the next year, the body changes dramatically. At one, children have just learned to stand erect and toddle, often losing their balance and abruptly sitting down. By two, they can take long strides with solid confidence and are learning to run, jump, and climb. The internal changes that make these new accomplishments possible are the accumulations of a larger mass and greater density of bone and muscle tissue. The changes are obvious in the figure below: Two-year-olds have lost much of their

One-year-old child and two-year-old child reduced to same height.

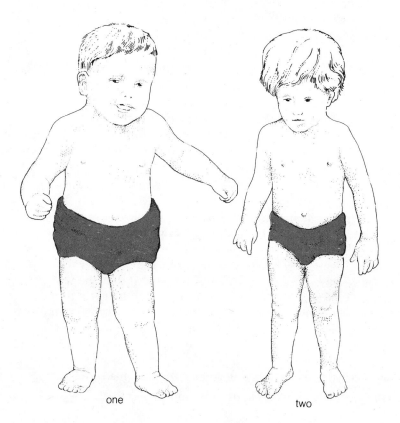

one   two

body fat; their muscles (especially in the back, buttocks, and legs) have firmed and strengthened, and the leg bones have lengthened and increased in density.

Thereafter the same trend—lengthening of the long bones and an increase in musculature—continues, unevenly and still more slowly, until adolescence. Growth comes in spurts; a six-year-old child may wear the same pair of shoes for a year, then need new shoes twice in the next four months.

A factor of importance is that there seems to be a period of rapid cell division in the fat tissue before the age of one or two. As with other critical periods, this is limited in time; later, cell division slows down and the proportion of fat cells becomes fixed. If a baby is overfed, the fat cell number may increase beyond the normal limit, leaving him with too many fat cells. If (and this is only theoretical) the number of fat cells is involved in hunger regulation in the adult, this may mean that the fat baby is destined to be fat for life.

The above hypothesis is not clearly established for human beings, but it is known that the obesity of childhood differs from adult-onset obesity in several respects. Excess weight in the early years places a demand on the skeletal and muscular tissues so that they too grow overly large. Obese children become adults whose fat tissues, skeleton, and muscles are all denser than those of slimmer children. The excess weight is less often successfully and permanently lost in such an adult.

Just before adolescence, the growth patterns of girls and boys begin to diverge. In girls, fat becomes a larger percentage of the total body weight, and in boys the lean body mass—muscle and bone—becomes much greater. Around this time, growth in height may seem to stop altogether for a while, as if the child were settling into a countdown before takeoff. This is the calm before the storm.

Nutritional Needs and Feeding   A one-year-old child needs perhaps 1,000 kcal a day; a three-year-old needs only 300 to 500 kcal more. Appetite decreases markedly around the age of one year, in line with the great reduction in growth rate. Thereafter, appetite fluctuates; a child needs and demands much more food during periods of rapid growth than during periods of quiescence. The nutrients that need emphasis continue to be protein, calcium, and phosphorus, and the food best suited to supply them continues to be milk.

The preadolescent period is the last one in which parental food choices have much influence. As children gather their forces for the adolescent growth spurt, they are accumulating stores of nutrients that will be needed in the coming years. When they take off on that growth spurt, there will be a period during which their nutrient intakes, especially of calcium, cannot meet the demands of rapidly growing bones; then they will be drawing on these stores. The denser their bones are before this occurs, the better prepared they will be.

The gradually increasing needs for all nutrients during the growing years are evident from the RDA table, which lists separate averages for each span of three years. To provide these nutrients, the Four Food Group Plan recommends:

- 3 servings of milk or milk products
- 2 servings of meat or meat substitutes
- 4 or more servings of fruits and vegetables
- 4 or more servings of breads and cereals

For meat, fruits, and vegetables, a serving is loosely defined as 1 tbsp per year of age. Thus a serving of any of these foods for a four-year-old would be 4 tbsp (1/4 c).

Following up on the crucial first year, there is much that a parent can do to foster the development of healthy eating habits. The goal is to teach children to like nutritious foods in all four categories.

Experimentation with children's food patterns shows that candy, cola, and other concentrated sweets must be limited in a child's diet if the needed nutrients are to be supplied. If such foods are permitted in large quantities, there are only two possible outcomes: nutrient deficiencies or obesity. The child can't be trusted to choose nutritious foods on the basis of taste alone; the preference for sweets is innate.[30] The possibility that overfeeding at critical times in children's lives can predispose them to lifelong obesity makes this especially important. On the other hand, an active child can enjoy the higher-kcalorie nutritious foods in each category: ice cream or pudding in the milk group, cake and cookies (whole-grain or enriched only, however) in the bread group. These foods, made from milk and grain, carry valuable nutrients and encourage a child to learn, appropriately, that eating is fun.

Children sometimes seem to lose their appetites for a while; this is nothing to worry about. The system of appetite regulation in children of normal weight guarantees that their kcalorie intakes will be right for each stage of growth. A child who wants to eat less is probably taking a normal "time off" from rapid growth. As long as the kcalories they do consume are from nutritious foods, they are well provided for during this time. (One caution, however: Wandering school-age children may be spending pocket money at the nearby candy store.) An overzealous mother, unaware that her one-year-old is supposed to slow down, may begin a lifelong conflict over food by trying to force more food on the child than the child feels like eating.

Nutrition at School While parents are doing what they can to establish favorable eating behavior during the transition from infancy to childhood, other factors are entering the picture. At five or so, the

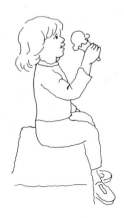

Calcium and riboflavin in a delicious form.

[30]R. B. Choate, Selling cavities—U.S. style, address presented at the American Dental Association annual meeting, October 11, 1977, Council on Dental Health, American Dental Association. According to the speaker, the taste for sweetness exists in the fetus, peaks at 14 years, and is more marked in blacks than in whites.

child goes to school and encounters foods prepared and served by outsiders.

The U.S. government funds several programs to provide nutritious, high-quality meals for children when they are at school. The National School Lunch Act stipulates that every public school must make lunches available to its children, and the federal government reimburses the schools for part or all the cost when families can't pay. School lunches are designed to meet certain requirements: They must include specified servings of milk; protein-rich food (meat, cheese, eggs, legumes, or peanut butter); vegetables; fruits; bread or other grain foods; and butter or margarine. The design is intended to provide at least a third of the RDA for each of the indicator nutrients. The school lunch program is available to about 90 percent of all U.S. school-children, and it represents several billion dollars a year in federal money. Every day, over 25 million lunches are served.[31]

Programs similar to the school lunch program operate in day care centers, settlement houses, and recreation programs. A school breakfast program, operating in many schools in every state, serves over 2 million youngsters, four-fifths of whom pay little or nothing for the food they receive.

The amount of federal money spent on child nutrition programs has risen explosively since the inception of these programs in the 1940s. To cut costs during the 1970s, experts have turned their attention to the problem of "plate waste." Food becomes nutrition only when it passes the lips—and children often refuse to eat the food they are served, thus wasting both food and money and defeating the effort to see that they are well fed. In response to children's differing needs and tastes, the school lunch program and others have been evolving toward better achievement of the objective of feeding the children both what they want and what will nourish them. The trend is toward (1) increasing the variety of offerings and allowing children to choose what they are served; (2) varying portion sizes, so that little children may take little servings; (3) involving students (in secondary schools) in the planning of menus; and (4) improving the scheduling of lunches so that children can eat when they are hungry and can have enough time to eat well.

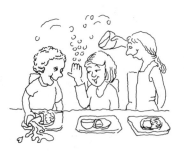

A step toward making school lunches more consistent with today's ideals of healthful food has been to drop the requirement for whole milk and to offer low-fat or skim milk instead. Another alteration has been to eliminate the requirement that butter or margarine be served. Both of these changes have the blessing of the American Dietetic Association, which monitors and offers its judgments about the child nutrition programs.[32]

[31]White House Conference on Nutrition, April 13, 1975, reported as A Tuesday at the White House, *Nutrition Today*, September/October-November/December 1975, pp. 20-25, 53-54.

[32]A. L. Galbraith, ADA's views on school lunch presented to Congress, *Journal of the American Dietetic Association* 70 (1977):630-632.

In many places, the mention of school lunch brings a grimace of dislike to the face of any child. However, some schools have responded to the children's attitudes in creative and imaginative ways that have increased student participation and reduced plate waste. A school in Colorado reports success in feeding its students breakfasts of sandwiches, fish sticks, and tuna salad.[33] A school in Massachusetts offers fast-food cuisine, and students fix their own. As a result, plate waste is greatly reduced, and student participation in the program is up 25 percent. No desserts are offered, but milk is available as milkshakes similar to those at the local fast-food chains. A California school has installed see-through walls so that the students can see the kitchen personnel at work. A school in Georgia offers health foods to meet popular demand. Other schools present ethnic meals and international cuisine on special occasions.[34]

While the schools strive to feed their young clientele nutritious meals, some also seek to educate them in nutritional matters. They are supported by some state programs that provide funds for nutrition education in the classroom. A 1978 public law (#95-166) provides federal funds that each state can apply for—50 cents per child—for nutrition education and training. As of 1980, nearly all 50 states had appointed Nutrition Education Coordinators and were developing nutrition education programs for the schools. Still, having read this book, you will probably know more about nutrition than many who teach it in the schools.

Television and Vending Machines For the most part, then, children learn about nutrition from parents or teachers who know very little about it. Meanwhile, they hear a great deal about foods from the television set. The very first year of life is probably the most crucial in establishing eating patterns that will persist throughout life, but a great deal is learned and internalized during the years that follow.

Many authorities are concerned that the influence of television commercials may be less than desirable. At a 1977 meeting of the American Dental Association, one speaker stated that the average U.S. child sees more than 10,000 commercials a year and that many more than half of them are for sugary foods. Hundreds of millions of dollars were being spent in the effort to sell the foods to children. Most of the concern centers on the issue of sugar. You may recall from Highlight 1 that public disapproval of sugar is not all based on scientific findings. However, there is widespread agreement on one point: Sticky, sugary foods left on the teeth provide an ideal environment for the growth of mouth bacteria and the formation of cavities.

A consumer group composed of concerned parents, Action for Children's Television, has urged the Federal Trade Commission to

[33]Breakfast: A second look, *School Foodservice Journal* 31 (March 1977):36-37.

[34]Type A served fast food style, *School Foodservice Journal* 31 (September 1977):19; San Jose: Moving more nutritious lunches, *Institutions/Volume Feeding Magazine* 81 (August 1, 1977): 42-43; and Fulton County school director plays a hunch on health food—and wins, *Institutions/Volume Feeding Magazine* 81 (September 15, 1977):33-34.

regulate television advertising of these foods. In 1977, this group petitioned the FTC to adopt four measures: (1) to stop the advertising of sticky, sugary foods on children's television programs; (2) to stop "unfair" selling techniques; (3) to require all advertisements to disclose the sugar contents of the products being advertised; and (4) to require the food industries to apply part of their advertising budgets to the support of public service announcements to promote desirable eating habits.[35] A precedent is provided by the Netherlands, where advertisers are required to exhibit an insignia within the last few seconds of every commercial for a sugared product. The insignia shows toothpaste being applied to a toothbrush. In the United States, as of 1980, no such regulations were in force, although there is widespread agreement that they would be effective in reducing demand for sugary foods.[36]

It thus remains up to us to determine which food commercials we will believe and which we will not. Dentists, especially, have the obligation to educate their patients individually as long as misleading claims continue to appear on national television. A model eating plan that favors dental health is shown in Table 5. Among the "bad guys" singled out by the dentists are granola bars—a grain food, but so sticky that the dentists consider them no different from candy bars—and fruit yogurt—which the dentists see as the equivalent of ice cream.[38]

Table 5   Eating Habits to Favor Good Dental Health[37]

Food group	Foods to eat	Foods to avoid
Milk and milk products	milk cheese plain yogurt	all dairy products with added sugar
Fruit	fresh fruit water-packed canned fruit	dried fruit sugar-packed canned fruit jams and jellies
Juice	unsweetened	sweetened
Vegetables	most vegetables	candied sweet potatoes glazed carrots
Grains	most grain products	grain products with added sugar

[35]P. Charren, Advertising of sugar-rich foods: What can the dental profession do? address presented at the American Dental Association annual meeting, October 11, 1977, Council on Dental Health, American Dental Association.

[36]J. T. Dwyer and J. Mayer, Beyond economics and nutrition: The complex basis of food policy, *Science* 188 (1975):566-570.

[37]L. P. DiOrio, Improving nutrition: What should we eat? A dentist's perspective, address presented at the American Dental Association annual meeting, October 11, 1977, Council on Dental Health, American Dental Association.

[38]N. L. Shory, School confection sale bans: What can the dental profession do? address presented at the American Dental Association annual meeting, October 11, 1977, Council on Dental Health, American Dental Association.

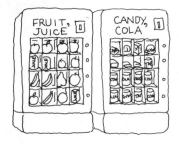

Television is not the only environmental force affecting children's food choices. Another factor that has an impact is vending machines, especially in the schools. The 1977 meeting of the American Dental Association concluded with the establishment of a National Task Force for the Prohibition of the Sale of Confections (sticky, sugary foods) in Schools and resolved that the Task Force should seek changes in the School Lunch Act to eliminate the sale of confections as snacks in schools.[39] A 1977 experiment in six Canadian schools showed that children would choose more nutritious snacks if they were offered side by side with the sugary foods. When apples were made available in vending machines, there was a 27 percent reduction in the selection of chocolate bars. When milk was made available, soft-drink use dropped by 42 percent.[40] A California school has eliminated all candy and soft drinks from its vending machines and is offering a mixture of orange juice and Hawaiian punch instead; acceptance is reported to be good.[41]

Soft drinks contain not only sugar but also caffeine, which is a matter of some concern to pediatricians. A cup of hot chocolate or a 12-oz cola beverage may contain as much as 50 mg caffeine; two or more are equivalent in the body of a 60-pound child to the caffeine in 8 c of coffee for a 175-pound man. Chocolate bars also contribute caffeine. Children and young adults who are troubled by irregular heartbeats or difficulty in sleeping may need to control their caffeine consumption.

Prevention of Future Health Problems   Parents look forward to being proud of strong, healthy, competent, and happy sons and daughters who function well in the adult world. To be on the safe side, parents may also think in terms of conditions to avoid. Some of the conditions they are concerned about are obesity, iron-deficiency anemia, cardiovascular disease, diabetes, cancer, and dental problems. In children, as in infants, eating habits help determine whether development takes place in a positive or in a negative direction.

To avoid obesity, the preschool child should be trained to "eat thin." This means that mealtimes should be relaxed and leisurely. The child should learn to eat slowly, to pause and enjoy her table companions, and to stop eating when she is full. The "clean your plate" dictum should be stamped out for all time. Parents who wish to avoid waste should learn to serve smaller portions or teach their child to serve herself as much as she truly wants to eat. Physical activity should be encouraged on a daily basis to promote strong skeletal and muscular development and to establish a habit that will undergird good health throughout life.

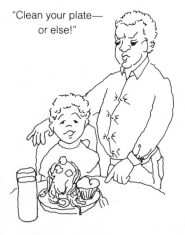

"Clean your plate— or else!"

[39]Shory, 1977.

[40]L. Crawford, Junk food in our schools? A look at student spending in school vending machines and concessions, *Journal of the Canadian Dietetic Association* 38 (July 1977):193; abstract cited in the *Journal of the American Dietetic Association* 71 (1977):572.

[41]San Jose, 1977.

The child who has already become obese needs careful handling. As in pregnancy, weight loss may easily have a harmful effect on growth. One expert who has worked extensively with obese children recommends that they be fed so as to maintain a constant weight while they grow. The object is to restrict the multiplication of fat cells while promoting normal lean body development. Thus the child can "grow out of his obesity."[42]

Of all nutritional disorders other than obesity found in children, the most common is iron-deficiency anemia. It is most prevalent in low-birthweight infants, babies from six months to two years of age, and children and adolescents from low-income families.[43]

Authorities recommend supplementing the diet of infants to ensure an iron intake of 7 mg a day and modifying their food intakes as they grow older so that they will receive 5.5 mg of iron or more per 1,000 kcal. To achieve this latter goal, milk must not be overemphasized in the diet, because it is a poor iron source. Too-high milk consumption causes a form of iron-deficiency anemia called milk anemia. If skim or low-fat milk is used instead of whole milk, there will be kcalories left for investment in such iron-rich foods as lean meats, fish, poultry, eggs, and legumes. Grain products should be whole-grain or enriched only, and children should be steered away from "dairy products (aside from the amount needed to ensure adequate calcium-riboflavin intakes), bakery goods unfortified with iron, candies and soft drinks."[44] Adolescent boys, with their high kcalorie intakes, can meet their iron needs (because they get 6 mg of iron with every 1,000 kcal) from their usual dietary intake. Adolescent girls, who need the same amount of iron and who consume fewer kcalories, probably need iron supplements in most cases.[45]

Most health professionals are aware of the need to promote ample iron intakes. Pediatricians recommend the use of iron-enriched foods for infants, the school lunch program uses enriched products, and obstetricians frequently prescribe iron supplements for pregnant women. But this is not enough. Teenagers are still left out, perhaps due to their use of "junk foods."[46] Nor does merely being male ensure immunity: 1 to 3 percent of the males in the United States and Canada

---

[42]J. L. Knittle, Obesity in childhood: A problem in adipose tissue development, *Journal of Pediatrics* 81 (December 1972):1048-1059.

[43]S. J. Fomon, T. A. Anderson, H. Y. W. Stephen, and E. E. Ziegler, *Nutritional Disorders of Children: Prevention, Screening, and Followup,* DHEW publication no. (HSA) 76-5612 (Washington, D.C.: Government Printing Office, 1976), p. 100.

[44]Fomon et al., 1976, p. 116.

[45]Fomon et al., 1976, p. 118.

[46]W. H. Crosby, Current concepts in nutrition: Who needs iron? *New England Journal of Medicine* 297 (1977):543-545; and Committee on Nutrition of the Mother and Preschool Child, Food and Nutrition Board, National Academy of Sciences, *Iron Nutriture in Adolescence*, DHEW publication no. (HSA) 77-5100 (Washington, D.C.: Government Printing Office, 1977).

are iron deficient.[47] "When simple iron deficiency anemia is observed in adolescent and adult males it is generally accepted that this is a reflection of iron stores never having attained adequate levels."[48] This points up the need to educate women of childbearing age, who are most critically affected by iron deficiency and who are responsible for the storage of iron in the bodies of their infants, both male and female.[49]

Cardiovascular disease is another condition to prevent, and many experts seem to agree that early childhood is the time to put practices into effect that until recently were recommended only for adults. Snacking on high-fat, high-sugar, and high-salt food items should be discouraged, because it sets a pattern that favors the development of atherosclerosis and hypertension.[50] Instead, foods of high nutrient density should be emphasized.

It seems that this recommendation might also help to prevent or retard the onset of diabetes in children who have the genetic tendency toward it.[51] Those who have been studying the effect of nutrition on cancer have reached the same conclusion. It is suggested that children should follow a "prudent diet," "since evidence is increasing that appropriate biological control in terms of fat and cholesterol may be set early in life."[52] The "prudent diet" is a diet originally developed for heart patients, but its outlines are the same as those recommended by nutritionists interested in the prevention of cancer.

Not everyone agrees that all children should be placed on diets strictly limited in sugar, salt, and fat and high in fruits, vegetables, and whole-grain cereals. However, even those who do not go this far recommend that children be screened early to determine what conditions each of them might be likely to develop. Then parents can pay appropriate attention to diet in each special case. (Figure 5 outlines the screening process.) Thus the child of parents who have high blood pressure should be raised on a diet relatively low in salt; the child whose parents are diabetic should avoid sugar and be encouraged to eat foods high in complex carbohydrate;[53] and the child whose parents

---

[47]P. C. Elwood, The enrichment debate, *Nutrition Today*, July/August 1977, pp. 18-24.

[48]Council on Foods and Nutrition, American Medical Association, Iron in enriched wheat flour, farina, bread, buns, and rolls (a Council statement), *Journal of the American Medical Association* 220 (1972):13-17.

[49]J. Mayer, ed., *U.S. Nutrition Policies in the Seventies* (San Francisco: W. H. Freeman, 1973).

[50]G. C. Frank, A. W. Voors, P. E. Schilling, and G. S. Berenson, Dietary studies of rural school children in a cardiovascular survey, *Journal of the American Dietetic Association* 71 (1977):31-35.

[51]K. M. West, Prevention and therapy of diabetes mellitus, in *Nutrition Reviews' Present Knowledge in Nutrition*, 4th ed. (Washington, D.C.: Nutrition Foundation, 1976), pp. 356-364.

[52]E. L. Wynder, The dietary environment and cancer, *Journal of the American Dietetic Association* 71(1977):385-392.

[53]West, 1976.

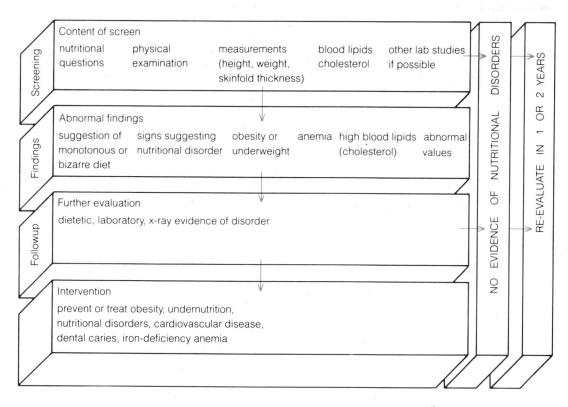

Figure 5 Nutritional screening of children.[54]

have coronary artery disease should eat foods that are low in fat, especially saturated fat and possibly cholesterol. Even acne is better prevented than treated, because success is much more likely if it is caught in the early stages,[55] although in this case the treatment is not primarily nutritional. In all these situations, the greatest success is likely to be achieved if the whole family, and not just the child, follows the recommended dietary guidelines.

There is widespread agreement that poor dental health is a preventable condition. The measures recommended for its prevention center around two objectives. First, there is a need to ensure adequate nutrition so that the mouth and teeth develop properly. This means providing an adequate diet, especially in terms of protein, calcium, vitamins A, C, and D, and fluoride. Where local water supplies are not fluoridated, direct application of fluoride to the teeth may be necessary. Second, it is important to restrict the supply of carbohydrate foods to the bacteria that cause tooth decay. This means brushing the teeth or washing the mouth after meals (especially meals high in carbohydrate), avoiding snacks that contain sticky carbohydrate that will linger

[54] Fomon et al., 1976, inside front cover.

[55] L. Goldman, Acne prevention in the family, *American Family Physician* 16 (August 1977):68-71.

along the teeth and gumlines, and dislodging persistent particles with dental floss or other devices.

It is desirable for children to learn to like nutritious foods in all of the food groups. With one exception, this liking usually develops naturally. Meats, breads and cereals, fruit, and milk are well accepted by children. The exception is vegetables, which young children frequently dislike and refuse. Even a tiny serving of spinach, cooked carrots, or squash may elicit an expression that registers the utmost in negative feelings (as well as great pride in the ability to make an ugly face). In light of the findings that people in the developed countries generally need to learn to eat more vegetables, the next few paragraphs are addressed to this problem.

Helping Children Like Vegetables   Do you remember how you felt when first offered a cup of vegetable soup, a serving of runny spinach, or a pile of peas and carrots? If the soup burned your tongue, it brought tears to your eyes. It may have been years before you were willing to try it again. As for the spinach, it was suspiciously murky looking. (Who could tell what might be lurking in that ugly dark-green liquid?) The peas and carrots troubled your sense of order: Before you could eat them, you felt compelled to sort the peas onto one side of the plate and the carrots onto the other. Then you had to separate, into a reject pile, all those that got mashed in the process or contaminated with gravy from the mashed potatoes. Only then might you be willing to eat the intact, clean peas and carrots one by one. You hoped your parents wouldn't notice your picking them up with your fingers. Peas, especially, were so hard to pick up with a fork; they kept rolling off.

Why children respond in this way to foods that look "off" or "messy" to them is a matter for conjecture. Parents need only be aware that this is how many children feel and then honor those feelings. Children prefer vegetables that are slightly undercooked and crunchy, bright in color, served separately, and easy to eat. They should be warm, not hot, because a child's mouth is much more sensitive than an adult's. The flavor should be mild (a child has more taste buds), and smooth foods such as mashed potatoes or pea soup should have no lumps in them (a child wonders, with some disgust, what the lumps might be). Irrational as the fear of strangeness may seem, the parent must realize that it is practically universal among children and may even have a built-in biological basis.

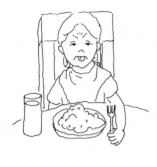

Little children like to eat at little tables and to be served little portions of food. They also love to eat with other children and have been observed to stay at the table longer and eat much more when in the company of their peers. A bright, unhurried atmosphere free of conflict is also conducive to good appetite. Parents who serve the food in a relaxed and casual manner, without anxiety, provide the emotional climate in which a child's negative emotions will be minimized.

Ideally, each meal is preceded, not followed, by the activity the child looks forward to the most. In a number of schools, it has been discovered that children eat a much better lunch if recess occurs

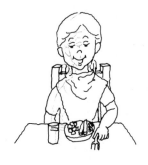

before, rather than after, the meal. With recess after, they are likely to hurry out to play, leaving food on their plates that they were hungry for and would otherwise have eaten. Before sitting down to eat, the small child should be helped to clean herself thoroughly, washing her hands and face so that she can enjoy her meal with "that clean feeling."[56]

Many little children, both boys and girls, enjoy helping in the kitchen. Their participation provides many opportunities to encourage good food habits. Family tradition often involves letting children help make cookies and lick the mixing bowl, but a child can also help with the preparation of main dishes. A little boy who helps his mother shell peas or cut green beans may eat so many of them raw, before the meal, that his rejection of the cooked equivalent at the dinner table will be a matter of no concern. A little girl who helps break up the lettuce and cut the carrots and celery for a salad may get absorbed in pretending to be a bunny rabbit and nibble a serving or two while she works. Vegetables are pretty, especially when fresh, and provide opportunities to learn about color, about growing things and their seeds, about shapes and textures—all of which are fascinating to young children. Measuring, stirring, decorating, cutting, and arranging vegetables on a plate are skills even a very small child can practice with enjoyment and pride.

When introducing new foods at the table, parents are advised to offer them one at a time—and only in small amounts at first. Whenever possible, the new food should be presented at the beginning of the meal, when the child is hungry. If the child is cross, irritable, or feeling sick, don't insist; withdraw the new food and try it again a few days later, just as you would with an adult. Remember, parents have inclinations and dislikes to which they feel entitled; children should be accorded the same privilege. Never make an issue of food acceptance. A power struggle almost invariably results in a confirmed pattern of resistance and a permanently closed mind on the child's part.

Psychological Growth of the Child   The key word (at one year) is *trust*; the parental behavior best suited to promote it is affectionate holding. At two years, the word is *autonomy*; parents should allow children to make their own choices, including giving them the right to say their favorite word (No!) to offered foods—at the same time providing, of course, other nutritious foods to choose from. (A child may also take great pride in saying no to toilet training by withholding a bowel movement for several days; this is not dangerous.) At four, when the development of *initiative* is their proudest achievement, children can be encouraged to participate in the planning and preparation of meals. At each age, food can be given and enjoyed in the context of growth in its largest, most inclusive sense. If the beginnings

[56]We are indebted to Dr. Joyce Williams of the Department of Home and Family Life, College of Home Economics, Florida State University, and coauthor (with M. Stith) of *Middle Childhood: Behavior and Development* (New York: Macmillan, 1974), for many of these suggestions.

are right, children will grow without the kind of conflict and confusion over food that can lead to nutritional problems.

At every age, there is a negative counterpart—distrust, shame, guilt, inferiority—to the desired development. These, too, can be promoted by unaware parents, even if they have the best of intentions. Mealtimes can be nightmarish for the child who is struggling with these issues. If, as she sits down to the table, she is confronted with a barrage of accusations—"Susie, your hands are filthy . . . get your elbows off the table . . . your report card . . . and clean your plate! Your mother cooked that food"—mealtimes may be unbearable. Her stomach may recoil, because her body as well as her mind reacts to stress of this kind.

In the interest of promoting both a positive self-concept and a positive attitude toward good food, it is important for mother and father to help Johnny or Susie remember that they are good kids. Their behavior may need correcting; what they do may sometimes be unacceptable; but what they are, on the inside, is normal, healthy, growing, fine human beings.

Summing Up

Growth is a major factor influencing the nutritional needs of developing infants and children. The growth rate is fastest during prenatal life, the first year, and the adolescent years. Growth patterns for different organs vary. Most are characterized by critical periods, during which cells divide and nutrition has greater importance than usual. Psychological growth accompanies and facilitates physical growth.

During pregnancy, changes in both the mother's and fetus's bodies necessitate increased intakes of the growth nutrients. A pregnant woman should gain about 24 pounds from high-nutrient-density foods. Malnutrition during pregnancy affects the developing fetus, and low-birthweight babies often fail to thrive. Alcohol, smoking, drugs, dieting, and unbalanced nutrient intakes of all kinds should be avoided for the duration of pregnancy. Salt and fluid intakes should be ample.

The breastfeeding mother needs additional kcalories from foods of high nutrient density and an ample fluid intake. Nicotine, caffeine, marihuana, alcohol, and other compounds are secreted into breast milk and so should be avoided during breastfeeding. The rapidly growing newborn infant requires milk, preferably breast milk, which provides the needed nutrients in quantities suitable to support the infant's growth. The advantages of breast milk over formula, especially in underdeveloped countries, are that it protects the infant against disease and that it is sanitary, economical, and premixed to the correct proportions. To avoid allergy, all infants should be breastfed at first, even in developed countries.

Additions to a baby's diet are selected according to the baby's readiness to handle them and its changing nutrient needs. Among the first nutrients needed in amounts beyond those provided by milk are iron and vitamin C. By a year of age, a baby can be eating foods from all four food groups. Normal weight gain, tooth development, and health can be promoted by feeding a balanced diet, avoiding empty-kcalorie foods, and encouraging infants to learn to like foods from all four food groups. Extremes are unwise at this critical period of development. The first year of life is the most important for setting future food habits, so attention to the emotional needs and developmental stage of the infant is well invested.

After the age of one, a child's growth rate slows, and with it, the appetite. However, all essential nutrients, especially the growth nutrients, continue to be needed in adequate amounts from foods with a high nutrient density. Milk remains important but should not exceed three servings a day, because it is a poor source of iron and vitamin C.

When children go to school, their nutritional needs are partly met by school lunches and other programs, which supply a third of the children's RDAs for each indicator nutrient. In recent years, school lunches have become flexible enough in many areas to meet children's preferences with imagination and creativity.

An influential factor in the lives of children is television, with its high proportion of advertisements for sugary foods; another is vending machines which limit choices to foods of low quality. Dentists and other health professionals are concerned that the advertisement and availability of sugary foods should be controlled; there may also be a need to control some children's caffeine consumption from cola beverages and cocoa products.

Sound nutritional practices may prevent future health problems to some extent. Obesity, iron-deficiency anemia, cardiovascular disease, and diabetes are conditions that may be retarded or prevented by nutritional and other measures; screening for these conditions helps early detection. Good dental health can be promoted by avoiding sticky, sugary foods and by adopting healthy eating habits as well as brushing teeth regularly.

It is desirable for children to learn to like nutritious foods in all of the food groups. This liking seems to come naturally, although some children have trouble liking vegetables. The person who feeds the child must be aware of the child's psychological and emotional development. With wise handling, children can learn eating habits that will continue to promote their good health and well-being after they have become adults.

To Explore Further

Many of the references suggested in Appendix J include good sections or chapters on nutrition for pregnant women, infants, and children. In addition, the following paperback book should be singled out for special mention:

Worthington, B. S., Vermeersch, J., and Williams, S. R., *Nutrition in Pregnancy and Lactation* (St. Louis: Mosby, 1977).

Also specially relevant to nutrition in pregnancy is:

Be Good to Your Baby before It Is Born, a pamphlet available from many local March of Dimes offices or from the National Foundation, March of Dimes, PO Box 2000, White Plains, NY 10602. The March of Dimes has been very active in working to prevent birth defects, and you might inquire what other materials they have available.

Inside My Mom is a set of about 80 slides with a cassette, a delightful presentation of pregnancy from the fetus's point of view. It is intended to motivate the pregnant woman to eat right. This is another March of Dimes resource.

The following teaching aids are available from the Nutrition Today Society (address in Appendix J), and each comes with an annotated syllabus.

James, L., and Hurley, L., *Diet and Birth Defects* (18 slides).

Shank, R. E., *Nutrition in Pregnancy: A Chink in Our Armor* (16 slides).

Many good references on breastfeeding are also available. We recommend:

Jelliffe, D. B., and Jelliffe, E. F. P., "Breast is best": Modern meanings, *New England Journal of Medicine* 297 (1977): 912-915. This presents the reasons why, in the authors' opinion, breastfeeding is best even in developed countries such as the United States.

Pryor, K., *Nursing Your Baby* (New York: Harper & Row, 1963). Although not especially notable for its scientific accuracy, this practical and emotionally warm paperback provides abundant encouragement and advice for the mother who wants to nurse.

Smith, G. V., Calvert, L. J., and Kanto, W. P., Jr., Breast feeding and infant nutrition, *American Family Physican* 17 (1978): 92-102. This is a fully up-to-date, well-illustrated, scientifically accurate article with useful tips on how to breastfeed.

On nutrition in the first year of life, Fomon, S. J., *Infant Nutrition*, 2nd ed. (Philadelphia: Saunders, 1974) is an excellent comprehensive reference. Small items that we have also found useful include:

Food: From Birth to Birthday, a 19-page pamphlet available from the National Dairy Council, Rosemont, IL 60018, publication number B205 (2), 1977.

Food with Love, a 56-page booklet available free from the Pennsylvania Department of Education, Division of Food Service, 8 South 13th Street, Pittsburgh PA 15203.

Parents Magazine makes available $58 worth of excellent filmstrip-cassette sets mostly for parental education. Write Department F, 52 Vanderbilt Avenue, New York, NY 10017.

On the rearing of children, Dr. Benjamin Spock's book remains a classic. The most recent paperback edition is:

Spock, B., *Baby and Child Care* (New York: Pocket Books, 1977). The original version is *The Common Sense Book of Baby and Child Care* (New York: Duell, Sloan and Pearce, 1958). The tolerance we recommend for contending with the antics of a young child originated with Spock.

On the nutrition of children:

Fomon, S. J., *Infant Nutrition*, 2nd ed. (Philadelphia: Saunders, 1974).

Pipes, P. L., *Nutrition in Infancy and Childhood* (St. Louis: Mosby, 1977). This 205-page paperback is an authoritative, clear, understandable text, one of the best in the field.

On the prevention of later health problems through good nutritional practices in childhood:

Breslow, L., and Somers, A. R., Lifetime health monitoring: A practical approach to preventive medicine, *New England Journal of Medicine* 296 (1977): 601-608. Breslow and Somers have studied the disorders most likely to appear at every age and have suggested an agenda for screening at intervals throughout life that would detect these disorders.

Fomon, S. J., Anderson, T. A., Stephen, H. Y. W., and Ziegler, E. E., *Nutritional Disorders of Children: Prevention, Screening, and Followup*, DHEW publication no. (HSA) 76-5612 (Washington, D.C.: Government Printing Office, 1976).

On teaching children to resist the allure of television commercials:

Seeing through Commercials: A Children's Guide to TV Advertising is a 1976 film available (for $220) from Vision Films, PO Box 48896, Los Angeles, CA 90048.

A booklet, *Buy and Buy*, to help 9- to 13-year-olds learn to see through cereal commercials is available for $.55 from MVR Hall, Cornell University, Ithaca, NY 14853.

A 12-page foldout, Children and television, can be obtained for $.50 by writing to Action for Children's Television, 46 Austin Street, Newtonville MA 02160. You might want to inquire what other resources they have.

For people concerned with the nutrition education of children, the National Nutrition Education Clearing House (address in Appendix J) puts out a listing of reference materials. For example:

Secondary Teaching Materials and Teacher References, rev. ed., Nutrition Education Resource Series 4 (Berkeley, Calif.: Society for Nutrition Education, 1977).

For people who feed children:

Goodwin, M. T., and Pollen, G., *Creative Food Experiences for Children* is available from the Center for Science in the Public Interest, PO Box 3099, Washington DC 20010. This paperback encourages children to participate in the preparation of healthful foods.

Lansky, V., *The Taming of the C.A.N.D.Y. Monster* (Wayzata, Minn.: Meadowbrook Press, 1978). This is an unusual cookbook (paperback) that encourages creativity in the kitchen and helps to solve such problems as what to put in the lunchbox.

Williams, J., and Stith, M., *Middle Childhood: Behavior and Development*, 2nd ed. (New York: Macmillan, 1979).

The *School Lunch Journal* and the *School Foodservice Journal* come out monthly with creative new ideas.

Frederick, L., *Fast Food Gets an "A" in School Lunch* (Boston: Cahner's Books, 1977) describes the fast-food style of serving school lunches, which has been proving successful in attracting children away from vending machines and off-campus eating places.

Hunger is a very personal matter. You cannot feel compassion and concern over a statistic—"X number of children go to school each day with no breakfast." Until that figure is translated in your mind into a child who must sit in a classroom and perform intellectual tasks on an empty stomach, it is difficult to comprehend the agony of hunger.

Hunger is hidden today. Every day, middle-class people drive on superhighways over and around the very poor and forget that the poor are there, because they reside on the back roads and in inner-city slums. In the Depression of the 1930s, the hungry were visible. They stood in long lines outside soup kitchens set up in church basements and said by their presence, "Look, I am hungry. I have no money to buy food." Today, based on newspaper reports of the immense sums spent on food stamps and welfare programs, people say to them-

With your neighbours and their child, the circumstances at their command supply a plenty and variety which embrace the whole quota of the vitamins. But the community at large has some of its children in sunless dwellings and some of their parents without the means of plenty.

SIR CHARLES SHERRINGTON

selves, "Surely, there are no hungry people in our country today!"

How do we know if there is hunger in our communities? What can we do to find out? And what do we mean by *hunger*? Are we speaking of the undernutrition of an empty stomach or of the malnutrition of imbalance? The nutritionist is concerned with both these defin-

itions of hunger; a nutrition survey is the only known way of discovering the hungry in a population. We wrote this Highlight to help you understand how a survey is conducted (by detailing one, the Ten-State Survey) and to demonstrate how to interpret results from a survey (by contrasting the Ten-State with two others).

Measuring Nutrients in the Body If you look at the route a nutrient follows from ingestion to metabolism, storage, or excretion, you can see that there are places where the nutrient or its metabolite is accessible to a diagnostician. When a nutrient comes into the body, the amount of the intake can be calculated; after digestion and absorption into the bloodstream, the nutrient level in the blood can be measured. Furthermore, if other tissues pick up the nutrient from the blood and metabolize it, the metabolites are put back into the bloodstream, filtered out by the kidney, and excreted in the urine; therefore both the unused nutrient and the metabolite can be detected in the urine. If the tissues of the body are able to store an excess of the nutrient, this storage form of the nutrient can also be measured. The level of the nutrient can therefore be measured on intake, in the blood, in the urine, and in the storage sites.

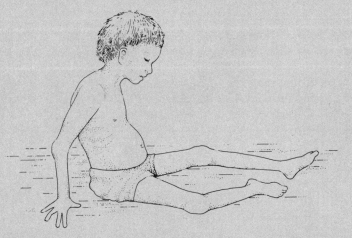

566

One of the methods of determining the nutritional status of a population is to study its food intake. The amount and kinds of food consumed by a person can be recorded either by keeping a diet record or in reply to an interviewer's questions. The usefulness of such measures depends on the honesty and memory of the people being interviewed and on the interviewer's skill. Tables of food composition are used to calculate the nutrient content of the diet, which is then compared to the recommended intakes. This method assumes that the recommendations apply to the people being studied. Individuals differ widely in their need for specific nutrients, so the larger the sample of the population, the more validity there is in using the recommendations as a yardstick. Two other assumptions are also made: that everyone absorbs the same amount of the nutrient and that the foods analyzed in the food composition tables have the same nutrient content as the food consumed by the people being studied. Remember too that the recommended intakes are based on the nutrient needs of healthy persons; thus a survey would need to include a medical examination for the presence of such conditions as intestinal parasites before it could properly compare nutrient intake with the recommendations.

In the same way that rec-ommended intakes have been established for most nutrients, standards for normal plasma and serum levels of many nutrients have also been established. Some of the blood tests require sophisticated equipment and techniques and so are unsuitable for field surveys, but many, such as the test for protein, are simple to perform and are widely used.

Means of assessing nutritional status:

Dietary history
Clinical tests
Physical examination
Anthropometric measures

A urine sample can furnish a wealth of information about what is happening in the cells, whether they have no need of a particular nutrient or hungrily use all they can get from the bloodstream. For example, a test load of thiamin can be given and the amount of it excreted in the urine can be measured. If a large percentage is excreted, the tissues can be assumed to have been saturated; thus the dietary intake must have been adequate. But if very little is excreted, the tissues must have been in need of it, and therefore the diet must have been inadequate. In children, excretion of less than 10 percent of a test load of thiamin indicates a dietary deficiency that has probably extended over many months. Sometimes the end product of the metabolism of the nutrient is measured instead of the nutrient itself. A higher level of excretion of the metabolite indicates a greater desaturation of the cells and a greater deficiency of the nutrient in the diet.

If a nutrient is one that is stored in the tissues, it may be possible to test for the nutrient in the storage sites. For example, there is no excretion route for iron, and one of the places it is stored is in the bone marrow. A test sample of the bone marrow, usually the marrow of the sternum (breastbone), will reveal the amount of iron present in storage form. (However, nutritional surveys would probably favor a simpler though less sensitive technique for discovering iron status, such as finding the level of hemoglobin, the iron-containing protein, in the blood.)

If a deficiency of a nutrient continues long enough or is very severe, the storage sites will be depleted. Eventually the damage will become evident in the tissues of the skin, eyes, hair, teeth, tongue, and mouth. The classical signs of deficiency include cracks at the corners of the mouth and glossitis, which the trained investigator looks for during a physical examination.

Thus the status of a nutrient can be determined by analyzing the actual nutrient intake and comparing it with the recommended intake or by testing biochemically the nutrient or its metabolites in the blood, urine, or storage sites and comparing the results with normal values. These tests can reveal the earliest signs of deficiency and are widely used for this purpose in nutritional surveys.

The Ten-State Survey The U.S. government mandated a nutritional survey for the United States between 1968 and 1970.[1] Dr. Arnold E. Shaefer, who had conducted many such surveys in other countries, was selected to head the project. Ten states (California, Kentucky, Louisiana, Massachusetts, Michigan, South Carolina, Texas, Washington, New York, and West Virginia) and New York City were chosen to represent geographic, ethnic, economic, and other features of the whole United States. In all, 62,532 people were surveyed.

The plan of the Ten-State Nutrition Survey (also called the National Nutrition Survey) incorporated the following essential basic measurements: clinical assessment including medical history, physical examination, various anthropometric measurements such

as height, weight, and subcutaneous fat, and X-ray measurements of bones; biochemical measurements of the levels of various substances in blood and urine; dietary assessment of nutrient and usual patterns of food consumption; dental examinations; and such related data as socio-economic status, food sources, and educational status.[2]

The results of this survey called forth protests from groups who believed that their states had been maligned by the reports. Such protests were probably due to a misunderstanding of the purpose of the survey and of the sampling techniques used. Any survey of a population as large as that of the United States must choose a sample of that population that will provide the data needed to meet the purposes of the survey. In the case of the Ten-State Survey, the purpose was to discover which segments were malnourished. It was assumed that malnutrition would be more likely to occur among low-income groups. Thus the entire population of each state was not surveyed but rather low-income groups within each state. The 1960 U.S. Census was used to identify the areas within the states that were most likely to con-

tain large numbers of people with income below the poverty line.

Whenever the results of a survey are used to make generalizations, they must be interpreted with caution. In the case of the Ten-State Survey, the population studied was a segment selected because it was especially likely to be malnourished. The Survey results do not reflect the nutritional status of the average citizen, but of the unfortunate citizen.

CAUTION WHEN YOU READ!

Before jumping to conclusions from survey results, be sure to understand the sampling method.

The HANES Another study, known as the HANES (Health and Nutrition Examination Survey), avoided the bias of the Ten-State Survey by adjusting for the effects of over-sampling among vulnerable groups. The U.S. National Center for Health Statistics in 1971-1974 conducted this study of over 20,000 people, aged 1 to 74, at 65 sampling sites in the

[1]U.S. Department of Health, Education, and Welfare, *Ten-State Nutrition Survey, 1968-1970,* publication no. (HSM) 72-8130 (Atlanta: Center for Disease Control, 1972).

[2]*Ten-State Nutrition Survey, 1968-1970.*

United States. Careful efforts were made to evaluate protein and kcalorie intakes in relation to height, sex, and age on an individual basis.

The HANES' principal usefulness was in identifying the subgroups most at risk and the nutrients most in need of attention. Whereas the Ten-State assumed at the outset that deficiencies would be more likely to occur in the poor, the HANES showed, through its broader sampling, that this was indeed true. Deficiencies in kcalories, protein, calcium, and iron were more extensive among people below the poverty line and generally more prominent among blacks than among whites. Infants, adolescents, and women of childbearing age were found to be especially vulnerable.

HANES II, undertaken in 1977 as a follow-up to HANES, was designed to collect biochemical and other data, with an emphasis on determining whether the low iron intakes found previously were reflected in a poor clinical picture. The findings showed that iron deficiency was a major public health concern.

Nutrition Canada   An illustration of how the purpose of a study determines the sample is provided by a study of food consumption patterns mandated by the Canadian government. Its purposes were to examine the con-

sumption of selected food groups, to examine patterns of food consumption and nutrient intake at certain times of the day, and to provide information on the changes in eating habits during pregnancy.[3] This study was intended to help the government to devise food legislation.

In Canada, the subcultures that needed to be identified were typically found in specific geographic regions—Atlantic, Quebec, Ontario, Prairies, and Pacific. Therefore, people were selected at random from the entire population of each region but were also identified as Indian or Eskimo if they happened to belong to either ethnic group. The Canadian survey did not specify regional income level, although individual socioeconomic level was determined. No clinical or physical characteristics, other than age and sex, were recorded.

You can see from the description of the Ten-State and Nutrition Canada that the results would be difficult to compare—like apples and oranges.

[3]Canada, Department of National Health and Welfare, *Food Consumption Patterns Report,* a report from Nutrition Canada by the Bureau of Nutritional Sciences Health Protection Branch, 1970-1972.

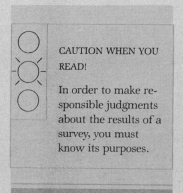

CAUTION WHEN YOU READ!

In order to make responsible judgments about the results of a survey, you must know its purposes.

Results of the Ten-State Survey   The results of the Ten-State Survey were broken down by age, sex, ethnic background, and location (whether the person resided in a low-income or high-income state). The following is a brief summary of the Ten-State Survey findings:

● *Clinical.*   Few severe deficiencies were established by the clinical examinations. This does not imply that there were no deficiencies present but rather that they were not prolonged or severe enough for the clinical signs to appear. (These are sometimes called subclinical deficiencies.)

● *Anthropometric.*   People with higher incomes had greater height, weight, fatness, and skeletal weight; larger head circumference; earlier skeletal maturation; and earlier tooth eruption. Blacks were taller than whites and were more advanced in skeletal and dental development. Obesity was more prominent in adult women, especially in black women (see Figure 1). One of the most significant findings was that the trends seen among the children persisted into adulthood, underscoring the effect of early poverty on later development.

● *Dental.* Among the children, Spanish-Americans were most in need of dental care. Among adults, Spanish-Americans and blacks had the greatest needs. There was a relationship between the intake of sugar and dental caries (cavities) among adolescents and between low income and dental caries in all groups.

● *Hemoglobin and related measurements.* Generally, higher dietary iron intakes correlated with higher hemoglobin levels. Black populations particularly showed a prevalence of low hemoglobin in all income groups.

● *Protein.* Protein deficiencies were not so widespread as for some of the other nutrients. The highest incidenc was found among blacks an(Spanish-Americans. Protein deficiency correlated with low income level. Pregnant and lactating women exhibited more dietary deficiency and lower serum values, but protein intake seemed to be generally adequate for most groups.

● *Vitamin A and carotene.* The data show that vitamin A nutritional status is a major public health concern, particularly among pre-

cents and Spanish-Americans (see Figure 2).

● *Vitamin C.* There seems to be no cause for concern regarding vitamin C nutritional status among the groups studied. There was, however, a greater incidence of low values for blacks in the low-income states and also a greater incidence, generally, among males than among females.

● *Riboflavin and thiamin.* Riboflavin status is a potential problem among young persons of all ethnic groups and particularly among blacks and Spanish-Americans in the low-income states. Thiamin status appears to be no cause for concern in the populations studied.

● *Iodine.* There does not seem to be a public health problem in regard to iodine nutriture. Iodinization of salt remains an important public health measure.

● *Multiple low biochemical values.* Generally, blacks and Spanish-Americans had a higher prevalence of multiple deficiencies. There was also a higher prevalence in the low-income states. One significant finding was that the fewer the years of school completed by the homemaker, the greater the prevalence of multiple low values (see Table 1).

● *Dietary intake.* In all states, intakes of nutrients were generally lower for

Figure 1 Comparison of obesity in white women and black women in low- and high-income states, Ten-State Survey, 1968-1970.

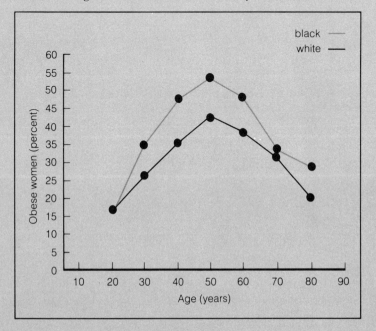

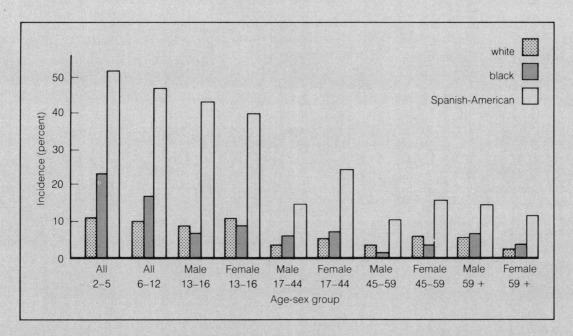

Figure 2   Incidence of deficient or low plasma vitamin A among various groups in low-income states, Ten-State Survey, 1968-1970.

blacks than for whites and Spanish-Americans, except that the latter had the lowest intakes of vitamin A. Foods rich in vitamin A were consumed on a daily basis by only 15 percent of all households, and 20 percent reported that they never or only rarely used them. Spanish-Americans were highest in their use of cereals and grains for kcalories; they received a substantially lower percentage of their kcalories from dairy products than did other groups. Over two-thirds of all households used fresh milk as a beverage daily; over 80 percent of all households reported never using dry skim milk as a beverage. (Evidently more education is needed in the use of economical dry skim milk.)

According to the data gathered in the Ten-State Survey, then, target groups who need help with their nutrition are blacks, Spanish-Americans, adolescents, and low-income groups. The greatest numbers of people

Table 1   Education and Biochemical Deficiencies*

Years of school completed by female head of family	Number of people tested	People with 2 or more deficient or low biochemical tests	
		Number	Percent
None	122	49	40.2
1-4	369	109	29.5
5-8	896	206	23.0
9-12	899	181	20.1
Post high school	24	4	16.7
College	49	8	16.3
Other	4	0	0.0
Total	2,363	557	23.6

*Deficiencies are expressed as a percentage of respondents under 17 years of age with deficient or low biochemical values in two or more of six biochemical tests. These figures are classified according to the education of the female head of the family or the wife of the head of the family. These data come from low-income states in the Ten-State Survey, 1968-1970.

were deficient in the nutrients iron, vitamin A, and riboflavin; and protein was a problem for pregnant and lactating women.

We have described the results of the Ten-State Survey in the style of scientific journals—concise, no frills, no telling you that something is an "Aha!" fact. We have done this with "malice aforethought." For one thing, we were able to squeeze more solid information into a space with this style, although this was only a minor consideration.

More important, we wanted you to have the fun of reading along in this dry, uninteresting report of survey results and then stumbling onto an "Aha!" fact by yourself. Did you? Did any of these statistics make your heart jump because you suddenly realized that they represented real, live people in trouble? Did you think maybe you could help? We hope so.

If it didn't happen anywhere else, surely reading about the effect of the mother's education on the nutriture of the child caused you to think. What exciting possibilities for the health of children lie in that dull sentence: The fewer the years of school

completed by the homemaker, the greater the prevalence of multiple low values. Service organizations, if they understood the implication of Table 1, would devise programs to encourage girls to stay in school: Helping them to dress better so they wouldn't drop out due to embarrassment, or providing an opportunity for pregnant teenagers to continue their education are two possibilities that come to mind. What do you think could be done? What effect might the trend for men to take a more active role in parenting have on children's nutrition?

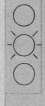

CAUTION WHEN YOU READ!

Don't put your brain in neutral when reading dull statistics. You miss a lot of excitement that way!

After the Ten-State Survey
There is good reason to believe that the poor are in worse shape now than when the Ten-State Survey was completed in 1970. Inflation and rising food prices have hurt the food-buying power of the poor much more than that of middle- and upper-income groups. In the first place, the poor spend a far

larger portion of their income on food. Also, the prices of the foods they eat have risen much faster than those of the foods middle-income and rich people eat. For example, a meal of rib roast, canned tomatoes, and broccoli with butter may increase by less than 30 percent during the same period in which a meal of pork sausage, dried beans, and rice with margarine increases in price by more than 100 percent. Probably one of the reasons for the great increase in prices of the poor person's choices of foods is that middle-income people, caught by inflation and rising prices, are able to lower their food costs by choosing less expensive foods, thereby increasing the demand for these foods and their price. But poor people cannot economize much more than they already do. Their only choices have been to go hungry or to go into debt.

Two groups in the United States have unique problems of poverty and thus of hunger—migrant farm workers and Native Americans. Migrant workers, essential to the food industry, have been excluded from the protective labor legislation that the rest of the U.S. labor force takes for granted. Since they move constantly with the harvest from state to state, they cannot obtain the social services available to other poor people. (Many of these services have a residence requirement, and their offices are located in the cities.) Typically, migrant workers don't even know they are eligible for these services; and if they did know, they would still have to lose a day's pay and find transportation to get to the offices. Their children, since they are rarely in school, cannot participate in school lunch programs.[4] All these circumstances lock the migrant farm worker into a cycle of poor education, poor nutrition, poor health, and poverty.

Native Americans, too, are locked into a virtually unbreakable cycle. A total of half a million live on reservations and about half are below the federal poverty line. They pay almost a third more for food than people in urban areas. Their median age is under 20 years, as compared to the U.S. median age of almost 30 years. Mortality of newborns is almost a quarter higher than the national rate. The death rate of older infants is almost three times the U.S. average. Several cases of kwashiorkor and marasmus have been reported. Obesity is seen in some tribes at a rate of 60 to 90 percent.[5] These statistics point to severe nutrition problems among the Indians.

Other groups in our society, such as the elderly and infants, are also in need of more and better food, but they are not easily identified because they are scattered throughout the well-nourished population. The elderly poor have multiple difficulties that affect their nutritional status, including no transportation to market, an inability to cook, no facilities for cooking, ill-fitting dentures, mental depression, and crippling diseases of old age.

Infants in poor families are increasingly at risk, nutritionally, because of the trend away from breastfeeding. A study in rural Mississippi discovered that the majority of mothers did not attempt to breastfeed. Of those who did, only 16 percent nursed the baby for longer than six months.[6] The ingestion of the kcalories and high-quality protein of breast milk during the critical first six months of life (when the brain is completing its development) could make a significant difference in the child's mental capacity.[7] The sterility of breast milk and the presence of its antibodies would help

to lower the incidence of infectious diseases among four- to six-month-old infants. The infant formulas so attractively advertised by the food industry cannot be used successfully without an uncontaminated water supply, education in how to prepare the formula, knowledge of the importance of sterile bottles and nipples, and refrigeration of the milk. To the very poor mother who is emulating the wealthier mothers in not using the milk provided by nature, the price of the formula may be such a large outlay that she will cut costs by overdiluting the milk.[8] The trend away from breastfeeding may be having more of an effect on nutritional status among the poor than can be shown in surveys or from income statistics.

Is there hunger in our communities? Yes. Painful as that answer is to face, it is true. There are pockets of hunger, hidden from the mainstream of society. The poor of whatever race, the migrant, the very old, and the very young are in need of nutritional help. The large middle-income group needs to be educated to the fact that the spiral of poverty— lack of education, more children than can be cared for, lack of good nutrition, ill health, poverty—must be broken. If the cycle is not broken for humanitarian reasons, then it must be broken

[4]U.S. Senate, Select Committee on Nutrition and Human Needs, Nutrition and Special Groups, *National Nutrition Policy Study, 1974 (Hearings)* (Washington, D.C.: Government Printing Office, 1974).

[5]*National Nutrition Policy Study,* 1974.

[6]R. E. Brown, Breast feeding in modern times, *American Journal of Clinical Nutrition* 26 (1973):556-562.

[7]M. Winick, P. Rosso, and J. Waterlow, Cellular growth of cerebrum, cerebellum, and brain stem in normal and marasmic children, *Experimental Neurology* 26 (1970):393-400.

[8]Brown, 1973.

because we need these people to contribute as healthy, mentally alert, productive, tax-paying citizens.

To Explore Further

An understanding of the part played by people's cultures and the food they select is prerequisite to improving the nutrition of a group:

Knutson, A. L., and Newton, M. E., Behavioral factors in nutrition education, *Journal of the American Dietetic Association* 37 (1960):222-225.

Wenkaw, N. S., Cultural determinants of nutritional behavior, *Nutrition Program News*, U.S. Department of Agriculture, July/August 1969.

The following articles deal with various aspects of culture and nutrition:

Inano, M., and Pringle, D. J., Dietary survey of low income, rural families of Iowa and North Carolina, III: Contribution of food groups to nutrients, *Journal of the American Dietetic Association* 66 (1975):366-370.

Schaefer, A. E., and Johnson, O. C., Are we well fed? The search for the answer, *Nutrition Today* 4 (1969):2 is based on Schaefer's experience with many surveys, including the Ten-State Survey in the United States.

Tizard, J., Early malnutrition, growth and mental development in man, *British Medical Bulletin* 30 (1974):169-174 combines the behavioral and nutrition sciences to gain an understanding of nutrition's role in human development.

Webb, T. E., and Oski, F. A., Iron deficiency anemia and scholastic achievement in young adolescents, *Journal of Pediatrics* 82 (1973):827-829 points up the dangerous combination of poor nutrition and poor environment.

Robson, J. R. K., Larkin, F. A., Sandretto, A. M., and Tadayyon, B., *Malnutrition: Its Causation and Control*, vol. 2 (New York: Gordon and Broach, 1972) contains an excellent chapter on food habits, taboos, parental attitudes, sociocultural factors, and the role of the educator in effecting change.

In Manocha, S. L., *Malnutrition and Retarded Human Development* (Springfield, Illinois: Charles C. Brown, 1972), several chapters are especially pertinent to the understanding of ways to fight the war against hunger: Chapter 7, "Fight against Prevalent Malnutrition"; Chapter 8, "Clinical Approaches to Fight Malnutrition"; and Chapter 9, "Nutrition Education."

A teaching aid, *Deficiency Disorders: How to Diagnose Nutritional Disorders in Daily Practice* by H. H. Sandstead, J. P. Carter, and W. J. Darby, contains 20 slides that show the clinical signs of nutritional deficiencies. These can be ordered from the Nutrition Today Society (address in Appendix J).

Malnutrition and Hunger in the United States and *Iron Deficiency in the United States* (reprints) can be ordered from the American Medical Association (see Appendix J).

A film, *Hunger in America*, can be ordered from the Audiovisual Center, Indiana University, Bloomington, IN 47401.

CHAPTER 16

CONTENTS

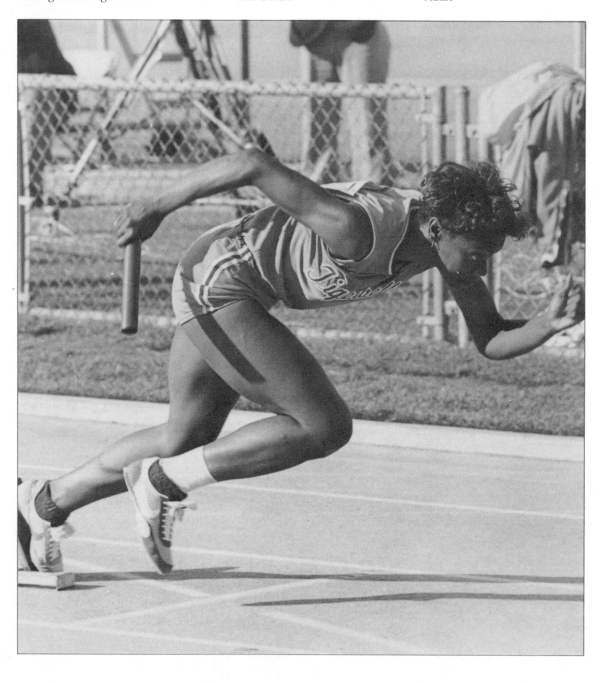

THE YOUNG ADULT

Young people want to develop their bodies, minds, and personalities. Middle aged and elderly people, if they are well, want to stay that way. . . . These objectives can be realized only if nutrition is superior.

ROGER J. WILLIAMS

Teenagers are not fed; they eat. For the first time in their lives, they assume responsibility for their own food intakes. At the same time they are intensely involved in day-to-day life with their peers and in preparation for their future lives as adults. Social pressures thrust choices at them: to drink or not to drink, to smoke or not to smoke, to develop their bodies to meet sometimes extreme ideals of slimness or athletic prowess. Few become interested in foods and nutrition except as part of a cult or fad, such as vegetarianism or crash dieting.

As adult life continues, many of the lifestyle patterns established during the growing years become fixed. Decades later, the cumulative impact of the habits of a lifetime becomes manifest. This chapter emphasizes the special nutritional factors that affect adult life for good or for ill.

The Teen Years: Growth and Nutrient Needs

At 12, Lynn was a stocky, solid, straight-legged child; at 15 she is a tall, curvaceous, glowing woman. Most of the boys in her class are shorter than she is; Mike is just beginning to shoot up but still has a boy's interests and the high-pitched voice of a girl. Just you wait, Lynn. Two years from now Mike will have reached and passed your height and may have become the man of your dreams. Keep your eye on him!

The adolescent growth spurt begins in girls at 10 or 11 and reaches its peak at 12, being completed at about 15. In boys it begins at 12 or 13 and peaks at 14, ending at about 19. In both sexes this intensive growth period brings not only a dramatic increase in height but hormonal changes that profoundly affect every organ of the body (including the brain) and that culminate in the emergence of physically mature adults within two or three years.

The same nutrition principles apply to this period as to the growth periods discussed in Chapter 15. The growth nutrients are needed in increased quantities, and there is an added need for iron, caused by the onset of menstruation in girls and by the great increase in lean body mass in boys. These changes, which are taking place in nearly adult-size people, may increase the total nutrient needs of adolescence more than at any other time in life. A rapidly growing, active boy of 15 may need 4,000 kcal or more a day just to maintain his weight. An inactive girl of the same age, however, whose growth is nearly at a standstill, may need fewer than 2,000 kcal if she is to avoid becoming obese. Thus there is a tremendous variation in the nutrient needs of adolescents.

Teenagers as a group do have nutritional problems, however. Nearly every nutrient can be found lacking in one or another group: iron in the girls, kcalories in young men (especially blacks), vitamin A in girls (especially Mexican- and Spanish-Americans), calcium, riboflavin, vitamin C, even protein. The insidious problem of obesity becomes more apparent, mostly in girls, especially in black girls. Some teenagers, usually girls, diet so violently that they become seriously ill (see p. 300). Serious nutritional deficiencies often arise in pregnant teenage girls.

Teenagers' Eating Patterns

Teenagers come and go as they choose and eat what they want when they have time. With a multitude of after-school, social, and job activities, they almost inevitably fall into irregular eating habits. The adult becomes a gatekeeper, controlling the availability but not the consumption of food in the teenager's environment. The adult can't nag, scold, or pressure teenagers into eating as they should, because they typically turn a deaf ear to coercion and often to persuasion. To "feed" effectively, the gatekeeper must make every effort to allow these young people independence while providing a physical environment that favors healthy development and an emotional climate that encourages adaptive choices.

In the home, a wise maneuver is to provide access to nutritious and economical energy foods that are low in sugar and fat and discouraging to tooth decay. Many parents have discovered independently the wisdom of welcoming their teenage sons and daughters and their friends into the kitchen with an invitation to "Help yourselves! There's plenty of food in the refrigerator" (cooked chicken, raw vegetables, milk, fruit juice) "and more on the table" (fruit, nuts, raisins, popcorn). The snacker—and a well-established characteristic of teenagers is that they are snackers—who finds only nutritious foods around the house is well provided for.

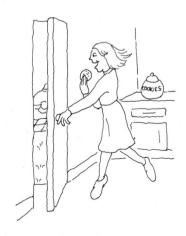

For the nutritive value of selected fast foods, see Appendix N.

Inevitably, teenagers will do a lot of eating away from home—at snack bars, hamburger stands, and corner stores. There, as well as at home, their nutritional welfare can be favored or hindered by the choices they make. A lunch of a hamburger, a chocolate shake, and french fries supplies some nutrients in substantial amounts, at a kcalorie cost of 780 (see Table 1). Except for vitamin A, these are sizable percentages of the recommended intakes at a kcalorie cost many teenagers can afford. Depending on how they adjust their breakfast and dinner choices, teenagers may serve their needs more than adequately with this sort of lunch. At the other meals, they need only obtain fruits and vegetables (for vitamins A and C), a good fiber source, and more good iron sources.

On the average, about a fourth of teenagers' total daily kcalorie intake comes from snacks. Their irregular schedules may worry adults who think they are feeding themselves poorly, but at least one study shows that the kcalories they eat are far from empty. They receive substantial amounts of thiamin, protein, riboflavin, and vitamin C. The nutrients found lacking in this study were calcium and iron and, to some extent, vitamin A.[1] This finding indicates that protein need not be stressed in the nutrition education of teenagers but that some should be encouraged to identify and consume more dairy products, for calcium, and more good vitamin A sources. Wherever vitamin A is lacking, folic acid is too, because both are found in green vegetables; so folic acid should also be stressed.

The teenager's iron needs are a special problem, caused by several factors. Two already mentioned are the burgeoning iron need at this age and the lack of iron in traditional snack foods. Other factors are the overemphasis on dairy products by some teenagers, vegetarianism, and the low contribution made by fast foods to iron intakes. A National Academy of Sciences committee, writing on this special problem, finds it doubtful that long-term administration of iron tablets is practical and advises against the measure of fortifying snacks and other foods with iron. Instead, the committee recommends that physicians and clinics screen all teenagers for low levels of iron in the blood. Their report stresses that fact that "the best dietary source of absorbable iron is meats of all varieties," a point that should in turn be stressed in the nutritional education of teenagers.[2] A later section of this chapter addresses the problem of teaching teens about nutrition.

Table 1 Nutrients in a Hamburger, Chocolate Shake, and Fries

Nutrient	Percentage of need*
Protein	42
Calcium	47
Iron	21
Vitamin A	3
Thiamin	25
Riboflavin	57
Vitamin C	21

*Calculated from the RDA for a teenage male.

The Pregnant Teenage Girl

A special case of nutritional need is that of the pregnant teenage girl. Even if she were not pregnant, she would be hard put to meet her own nutrient needs at this time of maximal growth. Nourishing the baby doubles her burden. Figure 1 shows that her needs for many nutrients double, although her kcalorie allowance increases by only a few

[1]J. A. Thomas and D. L. Call, Eating between meals: A nutrition problem among teenagers? *Nutrition Reviews* 31 (May 1973):137-139.

[2]Committee on Nutrition of the Mother and Preschool Child, Food and Nutrition Board, National Academy of Sciences, *Iron Nutriture in Adolescence*, DHEW publication no. (HSA) 77-5100 (Washington, D.C.: Government Printing Office, 1977).

Figure 1 Comparison of the nutrient needs of a 10-year-old girl with those of a pregnant 15-year-old girl. These values were calculated by adding the difference between the RDAs for a 10-year-old and a 14-year-old to the difference between the RDAs for a 14-year-old and a pregnant woman (see inside front cover).

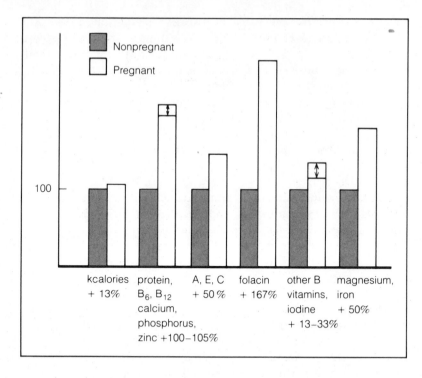

percent. In the case of a girl who begins pregnancy with inadequate nutrient stores or who lacks the education, resources, and support she needs in order to provide for herself, these problems are compounded.

The complications of pregnancy were briefly discussed in Chapter 15, where it was made obvious that the consequences of poor nutrition are acute and long-lasting. Sickness is common in pregnant teenagers, with toxemia occurring in about one out of every five girls under the age of 15. If one pregnancy is followed by another, "the conditions are established for a rapid and irreversible slide from simple toxemia to renal damage and hypertensive disease."[3]

Toxemia: see p. 537.

Teenage pregnancy is more common now than it was earlier. About one out of every five babies is born to a mother under 19 years of age, and more than a tenth of these mothers are 15 or younger. The importance of preparing young girls for future pregnancy needs emphasis in public schools and public health programs. Faced with her parents' and classmates' often insensitive reactions, a pregnant girl is likely to wind up alone, with little or no money to buy food and no motivation to seek prenatal care. Programs addressed to all her problems are urgently needed, including medical attention, nutritional guidance, emotional support, and continued schooling.[4] A model

[3]B. S. Worthington, Nutritional needs of the pregnant adolescent, in *Nutrition in Pregnancy and Lactation*, ed. B. S. Worthington, J. Vermeersch, and S. R. Williams (St. Louis: Mosby, 1977), pp. 119-132.

[4]B. Lucas, Nutrition and the adolescent, in *Nutrition in Infancy and Childhood*, ed. P. L. Pipes (St. Louis: Mosby, 1977), pp. 132-144.

program for giving nutritional help to teenage mothers, among others, is the WIC (Women's, Infants' and Children's) Program, which gives low-income pregnant girls coupons with which to buy foods. The coupons can be redeemed only for foods selected especially for their nutritional value.

Complicating Factors: Alcohol and Others

In the midteens comes a choice point: whether to drink alcohol or to abstain. A 1975 study showed that more than half of all seventh graders nationwide had tried alcohol at least once within the previous year; nine-tenths of all high school seniors had had experience with alcohol.[5]

The year between the ages of 13 and 14 seems to mark the decision point for most white teenagers; and the year between 15 and 16 is critical for blacks. Another transitional stage occurs between the ages of 17 and 18, when infrequent drinkers apparently make a decision either to abstain or to drink more heavily. The highest population of heavy drinkers by ethnic group is found in American Indian youth (16.5 percent), followed by Orientals (13.5) and Spanish (10.9). For white Americans, the proportion is 10.7 percent, and for black Americans 5.7 percent. Those receiving high grades in school are less likely to become alcohol drinkers; the heavy drinkers characteristically spend more time with peers who also drink.[6]

By the time students get to college, alcohol abuse is common and considered part of normal college life. About 90 percent of all college students use alcohol, and heavy drinking is common, with a third or more of all students getting drunk more than once a month.[7] Only a few college students are alcoholics, but 5 to 10 percent will experience serious complications as a result of drinking, and 1 in 12 will go on to become an adult problem drinker or an alcoholic.[8] This represents about 3 or 4 out of a college class of 50 people.

Alcohol is by far the most widely used drug in the United States. About 100 million adults drink, and 9 million are estimated to be alcoholics. Because alcohol drinking is more socially acceptable than taking other drugs, alcohol abuse is our most common form of drug abuse.

[5]Young people and alcohol, *Alcohol Health and Research World,* Summer 1975, DHEW publication no. (ADM) 75-157 (Washington, D.C.: Government Printing Office, 1975), pp. 2-10.

[6]Drinking motivations: Habits of youth illuminated by national survey results, *NIAAA Information and Feature Service* 18 (26 November 1975), DHEW publication no. (ADM) 75-151 (Washington, D.C.: Government Printing Office, 1975).

[7]D. P. Kraft, College students and alcohol: The 50 + 12 project, *Alcohol Health and Research World,* Summer 1976, DHEW publication no. (ADM) 76-157 (Washington, D.C.: Government Printing Office, 1976), pp. 10-14.

[8]G. Globetti, as quoted in Young people and alcohol, Summer 1975.

addiction: a state of physiological dependence on a drug; withdrawal of the drug causes toxic symptoms that can only be relieved by administering the drug. We choose to call alcoholics *alcohol addicts*, because their need for alcohol is a true addiction and because the term is less of a stigma than the term *alcoholic*.

The nutritional implications of alcohol use and the consequences of its abuse were described in Highlight 9. To sum them all up in a single sentence, alcohol must be used with moderation, because it is an empty-kcalorie beverage and can displace needed nutrients from the diet while simultaneously increasing the demand for them. Those who are unable to use it with moderation must abstain completely from its use if they are to maintain good health.

Much remains to be learned about people's use of alcohol, especially why some people become uncontrolled drinkers (alcohol addicts) whereas others can drink frequently or even daily with moderation. But much is already known and is worth passing on. The student of nutrition is entitled to know the important new findings about this disease which so complicates the nutrition picture.

What we know suggests that there should be no stigma attached to alcoholism. There is a great need for the public to realize that being an alcoholic is not a sign of inferiority or something to be ashamed of. It does not reflect failure as a person or moral degeneracy. Like diabetes, alcoholism is now recognized as a disease—a definite process having a characteristic train of symptoms. Although the causes are not yet known, the symptoms have been extensively studied, and the criteria for diagnosis have been completely defined. To identify the person with this disease more accurately, we will use the term *alcohol addict* in the rest of this discussion.

Being an alcohol addict, like being a diabetic, is probably determined at least to some extent by a person's genes, which give him a predisposition toward alcohol addiction. People who have every reason to be proud of themselves, their potential, and their achievements may be alcohol addicts. The typical addict is not a Skid Row bum. He or she is just as likely to be a doctor, a nurse, a Hollywood star, or a prestigious local businessperson. In fact, there is no such thing as "the typical alcoholic."

The only statement that can be made with certainty about the addict is that she has lost control over alcohol. Intending to drink moderately and responsibly, she repeatedly overconsumes alcohol to the point where it damages her family relationships, her job, her social functioning, and her self-esteem. Broken resolutions are a hallmark of the addict. Such a person cannot drink at all: The first drink too often becomes the first of too many.

Many myths and misconceptions surround the public's picture of the disease alcoholism. Four of the most common wrong ideas are:

- A person who gets drunk has the disease. This is not true. Anyone who loses control over his reactions and behavior while drinking alcohol is drunk. This is a temporary state. But an alcohol addict is a person who must have alcohol in order to function or who, in giving it up, suffers severe withdrawal reactions.

- An alcohol addict is a drunk. This is also not true. An addict may appear to be functioning normally while drinking large quantities of alcohol. His problem is likely to become apparent when he is not drinking, and feeling the craving that indicates withdrawal, rather than when he is drinking.

- A person who never passes out is not an addict. This too is not true. Passing out is the result when the anesthetic effect of alcohol has reached the part of the brain that controls wakefulness. An alcohol addict may drink to this end point no more often than a non-addict. What the addict experiences at a certain stage in her progress toward serious addiction is the blackout. This is temporary loss of memory, not loss of consciousness. No one notices that anything is wrong while the person is drinking—she behaves normally—but the next day she can't remember what she was doing beyond a certain point the day before. Blackouts are one of the distinguishing characteristics of alcohol addiction.

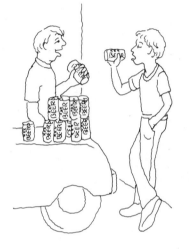

- A beer drinker can never become an addict. Because beer contains alcohol, it is just as capable of contributing to alcoholism as is wine or "hard" liquor (whiskey, gin, vodka, and the like). It is not the beverage but the constitution of the consumer that determines whether a person will become addicted to alcohol.

Some beer drinkers protest that beer has some redeeming features. It makes people drunk less quickly, and it provides valuable nutrients. True, because the alcohol in beer is diluted, it will reach the bloodstream more slowly than the same amount of alcohol taken straight. But the carbonation in beer stimulates the stomach, hastening the entry of the alcohol into the intestine, where it will immediately be absorbed. As for the nutrient content of beer, an adult male would have to drink at least a six-pack of 12-oz cans to meet his niacin needs and nine six-packs to meet his protein needs.

Some people choose to abstain from alcohol consumption because they are alcohol addicts; others make the same choice for other reasons. Such people have a hard time in some social settings, because drinking is often not only accepted but even almost demanded of all comers. It is to be hoped that this discussion will have shown why it is desirable not to pressure other persons to drink. Considerate hosts or social groups will welcome the nondrinker and provide nonalcoholic beverages for his enjoyment just as they would provide nonmeat food for a guest who is a vegetarian.

Prescription Drugs   The dictionary defines a drug as any chemical compound given to humans to help with the diagnosis or treatment of a disease or the relief from its symptoms. It is thus different in important ways from a nutrient, which only functions to prevent disease caused by a deficiency of that nutrient. Drugs are not natural compounds found in the body when it is functioning normally, and no drug has been shown to be completely without ill effects.

Many drugs affect the body's need for and use of nutrients. Alcohol is a prime example of these effects. Prescription medications, like alcohol, can affect nutritional status by:

- Increasing or decreasing appetite
- Causing nausea, vomiting, or an altered sense of taste
- Inhibiting the synthesis of nutrients
- Reducing the absorption or increasing the excretion of nutrients
- Altering the transport, use, or storage of nutrients

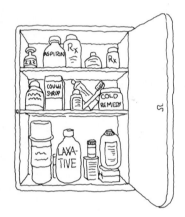

Foods and nutrients can also affect the drugs in the body. For example, some foods interfere with the absorption of medications taken with them, so the medications should be taken between meals. In other cases, the presence of food in the intestine prevents the nausea that might otherwise be caused by the drug; such a drug should be taken with meals. The doctor doesn't always tell you, but your pharmacist will probably be glad to inform you which is which.

Prolonged use of almost any prescription medication can result in gradual nutrient depletion. Aspirin can irritate the intestine and cause bleeding, vitamin C deficiency, and anemia. Antibiotics inhibit iron absorption. Antacids can cause increased excretion of calcium, leading to adult bone loss. Mineral oil depletes fat-soluble vitamins and can cause rickets in children; other laxatives cause multiple nutrient deficiencies. Many other such effects are known.[9]

The special case of the woman taking oral contraceptives deserves a moment's attention. The Pill alters blood levels of several nutrients, raising some (vitamin A and iron) and lowering others (B vitamins and vitamin C). Women often wonder what vitamin supplements, if any, they should take while on the Pill. The answer in general seems to be: "None. You are risking a nutritional deficiency only if your diet is grossly inadequate, especially in folic acid. And if it is, you need diet counseling more than you need a vitamin pill."[10] However, a problem sometimes seen in oral contraceptive users is an alteration in the metabolism of the amino acid tryptophan which can be corrected by moderate vitamin B_6 supplementation; researchers think this effect may be linked to depression. A 1979 review of the findings to date concluded cautiously that oral contraceptive users should take vitamin B_6 supplements to bring their vitamin B_6 intake up to 5 mg/day (the RDA is 2 mg/day).[11]

---

[9]A. K. Sim, Ascorbic acid: A survey, past and present, *Chemistry and Industry* (19 February 1972), pp. 160-165; N. J. Greenberger, Effects of antibiotics and other agents on the intestinal absorption of iron, *American Journal of Clinical Nutrition* 26 (1973):104-112; H. Spencer, C. Norris, F. Coffey, and E. Wiatrowski, *Gastroenterology* 68 (1975):990, abstract cited in Diet-drug interactions (reviewed by D. A. Roe), *Dairy Council Digest* 48 (March/April 1977); D. A. Roe, Drugs, diet and nutrition, *Contemporary Nutrition* 3 (June 1978); and J. A. Visconti, ed., Drug-food interaction, in *Nutrition in Disease* (Ross Laboratories, May 1977).

[10]Roe, 1978.

[11]The vitamin B_6 requirement in oral contraceptive users, *Nutrition Reviews* 37 (1979):344-345.

On the other hand, the person who has taken prescription medications for a long time may well have developed nutrient deficiencies. This is most likely in older people who are taking a combination of medications or who abuse laxatives, in long-time alcohol users, and in children during the period of active growth.

In addition, many drugs (medications) interact with one another, further complicating the picture. A prime example is the interaction of alcohol with other "downer" drugs, such as barbiturates and tranquilizers. The body adapts at first to prolonged alcohol consumption by increasing the rate at which it breaks down alcohol. This adaptation involves increasing the amount of liver machinery (enzymes) maintained for alcohol metabolism. Many drugs are processed by that same machinery, so that a dose of these drugs given to an alcohol user may be ineffective; the liver may break it down before it has a chance to reach effective levels in the body. On the other hand, if the user takes alcohol with the drug, he may swamp his liver metabolizing system, so that it can't handle the drug at all, and the drug may reach unexpectedly high, even toxic, levels in the body. The physician prescribing medications that interact with the body's alcohol system should be fully informed about the patient's use of alcohol.

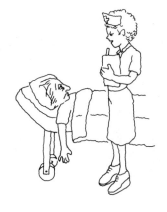

Hundreds of millions of prescriptions are written for mind-altering drugs each year, and billions for other drugs. To protect against the risks of nutrient-drug and drug-drug interactions, one writer on the subject urges:

- Avoidance of unnecessary prescriptions
- Limitation of multiple-drug regimens
- Support for control of over-the-counter drug sales
- Education of medical and other health personnel, as well as patients, regarding the nutritional effects of drugs.[12]

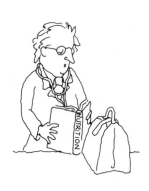

"The physician" has been mentioned several times in this chapter, sometimes with the implication that she is not always aware of the contributions nutrition makes to health and disease. Whenever we have spoken of a medical problem, such as diagnosis and treatment of abnormal conditions, we hae urged you to ask your doctor. However, when we have dealt with nutrition-related problems, we have sometimes intentionally suggested that the doctor may not be the most reliable authority. Medical schools often neglect nutrition in their course offerings, and many doctors know as little as or less than the average layperson when it comes to the nutrients, the nature of foods, and the adequacy of diets.

[12] D. A. Roe, *Drug-Induced Nutritional Deficiencies* (Westport: Avi Publishing, 1976), as cited in Diet-drug interactions (reviewed by D. A. Roe), 1977.

We have also tried to convey the notion that, like automobile mechanics, doctors come in all varieties: competent and incompetent, honest and dishonest. In choosing a doctor to consult, you might well want to investigate the reputation, training, and experience of several in relation to the particular problem you have in mind. The questions of how much doctors know about nutrition and what should perhaps be done to alter their training are important ones in this society, which spends billions of dollars each year on medical care. Highlight 16 addresses these questions.

marihuana: alternative spelling
marijuana

Marihuana   Like alcohol, marihuana has characteristic effects on the body, and like alcohol, it has not been shown to have many pronounced harmful effects even with long-term use, unless the use is heavy (daily for extended periods). The active ingredients are rapidly and completely (90 percent) absorbed from the lungs.[13] Then, being fat-soluble, they are packaged in protein (possibly in lipoproteins[14]) before being transported by the blood to the various body tissues. They are processed by many tissues (not just by the liver), and they persist for several days in body fat, being excreted over a period of a week or more after the smoking of a single cigarette.[15]

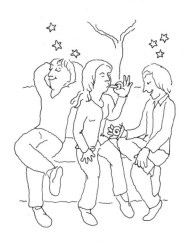

Smoking a marihuana cigarette has characteristic effects on hearing, touch, taste, and smell and on perceptions of time, space, and the body; it also produces changes in mental sensations and alterations in the nature of sleep. Among the taste changes apparently induced is a great enjoyment of eating, especially of sweets, but it is not known how this effect occurs.[16] The drug apparently does not change the blood glucose level.[17] Investigators speculate that the so-called hunger induced by marihuana is actually a social effect caused by the suggestibility of the group in which it is smoked.[18] Prolonged use of the drug does not seem to bring about a weight gain; one small sample of regular users (30 smokers) has been observed to weigh less than comparable nonsmokers by about seven pounds.[19]

[13]L. J. King, J. D. Teale, and V. Marks, Biochemical aspects of cannabis, in *Cannabis and Health*, ed. J. D. Graham (New York: Academic Press, 1976).

[14]L. E. Hollister, Marihuana in man: Three years later, *Science* 172 (1971):21-29.

[15]King, Teale, and Marks, 1976; and Hollister, Marihuana, 1971.

[16]E. L. Abel, Effects of marihuana on the solution of anagrams, memory and appetite, *Nature* 231 (1971):260-261; and C. T. Tart, Marijuana intoxication: Common experiences, *Nature* 226 (1970):701-704.

[17]L. E. Hollister, Hunger and appetite after single doses of marihuana, alcohol, and dextroamphetamine, *Clinical Pharmacology and Therapeutics* 12 (1971):44-49; and J. D. P. Graham and D. M. F. Li, The pharmacology of cannabis and cannabinoids, in *Cannabis and Health*, 1976.

[18]Hollister, Hunger and appetite, 1971.

[19]Marijuana: Truth on health problems, *Science News* 107/108 (22 February 1975):117.

Many young people in the United States are turning to marihuana as an alternative to alcohol. The number of individuals using it at least once a day had grown from half a million in 1971 to over 3 million by 1980.[20] There is much disagreement about the desirability of this trend. Despite much current research, little is known about the possible risks of regular smoking.

It has become clear, however, that even in "socially acceptable" concentrations, the drug brings about a deterioration in some aspects of driving performance. Another effect widely agreed on is that it causes alterations in heart action, including rapid and sometimes irregular heartbeat.[21] It also reduces the body's immune response and, in young men, reduces the sex hormone level and sperm count after a lag period of about six weeks. Reporting on this effect, an investigator points out that marihuana "is much like other drugs, such as tobacco and liquor, in that the greatest potential hazard exists for those who abuse it. . . . There is still no convincing evidence that casual, infrequent use of marihuana produces any ill effects."[22]

The potency of marihuana preparations reaching the United States has been increasing. Before 1970, most marihuana used was a very weak domestic variety with an average THC content of about 0.2 percent. During the 1970s, users shifted to a Mexican variety (about 1.5 percent), then to Jamaican and Colombian marihuana (3 to 4 percent). The present trend is toward even higher concentrations. Users looking for a greater "high" then sometimes shift to hashish oil, a much more concentrated form of the active drug (about 40 to 50 percent THC and up to 90 percent), at which point the risks probably increase dramatically.[23]

THC, or **tetrahydrocannabinol** (tet-ra-high-dro-can-NAB-in-ol): the primary active ingredient of marihuana.

Most investigators agree that with moderate use the hazards of marihuana smoking are few and small. However, it should be remembered that because possession and use of the drug is not legal, no controls are exerted by any agency, such as the FDA, on the content of preparations sold as marihuana. There is a significant hazard associated with the possibility that they may be contaminated with pesticides or that they may contain "hard" (addictive) drugs such as heroin, concealed in them by the pusher in order to create a demand for a product he can sell for greater profits. Also, when marihuana use escalates into the use of "hard" drugs, the nutrition and health effects become pronounced, as the next section illustrates.

"Hard" Drugs and Drug Abuse The term *drug* has a second meaning, as familiar to most people as the first: a narcotic, especially

[20]T. H. Maugh II, Marihuana: New support for immune and reproductive hazards, *Science* 190 (1975):865-867.

[21]Graham and Li, 1976; and Pot update: Possible motor effects, *Science News* 113 (4 February 1978):71.

[22]Maugh, 1975. Infrequent use might be defined as three cigarettes a week or less.

[23]Maugh, 1975.

one that is addictive. Among the hard drugs in most common use today are heroin, morphine, LSD, PCP, and cocaine. Users of these drugs face multiple problems, not the least of which are nutritional. Their nutrition suffers severely for a multitude of reasons:

● They spend their money for drugs rather than for food.

● They lose interest in food during "high" periods on drugs.

● Some drugs (for example, amphetamines) induce at least a temporary depression of appetite.

● Their lifestyle lacks the regularity and routine that would promote good eating habits.

hepatitis (hep-uh-TIGHT-us): a severe viral liver disease transmitted from person to person either through contaminated water or (as in the case of drug addicts) by way of contaminated needles.

● They often have hepatitis which causes taste changes and loss of appetite.

● They often depend on alcohol, especially when withdrawing from drug use.

● They often become ill with infectious diseases that increase their need for nutrients.

During their withdrawal from drugs, one of the most important aspects of treatment is to identify and correct these nutritional problems while teaching and supporting adaptive eating habits.[24]

Caffeine   Like alcohol use, the use of caffeine-containing beverages becomes common during the teens. Coffee, tea, and especially cola beverages become permitted drinks.

Caffeine is less likely to be dangerously abused than alcohol, perhaps because its use neither dulls the senses nor impairs judgment. Caffeine is a true stimulant drug, increasing the respiration rate, heart rate, blood pressure, and secretion of the stress and other hormones.[25] Its "wake-up" effect is maximal within an hour after the dose. In moderate amounts (50 to 200 mg a day), caffeine seems to be a relatively harmless drug. See Table 2 for amounts of caffeine in familiar beverages and medicines.

Every human society has made a caffeine-containing food or beverage a staple in its diet: the habitual tea of the English and many other cultures; the coffee of Arabia, Indonesia, Brazil, and others; cola beverages in many South American countries; and many exotic-sounding drinks, chewing gums, and foods elsewhere. The universal human use of caffeine shows that at least as subjectively perceived, it does something for the user.

Table 2   Caffeine Sources[26]

Source	Caffeine (mg)
Brewed coffee (1 c)	85
Instant coffee (1 c)	60
Brewed black tea (1 c)	50
Brewed green tea (1 c)	30
Instant tea (1 c)	30
Decaffeinated coffee (1 c)	3
Cola beverage (12 oz)	32-65
Aspirin compound (pill containing aspirin, phenacetin, and caffeine)	32
Cope, Midol, etc.	32
Excedrin, Anacin (tablet)	60
Pre-Mens	66
Many cold preparations	30
Many stimulants	100
Cocoa (1 c)	6-42
No Doz (tablet) or Vivarin	100-200

[24]R. T. Frankle and G. Christakis, eds., Some nutritional aspects of "hard" drug addiction, *Dietetic Currents, Ross Timesaver* 2 (July/August 1975).

[25]D. Robertson, J. C. Frölich, R. K. Carr, J. T. Watson, J. W. Hollifield, D. G. Shand, and J. A. Oates, Effects of caffeine on plasma renin activity, catecholamines, and blood pressure, *New England Journal of Medicine* 298 (1978):181-186.

[26]"Food allergy," *Nutrition and the MD*, July 1978; and P. E. Stephenson, Physiologic and psychotropic effects of caffeine on man, *Journal of the American Dietetic Association* 71 (1977):240-247.

Caffeine is not addictive, but it is habit forming, and the body adapts to its use to some extent. A dose greater than what the body has adapted to causes jitteriness, nervousness, and intestinal discomfort. Sudden abstinence from the drug after long (even moderate) use causes a characteristic withdrawal reaction; the most frequently observed symptom is a headache. If a person has adapted to a much higher dose level than 50 to 200 mg caffeine, then dropping back to this level may cause the same withdrawal reaction.

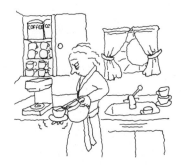

An overdose of caffeine produces reactions in the body that are indistinguishable from those of an anxiety attack.[27] People who drink between 8 and 15 cups of coffee a day, for example, have been known to seek help from doctors for complaints such as "dizziness, agitation, restlessness, recurring headaches, and sleep difficulties." Before prescribing a tranquilizer, the doctor would do well to inquire about the caffeine consumption of such patients.

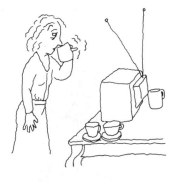

A large dose of caffeine can also cause extra heartbeats and is believed to have caused heart attacks in people whose hearts were already damaged by degenerative disease. However, neither caffeine nor its vehicle, coffee, can be considered a risk factor for the development of atherosclerosis. Neither the Framingham Study (see p. 212) nor a study of 7,705 Japanese showed any correlation between coffee drinking and heart attack risk.[28]

Of all people who drink coffee, the pregnant woman is most strongly advised to curtail her consumption (see p. 536). Another type of person who should perhaps be warned against caffeine, and coffee in particular, is the ulcer patient. It has been shown that even decaffeinated coffee stimulates the secretion of stomach acid. There must be compounds in coffee besides caffeine that aggravate ulcers.

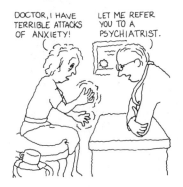

Caffeine tolerance decreases with age. As you grow older, you are advised to reduce your caffeine intake gradually. The morning cup of coffee is all right as a "pick-me-up," but the afternoon or evening cup may seriously interfere with your ability to sleep at night. People vary greatly in their responses to caffeine, however; if you think your consumption of caffeine may be causing insomnia, try cutting it down (especially in the afternoon) and see if you sleep better. If you do, better keep it down.

Nutrition for Athletes

A question often asked by young people interested in nutrition is whether there is any special diet that will enhance their athletic performance. In particular, they want to know whether athletes need diets higher in protein than nonathletes.

[27]"Food allergy," 1978.

[28]Coffee: Downs and ups, *Nutrition and the MD,* April 1978; and K. Yano, G. G. Rhoads, and A. Kagan, Coffee, alcohol, and risk of coronary heart disease in Japanese-Americans, *New England Journal of Medicine* 297 (1977):405-409.

Actually, it has been known since 1904 that protein is not the fuel of muscular work. People engaged in hard physical labor excrete only slightly more nitrogen than others do. They are able to perform just as well for weeks or months on 50 g of protein a day as on 75, 100, or 150. (Two quarter-pound hamburgers can supply 50 g of protein in a single meal.) No athlete is likely to consume a diet that is marginal or deficient in protein, and no evidence exists, despite many experiments, that added protein confers any advantage to the athlete in terms of strength, endurance, or speed.[29]

On the other hand, an athlete does need more fuel during training and athletic events than he does when he's sitting around. Protein can be used for fuel, of course, but this is an expensive and unnecessary use of protein. A mixture of carbohydrate and fat kcalories serves the same function more efficiently. Short-duration, high-intensity activities, such as the 440-yard run or the 100-yard swim, depend primarily on carbohydrate for fuel, specifically as glucose from glycogen stored in the muscles themselves. Long-duration, endurance activities, such as marathon races, also depend on muscle glycogen, and low-carbohydrate, high-fat diets have been found to hamper seriously the athlete's ability to perform in these events.[30]

Muscle glycogen: see Chapter 1.

A special advantage is conferred on long-distance runners by glycogen loading, a technique based on manipulation of dietary carbohydrate. First the athlete reduces carbohydrate intake for several days and exercises heavily to deplete muscle glycogen stores. Then abruptly she begins consuming a lot of carbohydrates. Muscle glycogen stores rebound to about twice the normal level, thus providing fuel that will last longer in an endurance event. This practice is now widespread; the hazards, if any, are unknown.[31]

glycogen loading: a technique of increasing muscle glycogen stores, used by athletes before athletic events. The athlete eats a low-carbohydrate diet, exercises to exhaustion, then eats a high-carbohydrate diet.

Whenever energy intake and expenditure are high, added B vitamins are needed. Provided that the added energy is from nutritious food, it will supply added B vitamins as well. Thus the need will be met automatically, without supplements.

Diet for Gaining Weight In preparation for the football season, an athlete may want to gain muscle mass and body weight. Some people believe that he should eat more protein (to gain muscle mass) rather than fat or carbohydrate (which would increase his fat stores). But adding protein to the diet turns out not to favor muscle growth. Muscles become larger in response to only one stimulus: muscle

---

[29]M. E. Shils, Food and nutrition relating to work and environmental stress, in *Modern Nutrition in Health and Disease*, 5th ed., ed. R. S. Goodhart and M. E. Shils (Philadelphia: Lea and Febiger, 1973), pp. 711-729; O. Mickelson, Nutrition and athletics, *Food and Nutrition News* 41 (April 1970), reprinted in *The Nutrition Crisis: A Reader*, ed. T. P. LaBuza (St. Paul: West, 1975), pp. 228-231; and M. H. Williams, *Nutritional Aspects of Human Physical and Athletic Performance* (Springfield, Ill.: Charles C Thomas, 1976).

[30]F. I. Katch and W. D. McArtle, *Nutrition, Weight Control, and Exercise* (Boston: Houghton Mifflin, 1977), p. 65.

[31]P. Slovic, What helps the long distance runner run? *Nutrition Today* 10 (3) (1975):18-21.

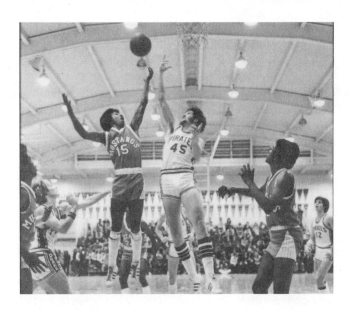

work.[32] Of course, the diet must be adequate in protein (and in all other nutrients), but to gain a pound of muscle mass an athlete must train—that is, exercise intensively. To gain a pound of muscle tissue, an additional 2,500 kcal are needed,[33] from a balanced assortment of foods. kCalories in excess of those needed to keep pace with the muscle growth induced by exercise will add only body fat—even if they come from protein. The weight gain therefore has to be gradual, and the increased food intake must be kept in line with the increased workload.

An athlete who wants to gain weight in a hurry and who doesn't care whether it is muscle or fat can add kcalories of any kind. Because fat in foods is more kcalorie-dense than protein or carbohydrate, he can most easily gain weight by eating a high-fat diet. This technique, "the most widespread nutrition-related abuse in American sports,"[34] also increases the risk of heart disease, to which athletes are not immune.

Lower kCalories for Weight Loss   After football season, the athlete may want to reduce his body weight for wrestling. Weight loss, too, can only take place at a limited rate. To achieve ideal body composition, "the maximum ratio of muscle strength to body weight," the athlete needs to reduce only body fat, and this cannot be done at a rate faster than about two pounds a week. Hurry-up techniques—such as sauna baths, exercising in a plastic suit, use of diuretics or cathartics, or

[32]G. Mann, Nutrition for athletes (a letter to the editor), *Journal of the American Medical Association* 237 (1977):1076-1077; and N. J. Smith, Gaining and losing weight in athletics, *Journal of the American Medical Association* 237 (1976):149-151.

[33]Smith, 1976.

[34]Smith, 1976.

induced vomiting—achieve faster weight loss only by dehydration. (The hazards of fasting and fad diets are discussed in Chapter 7 and Highlight 8.)

Hormones for Adding Muscle   Another technique used to increase muscle mass is to take hormone preparations designed to duplicate the hormones of puberty, which favor muscle development in growing boys. The evidence on their effectiveness has been reviewed, and the consensus seems to be that they are ineffective when used alone. They may seem to enhance muscle development when used in conjunction with hard physical conditioning and increased food intake, but the effects seen under these conditions are more probably due to the increased exercise and food.[35]

These hormones are the **anabolic** (ann-uh-BAHL-ic) **steroids**.

ana = up
ballein = to change

Hormones have profound and far-reaching effects on many target tissues, and these are no exceptions. Hazards associated with their use include disturbed spermatogenesis and testicular degeneration in older athletes. Younger athletes may stop growing early, because the bones of the lower back fuse to terminate growth in response to the hormones of puberty.[36]

spermatogenesis: the making of sperm.

testicular: of the testicles.

degeneration: atrophy, wasting away.

Protein for Hard Work at High Temperatures   Although athletes need no added protein, either as fuel or to support muscle growth, there is one situation in which added protein may be needed. Both protein and kcalorie needs increase tremendously when heavy exercise is performed at very high temperatures and sweat losses are extremely high. Such stresses are not experienced by athletes under most conditions.[37]

Salts and Water for Fluid Losses   One nutritional measure on which all experts agree is maintenance of the water balance during an athletic event. The main symptom of dehydration is fatigue, which impairs an athlete's performance. Sir Edmund Hilary is said to attribute his success in the conquest of Mount Everest to the fact that he and his team took along enough fuel to melt about 3 qt of water a day for each person during the final stages of the ascent.[38] A rapid water loss equal to 5 percent of the body weight can reduce muscular work capacity by 20 to 30 percent.[39]

If you lose more than about 4 qt of water in sweat, you need to replenish your body's sodium as well as its water. For guidelines, see Chapter 14.

The Pregame Meal   There seems to be no special food that should be eaten before an athletic contest. A meal of steak may boost morale, but

[35]Smith, 1976; and D. R. Lamb, Androgens and exercise, *Medicine and Science in Sports* 7 (1975):1-5.

[36]Smith, 1976.

[37]D. M. Watkin, J. B. Das, and M. C. McCarthy, Protein for strenuous physical work (abstract) *Federation Proceedings* 23 (1964):399; and Mickelson, 1970.

[38]Mickelson, 1970.

[39]J. Bergstrom and E. Hultman, Nutrition for maximal sports performance, *Journal of the American Medical Association* 221 (1972):999-1006.

a meal so high in fat may also stay on the stomach long enough to hinder the athlete's performance. Olympic training tables abound with carbohydrate foods such as fruit. To avert pregame excitement and nausea, some athletes find they tolerate a liquid pregame meal best. Whatever is chosen is probably fine, as long as the total diet balances well.

In the final analysis, many athletes agree that what really wins athletic contests is the feeling of being "up for it" and the "will to win." Contestants will go through extraordinary rituals to get into the winning frame of mind. If among these rituals is the taking of some unusual mixture of foods or nutrients, and if they do no physical harm, perhaps there is nothing to be said against them. On the basis of the evidence, however, there seems to be no physical advantage in most of these practices. The conclusion shared by most authorities is clearly expressed by O. Mickelson: "A nutritious, normal diet should be adequate for extremely active athletes. The increased caloric intake of such individuals is likely to insure an adequate supply of all essential nutrients. The primary concern of athletes should be their water intake."[41]

Some foods and supplements are wrongly believed by athletes to be **ergogenic** (energy-enhancing):

> wheat germ
> wheat germ oil
> vitamin E
> vitamin C
> lecithin
> honey
> gelatin
> phosphates
> sunflower seeds
> bee pollen
> kelp
> brewers yeast

Actually, no food or supplement is ergogenic.[40]

The Self-Determining Young Adult

Adolescence is well known as a time of rebellion. This rebellion extends to foods as well as to all other aspects of lifestyle. The choice of what to eat is up to teenagers themselves. Access points already mentioned include the refrigerator, the school lunchroom, and vending machines, but other than controlling the contents of these, adults can hope to have little impact on the nutrient intakes of adolescents—especially by such conventional means as education. Still, most young adults are well fed, for reasons perceptively stated by R. M. Leverton: They get hungry; they like to eat; they want energy, vigor, and the means to compete and excel in whatever they do; and they have many good habits, which are just as hard to break as the bad ones.[42]

Nutrition educators who wish to reach the teenager and young adult with nutrition information must find out and pay attention to two factors: why they sometimes are poorly nourished or develop poor food habits and what means of communicating turns them on.

The young person with a negative attitude toward food and poor food habits is likely to have at least one of the following characteristics:

[40]American Dietetic Association, Nutrition and physical fitness (a statement), *Journal of the American Dietetic Association* 76 (1980):437-443.

[41]Mickelson, 1970.

[42]R. M. Leverton, The paradox of teen-age nutrition, *Journal of the American Dietetic Association* 53 (1968):13-16.

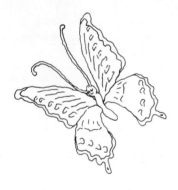

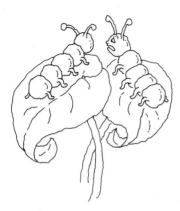

"You'll never get me up in one of those things."

- He thinks nutrition means eating what you don't like because it's good for you.
- He has been criticized for his eating pattern but feels fine and sees no ill effects.
- He is uninterested in food, and it plays a negligible role in his very busy life.
- The people he is most likely to listen to are not knowledgeable about nutrition.[43]

Let's suppose for a moment that you are the parent or teacher of a teenager, concerned about his food habits. What can you do to promote accurate nutritional knowledge and adaptive eating behavior? How can you avoid provoking a negative reaction against the very standards you feel are most important to convey?

First of all, be aware of what teenagers feel about themselves (some reflection into your own past may recall painful memories in this regard). They crave acceptance, especially from their peers. They need to fit in. In many cases they are greatly dissatisfied with themselves as they are. One of the most important aspects of their image is the body image. Young men want larger biceps, shoulders, chests, and forearms; young women want smaller hips, thighs, and waists. One study of U.S. teenagers revealed that 59 percent of the young men wanted to gain weight, although only 25 percent actually needed to do so. Similarly, 70 percent of the girls wanted to lose weight, but no more than about 15 percent were obese.[44] Words to the effect that "you look fine as you are" fall on deaf ears. (The same can be said of adults in some cases, up to the age of about 99.) To be effectively conveyed, nutrition information can be sold as part of a package that will bring about these desired changes. Fortunately, it happens to be true that nutrient-dense, low-kcalorie foods favor the development of strong biceps in men and a trim figure in women.

When the young person who is the target of your campaign possesses and cherishes nutrition misinformation, one of the first questions to ask yourself is "whether the practice is beneficial, neutral, or harmful."[45] Opposing a loved ideal is more likely to polarize than to convert the opposition. A practice such as vegetarianism, dieting, or consuming a "muscle-building diet" can be encouraged—with modifications—rather than condemned: "Nancy, that diet looks like a good idea. . . . I wonder if you can make it still better by including some skim milk and cutting down your meat intake a little. . . . Look at the kcalorie difference. . . . Did you know that meat contains no calcium at all? Or vitamin A? And that vitamin A is one of the most important vitamins for the health of your skin?" Or try: "Mike, you look taller and stronger this week than you did last week. You must be doing something right with all those hamburgers. . . . I wonder if your

[43]Leverton, 1968.

[44]Lucas, 1977.

[45]Lucas, 1977.

complexion would be clearer, though, if you ate more fruits and vegetables. Do you know what fiber is believed to do for a man's health?"

One of the most effective ways to teach nutrition is by example. When nutrition teachers are moralists who fail to practice what they preach, their words of wisdom fall on deaf ears. The coach and gym teacher, the friendly young French teacher, the admired city recreation director—those who enthusiastically maintain their own health—can have a great impact on teenagers, who seek to emulate those they admire. Remember, this is the period of identity formation, the time of seeking and imitating models.

When communicating nutrition information, above all be sure that you have it straight. We make fools of ourselves when we (for example) admonish our students to follow restrictive patterns when their own choices are already as good as ours or better. There may be no harm in using candy bars to meet part of the kcalorie allowance of an active young adult. It may not be necessary to drink milk if the calcium, vitamin D, and riboflavin needs are being met by cheese or other food sources. Satisfactory diets can be designed on a great variety of different foundations. It is the nutrient content and balance of foods, not the specific foods consumed, that make the difference between "good" and "bad" diets.

Much of the work of teaching nutrition can be delegated to the teenagers themselves. Those who are interested and motivated can be guided to reliable sources and allowed to indulge their own desire to benefit their friends and classmates. Among the best materials prepared to convey to teenagers the importance of good nutrition are those made by teenagers themselves.

Finally, hard as it is to accept sometimes, remember that teenagers have the right to make their own decisions—even if they are ones you violently disagree with. You can set up the environment so that the foods available are those you favor and you can stand by with reliable nutrition information and advice, but you will have to leave the rest to them. Ultimately they are the ones who make the choices.

Summing Up

The teen years mark the transition from a time when children eat what they are fed to a time when they choose for themselves what to eat. Nutrition education becomes important as a means of encouraging healthy food habits. Teenagers' snacking patterns and lifestyles predispose them to certain nutritional inadequacies, notably a lack of iron, but teenagers vary so widely that generalizations are difficult. Screening for problems would be a way to detect them early.

The pregnant teenage girl, whose nutrient needs are higher than those of any other person, needs medical attention, nutritional guidance, and emotional support; teenage pregnancies now represent about 20 percent of all pregnancies in the United States. The WIC (Women's, Infants' and Children's) Program reaches many of these pregnant girls with nutritional help.

Alcohol use is common among teenagers, and 90 percent of U.S. college students use alcohol. About 1 out of every 12 alcohol users becomes an addict (alcoholic). Alcohol addiction (alcoholism) is now known to be a disease, requiring early diagnosis for the best chance of recovery. About 9 million U.S. adults are alcoholic persons. Alcoholism is not the same as drunkenness. It is distinguished by symptoms characteristic of addiction, including blackouts (temporary losses of memory). Beer, as well as hard liquor, can be abused and lead to alcoholism.

Prolonged use of prescription drugs in the young adult and adult may affect appetite, nutrient synthesis, and other aspects of the body's handling of nutrients. Drugs also interact with one another and with alcohol, causing nutritional problems. Awareness of this and attention to diet planning provides safeguards against health hazards. In the case of oral contraceptives (the Pill), many nutritional effects are known, but none seem hazardous provided that the diet is adequate and balanced.

Marihuana has characteristic effects on taste and appetite, but the long-term effects of heavy use of this drug are not well understood. There is some concern that the potency of marihuana preparations reaching this country has been increasing. "Hard" drug users suffer profound health damage. An important part of the rehabilitation process is the identification and correction of nutritional problems.

Caffeine use also becomes common in the teen and adult years. Caffeine is a stimulant drug, habit-forming but not addictive, whose moderate use is not harmful. But excessive caffeine consumption may be the cause of anxiety symptoms; lack of sleep; and, in the ulcer patient, excessive stomach acid secretion. Pregnant women should curtail their caffeine and coffee consumption.

Teenagers and adults, being self-determining, make their own choices. The nutrition educator must be aware of the sources of their motivation and convey important information in a way that honors their individuality.

To Explore Further

Good books for the young adult and adult have been referred to throughout the preceding chapters, in Appendix J, and in this chapter's notes. In addition, the American Health Foundation makes available a set of four pamphlets at a reasonable cost (write to 1370 Avenue of the Americas, New York, NY 10019):

Diet for Life I (AC-N1-4/76) — $.40 (on risk factors).
Diet for Life II (AC-N2-6/76) — $.60 (for weight loss).

Diet for Life III (AC-NCB-76) — $.60 (a cookbook).

Diet for Life (Diet Plan) (AC-N-76) — $.30 (a diet plan).

The American Dietetic Association (address in Appendix J) makes available cassettes on adolescent pregnancy and on women and oral contraceptives:

King, J., Nutrition during oral contraceptive treatment and pregnancy, *Cassette-a-Month*, June 1975.

Ritchey Jordan, S., and Faulkner, S., Adolescent pregnancy: The influence of growth, nutrition and the environment, *Cassette-a-Month*, April 1974.

On alcoholism:

Alcoholism, a 1975 pamphlet making clear some aspects of the problem, is available free from Metropolitan Life (offices in many cities).

Criteria for the diagnosis of alcoholism, *American Journal of Psychiatry* 129 (August 1972):127-135 is a highly technical article, intended for use by the diagnosing physician.

What are the signs of alcoholism? can be obtained from the National Council on Alcoholism, 733 3rd Avenue, New York, NY 10017. This is a 20-question quiz that enables the alcohol addict to diagnose himself. Similar pamphlets are available at local alcohol information centers in most cities and towns.

For athletes, the following booklet is excellent for exploding myths about eating:

Nutrition for Athletes, available from the American Alliance for Health, Physical Education, and Recreation, 1201 16th Street NW, Washington, DC 20036.

Four excellent articles on nutrition for the athlete appeared in *Nutrition Today*, November/December 1979:

Hanley, D. F., Jr., Athletic training—and how diet affects it; Vitousek, S. H., Is more better?; Hursh, L. M., Practical hints about feeding athletes; and Hanley, D. F., Jr., Basic diet guidance for athletes (editorial).

Nutrition Counseling

"The treatment of disease by diet is as much determined by myth . . . as it is by research."

PENELOPE EASTON

This Highlight was written out of our concern for people who turn to amateurs for the nutrition advice they need. Some of these amateurs are people who have studied this book, and we feel a responsibility to give them guidance. Other "amateurs" they may consult are doctors; we want to give a progress report on the state of nutrition education in the medical profession. Following are three representative kinds of requests people who have studied nutrition receive:

My daughter is pregnant. Her doctor says she must not cut down on calories. But you know doctors don't know anything about nutrition. You tell me what she should eat.

Our son has been injured in a football game. He is facing a long hospitalization. I've been reading about hospital malnutrition, and I'm scared he won't be fed right and then won't heal properly. Tell me how I can help him.

My husband has just been told he has cancer and will have radiation therapy. I asked the doctor what he should be eating, and he said for me not to worry my head about that. But I know proper food is important now. You tell me what I should feed him.

You can tell these people have read that medical schools don't teach doctors nutrition or that someone became well after checking himself out of the hospital so he could get the right food. Now, a loved one is in a doctor's care, and they are frightened because they don't feel secure that the doctor will attend to the nutritional problems.

If you explore these cries for help on a deeper level, you will hear another human plea: Tell me what to do! Stress calls for fighting or running (see Highlight 5). These people are under stress of the first order and need to be able to plan an active role. The oldtime country doctor knew about this need. When he arrived at a home to deliver a baby, he had the husband put on lots of water to boil. The distraught father worked off his stress pumping water from the well and keeping the fire stoked in the kitchen stove.

In responding to people in stress situations, you (the nutrition adviser) have some clear responsibilities. First, you have a responsibility to give support, not to make the situation worse. Find areas in which you can reinforce the patient's confidence in the medical team; faith has a healing effect. We are not proposing that you pat the person on the head and say soothingly, "Now don't you worry, everything is going to be all right." That is an insult. But do refrain from the compulsion to share all the horror stories that you are reminded of. Remember that it won't help the medical problem to add to the stress the patient or relative is suffering. One of the best supportive techniques, sometimes, is to say nothing. Supportiveness should filter into everything you recommend.

Second, know your own limits. It is tempting to rush in with your nutrition knowledge and play expert, yielding to the very human desire to be important and effective in a crisis. (The role of nutrition adviser may be thrust upon you when your friends learn that you have taken a nutrition course.) But remember, you are only a novice. It takes years of training to learn the correct diet recommendations for each specific medical case. In many instances, the best help you can give is not to play expert yourself but to refer the questionner to a real expert: a competent registered dietitian or nutritionist. Your role, after that, is to help the questionner to understand the nutrition advice given, to translate terms, explain, interpret, and offer strategies.

In replying to the expressed concern about doctors' knowledge about nutrition, be careful to stay within the bounds of what is known and to exclude anything that is merely hearsay or conjecture. Let us sift through what is being said in reliable literature and see if we can determine what is known.

Is It True What They Say About Doctors, Hospitals, and Nutrition? "Often doctors are trained in nutrition by doctors who heard it from another doctor who made it up."[1] This statement is typical of many being made today. Dr. Philip R. Lee (director of the Health Policy Program, School of Medicine, University of California at San Francisco) has commented:

> I would guess 90 percent of the graduates of our medical schools couldn't describe an adequate, nutritious diet.[2]

According to Dr. Myron Winick (professor of pediatrics, professor of nutrition, and director of the Institute of Human Nutrition, Columbia University College of Phy-

---

Mini-Glossary

Experts in Nutrition, Dietetics, and Food Sciences

nutritionist: a person trained by education and experience in the science and practice of nutrition. The education involves a graduate program leading to a degree (such as M.S. or Ph.D.) that includes basic sciences and professional courses to develop at least minimum competencies in nutrition and allied sciences. This person can answer questions on nutrition.

dietitian: a person who has earned a B.A. or B.S. degree and has met basic academic and training requirements for eligibility to pass the qualifying examination for professional registration in dietetics. The registration program is maintained by the American Dietetic Association; on passing the examination a person becomes an R.D. (Registered Dietitian). This person can answer questions on special diets, menu planning, and related topics.

food scientist: a person who has earned a B.A. or B.S. degree and whose college program has included basic sciences (chemistry, biology) and food science courses that qualify him/her to work in a laboratory of food research. This person can answer questions on food processing, food chemistry, and the like.

---

sicians and Surgeons, New York):

> The state of nutrition education in this country as it relates to health is in complete chaos. . . . One cause of that chaos is the medical profession's failure to take responsibility for this area.[3]

Statements like these are upsetting to people who feel that doctors are supposed to know everything and make no mistakes. After all, not only our health but also our life and death are in their hands. Whenever a story is told of a doctor's incompetence, it hits the front page of the newspapers and rapidly travels the grapevine. Often the incompetence is medical or surgical, but sometimes it is nutritional. A 23-year-old recently collected $50,000 in damages when his lawyer proved to the court's satisfaction that his doctor caused his mental retardation by putting his mother on a rice-fruit diet during her pregnancy.[4] The public is outraged by stories like this— and rightly so, if the stories are true. But are they? What is the true state of nutritional knowledge among doctors?

Half a century ago, it was routine to teach medical students that starvation of a mother during her pregnancy

---

[1] J. B. Schorr, as quoted by L. Hofmann, ed., *The Great American Nutrition Hassle* (Palo Alto, Calif.: Mayfield, 1978), p. 399.

[2] P. R. Lee, quoted by L. Hofmann, ed., *The Great American Nutrition Hassle* (Palo Alto, Calif.: Mayfield, 1978), p. 321.

[3] M. Winick, as quoted by R. Kotulak, Many doctors ignorant of nutrition, *Chicago Tribune*, May 1977.

[4] Tidbits and morsels, *Nutrition and the MD*, January 1978.

was a desirable practice, because it produced a tiny baby that was easy to deliver.[5] Medical schools also taught their students that women should drastically restrict their salt intake during pregnancy to avoid developing toxemia. Both of these harmful teachings (see Chapter 15) persisted by tradition and were still being perpetuated by some medical schools in the late 1960s, with little else about nutrition being taught. Only the postgraduate medical training of one class of doctors— pediatricians—emphasized nutrition, and only one medical society— the American Association of Pediatrics— has for decades made efforts to educate the public on nutrition, specifically that of infants.

One of the first popular nutrition writers to make this unfortunate situation known to the public was Adelle Davis, whose *Let's Eat Right to Keep Fit* (first edition, 1946) and other books have sold millions of copies. They have contributed greatly to the public's awareness of the importance of nutrition. She also made people aware that an M.D. degree is not evidence of nutritional know-how.[6] In the 1970s it was not uncommon for a doctor to adopt for himself a nutritionally unsound low-carbohydrate diet or for a psychiatrist to treat a woman for anxiety and depression with tranquilizers while forgetting to inquire about her daily intake of food and drink. In one instance, for example, a psychiatric patient habitually drank 28 cups of coffee a day, yet the psychiatrist kept prescribing tranquilizers, unaware of her caffeine intake.

The public has been becoming increasingly aware that it is not traditional to teach nutrition in medical schools, and that awareness has been bringing about change. Still, a survey of 42 medical schools in 1976, reported in the *Journal of the American Medical Association*, showed that 7 of them offered no nutrition instruction of any kind and that 13 more offered fewer than 11 hours in their four-year curriculum. Only 3 offered more than 20 hours, and only 1 had a nutrition department.[7] However, the situation appeared to be changing rapidly. A year later, a survey of 102 medical schools reported by the *Journal of Nutrition Education* showed that nutrition training was increasing in the medical schools, a trend reported by another journal to be "a groundswell."[8] As of the beginning of 1977, perhaps one out of every ten medical schools was teaching nutrition adequately.[9]

Nutrition is a relatively new science; medicine is an ancient art. Medicine has been practiced for hundreds of years without knowledge of nutrition. Before that situation would change, there had to be a demand for change, and that demand now exists. The *Journal of the American Medical Association* began publishing articles on nutrition issues in 1973.[10] Efforts are being made to provide nutrition education for doctors who are already practicing, by way of public service announcements and courses on television. About 5,000 doctors took such a course in in-

[5]S. R. Williams, Nutritional guidance in prenatal care, in *Nutrition in Pregnancy and Lactation*, eds. B. S. Worthington, J. Vermeersch, and S. R. Williams (St. Louis: Mosby, 1977), p. 55.

[6]A. Davis, *Let's Eat Right to Keep Fit* (New York: Harcourt Brace Jovanovich, 1946).

[7]E. S. Nelson, Nutrition instruction in medical schools, 1976, *Journal of the American Medical Association* 236 (1976):2534.

[8]C. K. Cyborski, Nutrition content in medical curricula, *Journal of Nutrition Education* 9 (1977):17-18; and W. J. Darby, The renaissance of nutrition education, *Nutrition Reviews* 35 (February 1977):33-38.

[9]Nelson, 1976.

[10]C. F. Enloe, Jr., For whom the bell tolls (editorial), *Nutrition Today*, July/August 1973, p. 14.

fant nutrition in 1978.[11] *Medical News* reports that "like sex, nutrition is increasingly discussed among physicians."[12]

New and excellent textbooks for medical students are also now available, and reading lists are being offered for them and for doctors already graduated from school.[13] An excellent newsletter for physicians, *Nutrition and the MD*, began coming out monthly in 1974 and was reaching over 900 physicians by the end of 1978.[14] A medical college reported the successful integration of nutrition education into its curriculum in 1975 and others were expected to follow suit.[15] It seems realistic to expect that within the next few decades, the public will be able to depend on its doctors to include nutrition in treatment and to rely on dietitians as part of the medical team.

But what about now? There must be many doctors now practicing whose nutrition education was inadequate and who have had no opportunity or made no effort to obtain this education on their own. They would be likely to overlook nutritional problems in their patients and might be unaware that the dietitian's specific instructions about changes in diet might promote good health and prevention of or recovery from disease. During the 1970s, as the gaps in medical school curricula were first being widely publicized, a serious situation in the nation's hospitals was also coming to light, which suggested that, at present, doctors often do fail in these respects.

In 1974 Dr. Charles E. Butterworth published an article in *Nutrition Today* titled "The Skeleton in the Hospital Closet."[16] In it he reported a high incidence of severe malnutrition in the hospital, which he called "physician-induced." He cited some of the causes: Patients are often deprived of food for days at a time so that they can be given medical tests; they are seldom given vitamin and mineral supplements; and they are often fed inadequate formulas (bottles of glucose and salts without protein, vitamins, or minerals) for long periods. Under these circumstances, they develop protein-kcalorie malnutrition

[11]J. Gutman, Physicians' exposure to health topics through mass media: An avenue for improving the dietitian's image, *Journal of the American Dietetic Association* 71 (1977): 505-509; and L. J. Filer and E. F. Calesa, Multi-media education about infant nutrition for physicians, *Journal of the American Dietetic Association* 72 (1978):404-406.

[12]Nutrition: No longer a stepchild in medicine (Medical News), *Journal of the American Medical Association* 238 (1977):2245-2248.

[13]For example, H. A. Schneider, C. E. Anderson, and D. B. Coursin, eds., *Nutritional Support of Medical Practice* (Hagerstown, Md.: Harper & Row Medical Department, 1977). Two such reading lists are *Education in Nutrition for Physicians and Dentists: An Annotated Bibliography* and *Selected Nutrition Reference Texts for Physicians and Medical Students*, both published by The Nutrition Foundation, Washington, D.C., 1976. The first is available for $2; the second is free on request.

[14]*Nutrition and the MD*, available from P.M., Inc., PO Box 2160, Van Nuys, CA 91405, at a subscription cost of $26 a year (as of 1978). Four to six pages of reading each month, this little newsletter features nutritional strategies in patient care, alerts the physician to new findings in the clinical literature (and cites its sources), notes important new publications, and provides authoritative answers to questions patients commonly ask.

[15]C. A. Hall, L. J. Howard, and J. A. Halsted, The clinical nutrition program at Albany Medical College, *Nutrition Today*, September/October-November/December 1975, pp. 31-33.

[16]C. E. Butterworth, The skeleton in the hospital closet, *Nutrition Today*, March/April 1974, pp. 4-8. Dr. Butterworth is professor of medicine and pediatrics and director of the Nutrition Program at the University of Alabama in Birmingham and chairman of the Council on Foods and Nutrition of the American Medical Association.

and iron-deficiency anemia, conditions that severely weaken them—delaying their recovery, prolonging their hospital stays, and increasing the cost of their treatment. Reasons for the neglect of their nutritional care, he reported, include failure to notice low weight and weight loss, frequent staff rotations, diffusion of responsibility, and lack of communication between doctors and dietitians.

Butterworth's report was promptly followed by a report from Boston by two hospital physicians who confirmed his findings. Drs. Blackburn and Bistrian reported that close to half of the patients in their hospitals showed evidence of protein-kcalorie malnutrition—often caused not by the diseases or conditions that had led to their admission to the hospital but by neglect of their nutritional needs while they were in the hospital.[17]

These findings have since been confirmed and extended by many other investigators. In 1977 the *Journal of the American Medical Association* published a strong statement on the subject, including this directive to physicians: "No patient should be hospitalized without an adequate nutritional profile." It included directions for monitoring patients' nutritional status while they are in treatment.[18]

Like the medical schools, the hospitals have responded to the outcry arising from public knowledge of this situation by conducting surveys and improvement programs of their own. One went to work to improve its height-weight data records.[19] Butterworth and Blackburn published a recommended procedure for detecting and correcting malnutrition in the hospital, and it was instituted with success at a Boston hospital.[20] The great im-

portance of nutrition in recovery from surgery was gaining recognition.[21] A chapter of a medical text published in 1977 was devoted to the management of protein-kcalorie malnutrition in the hospital.[22]

In answer to the question, "Is it true what they say about doctors, hospitals, and nutrition?," we reluctantly answer, "Yes." The situation is changing, and rapidly, but it is still far from ideal. Physicians are being trained better and dietitians are being given greater initiative and responsibility in the care of hospital patients, but there is much room for improvement.

Providing Nutrition Advice Meanwhile, what do you say to the three frightened people who expressed concern about the nutritional needs of their family members? Do you tell them their doctor may be ignorant in nutrition? Absolutely not. If the patient is in the process of selecting a physician, then

[17]G. L. Blackburn and B. Bistrian, A report from Boston, *Nutrition Today*, May/June 1974, p. 30. Dr. Blackburn is assistant professor of surgery, Harvard University; research associate, Department of Nutrition and Food Science, Massachusetts Institute of Technology; and director of the Intensive Care Unit and Nutritional Services, Boston City and New England Deaconess Hospitals. Dr. Bistrian is research associate, Department of Nutrition and Food Science, Massachusetts Institute of Technology; visiting physician, Department of Medicine, Boston City Hospital; and research assistant, New England Deaconess Hospital.

[18]A. Fonaroff, Undernutrition (letter to the editor), *Journal of the American Medical Association* 237 (1977):1825-1826.

[19]Veterans Administration Hospital, New York City, Height and weight data in the patient's medical record, *Journal of the American Dietetic Association* 72 (1978):409-411.

[20]C. E. Butterworth and G. L. Blackburn, Hospital malnutrition, *Nutrition Today*, March/April 1975, pp. 8-18; and J. E. Wade, Role of a clinical dietitian specialist on a nutrition support service, *Journal of the American Dietetic Association* 70 (1977):185-189.

[21]This view was expressed in a letter to the editor of the *Journal of the American Medical Association*, suggesting that the recognition of the importance of nutrition in surgery was the fourth major advance in the field: J. C. Stevens, Surgical nutrition: The fourth coming, *Journal of the American Medical Association* 239 (1978):192.

[22]G. L. Blackburn and B. R. Bistrian, Curative nutrition: Protein-calorie management, in Schneider, Anderson, and Coursin, 1977.

you might help him discover the doctor's orientation and perhaps suggest one who is aware of the importance of nutrition. If the patient is already hospitalized and, let's say, in a coma, there is nothing that the outsider (nutritionist or relative) can contribute except moral support—and that is even more important at this time than usual.

Between these two extremes, there are many medical situations in which you are aware that nutrition plays an active part in recovery, and you have the responsibility to communicate that knowledge. You may not know specifically what to do, but you should steer the family in the direction of getting not only medical but also nutritional help.

Both prevention of and recovery from some major diseases have strong nutritional components. The four leading causes of death in the United States are cardiovascular disease, cancer, diabetes, and alcoholism. For cardiovascular disease, control of fat and salt intake often is helpful. For cancer, aggressive nutritional therapy, if introduced early enough, often makes the difference between life and death. Diabetes can often be controlled by diet alone. Alcoholism requires abstinence, but recovery is greatly enhanced by the adoption of healthful eating habits. Among other major causes of hospitalization are wounds,

fractures, and burns; in these, too, nutritional therapy greatly speeds the recovery process, whereas poor nutrition delays and prolongs it. In these kinds of cases you can help by explaining the need for dietary management and by referring the family to an expert trained in nutrition and dietetics. In the hospital a dietitian is in charge and can be sought out to answer questions.

There are also some generalized strategies to offer the hospitalized patient. Recall that the relative needs action. What will you tell the relative to do? First, explain to the relative the nutritional factors involved in the situation so that he, in turn, can instruct the patient. Once the patient understands, he will cooperate in the fight for recovery. If he is hospitalized, he should vigorously follow the doctor's and the dietitian's orders.

But patients in the hospital often do not eat, and it is important to understand why. Perhaps the patient objects to the taste of the food. He needs to be reminded that institutional food cannot be cooked to his individual taste specifications, but that the nutrients that he needs are present nevertheless. As an adjunct, the relative, with the dietitian's approval of course, can bring some seasonings from home to dress up the hospital diet. A patient often enjoys food that a relative prepares at home and brings to him. (Again the warning:

Be sure the dietitian approves what is brought.)

There may be other reasons for the patient's anorexia. He may be in pain—and who feels like eating when he is hurting? Or one of his medications may be interfering with his appetite or altering his taste sensations. Medications and illness can also depress the patient to the point where he does not have the energy to eat. The staff person who delivers the tray may not be trained to recognize the patient's need to have the bed raised, the tray moved closer, a milk carton opened, or the food cut into bite-size pieces. In some of these instances the relative can play an important role by being present at meal time to help.

It is especially important to be aware that there may be an underlying psychological cause for the refusal of food. General depression and hostility over his situation could be finding expression through refusal to eat. The patient may recognize that he needs to cooperate and be pleasant with the doctors and nursing staff but rebel against someone telling him the food tastes good. He releases all his pent-up feelings in diatribes against that "awful hospital food." If this is the problem, there is a dilemma. The patient needs nutrients for his recovery but also needs a sense of autonomy or control over his life. This situation requires the cooperative efforts of doctor and dietitian with the relative playing a sensitive, supporting role. Badgering and arguing are out of place.

You recognize that we are "dabbling" in psychology and that this is not our field. However, we are not repeating pronouncements from psychologists but are telling you what patients have said to us. They often say that the most demoralizing person to have in the hospital room is the disgustingly healthy "general-in-command-of-the-situation" kind of person. Every remonstrance of the patient is quickly mowed down with reasonable arguments. The patient is left feeling inadequate, lonely, and isolated. "Isn't there anyone out there who thinks of me as capable of guiding my life?" they cry. "I didn't lose all my intelligence when I became flat on my back in this bed." The elderly especially complain of this.

We hope that you will see from this discussion that nutrition counseling is more than telling someone to eat a certain diet. As we've said many times, food and emotions are intertwined and the counselor who fails to honor this fact may be ineffective.

Now let's look at the three cases mentioned at the beginning and see what these patients' relatives need to understand about their nutritional support. The mother of the pregnant girl has not kept up with the newer knowledge about diet during pregnancy. Her daughter's doctor, on the other hand, shows that he has kept up (see Chapter 15). Pregnant women are no longer advised to control their weight so rigorously as they were a generation ago; they are advised to gain about 25 pounds during pregnancy. You can explain to the mother that enough food needs to be eaten to provide ample nutrients. Perhaps in the conversation you will be able to hint gently that she should let her daughter and her doctor work this problem out together.

What we said about helping patients cooperate with the dietitian in the hospital would be good general advice for the parent of the football player. One problem he may have is that his appetite may not be a proper guide to the amount of food he now needs. He may be saddled with a large appetite, in the same way a retired athlete is. Without vigorous exercise to use the kcalories, he may gain fat tissue and weight as many former athletes do. If the hospital diet is supplemented with food from home, it should be low-kcalorie, nutrient-dense food such as fruit. If he receives

candy and cakes, suggest that he "bribe" the hospital staff with them. He will get more benefit from them that way than when they are stored in his fat tissue.

The third question concerned a cancer patient. We are using this case to illustrate the complexities in disease treatment that make it imperative for the amateur to know when *not* to take on himself the task of directing nutritional therapy. There are additional problems here that the other two cases did not have to contend with—nausea and anorexia at a time when supplemental nutrients are especially needed. Radiation therapy often causes anorexia even when the cancer does not affect the digestive system. Dr. E. M. Copeland, professor of surgery at the University of Texas System Cancer Center, writes:

> Malnutrition results from the intensive effort to eradicate the tumor either by surgery, radiation therapy or chemotherapy. Each of these therapeutic steps is predicated upon recovery from the preceding step and unless adequate nutrient intake is ensured, the patient is at risk for protein-calorie malnutrition.[23]

The best way for anyone to obtain nutrients is from food, but the cancer patient often

[23]E. M. Copeland, Nutritional concepts in the treatment of cancer, *Journal of the Florida Medical Association* 66 (1979):373-378.

has poor appetite, pain, nausea, and diarrhea, which make eating a normal diet almost impossible.

The medical team will closely monitor the weight and other parameters of the hospitalized cancer patient. They may institute intravenous hyperalimentation, the feeding of a carefully prescribed mixture of vitamins, minerals, amino acids, and glucose through a tube inserted directly into a large central vein. Patients can be kept on this mixture for a number of weeks, but most only need to be on it for 10 to 20 days. Tumor growth is not stimulated with this extra nourishment, and the patient's immune response is greatly enhanced.[24]

If the patient can eat, whether he is in the hospital or at home, he needs all the encouragement that relatives can give. If he can grasp the picture of his need for the nutrients, he will try to cooperate. However, the people who are helping him should be aware that he may develop an aversion to some of

[24]Copeland, 1979.

his favorite foods. For example, he may take extra nourishment in the form of milkshakes for several days and then refuse the shakes abruptly. This is like becoming nauseous one time when you ate a certain food and ever more being repulsed by that food. For this reason, many small servings should be offered. One wife recalls preparing 10 to 20 items for a meal and expecting her cancer-patient husband to do no more than taste each one. With constant care like this, although he lost close to forty pounds in a few weeks, he received just enough food to sustain him while the radiation treatments conquered the cancer.

Another discomfort that the patient receiving chemotherapy or radiation may have is a dry mouth. Fresh lemon juice or lemonade may help. Sourball candy may also help relieve this discomfort. There are also altered taste sensations, apart from the aversion developed toward specific foods, especially if the neck and upper chest are treated with radiation. For patients to detect a

sweet taste, the concentration of sugar may have to be increased. Bitter tastes are more easily noted, especially in protein foods. Encourage the patient to take an active role in planning his diet; he is the one who is most affected and the one who knows how certain foods taste.[25]

In summary, relatives can furnish or augment nutritional support for many patients. But the person who counsels the family about nutrition should be aware of the psychological needs of the patient as well as his nutritional needs and be knowledgeable about hospital and medical procedures. The amateur nutritionist should tread lightly and be aware of his own limitations of knowledge and experience. Counseling in nutrition of the kind presented here is supplemental and should support the medical team of doctor and dietitian.

[25]D. L. Ponder and H. Van Slyke, Home management of nutrition for patients receiving cancer therapy, *Journal of the Florida Medical Association* 66 (1979):378-389.

CHAPTER 17

CONTENTS

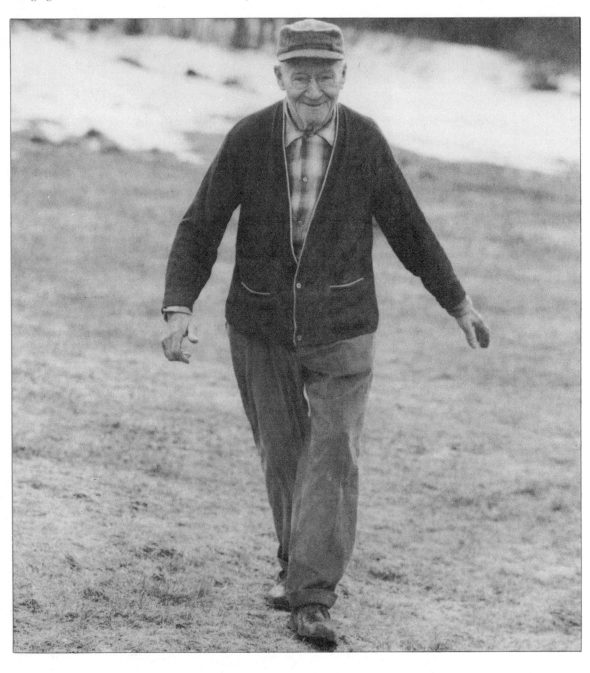

THE OLDER ADULT

Today the care of the fastest growing minority, the aged, presents the greatest challenge—to create health to correspond with the duration of life.

A. A. ALBANESE

Aging begins at birth but becomes most apparent after growth has stopped at adulthood. Thereafter, the rate of aging and the quality of life depend partly on prior nutrition. At each stage, the health of the individual is based on the foundations laid down in the previous stage. But there are some givens: Aging will occur in all people. To adapt successfully, a person needs to know what he can change and what he must accept. This chapter begins with what is known about the process itself: What we must accept.

The Aging Process

We humans have not comprehended what is involved in the aging process, nor have we figured out how to prevent or postpone it. Even our definitions of the process are vague. One writer calls aging a certain kind of change in living systems due to the passage of time—the increased probability of death with increased chronological age. Another calls it a decrease in viability and an increase in vulnerability.[1] However aging is defined, research on it has been scarce. Much is known about the growth, development, and nutritional needs of the human body from the time of conception until it reaches maturity. But only in recent times has the scientific community become interested in the mechanism by which the human organism ceases to grow once it reaches maturity and then "runs down" and dies. Current interest is increasing, due in large part to the rising numbers of older people and the impact they are having on our social and government institutions, but answers are still few and far between.

It is clear, however, that most people do die around the age of 70, if not before, just as they always have. You may have heard that people are living longer than in the past, but there is a fallacy in this statement.

[1]These statements come, respectively, from B. L. Strehler, *Time, Cells, and Aging,* 2nd ed. (New York: Academic Press, 1977); and A. Comfort, *A Good Age* (New York: Crown, 1976).

The "increased life span" of people in the twentieth century does not reflect a longer total life expectancy but rather a greater survival rate among the very young. Infant mortality has been sharply reduced, thanks to the defeat of many infectious diseases, so more infants can be expected to reach the age of 20 now than 100 years ago. But there has been no recent increase in life expectancy for people who have reached the age of 20. It seems that something built into the human organism—the something we call aging—cuts off life at a rather fixed point in time.[2]

Natural selection has not operated in favor of genes that promote longevity. But the human race, with its superior brain, can collect and store information that helps keep individuals alive after they have reproduced. Thus longevity can be said to result from evolution only in the sense that the brain has evolved. In today's world, however, people are valued for the accumulated wisdom and experience that they can contribute to society, and so they are important to us long after they have passed their reproductive years and the time when they would contribute genes to their offspring.

longevity (lawn-JEV-ih-tee): long life.

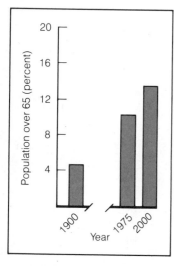

One out of every ten citizens in the United States is above 65 years of age, and the percentage is increasing.

Aging of Cells   Cells seem to undergo a built-in (genetic) aging process and also to age in response to outside (environmental) forces. Environmental stresses that promote aging include extremes of heat and cold, disease, lack of nutrients, the wear and tear of hard physical labor, and the lack of stimulation caused by disuse, for example, of the muscle cells in the legs of a cripple who can't exercise. But even in the most pleasant and supportive of environments, inevitable changes in the structure and function of the body's cells make them increasingly vulnerable to these environmental stresses.

All theories of aging have one element in common. They agree that at some point the cells become incapable of replenishing their constituents. In a complex organism such as the human body, the cells are interdependent. When some cells die and their function is lost, other cells dependent on the first ones suffer and also eventually die. A consequence of the gradual slowing down of cell function over the years is reduced cell metabolism, which results in reduced energy needs of older people.

A second common element seems to be that aging cells are programmed to stop reproducing once a certain stage of development has been reached.[3] Cells have different timetables for reproduction, but each type of cell seems to come to a natural end somehow. For example, red blood cells undergo division only as long as they are in the marrow of the long bones. When they are mature, they move out of the marrow to perform their function in the bloodstream. In the blood, they no longer reproduce; they work for three to six months and then die.

[2] J. Mayer, Aging and nutrition, *Geriatrics* 29 (5) (1974):57-59.
[3] Strehler, 1977.

The brain cells are also programmed to stop reproducing, but they all stop within the first two years of life. Many of them maintain themselves without further cell division for about 70 years. Thus at about 14 months of age, the human organism already has all the brain cells it will ever have. Thousands die daily, but the daily loss is not noticeable. The accumulated loss over a lifetime is felt only in the slowing of reflexes and in garbled messages going to other organs. It seems strange that the human species should have evolved such a magnificent instrument for receiving, storing, interpreting, and retrieving information and yet not have evolved a method of repairing it.[4] Some scientists view this evolutionary mishap as a "self-destruct" mechanism for the human body.

Some cells seem never to die but only to reproduce. They take in nutrients from their environment and grow; profound changes take place in their internal structure; and the living material within them then divides itself equally between two poles while the cell splits down the middle. Each new daughter cell is an exact replica of the parent cell and contains the same material. Thus the parent cell still lives, in a sense, as two replicas of itself. However, even in optimal conditions the cells of a multicellular organism seem unable to go on dividing in this manner forever. About 50 to 55 replications seem to be the maximum.

A third factor in the aging process seems to be that with the passage of time, cells become cluttered with debris—partially completed proteins that are never totally dismantled. This intracellular "sludge" interferes with the efficiency of operations within the cells. The material that accumulates in the cells is known as the pigment of old age.[5]

The aging pigment is **lipofuscin** (lip-oh-FEW-sin).

Another factor may be that cells lose their ability to interpret the DNA genetic code words and thus make their proteins incorrectly. As reduced amounts of protein or wrong proteins are produced, cell and organ functions that depend on those proteins also falter. Organs elsewhere in the body may also be adversely affected. A theory that is somewhat allied to this one is that through some environmental stress, such as the continuous bombardment of cosmic rays that penetrate the earth's atmosphere, the DNA code itself may become altered. This too would lead to the production of wrong proteins.

If wrong proteins are produced for any reason, another theory states, the body's immune system will react to them as if they were foreign proteins from outside and will produce antibodies to counteract them. Complexes then form between the antibodies and these proteins and accumulate in and among cells as useless debris. The autoimmune theory may account in part for the accumulation of deposits in joints, which causes arthritis.

Finally, another theory of aging suggests that cosmic rays bombard molecules in the cells and split them into highly reactive compounds

[4]Strehler, 1977.

[5]Strehler, 1977; and M. Puner, *To the Good Long Life* (New York: Universe Books, 1974).

For a picture of the disulfide bridges in insulin, a protein molecule, see Chapter 3.

known as free radicals. These free radicals then bind rigidly to other cellular molecules by way of disulfide bridges. This disrupts the informational content of important molecules and so impairs their function. As in other cases, the cells this occurs in, as well as others that depend on them, then die. (Some investigators have suggested that the formation of free radicals might be retarded by taking vitamin E supplements.)

Just as a chain is only as strong as its weakest link, so also is an organism only as long-lived as the least stable of its vital cells. The ability of cells to replenish the substances they need for life or to make fresh copies of themselves after they have reached maturity determines their life spans and ultimately the life span of the entire organism.

An analogy may help to show how all these processes work together to cause aging. A shipbuilding firm must have an office where the plans and specifications for all the various boats are kept and a warehouse where the materials to carry out these orders are stored. There must also be a site where the actual construction takes place. When an order is received for a particular boat to be constructed, the plans on file are duplicated for a working copy, and messengers are sent to bring the materials to the construction site. Following the instructions, workers then build the boat.

If, through years of heavy use, the warehouse becomes cluttered and disorganized, then it will become increasingly difficult to fill the orders efficiently. (This parallels the theory that with age the cell fluid becomes cluttered with debris.) If some of the messengers take the wrong orders from the files or bring the wrong materials, this too will cause production to slow down or cease. (This parallels the cells' loss of ability to read the genetic code words.) With rain or fire damage to the files themselves, some of the specifications will become unavailable or illegible (like the cellular DNA becoming altered by cosmic ray bombardment). Should one worker be instructed to burn the trash, he might lazily leave behind marred instructions or parts (as in the autoimmune theory). Vandalism (free radicals) might do further damage. With inefficient management of the warehouse, there might be delays in getting supplies. (For the cell, the nutrients might not be present in the blood because they were not taken in, or there might be a breakdown in the ability of the intestinal cells to absorb the nutrients.) Finally, the warehouse might have been set up for a limited order—its destruction, once it had produced a certain number of boats, might have been planned from the beginning. (This represents the idea that cells are programmed to self-destruct after a certain number of generations.)

None of the theories of cellular aging are more than theories, but some interesting work has been done in the attempt to solve the riddle of why cells age. One such experiment was conducted as early as the 1930s. Rats were fed a diet balanced in every respect except that it was severely restricted in kcalories. A control group was fed the same diet but with ample kcalories. When the control group had reached maturity, the starved rats were still immature. They were then permitted to catch up, by being fed ample kcalories. Surprisingly, the previously starved rats outlived the controls, averaging 1,465 days as compared with the controls' 969 days.[6] Similar experiments have since yielded similar results with many different species, and a tentative conclusion is that the key to success is keeping the animals in a juvenile state for longer than the normal period. Obviously this experiment could not be carried out on human beings, but it suggests some interesting possibilities for explaining longevity.

Aging of Organs   The aging of cells is reflected by changes in the organs they are a part of. The most visible changes take place in the skin. As people age, wrinkles increase, partly because of a loss of the fat that underlies the skin and partly because of a loss of elasticity. The scars that have accumulated from many small cuts roughen the texture of the skin. Exposure to sun, wind, and cold hasten the drying process and contribute to wrinkling. The hair disappears also, particularly from the head and face of males.

Another obvious and traumatic change, in the digestive system, is painful deterioration of the gums and subsequent loss of teeth. According to the Ten-State Survey, gum disease increases with age and exists in 90 percent of the population by age 65 to 74.[7] In addition, the senses of taste and smell diminish, which reduces the pleasure of eating.

In other parts of the digestive system, secretion by the stomach of hydrochloric acid and enzymes decreases with age, as does the secretion of digestive juices by the pancreas and small intestine. The large intestinal muscles weaken with reduced use, thus allowing the walls to form outpocketings, a condition called diverticulosis (see p. 121).

The liver is somewhat different. Liver cells regenerate themselves throughout life, so with normal aging the loss of liver cells is not a major problem. However, even with good nutrition, fat gradually infiltrates the liver, reducing its work output.[8] The response of the liver to moderate blood glucose levels is not appreciably altered with age, but the response to a large glucose load, as in the glucose tolerance test, is reduced. There may be two reasons for this: First, the blood may not be pushed strongly enough by the heart to reach the pancreas, so that it does not send its insulin message to the liver; second, there may be a reduction in the number of glucose-responsive cells in the pancreas.

Glucose tolerance test: see Chapter 1.

As the heart and blood vessels age, the volume of blood that the heart can pump decreases. The arteries lose their elasticity. The amount of blood going into the networks of capillaries in the various organs

[6]Puner, 1974.

[7]*Ten-State Nutrition Survey, 1968-1970*, DHEW publication no. (HSM) 72-8130-8133 (Atlanta, Ga.: Center for Disease Control, 1972).

[8]Mayer, 1974.

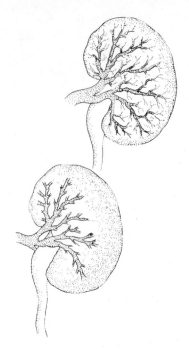

As the heart pumps less blood into an organ, the capillary trees within that organ recede, leaving some of the cells without nourishment.

Osteoporosis: see also Chapter 12.

decreases. There are deposits of fat in the walls of the arteries, and these deposits may be invaded by calcium salts, which make them hard and inflexible. Because all organs and tissues depend on the circulation of nutrients and oxygen, degenerative changes in this system critically affect all other systems.

The decrease in blood flow through the kidneys makes them gradually less efficient at their task of removing nitrogen and other wastes from the blood and maintaining the correct amounts of salts, sugar, and other valuable nutrients in the body fluids. As the heart pumps less blood into the capillary trees of the kidneys, the capillary trees diminish in size, causing some kidney cells to be deprived of their nutrient and oxygen supply. Cells formerly fed by these capillaries then die. Both the heart rate and the volume of blood pumped into the kidneys depend on the muscular activity of the person, so this degenerative process can be retarded by regular exercising.

The ability of the brain to direct the activities of the body decreases during aging. However, the older person compensates for this with a greater amount of stored information and wisdom. The nerve cells are not replaceable, so any damage by accident permanently diminishes mental ability. This is probably the greatest cause of unhappiness among older people and their relatives, because it decreases the ability to enjoy life. Visual impairment, hearing loss, loss of the senses of smell and taste, and loss of the sense of balance are all evidence of impaired nerve cell function.

Finally, the skeletal system is subject to change. Bone is a structure composed of salts of calcium, phosphorus, and other minerals. Bone is not made of cells but is continuously being laid down by bone-building cells and dissolved or reabsorbed by bone-dismantling cells. With the passage of years, for unknown reasons, the balance shifts in favor of destructive activity, resulting in thinning of the bone and adult bone loss (osteoporosis).

Osteoporosis is more common in women than in men by a ratio of four to one. In our population, it may be severe enough to produce fractures in as many as 30 percent of the people over age 65.[9] A hip fracture caused by osteoporosis may not be a clean break but a shattering of the bone into fragments that can't readily be reassembled. Surgical repair often requires replacement of the broken bone with an artificial substitute.

The causes of osteoporosis seem to be multiple. Because it occurs more often in women than in men and because it occurs more predictably after menopause, the cessation of female hormone secretion is thought to be a contributing factor. But it can't be the only factor. If it were, the excretion of calcium would increase after menopause, and this is not the case.[10] Gradual calcium loss may occur

[9]L. Lutwak, Symposium on osteoporosis: Nutritional aspects of osteoporosis, *Journal of the American Geriatrics Society* 17 (2) (1969):115-119.

[10]Lutwak, 1969.

because of dietary deficiency, but it would take a large daily deficit (50 mg a day) for a long period of time (20 years) before clinical signs of osteoporosis would appear.[11]

The mass of the skeleton seems to be greatly influenced by the amount of use or the pressure put on the bones. Pressure on the long bones, particularly, causes an increase in the activity of the bone-building cells. Given this stimulation, the skeletal system seems able to repair itself remarkably well into great old age, even though it is subjected to a great deal of wear and tear.[12] However, idleness promotes bone dissolution. Probably the lessened activity of old age combined with long hospitalizations for age-related problems contributes to osteoporosis.

Perhaps the factors that promote or prevent the develoment of osteoporosis can be traced back to the growing years at the beginning of life. The higher the density of the bones at maturity, the later will be the development of osteoporosis. Heredity also plays some part. Men have denser bones than women, and Mediterranean, Latin American, and African populations have denser bones than Northern European and Asian peoples. Still, the rate at which bone minerals are lost is about the same for all populations.[13] The initial deposit of minerals into bones is responsive to early nutrition, pointing up the importance of prevention of adult bone loss early in life. It may be that once osteoporosis has developed it cannot be reversed by taking extra calcium.[14] Lifelong adequate intakes of both calcium and fluoride doubtless protect against osteoporosis; the condition is not usually seen in a person who has had a consistently high calcium intake. In fact, patients with osteoporosis give a lifetime history of exceptionally low calcium intakes.[15]

During movement, the bones must rub against each other at the joints. The ends are protected from wear by cartilage and by small sacs of fluid that act as cushions. With age, the ends of the bones become pitted or eroded as a result of wear or of diseases such as arthritis. The cause of arthritis, a painful swelling of the joints, is unknown, but it affects millions around the world and is a major problem of the elderly.

The aging of every body system can be accelerated by reducing the flow of nutrients and oxygen to the system. To put this statement more positively, the process of aging can be retarded by maintaining a strong cardiovascular and respiratory system. Exercise, regular and active enough to increase the heartbeat and respiration rate, is one of the keys

[11]I. Dallas and B. E. C. Nordin, The relation between calcium intake and roentgenologic osteoporosis, *American Journal of Clinical Nutrition* 11 (1962):263-269.

[12]Strehler, 1977.

[13]Lutwak, 1969.

[14]Mayer, 1974.

[15]A. F. Morgan, Nutrition of the aging, *The Gerontologist* 2 (1962):77-84; Lutwak, 1969; and Dallas and Nordin, 1962.

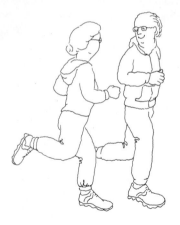

to good health in the later years. An added benefit of exercise, as you already know, is to prevent the atrophy of all muscles (not only the heart), which would take place with inactivity. A good flow of blood requires a strong heartbeat and strongly flexing muscles to press expelled lymph back into the bloodstream for recirculation. Many older persons believe that they can't participate in strenuous exercise, but studies have shown that they can do more than they think they can. Even modest endurance training can improve the cardiovascular and respiratory function and promote good muscle tone while controlling the accumulation of body fat.[16]

Nutritional Implications of Aging

Good health habits, including good nutrition throughout life, are the best guarantee of healthy and enjoyable later years. Many of the nutrient needs of the elderly are the same as for younger persons, but some special considerations deserve emphasis.

Energy   kCaloric needs decrease with advancing years—because of the decreased metabolism of all cells and because of decreased muscular activity. About a 5 percent reduction per decade in energy intake is suggested. One study showed that of older persons living alone, 35 percent of the men and 52 percent of the women exceeded their kcalorie allowances. The kcaloric needs of each individual vary with metabolic activity, but a rule of thumb for older adults is 1,500 kcal for women and 2,000 for men.[17] This may seem a little low, but because overweight is well recognized as a shortener of the life span, it seems to be a life-sustaining recommendation.

Protein foods should contribute about 20 to 25 percent of the kcalories in the older person's diet, fats no more than 20 percent, with the remainder coming from complex carbohydrates[18] (see Table 1). On such a limited kcalorie allowance, all foods must be nutrient-dense. There is little leeway for such empty-kcalorie foods as sugar, sweets, fats, oils, or alcohol.

One side of the energy budget is for kcalories to be taken in, and the other side is for the expenditure of those kcalories. Increase in activity should be emphasized for any person interested in maintaining good health in the later years. Not only would this help control overweight, but also (as already mentioned) it would increase blood flow into all

Table 1   Eating Pattern Supplying the Recommended Proportions of Protein, Fat, and Carbohydrate for Older People

Food group	Number of exchanges	
	Woman (1,500 kcal)	Man (2,000 kcal)
Milk (skim)	3	3
Vegetable	2	3
Fruit	3	4
Bread	10	10
Meat (lean)	4	7
Fat	4	4

[16]K. H. Sidney, R. J. Shephard, and J. E. Harrison, Endurance training and body composition of the elderly, *American Journal of Clinical Nutrition* 30 (1977):326-333.

[17]J. S. Lyons and M. F. Trulson, Food practices of older people living at home, *Journal of Gerontology* 11 (1956):66-72.

[18]D. B. Rao, Problems of nutrition in the aged, *Journal of the American Geriatrics Society* 21 (8) (1973):362-367.

the organs of the body, keeping them more vigorous. One investigator designed an experiment to find out if the trainability of older men depended on their physical prowess in their youth. The answer was no. He decided that their increase in muscle strength during the training was not due to the improvement in their muscles but to the improvement in the nervous system that resulted from the increased blood flow to the brain engendered by the exercise.[19]

Physical activity like walking increases the deposit of calcium in the bones, thus forestalling the development of osteoporosis. People responsible for the care of older adults should encourage more activity of all kinds and shorter recuperation periods in bed following illnesses.

Protein The need for essential amino acids is the same for older adults as it is for younger adults. However, the older person needs to get these essential nutrients from less food, so care should be taken to assure that the protein is of high quality. The protein should also be protected from being used for energy by including complex carbohydrates in the diet.

It has been shown that older persons living at home most often omit milk or its equivalent in cheese from their diet.[20] Another protein food, meat, is often omitted because it is difficult to chew; in one study, only those with excellent teeth had a high protein intake.[21] Both milk and meat may also be omitted because of difficulties with purchasing and storage. Low hemoglobin levels have been shown to correlate with protein (and iron) content of the diet.[22] Low hemoglobin levels may be the cause of the fatigue and apathy so often mentioned as a problem by older persons. It has been recommended that the protein allowance for those over 65 be increased to 2 g per kilogram of ideal weight.[23]

Fat For many reasons, fat should be limited in the older person's diet. Cutting fat helps cut kcalories and may also help retard the development of atherosclerosis. On the limited kcalorie allowance recommended for older adults, it would be difficult to obtain the many vitamins and minerals that come from protein-rich and complex-carbohydrate foods if too high a percentage of the kcalories came from fat. Moreover, high fat interferes with calcium absorption, promoting osteoporosis.

---

[19]H. A. deVries, Physiological effects of an exercise training regimen upon men aged 52 to 88, *Journal of Gerontology* 25 (1970):325-336.

[20]Lyons and Trulson, 1956.

[21]P. Swanson, Adequacy in old age, part 2: Nutrition programs for the aging, *Journal of Home Economics* 56 (1964):728-734; and C. S. Davidson, J. Livermore, P. Anderson, and S. Kaufman, The nutrition of a group of apparently healthy aging persons, *American Journal of Clinical Nutrition* 10 (1962):181-199.

[22]Morgan, 1962.

[23]Rao, 1973.

On the other hand, if fat kcalories are restricted too much, the fat-soluble vitamins and linoleic acid may be deficient. Of the 20 percent of the kcalories to come from fat, most should be polyunsaturated to contribute linoleic acid, and to displace the saturated fat thought to contribute to high levels of cholesterol in the blood.

Carbohydrate   Another emphasis in the older person's diet should be on securing a wide variety of complex-carbohydrate foods to provide the associated vitamins and minerals. Older people often omit fruits and vegetables from their diets. It is not known whether this arises from lifelong habits or is due to their finding fruits and vegetables too expensive or too difficult to store and prepare. Any educational campaign designed to improve the diets of the elderly should emphasize the great nutritional value of fruits, vegetables, and grains. One congregate-meals group furnishes extra fruit for the participants to take home, in order to promote its use.[24]

Vitamins   Many of the problems seen in the elderly may result from decreased vitamin intakes. Vitamin deficiency is likely unless great care is taken to include foods from each of the food groups. Studies have shown that the one food group omitted most often by the elderly is the vegetable group, which would contribute vitamin A.[25] About 18 percent of older people are reported to eat no vegetables at all. Fruit, a contributor of vitamin C, is lacking in many diets (see Table 2), and 34 percent in one study reported never eating fruit.[26] Some men and women do not eat whole-grain breads and cereals, which would donate the B vitamins; the mental confusion sometimes exhibited by the elderly may be caused not by a loss of brain function but by a B-vitamin deficiency.[27] The destruction of vitamin E by heat processing and oxidation is well known; the processed and convenience foods so often used by the elderly and nursing homes may contribute to a vitamin E deficiency if their use continues over several years.[28] These statistics have somber implications for the health of older persons.

Not only the omission of food groups that contribute vitamins but also other conditions contribute to vitamin deficiency in the elderly. Many are house- or hospital-bound and thus are deprived of the vitamin D they would get from sunshine on their skin. Many take laxatives regularly (one study says 55 percent[29]), and this causes such a

Table 2   Vitamin C Intake of People 60 Years and Older (Ten-State Survey)

Category	Vitamin C intake (mg)
White males	30
White females	46
Black males	37
Black females	52
Spanish-American males	28
Spanish-American females	47

U.S. RDA for vitamin C: 60 mg

[24]J. Pelcovits, Nutrition to meet the human needs of older Americans, *Journal of the American Dietetic Association* 60 (1972):297-300.

[25]Lyons and Trulson, 1956.

[26]Pelcovits, 1972.

[27]Mayer, 1974.

[28]Morgan, 1962; and H. H. Koehler, H. C. Lee, and M. Jacobson, Tocopherols in canned entrees and vended sandwiches, *Journal of the American Dietetic Association* 70 (1977):616-620.

[29]M. Jordan, M. Kepes, R. B. Hayes, and W. Hammond, Dietary habits of persons living alone, *Geriatrics* 9 (1954):230-232.

rapid transit time through the intestine that many vitamins do not get absorbed. The use of mineral oil as a laxative robs the person of the fat-soluble vitamins in particular. Some drugs regularly taken by older adults interact with vitamins: Some antibiotics kill bacteria in the intestine that produce vitamin K, and anticonvulsant drugs produce a folic-acid deficiency.[30]

The recommended intakes for many of these vitamins are thought by some nutritionists to be too low for the over-65 group. They suggest supplements, particularly for the B vitamins and vitamin C, because toxicity from large amounts does not pose a great threat.[31] However, other nutritionists feel that recommending vitamin supplements is a "cop-out," laying the elderly open to exploitation by quacks.[32] Money is better spent, they say, on food of greater nutrient density.

Minerals   Calcium and iron are the minerals most often low in older adults' diets. Low hemoglobin levels, which correlate with low iron intake,[33] could be the cause of much of the fatigue and apathy experienced by the elderly. Decreased stomach acidity may also contribute, because iron is best absorbed in an acid environment. Serious loss of calcium from the bones, enough to cause osteoporosis, is probably best prevented by an adequate intake of calcium from infancy. Calcium excretion occurs every day throughout life, so the need for calcium remains constant with advancing age.[34]

Salt, which contains the mineral sodium, should be curtailed, not only by those with hypertension, congestive heart failure, or cirrhosis of the liver but by all older people.[35] Salt is conducive to the retention of fluid, which results in raised blood pressure. Convenience and processed foods are high in salt content and are widely used by older persons living alone, thus making it difficult for them to restrict their salt intakes. Wherever possible, fresh foods should be eaten instead.

To supply the needed minerals, the same rcommendation holds as for vitamins: Every food group should be represented in the diet every day. Milk especially should be included in some form. If liquid milk causes flatulence (gas), as some older people report,[36] then cheese should be included and dry skim milk should be incorporated into other foods.

---

[30]M. Balsley, M. F. Brink, and E. W. Speckman, Nutrition in disease and stress, *Geriatrics* 26 (1971):87-93.

[31]Lutwak, 1969; and Morgan, 1962. (Ratios to look for in B vitamin supplements are thiamin, 1.0 mg; riboflavin, 1.1; pyridoxine, 0.8; niacin, 9.0; pantothenic acid, 5.3. Morgan, 1962.)

[32]Mayer, 1974.

[33]Morgan, 1962.

[34]Mayer, 1974.

[35]Mayer, 1974.

[36]Swanson, 1964.

Fiber The fiber recommendations for the general population should be stressed to older citizens as well: Increase the use of fruits, vegetables, and whole-grain cereals. The fiber content of these food groups is important to the health of the muscles of the intestinal tract. If there is bulk for these muscles to work against, it will be less necessary to resort to the use of laxatives. In addition, some fibers (except wheat bran) bind cholesterol and carry it out of the body.

Water The elderly need to be reminded to drink fluids. They should drink six to eight glasses a day, enough to bring their urine output to about 1,500 ml (6 c) per day.[37] A large percentage of foster home operators note that one of the biggest problems with elderly patients is getting them to use more water and fruit juices.[38]

Those older adults most at risk nutritionally are those who overemphasize one food group to the exclusion of another and this is an especially common failing of older people. Whenever one food group is excluded, the vitamins and minerals donated by that group become deficient in the diet. Even small amounts of food from each food group may protect from an overt deficiency. An example of such a skewed diet would be that of a person who, for whatever reason, omits milk and dairy products. Calcium deficiencies would be expected, and osteoporosis would be likely to develop if the omission had been continuing for most of the adult years. In the same manner, someone who excludes meat and cereals might be expected to develop a zinc deficiency, which would impair the sense of taste. The familiar maxim holds throughout the life cycle: The best dietary guideline is to eat a balanced and varied selection of foods.

All of the above objectives may seem worthwhile, but they may be hard to achieve, especially for the person living alone who has difficulty buying groceries and preparing meals. Packages of meat and vegetables are often prewrapped in quantities suitable for a family of four or more, and even a head of lettuce will perish before one person can use it all. A large package of meat is often a good buy, but dividing and wrapping it in individual portions to be put away in the freezer is time-consuming and hardly seems worth the effort—especially when the packets may get "lost" in the freezer and ruined by freezer burn. For the person who has little or no freezer space, the problem of storage is further compounded. These problems can all be overcome (see Highlight 14 for many practical suggestions), but they can be overwhelming if morale is low—and nothing affects morale so profoundly as the loneliness of a person living in isolation.

[37]Rao, 1973.

[38]B. R. Bradshaw, W. P. Vonderhaar, V. T. Keeney, L. S. Tyler, and S. Harris, Community-based residential care for the minimally impaired elderly: A survival analysis, *Journal of the American Geriatrics Society* 24 (1976):423-429.

The Effect of Loneliness on Nutrition

Old age is a time of losses. Old friends are lost due to death or their moving away; offspring move away also and are too busy to write; there is loss of income on retirement and loss of status in the community. There is loss of control over the environment, as when the home that was to be a haven in retirement now sits in the middle of a high-crime area so that one can no longer walk the streets or visit with neighbors. The familiar shops and fruit stands, where a person knows the owner and is known by him, may close. The aging person develops a feeling of deep loneliness as the familiar environment constantly shifts. But what place, you may well ask, does such a discussion have in a book on nutrition?

Many authorities believe that malnutrition among the elderly is most often due to loneliness.[39] For the 6 million adults over 65 who live alone, the pressing need seems to be for companionship first, then for food. Without companionship, appetite decreases. The association of food with human companionship is built into our genes, and our very first experience with food was combined with human body contact. The social life of the adult is built around food. Most invitations into adults' homes are accompanied by an offer of food or drink. We must admit that feeding is, for human beings, as much a social and psychological event as a biological one.

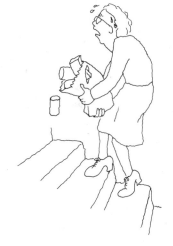

Having spent a lifetime internalizing the concept of food as part of a social activity, the older adult, alone all day every day, must exert a wrenching effort to place enough importance on the nutrient content of food to prepare it and eat it alone. The purchase, storage, and preparation of food and kitchen cleanup take a tremendous amount of energy. When the lonely, depressed person looks at the task, he forgets about his body's needs and says, "What's the use?"

Dr. Jack Weinberg, professor of psychiatry at the University of Illinois, wrote perceptively of this:

> In our efforts to provide the aged with a proper diet, we often fail to perceive it is not *what* the older person eats but *with whom* that will be the deciding factor in proper care for him. The oft-repeated complaints of the older patient that he has little incentive to prepare food for only himself is not merely a statement of fact but also a rebuke to the questioner for failing to perceive his isolation and aloneness and to realize that food . . . for one's self lacks the condiment of another's presence which can transform the simplest fare to the ceremonial act with all its shared meaning.[40]

[39]Mayer, 1974; Rao, 1973; Pelcovits, 1972; J. Weinberg, Psychologic implications of the nutritional needs of the elderly, *Journal of the American Dietetic Association* 60 (1972):293-296; L. M. Williams, A concept of loneliness in the elderly, *Journal of the American Geriatrics Society* 26 (1978):183-187; and J. Pelcovits, Nutrition for older Americans, *Journal of the American Dietetic Association* 58 (1971):17-21.

[40]Weinberg, 1972.

The lack of social interaction is no respecter of income. It is equally important in the lives of the financially secure and in the lives of the poverty-stricken. Newspapers occasionally carry stories of wealthy older persons being discovered in their mansions, alone and without food. The story is newsworthy because people wonder why the victim did not ask for help or make arrangements for someone to take care of her, since she had plenty of money. The answer is simple. Apathy evolves from loneliness; apathy is expressed in no action. The victim sits for long hours in a chair without the energy even to lift her arms. There is no energy to eat, even when food is just a phone call away. Without adequate food, nutrient deficiencies develop that increase the apathy and depression and eventually result in mental confusion. The downward spiral continues, unless the interference of neighbors or friends breaks it at some point.

Let's look at what happens when a person receives too little food. In the first place, the body can't tell why it is receiving too few nutrients or kcalories. The situation is the same for a child dying in a famine in Cambodia as for a wealthy solitary person who is depressed and refusing food. The B vitamins and vitamin C are quickly depleted, because they are needed daily. The first organ to suffer from deprivation is the brain. The B vitamins are necessary for the metabolism of the glucose energy that the brain requires. The brain responds by slowing down all muscular functions. This explains some of the apathy exhibited by the elderly who do not eat. If the carbohydrate kcalories and the B vitamins are not restored, mental confusion that resembles senility will be manifest and may even progress to hallucinations and insanity.

If protein foods, protected by complex carbohydrates, are insufficient, then enzymes to digest food and antibodies to protect against infection cannot be synthesized. When iron and vitamin C are absent, the protein hemoglobin cannot be made for the delivery of oxygen, so the feeling of weakness and tiredness grows. With tiredness due to lack of food added to the apathy from loneliness, there is even less energy with which to make the effort to secure nourishment. If the confusion of vitamin deficiency is diagnosed as senility, the elderly person may wrongly be confined to a nursing home.[41]

The story is told of a woman who took her mother-in-law to live with her while the older woman waited for a place in a nursing home. The mother-in-law had exhibited the classic signs of senility—mental confusion, inability to make decisions, forgetting to perform important tasks such as turning off a stove burner—so the family had decided she needed institutional care. After several weeks in the daughter-in-law's home—eating good meals and enjoying social stimulation—she became her old self again and returned to her home. This story has been repeated with many variations and serves to remind us to seek a

[41] Mayer, 1974.

careful medical diagnosis before concluding that a person is senile and needs institutional care. What harm could there be in first trying good, balanced meals served with plenty of tender, loving care?

Money and Other Worries

Most older citizens are in reasonably good health and have enough money to support themselves, if not in luxury at least not in poverty. When we look around us and see the great needs of some people, we sometimes overlook those who are enjoying their later years. They have leisure to pursue some of their favorite activities and are unencumbered for the first time in their lives by family responsibilities. These facts contradict the popular belief that older people are all poor, lonely, and ill. They are not; they are as individual as all other age segments. Grouping them into a stereotype is a disservice to everyone, especially to young adults who might project into their futures a depressing view of old age. Just as only a few teenagers are reckless drivers and only a minority of middle-age men are "squares," so only a third of the elderly are "poor" with the "typical problems" attributed to them. Aunt Charlotte at 77 jets every winter to Europe to enjoy the social life of Paris; Uncle James at 84 is out early every morning in his vegetable garden hoeing his cabbages; and it is only Grandma Sadie who at 82 is lonely, withdrawn, ill, and forgetful, a problem to her family. Two-thirds of the elderly are relatively free of major problems.

However, the one-third who live at or below the poverty line deserve our attention. In 1975, the average income of all older single people in the United States was $75 a week. Of aged black women, nearly half had a yearly income of under $1,000.[42] These people clearly need help in many areas, one of them being nutrition.

Most retired persons have a loss of real income that occurs because the retirement check is fixed while all other expenses are increasing. This has a direct effect on the amount of money spent on food, because food (and clothing) purchases are among the few flexible items in the budget. Costs of shelter, utilities, and medical care must be paid, and then the amount left over is stretched to cover food and other needs.

Forced to practice economy, the older person usually first eliminates so-called luxury items such as fresh fruit, vegetables, and milk. In some cases, transportation to and from the market is both expensive and difficult, so that use is made of a nearby convenience store. The foods offered there are limited in variety and are for the most part more expensive than the same items in the larger markets. The amount of food that can be purchased is thus curtailed even further, and eating,

---

[42] *Money, Income and Poverty Status of Families and Persons in the United States,* 1974-1975, Bureau of the Census, U.S. Department of Commerce.

one of the few pleasures left to the older person, becomes another reminder of reduced status.

Sometimes older people fall prey to food fads and fallacies. Led by false claims to believe that health can be improved, aging forestalled, and illness cured by magical food and nutrient preparations, they spend money needlessly on fraudulent health-food products, thus depleting their already limited funds.

Food Stamps

Two programs are helpful with older people's money problems, although they are not designed specifically for older people but for the poor of all ages. The Food Stamp program enables people who qualify (by way of showing low income or high expenses for dependent children or for medical bills) to stretch their food budgets. A part of the relief money is exchanged for food stamps which will buy more food than the money could have purchased. The Supplemental Security Income (SSI) program is aimed at directly improving the financial plight of the very poor, by increasing a person's or family's income to the defined poverty level. This sometimes helps older people retain their independence.

Supplemental Security Income

Besides loneliness, loss, and limited income, the older person faces an increased likelihood of illness and invalidism. Poor dental health, mental illness, and chronic alcoholism are other problems prevalent among the elderly. With all of these problems to live with and with the increasing numbers of people in the older age group, it is not surprising that at least a few individuals and agencies are concerned enough to ask what can be done to help.

Assistance Programs

In recent years we have come to recognize that the responsibility for support in old age cannot be left entirely to the individual. Two programs arising from this awareness have already been mentioned (the Food Stamp and Supplemental Security Income programs). The first venture into help for older persons grew out of the experiences of the Depression years of the 1930s. The Social Security Act was put into effect in 1935. Under this act, employees and employers pay into a fund that the employee collects benefits from when he retires.

Social Security

Title VII of the Older Americans Act

A second major political move to benefit the elderly was the Older Americans Act of 1965. Title VII of this act is an amendment, the Nutrition Program for the Elderly, which was signed into law by President Nixon in 1972. The major goals of this amendment are:

- Low-cost nutritious meals
- Opportunity for social interaction
- Auxiliary nutrition, homemaker education, and shopping assistance
- Counseling and referral to other social and rehabilitative services
- Transportation services

The nutrition program of Title VII was based on the belief that people living alone are apt to have poor nutrition. If their nutritional status could be improved, they might avoid medical problems, continue to live in communities of their own choice, and stay out of institutions. The program was not designed as charity, but during its first years, it was found that 80 percent of the participants had incomes less than $200 a month and 34 percent had incomes under $100 a month.[43]

Sites chosen for congregate meals under this program must be accessible to most of the target population. Church or school facilities are often used when they are conveniently located. Providing transportation increases the cost of meals by 20 to 30 percent, but often it is indispensable to the existence of a project. Some projects have been successful in recruiting volunteers to help with the transportation. Volunteers may also deliver meals to those who are homebound either permanently or temporarily: These efforts are known as Meals on Wheels. In 1977 there were about 350 such Meals on Wheels programs in the United States.[44]

Meals on Wheels

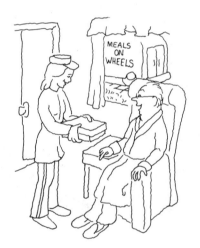

Every effort is made to persuade the elderly person to come to the congregate meal sites. The social atmosphere at the sites is as valuable as the nutrition. One participant was heard to remark, "It is better to come to the congregate meal and eat at a table with others, even if no one speaks to me, than it is to sit at home and stare at a wall while I eat."[45]

Independence is rated high by those over 65, and this is usually equated with staying in the home where they have lived many years. But this aloneness may not be a wise choice from a nutritional standpoint. There are alternatives that would enhance the elderly person's health without threatening independence. One alternative is covenant living, a lifestyle gaining in popularity. It is patterned after the communes of the young people of the 1960s, although the participants probably would deny this. A number of congenial people, wishing to live in a family group but having no family of their own, agree to live together. Sometimes they buy a house together or rent a house or, in some cases, rent the house of one of the members. The word *covenant* refers to the contractual agreements made among the parties before the arrangement begins. Sometimes it takes several months of talking to hammer out the details of problems that may arise.

The general work of running the house is shared. Either everyone shares equally, taking turns at various jobs, or there is a division based on what each person likes to do or can do well. There are definite economic advantages, but from a nutritional standpoint the main advantage is the sharing of meals and the relief from loneliness. One person described covenant living as coming out of solitary confinement into a warm family with the sound of laughter and people to touch.

[43] Pelcovits, 1972.

[44] Pelcovits, 1972.

Another way of gaining sociability while remaining independent is for several older persons to remain in their own homes but to meet together regularly for meals, each one taking a turn at preparing the food. Socialization encourages better food intake, and the one who prepares the food has leftovers to enjoy the next day. Some of the participants in the congregate meal programs have formed what they call a "diner's club" and go to restaurants in a group on the days when the congregate meal is not served. This kind of arrangement among friends helps improve the dietary intake of many older persons.

Another alternative is to move into a retirement community. Some of these are very expensive, but some have a rule that no one who has an income above a certain moderate amount is eligible. In these, a variety of living arrangements are available, from nursing home space to luxury apartments or separate homes on the grounds. In most, several services are maintained on the premises: an infirmary for slight illnesses, a restaurant, barber shops, and beauty salons. A daily check on persons who live alone is one of the valuable services.

Foster home care has proved to be an alternative for people who need some supportive care but do not need medical supervision. Foster homes have the advantage of being located within the community where the older person has lived, so that contact with friends and relatives can be maintained easily. The operators of such homes have no special qualifications and need help from nutritionists for some of their problems. One study of the problems of foster homes, involving 183 operators and 422 residents, showed the biggest problem they faced was the residents' lack of interest in food and their special diet needs. Guidance from nutritionists might help alert them to deteriorations that, if allowed to continue, would necessitate more expensive medical care.[46]

Churches and synagogues are ideal organizations to help with the problems of the elderly for a number of reasons: (1) they have neighborhood facilities that lie idle a good portion of the week, (2) they are "caring" organizations, (3) they have a target population, either among their own members or in their neighborhood, and (4) they have a reservoir of volunteers to help cut down on labor costs. Many religious organizations have taken the lead in establishing retirement and nursing homes. However, these facilities are very expensive and usually necessitate the resident's leaving her own community, which means leaving behind the people who care about her. In addition, a nursing home is a medical solution to what in many cases is a social problem.[47]

A group of churches in Kansas City discovered the many needs of older people when they started plans to establish a retirement

[45]Pelcovits, 1971.

[46]Bradshaw et al., 1976.

[47]R. L. Kane and R. A. Kane, Care of the aged: Old problems in need of new solutions, *Science* 200 (1978):913-919.

community.[48] Seven churches met together to build a nursing and retirement home and learned that what was really needed was a community service group capable of helping people remain in their own homes. The Shepherd's Center was the result of their planning. This center is now operated by 22 churches in the Kansas City area and has available eight home services, with new ones being made available as the need becomes apparent. The services are congregate meals in neighborhood churches; home delivery of hot meals; a shopping service that takes people to buy groceries or makes purchases for them; a transportation service to take persons to medical appointments; a visitation program in which volunteers keep in personal touch with truly isolated persons; a handyman service to make minor repairs to the home; a crime assistance program; and a team that responds to emergencies at any hour.

In addition to these home services, the Shepherd's Center offers classes on a wide range of topics that are taught by skilled or scholarly retired persons. Some 800 are currently enrolled, and there are long waiting lists for these classes. The discovery that retired persons are eager to learn new skills and explore new areas of knowledge has been the experience of many other such groups as well. Health care is one topic of prime importance to older persons, and they are especially eager to study nutrition.[49]

Only 5 percent of those over 65 live in nursing homes, but for those who need constant medical care, homes provide a less expensive facility than hospitals. Nursing homes are patterned after hospitals in their approach to the patient. Sometimes this is detrimental to the patient's attitude toward herself and her future. However, for some, especially the crippled, paralyzed, or bedridden, the nursing home offers a valuable service. There has been a great deal of unfavorable publicity about some substandard homes, which makes many older people frightened at the prospect of having to enter one. But investigation by relatives can identify a home that provides the kind of service the individual needs.

The relative inquiring into nursing homes should ask the director or dietitian some questions about the food service. Is a choice given the patient in the selection of food? How often are fresh fruits and vegetables served? Is a plate check conducted regularly, at least once a week, to discover what the patient is consuming? Alternatively, is there good communication between the nursing staff and the dietitian so that what a patient is not eating will be known by the dietitian? Is the patient encouraged and helped to go to the dining room to eat so that some socialization will occur? Are minced meats offered to those who have problems with their dentures? Are religious dietary restrictions

---

[48]E. C. Cole, An alternative to institutional care, *The Interpreter*, March 1975.

[49]Cole, 1975; and D. Boss, Reaching out: Diet and senior Americans, *Food Management* 12 (November 1977):70-73, 89, 91-93.

honored? How high a proportion of the foods are prepackaged? (No guide can be given for what proportion is desirable, but it should be remembered that processed foods are low in vitamin content and high in salt.) Other questions that the investigator will want to ask have to do with the general atmosphere of the nursing home, in recognition of the effect of social climate on a person's appetite. A nursing home that views residents as persons, not as patients, gets a mark in its favor.

Preparing for the Later Years

The programs just described can do much to help older people adjust to their changing circumstances, but the very best help we could give our elderly citizens would be a change of attitude. As a nation, we value the future more than the present, putting off enjoying today so that tomorrow we will have money or prestige or time to have fun. The elderly feel this loss of future. The present is their time for leisure and enjoyment, but they have no experience in the use of leisure time.

Our culture also values the doers, those concerned with action and achievement. The Mexican mother may enjoy her child because he is sitting in her lap and laughing in her face, but the mother in our culture is more likely to be preoccupied with asking herself how well he is preparing for tomorrow. The elderly are aware of the status given those who are doing something and of the disrespect given those who lead a contemplative life in retirement.

It would take a near miracle to change these attitudes, but there is a change each person can make in his attitude toward himself as he ages. Preparation for the later years should of course include financial planning, but other lifelong habits should be developed as well. Each adult needs to learn to reach out to others, to forestall the loneliness that will otherwise ensue. Each needs to learn some skills or activities that can continue into the later years—volunteer work with organizations, reading, games, hobbies, or intellectual pursuits—which will give meaning to the activities of the days. One also needs to develop the habit of adjusting to change, especially when it comes without consent, so that it will not be seen as a loss of control over life. The goal is to arrive at maturity with as healthy a mind and body as it is possible to have, and this means cultivating good nutritional status and maintaining a program of daily exercise.

Preparation for the later years begins early in life, both psychologically and nutritionally. Everyone knows older people who have gathered around themselves many contacts—through relatives, church, synagogue, or fraternal orders—and have not allowed themselves to drift into isolation. Upon analysis, you will see that their favorable environment came through a lifetime of effort. They spent their entire lives reaching out to others and practicing the art of weaving themselves into other people's lives. Likewise, a lifetime of effort is

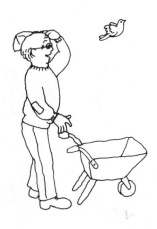

required for good nutritional status in the later years. A person who has eaten a wide variety of foods, has stayed lean by using nutrient-dense foods, and has remained physically active will best be able to withstand the assaults of change.

Summing Up

With adulthood comes aging. The aging process is natural and in some ways cannot be prevented. Life still ends at about 70 for most people; the increase in the number of older people seen in U.S. Census reports does not reflect an increase in life expectancy but an increase in the number of people surviving the early years.

Cells may age for any of several reasons: They may accumulate debris; they may lose the ability to read the genetic code words that specify their functions; they may make wrong proteins, to which the body reacts by producing antibodies; or they may be programmed to divide a definite number of times before they die. Cellular aging is reflected in such familiar phenomena as the wrinkling of the skin, loss of digestive functions, loss of responsiveness to such change as increased blood glucose, loss of elasticity of blood vessels, and loss of function of the kidneys. The brain and nervous system lose cells, and those that remain slow down in reaction time. To some extent these changes can be slowed by maintaining a strong cardiovascular and respiratory system by means of regular exercise. Adult bone loss (osteoporosis) is least likely in those whose bones were dense at maturity, thanks to good mineral and vitamin nutrition in the early years. Some calcium loss does occur in aging, however. For many, arthritis makes movement difficult and painful.

Nutritional requirements of the older person are for fewer kcalories, increased protein, reduced fat, sufficient complex carbohydrates, sufficient vitamins and minerals (especially vitamin C, iron, and calcium), adequate water intake (six or seven glasses a day), and ample fiber (roughage) from fruits, vegetables, and whole grains. Meals should be regular and, as far as possible, prepared from fresh ingredients. The enjoyment of food is enhanced if loneliness—a major problem of older people living alone—can be alleviated. Eating with others often restores the appetite and health that may seem to be failing due to degenerative disease.

Having enough money is basic to coping with the nutritional problems of the later years. Government programs designed to help by providing money, either directly or for food, include Social Security, the Food Stamp program, and the Supplemental Security Income program. A government program that provides both food and settings to enjoy it in is the Nutrition Program for the Elderly, which includes both congregate meals and Meals on Wheels. Alternatives to institutional care are desirable to preserve the older person's independence; among the possibilities are covenant living, diners' clubs, retirement communities, and foster home care. When a nursing home is chosen, its food service should be examined for characteristics that will facilitate good nutrition and appetite.

Old age need not be a time of despair, isolation, and ill health. Preparation for enjoyable later years should include financial planning, the establishment of lasting social contacts, the learning of skills and activities that can be pursued into later life, the maintenance of a program of regular physical activity, and the cultivation of healthy nutritional status throughout life.

To Explore Further

We recommend highly these books on aging:

Comfort, A., *A Good Age* (New York: Crown, 1976).

Puner, M., *To the Good Long Life* (New York: Universe Books, 1974).

A book that helps the reader understand the medical-social problems that develop with aging is:

Field, M., *The Aged, the Family, and the Community* (New York: Columbia University Press, 1972), which emphasizes the need to preserve the older individual's feelings of worth and to safeguard his dignity.

The *Journal of the American Geriatrics Society* and *The Gerontologist* make good reading for the general reader.

A short article that takes a positive approach toward the nutritional problems of older people and presents up-to-date information on them is:

Rowe, D., Aging: A jewel in the mosaic of life, *Journal of the American Dietetic Association* 72 (1978):478-486.

Some persuasive arguments in favor of older people's needing higher RDAs than young adults are advanced by Munro, H. N., Major gaps in nutrient allowances, *Journal of the American Dietetic Association* 76 (1980):137-141.

Practical pointers on buying, preparing, and cooking food can be found in:

Peterkin, B., *Your Money's Worth in Foods*, a 29-page pamphlet available for $.60 from Home and Garden Bulletin, U.S. Government Printing Office, Washington, DC 20402.

Although originally intended for dieters, Nidetch, J., *Weight Watchers Program Cookbook* (Great Neck, N.Y.: Hearthside Press, 1973) is useful for older people. Many of the recipes are for one or two servings. And they are low in saturated fat and sugar, which enhances their value. Nidetch has experimented with standard "down home" recipes to lower saturated fat and sugar content. Her dessert recipes using dry skim milk are especially recommended.

For help in detecting and avoiding fraudulent products and claims, see U.S. Senate, Special Committee on Aging, *Frauds and Deceptions Affecting the Elderly*, a 1965 publication available from the U.S. Government Printing Office, Washington, DC 20402.

For help in finding all the retirement communities in your area, contact Retirement, Research, and Welfare Association, Andrus Building, 215 Long Beach Boulevard, Long Beach, CA 90802.

A technique for assessing the nutritional care offered by a nursing home is outlined in Davies, L., and Holdsworth, M.D., A technique for assessing nutritional 'at-risk' factors in residential homes for the elderly, *Journal of Human Nutrition* 33 (1979): 165-169.

The Space Age has brought the development of convenience foods, originally intended for use by astronauts but remarkably tasty and handy for the older person living alone. You can obtain freeze-dried meals for one person—containing a quarter pound of meat, vegetable, fruit, dessert, and beverage—from Easy Meal, Oregon Freeze Dry Foods, Inc., PO Box 1048, 770 West 29th Avenue, Albany, OR 97321. The 1978 price was five for $10. These meals, which require no refrigeration, can be converted into hot meals in ten minutes.

Among the many films and teaching aids that promote understanding of aging are:

Pelcovits, J., Nutrition education for older Americans, *Cassette-a-Month*, February 1977, available from the American Dietetic Association (address in Appendix J).

The String Bean, a 15- to 20-minute long film, a hauntingly poetic masterpiece portraying an old lady's devotion to life, love, and beauty. Available from McGraw-Hill Films, in care of Association Films, Inc., 600 Grand Avenue, Ridgefield, NJ 07657.

APPENDIX A

History of Discoveries in Biochemistry and Nutrition

As early as 1500 B.C., scurvy was described by the Egyptians in the Ebers papyrus, discovered at Thebes. All peoples since that time (and perhaps before) have attempted to diagnose and treat diseases. Understanding of the scientific principles underlying health and the life process followed speculation by da Vinci in the 16th century and Van Helmont in the 17th century that animal nutrition was in some way similar to the burning of a candle. Real progress in the history of biochemistry and nutrition began to be made in the latter half of the eighteenth century and has been accelerating ever since.[1] The following are a few selected major events in that history, up to 1953. Since then, significant events have become too numerous to mention.

1753	Lind used limes to prevent scurvy in British sailors.
1770-1774	Priestley discovered oxygen and showed that it was produced by plants and consumed by animals.
1770-1786	Scheele first isolated an organic compound, glycerol, from natural sources, as well as citric, malic, lactic, and uric acids.
1773	Rouelle isolated urea from urine.
1780-1789	Lavoisier demonstrated that animal life depends on oxygen, showed that respiration is oxidation, and first measured oxygen consumption in a human being.

[1]Dates and events are those given in A. L. Lehninger, *Biochemistry* (New York: Worth, 1970); and in M. G. Wohl and R. S. Goodhart, eds., *Modern Nutrition in Health and Disease*, 4th ed. (Philadelphia: Lea and Febiger, 1968).

1783	Spallanzani proposed that gastric digestion of proteins is a chemical process.
1806	Vauquelin and Robiquet first isolated an amino acid, asparagine.
1807	Bardsley reported that cod liver oil was effective against osteomalacia.
1811	Courtois discovered iodine while preparing saltpeter from seaweed for Napoleon's army.
1820	Coindet reported curing goiter with iodine.
1828	Wöhler synthesized the first organic compound, urea.
1833	Payen and Persoz purified the enzyme diastase (amylase) from wheat.
1838	Schleiden and Schwann theorized that the basic unit of life was the cell.
1838	Mulder initiated systematic study of proteins.
1850-1855	Bernard isolated glycogen from the liver and showed that it is a source of blood glucose.
1862	Sachs showed that photosynthesis results in the production of starch.
1864	Hoppe-Seyler crystallized a protein, hemoglobin.
1867	Huber purified nicotinic acid (niacin).
1872	Pfluger proved that oxygen is used in all animal tissues, not only blood or lungs.
1877	Kühne proposed the term *enzyme*.
1882	Takaki cured beriberi in the

A

Japanese army by substituting natural and whole-grain foods for polished rice.

1890   Lam suggested that sunlight was effective against rickets.

1893   Ostwald proved that enzymes are catalysts.

1894   Fischer showed the specificity of enzymes and enunciated the lock-and-key model as the way enzymes fit their substrates.

1897   Eijkman reported causing polyneuritis (beriberi) in hens by feeding them polished rice.

1901   Grijns originated the idea of a deficiency disease, suggesting that polyneuritis was due to the lack of something.

1902   Fischer and Hofmeister showed that proteins are polypeptides.

1905   Harden and Young isolated the first coenzyme (NAD).

1905   Knoop reported details of the oxidation of fatty acids.

1906   Eijkman showed that a water-soluble extract from rice polishings can cure beriberi.

1911   Funk isolated niacin from rice polishings and coined the word *vitamine.*

1912   Warburg showed that iron is required for respiration.

1915   McCollum and Davis first described "fat-soluble A," later named vitamin A.

1916   McCollum and Kennedy further purified "water-soluble B" from rice polishings that contained the antiberiberi substance.

1917   McCollum and Simmonds demonstrated that xerophthalmia was due specifically to lack of a fat-soluble vitamin.

1917-1918   Marine confirmed that iodine deficiency caused goiter.

1919   Huldchinsky cured rickets with ultraviolet rays from a mercury vapor lamp.

1920   Rosenheim and Drummond showed that carotene in plants had a biological activity similar to that of vitamin A.

1922   McCollum proved that cod liver oil contains two vitamins (A and D) and showed that vitamin D deficiency causes rickets.

1923-1924   Evans, Bishop, and others showed a dietary fat-soluble factor (vitamin E) to be essential for reproduction in the rat.

1926   Smith and Hendrick divided "water-soluble B" into antiberiberi and antipellagra fractions; Jansen and Donath isolated vitamin B_1 (thiamin).

1927   Windaus showed that ergosterol is a vitamin D precursor.

1928   Euler isolated carotene.

1928   Szent-Györgyi isolated hexuronic acid from orange juice, cabbage juice, and the adrenal glands of oxen. In the same year, Waugh and King showed that it was identical to the antiscorbutic substance, vitamin C, which they had isolated from lemon juice. Haworth determined its structure and Reichstein synthesized it.

1929   Dam described a hemorrhagic disease in chicks fed a fat-free diet and later showed this to be due to vitamin K deficiency.

1930   Moore showed that carotene is converted to vitamin A in animal tissues.

1930-1933   Northrup crystallized pepsin and trypsin and showed they were proteins.

1932   Warburg and Christian identified a yellow enzyme needed for respiration.

1934   Szent-Györgyi recognized and named vitamin B_6.

1935   Williams and his colleagues determined the structure of vitamin B_1.

1935   Rose discovered the last amino acid, threonine.

1935	Best showed choline essential in animals.	1939-1941	Lipmann suggested that ATP plays a central role in energy metabolism.
1935	Kuhn discovered that riboflavin (vitamin B_2) is part of the yellow enzyme discovered by Warburg and Christian.	1940	Williams and Major synthesized pantothenic acid and showed it cures the deficiency disease dermatitis in chicks.
1936	Williams established the structure of thiamin (vitamin B_1).	1945	Tucker and Eckstein showed that choline and methionine are methyl donors in transmethylation reactions.
1936	Evans, Emerson, and Emerson isolated pure vitamin E from wheat germ oil.	1945	Angier and his associates synthesized folacin.
1937	Krebs reported details of the tricarboxylic acid cycle (Krebs cycle or TCA cycle).	1947-1950	Lipmann and Kaplan isolated and characterized coenzyme A.
1938	Elvehjem, Madden, Strong, and Wooley's work led to recognition that nicotinic acid (niacin) is a vitamin and cures a deficiency disease, blacktongue, in dogs. Soon after, niacin was confirmed as the human antipellagra vitamin.	1948	Rickes and associates isolated crystalline vitamin B_{12}.
		1951	Lehninger showed that ATP is generated from the electron transport chain.
1938	Karrer, Fritzsche, Ringier, and Salomon reported the structure and synthesis of vitamin E.	1951	Pauling and Corey postulated the alpha-helical structure of proteins.
1938	Braunstein and Kritzmann discovered transamination reactions.	1953	Sanger deduced the amino acid sequence of a protein, insulin.
1938	Williams isolated pantothenic acid.	1953	Watson and Crick published the structure of DNA.
1939	Doisy and Dam independently announced the isolation of vitamin K.		

APPENDIX B

Summary of Basic Chemistry Concepts

CONTENTS

This appendix is intended to provide the background in basic chemistry that you need to understand the nutrition concepts presented in this book.

Chemistry is the branch of natural science that is concerned with the description and classification of matter, with the changes that matter undergoes, and with the energy associated with these changes. **Matter** is anything that takes up space and has mass. **Energy** is the ability to do work.

Matter: The Properties of Atoms

Every substance has characteristics or properties that distinguish it from all other substances and thus give it a unique identity. These properties are both physical and chemical. The physical properties include such characteristics as color, taste, texture, and odor, as well as the temperatures at which a substance changes its state (changes from a solid to a liquid or from a liquid to a gas) and the weight of a unit volume (its density). The chemical properties of a substance have to do with how it reacts with other substances or responds to a change in its environment so that new substances with different sets of properties are produced.

A physical change is one that does not change a substance's chemical composition. For example, when ice changes to liquid water and to steam, two hydrogen atoms and one oxygen atom remain bound together in all three states. However, a chemical change does occur if an electric current is passed through water. The water disappears, and two different substances are formed: hydrogen gas, which is flammable, and oxygen gas, which supports life. Chemical changes are also referred to as **chemical reactions**.

Substances: Elements and Compounds

Molecules are the smallest particles of a substance that retain all the properties of that substance. If the molecules of a substance are composed of atoms that are all alike, the substance is an **element.** If the molecules are composed of two or more different kinds of atoms, the substance is a **compound**.

Just over 100 elements are known, and these are listed in Table 1. A familiar example is hydrogen, whose molecules are composed only of hydrogen atoms linked together in pairs (H_2). On the other hand, over a million compounds are known. An example is the sugar glucose: Each of its molecules is composed of 6 carbon, 6 oxygen, and 12 hydrogen atoms linked together in a specific arrangement (as described in Chapter 1).

The Nature of Atoms   Atoms themselves are made of smaller particles. The atomic nucleus contains **protons** (positively charged particles);

Table 1   Chemical Symbols for the Elements

Number of protons (atomic number)	Element	Number of electrons in outer shell	Number of protons (atomic number)	Element	Number of electrons in outer shell
1	Hydrogen (H)	1	52	Tellurium (Te)	6
2	Helium (He)	2	53	Iodine (I)	7
3	Lithium (Li)	1	54	Xenon (Xe)	8
4	Beryllium (Be)	2	55	Cesium (Cs)	1
5	Boron (B)	3	56	Barium (Ba)	2
6	Carbon (C)	4	57	Lanthanum (La)	2
7	Nitrogen (N)	5	58	Cerium (Ce)	2
8	Oxygen (O)	6	59	Praseodymium (Pr)	2
9	Fluorine (F)	7	60	Neodymium (Nd)	2
10	Neon (Ne)	8	61	Promethium (Pm)	2
11	Sodium (Na)	1	62	Samarium (Sm)	2
12	Magnesium (Mg)	2	63	Europium (Eu)	2
13	Aluminum (Al)	3	64	Gadolinium (Gd)	2
14	Silicon (Si)	4	65	Terbium (Tb)	2
15	Phosphorus (P)	5	66	Dysprosium (Dy)	2
16	Sulfur (S)	6	67	Holmium (Ho)	2
17	Chlorine (Cl)	7	68	Erbium (Er)	2
18	Argon (Ar)	8	69	Thulium (Tm)	2
19	Potassium (K)	1	70	Ytterbium (Yb)	2
20	Calcium (Ca)	2	71	Lutetium (Lu)	2
21	Scandium (Sc)	2	72	Hafnium (Hf)	2
22	Titanium (Ti)	2	73	Tantalum (Ta)	2
23	Vanadium (V)	2	74	Tungsten (W)	2
24	Chromium (Cr)	1	75	Rhenium (Re)	2
25	Manganese (Mn)	2	76	Osmium (Os)	2
26	Iron (Fe)	2	77	Iridium (Ir)	2
27	Cobalt (Co)	2	78	Platinum (Pt)	1
28	Nickel (Ni)	2	79	Gold (Au)	1
29	Copper (Cu)	1	80	Mercury (Hg)	2
30	Zinc (Zn)	2	81	Thallium (Tl)	3
31	Gallium (Ga)	3	82	Lead (Pb)	4
32	Germanium (Ge)	4	83	Bismuth (Bi)	5
33	Arsenic (As)	5	84	Polonium (Po)	6
34	Selenium (Se)	6	85	Astatine (At)	7
35	Bromine (Br)	7	86	Radon (Rn)	8
36	Krypton (Kr)	8	87	Francium (Fr)	1
37	Rubidium (Rb)	1	88	Radium (Ra)	2
38	Strontium (Sr)	2	89	Actinium (Ac)	2
39	Yttrium (Y)	2	90	Thorium (Th)	2
40	Zirconium (Zr)	2	91	Protactinium (Pa)	2
41	Niobium (Nb)	1	92	Uranium (U)	2
42	Molybdenum (Mo)	1	93	Neptunium (Np)	2
43	Technetium (Tc)	1	94	Plutonium (Pu)	2
44	Ruthenium (Ru)	1	95	Americium (Am)	2
45	Rhodium (Rh)	1	96	Curium (Cm)	2
46	Palladium (Pd)	—	97	Berkelium (Bk)	2
47	Silver (Ag)	1	98	Californium (Cf)	2
48	Cadmium (Cd)	2	99	Einsteinium (Es)	2
49	Indium (In)	3	100	Fermium (Fm)	2
50	Tin (Sn)	4	101	Mendelevium (Md)	2
51	Antimony (Sb)	5	102	Nobelium (No)	2

B

and **electrons** (negatively charged particles) surround the nucleus. Because opposite charges attract, the number of protons (+) in the nucleus of an atom determines the number of electrons (−) around it. The positive charge on a proton is equal to the negative charge on an electron, so that the charges cancel each other out and leave the atom neutral.

The nucleus may also include **neutrons**, subatomic particles that have no charge. Protons and neutrons are of equal mass, and together they give an atom its weight. Electrons are of negligible mass but represent the atom's chemical energy.

Each type of atom has a characteristic number of protons in its nucleus. The hydrogen atom (symbol H) is the simplest of all. It possesses a single proton, with a single electron associated with it:

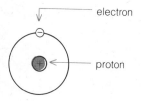

Hydrogen atom (H), atomic number 1.

Just as hydrogen always has one proton, helium always has two, lithium three, and so on. The **atomic number** of each type of atom represents the number of protons it contains. The atomic number never changes; it gives the atom its identity. All of the known atomic elements are listed in Table 1, and their atomic numbers are shown.

All atoms except hydrogen also have neutrons in their nuclei, and these contribute to their atomic weight. Helium, for example, has two neutrons in its nucleus in addition to its two protons, for a total of four nuclear particles and an atomic weight of 4. However, only the two protons are charged, and these determine the number of electrons the atom has. The number of electrons determines how the atom will chemically react with other atoms. Hence the

atomic number, not the weight, is what gives an atom its chemical nature.

Besides hydrogen, the atoms most common in living things are carbon (C), nitrogen (N), and oxygen (O), whose atomic numbers are 6, 7, and 8 respectively. Their structures are more complicated than that of hydrogen. Each possesses a number of electrons equal to the number of protons in its nucleus. These electrons have two energy levels, symbolized in the following diagrams as two orbits, or shells:

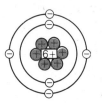

Carbon atom (C), atomic number 6.

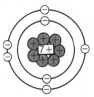

Nitrogen atom (N), atomic number 7.

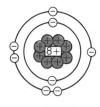

Oxygen atom (O), atomic number 8.

In this and all diagrams of atoms that follow, only the protons and electrons are shown. The neutrons, which contribute only to atomic weight, not to charge, are omitted.

The shells closest to the nucleus are occupied by electrons of lesser energy. Thus the two electrons in the first shells of carbon, nitrogen, and oxygen have less energy than the electrons in their second or outer shells. Also, the first shell can hold only two electrons; when it is full, it is in a very stable energy state, or a state of lowest energy.

The most important structural feature of an atom for determining its chemical behavior is the number of electrons in its outer shell. The first shell is full when it is occupied by two electrons, so an atom with three protons has a filled first shell. Its third electron posssesses greater energy and has a greater probability of being farther from the nucleus. In other words, the third electron is not so tightly bound as the first two and has a high probability of flying off to join other substances in chemical reactions. As a matter of fact, lithium, atomic number 3, is just such a highly reactive element.

The second shell is completely full when it has eight electrons. A substance that has a full outer shell tends to enter into no chemical reactions. Atomic number 10, neon, is a chemically inert substance, because its outer shell is complete. Fluorine, atomic number 9, has a great tendency to draw an electron from other substances to complete its outer shell and thus is highly reactive. Carbon has a half-full outer shell, which helps explain its great versatility; it can combine with other elements in a great variety of ways to form a large number of compounds.

Atoms seek to reach a state of maximum stability or of lowest energy in the same way that a ball will roll down a hill until it reaches the lowest place. An atom achieves a state of maximum stability by two means:

● By having a filled outer shell (occupied by the maximum number of electrons it can hold)

● By being electrically neutral

In order to achieve this stability, an atom may become bonded to other atoms.

Chemical Bonding

Atoms often complete their outer shells by sharing electrons with other atoms. In order to complete its outer shell, a carbon atom requires four electrons. A hydrogen atom requires one. Thus when a carbon atom shares electrons with four hydrogen atoms, each completes its outer shell:

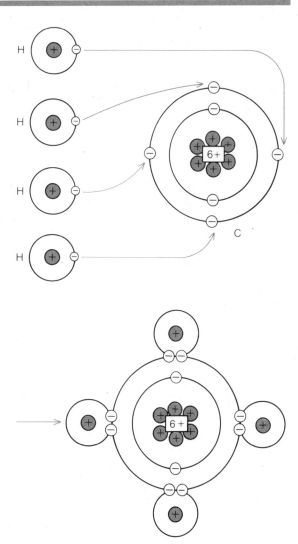

Methane molecule. The **chemical formula** for methane is CH_4. (Note that with the sharing of electrons, every atom has a filled outer shell.)

This electron sharing binds the atoms together and satisfies the conditions of maximum stability for the molecule: The outer shell of each atom is complete, since hydrogen effectively has the required two electrons in its first and outer shell and carbon has eight electrons in its second and outer shell; and the molecule is electrically neutral, with a total of ten protons and ten electrons.

Bonds that involve the sharing of electrons, like the bond between carbon and hydrogen, are the most stable kind of association that atoms can form with one another. They are sometimes called **covalent bonds**, and the resulting combinations of atoms are called molecules. A single pair of shared electrons forms a **single bond**. A simplified way to represent a single bond is with a single line. Thus the structure of methane could be represented (ignoring the inner-shell electrons that do not participate in bonding):

$$\begin{array}{c} H \\ | \\ H-C-H \\ | \\ H \end{array}$$

Methane (**chemical structure**).

Similarly, one nitrogen atom and three hydrogen atoms can share electrons to form one molecule of ammonia:

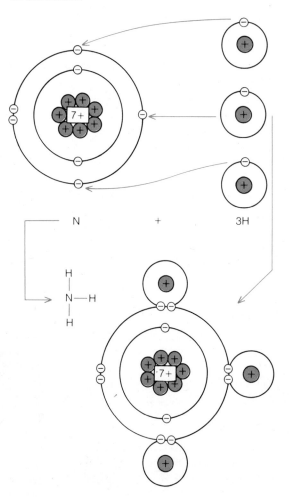

Similarly, one oxygen atom may be bonded to two hydrogen atoms to form one molecule of water:

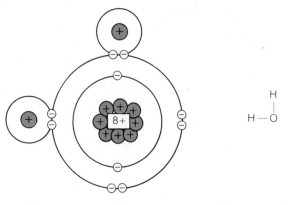

$$\begin{array}{c} H \\ | \\ H-O \end{array}$$

Water molecule (H_2O).

When two oxygen atoms form a molecule of oxygen, they must share two pairs of electrons. This **double bond** may be represented as two single lines:

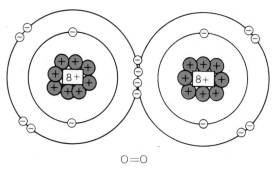

$$O=O$$

Oxygen molecule (O_2).

Small atoms form the tightest, most stable bonds. H, O, N, and C are the smallest atoms capable of forming one, two, three, and four electron-pair bonds (respectively). This fact is the basis for the simple statement in Chapter 1 that when you draw compounds containing these atoms, hydrogen must always have one, oxygen two, nitrogen three, and carbon four lines radiating to other atoms:

Ammonia molecule (NH_3). (Count the electrons in each atom's outer shell.)

$$H-\quad -O-\quad \overset{|}{\underset{|}{N}}-\quad \overset{|}{\underset{|}{C}}-$$

The stability of the associations between these small atoms and the versatility with which they can combine make them very common in living things. Interestingly, all cells, whether they come from animals, plants, or bacteria, contain the same elements in very nearly the same proportions.[1] The atomic elements found in living things are shown in Table 2.

Formation of Ions

An atom such as sodium (Na, atomic number 11) is more likely to lose an electron than to share electrons. Sodium possesses a filled inner shell of two electrons and a filled second shell of eight; there is only one electron in its outermost shell:

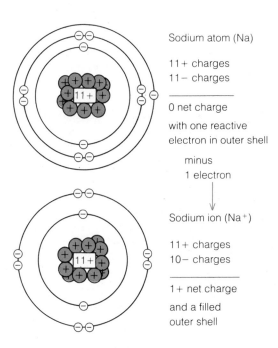

Sodium atom (Na)

11+ charges
11− charges
_____
0 net charge

with one reactive
electron in outer shell

minus
1 electron
↓
Sodium ion (Na⁺)

11+ charges
10− charges
_____
1+ net charge
and a filled
outer shell

[1]V. Rodwell, Appendix: Organic chemistry (a brief review), in *Review of Physiological Chemistry*, ed. H. Harper (Los Altos, Calif.: Lange Medical Publications, 1971), p. 499.

If sodium loses this electron, it satisfies one condition for stability: a filled outer shell (now its second shell counts as the outer shell). However, it is not electrically neutral. It has 11 protons (positive) and only 10 electrons (negative). It therefore is positively charged. Such a structure is called an **ion**—an atom or molecule that has lost or gained one or more electrons and so is electrically charged.

An atom such as chlorine (Cl, atomic number 17) is likely to gain an electron for a similar reason. It possesses filled inner shells of two and eight electrons and has seven electrons in its outermost shell. Gaining one electron makes its outer shell complete and thus makes it a negatively charged ion:

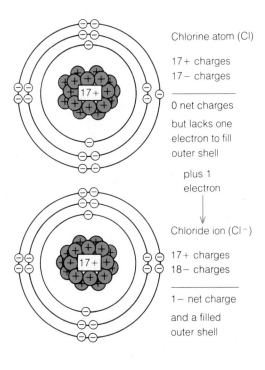

Chlorine atom (Cl)

17+ charges
17− charges
_____
0 net charges

but lacks one
electron to fill
outer shell

plus 1
electron
↓
Chloride ion (Cl⁻)

17+ charges
18− charges
_____
1− net charge
and a filled
outer shell

A positively charged ion such as a sodium ion (Na⁺) is a **cation**; a negatively charged ion such as chloride ion (Cl⁻) is an **anion**. Cations and anions attract one another to form **salts**:

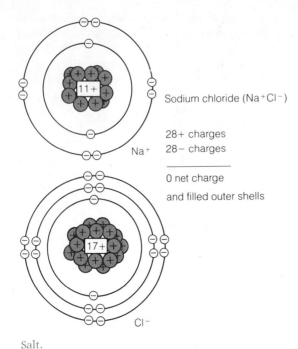

Sodium chloride (Na^+Cl^-)

28+ charges
28− charges
_____
0 net charge

and filled outer shells

Na^+

Cl^-

Salt.

Table 2 Elemental Composition of Living Cells

Element	Chemical symbol	Composition by weight (%)
Oxygen	O	65
Carbon	C	18
Hydrogen	H	10
Nitrogen	N	3
Calcium	Ca	1.5
Phosphorus	P	1.0
Sulfur	S	0.25
Sodium	Na	0.15
Magnesium	Mg	0.05
TOTAL		99.30*

*The remaining 0.70 percent by weight is contributed by the trace elements: copper (Cu), zinc (Zn), selenium (Se), molybdenum (Mo), fluorine (F), chlorine (Cl), iodine (I), manganese (Mn), cobalt (Co), iron (Fe). There are also variable traces of some of the following in cells: lithium (Li), strontium (Sr), aluminum (Al), silicon (Si), lead (Pb), vanadium (V), arsenic (As), bromium (Br), and others.

With all its electrons, sodium is a shiny, highly reactive metal; chlorine is the poisonous greenish-yellow gas that was used in World War I. But after they have transferred electrons, they form the harmless white salt familiar to you as table salt, or sodium chloride (Na^+Cl^-). The dramatic difference illustrates how profoundly the electron arrangement can influence the nature of a substance. The wide distribution of salt in nature attests to the stability of the union between the ions. Each meets the other's needs (a good marriage).

When dry, salt exists as crystals; its ions are stacked very regularly into a lattice, with positive and negative ions alternating in a sort of three-dimensional checkerboard structure. In water, however, the salt quickly dissolves, and its ions separate from each other, forming an electrolyte solution in which they move about freely. Covalently bonded molecules do not dissociate like this in water solution. Molecules and ion pairs (salts) behave very differently in many ways.

An ion can also be a group of atoms bound together in such a way that the group has a charge and enters into reactions as a single unit. Many such groups are active in the fluids of the body: The bicarbonate ion is composed of five atoms—one H, one C, and three Os—and has a net charge of −1 (HCO_3^-). Another important ion of this type is a phosphate ion with one H, one P, and four Os, and a net charge of −2 (HPO_4^{-2}). (For a description of the behavior of salts in water, electrolytes, and osmosis, which follows from this, see Chapter 14.)

Whereas many elements have only one configuration in the outer shell and thus only one way they can bond with other elements, some elements have the possibility of varied configurations. Iron is such an element. Under some conditions iron has two electrons in its outer shell, and under other circumstances it has three. If iron has two electrons in its outer shell and loses them, it then has a net charge of +2, and we call it ferrous iron. If it has three electrons in its outer shell and donates them, it becomes the +3 ion, or ferric iron.

(Note: It is important to remember that a positive charge on an ion means that negative charges—electrons—have been lost and not that positive charges have been added. If you could add two protons to an iron atom, they would go to the nucleus, adding 2 to its atomic number. Then it would no longer be iron, atomic number 26, but nickel, atomic number 28—and it would gain two more electrons to balance its positive charges.)

Ferrous iron.

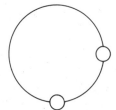

Ferrous iron (Fe^{++})
(had 2 outer-shell
electrons but has
lost them)

26+ charges
24− charges
_____
2+ net charge

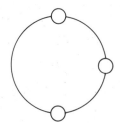

Ferric iron (Fe^{+++})
(had 3 outer-shell
electrons but has
lost them)

26+ charges
23− charges
_____
3+ net charge

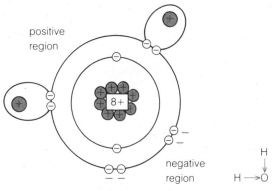

A polar molecule

The arrows show displacement of electrons toward the O nucleus, so the negative region is near the O, the positive region near the Hs.

Water (H$_2$O).

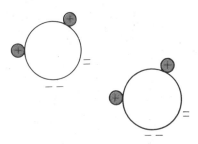

Water, Acids, and Bases

The water molecule is electrically neutral, having an equal number of protons and electrons. However, if the hydrogen atom is to share its one electron with oxygen, that electron must spend most of its time near the large positively charged oxygen nucleus on the oxygen side of the hydrogen atom. This leaves the positive proton (nucleus of the hydrogen atom) exposed on the outer part of the water molecule. We know, too, that the two hydrogens both bond toward the same side of the oxygen. These two ideas explain the fact that water molecules are **polar**: They have regions of more positive and more negative charge.

Polar molecules like water are drawn to one another by the attractive forces between the positive polar areas of one and the negative poles of another. These attractive forces, sometimes known as polar or **hydrogen bonds**, occur among many molecules and also within the different parts of single large molecules. Although very weak in comparison to covalent bonds, polar bonds may occur in such abundance that they become exceedingly important in determining the structure of such large molecules as proteins and DNA.

Water molecules have a slight tendency to ionize, separating into positive and negative ions. In any given amount of pure water, a small but constant number of these ions is present, and the number of positive ions exactly equals the number of negative ions.

An **acid** is a substance that releases H$^+$ ions (protons) in water solution. Hydrochloric acid (HCl) is such a substance, because it dissociates in water solution into H$^+$ and Cl$^-$ ions. Acetic acid is also an acid, because it ionizes in water to acetate ions and free H$^+$:

B

(structural formula showing acetic acid dissociation:)

$$H-\underset{\underset{H}{|}}{\overset{\overset{H}{|}}{C}}-\overset{\overset{O}{\|}}{C}-O-H \longrightarrow H-\underset{\underset{H}{|}}{\overset{\overset{H}{|}}{C}}-\overset{\overset{O}{\|}}{C}-O^- \;+\; H^+$$

Acetic acid dissociates into an acetate ion and a hydrogen ion.

The more H^+ ions free in a water solution, the stronger the acid.

Chemists define degrees of acidity by means of the **pH scale.** The pH scale runs from 0 to 14. A pH of 1 is extremely acidic, 7 is neutral, and 13 is very basic. There is a tenfold difference between points on this scale. A solution with pH 3, for example, has *ten times* as many H^+ ions as a solution with pH 4. At pH 7, the concentrations of free H^+ and OH^- are exactly the same, 1/10,000,000 moles per liter (10^{-7} moles per liter).[2] At pH 4, the concentration of free H^+ ions is 1/10,000 (10^{-4}) moles per liter. This is a higher concentration of H^+ ions, and the solution is therefore acidic.

A **base** is a substance that can soak up or combine with H^+ ions, thus reducing the acidity of a solution. The compound ammonia is such a substance. The ammonia molecule has two electrons that are not shared with any other atom; a hydrogen ion (H^+) is just a naked proton with no shell of electrons at all. Thus the proton readily combines with the ammonia molecule to form an ammonium ion and so is withdrawn from the solution as a free proton and no longer contributes to its acidity. Many

(structural formula showing ammonia capturing a hydrogen ion:)

$$:\underset{\underset{H}{|}}{\overset{\overset{H}{|}}{N}}-H \;+\; H^+ \longrightarrow H-\underset{\underset{H}{|}}{\overset{\overset{H}{|}}{N^+}}-H$$

The two dots here represent the two electrons not shared with another atom. These are ordinarily not shown in chemical structure drawings. Compare this with the earlier diagram of an ammonia molecule.

Ammonia captures a hydrogen ion from water.

[2] A mole is a certain number (about 6×10^{23}) molecules. The pH of a solution is defined as the negative logarithm of the hydrogen ion concentration of the solution. Thus if the concentration is 10^{-2} (moles per liter), the pH is 2; if 10^{-8}, the pH is 8; and so on.

compounds containing nitrogen are important bases in living systems. Acids and bases neutralize each other to produce substances that are neither acid nor base.

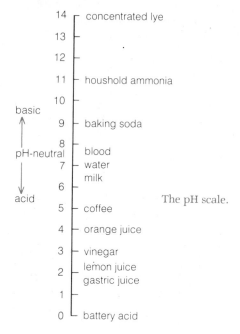

The pH scale.

Note: Each step is ten times as concentrated in base (1/10 as acid) as the one below it.

Chemical Reactions

A chemical reaction or chemical change is one that results in the disappearance of substances and the formation of new ones. Almost all such reactions involve a change in the bonding of atoms: Old bonds are broken, and new ones are formed. The nuclei of atoms are never involved in chemical reactions—only their outer-shell electrons. At the end of a reaction there is always the same number of atoms of each type as there was at the beginning. For example, two hydrogen molecules can react with one oxygen molecule to form two water molecules. In this reaction two substances (hydrogen and oxygen) disappear, and a new one (water) is formed, but at the end of the reaction there are still four H atoms and two O atoms, just as there were at the beginning. The only difference is in how they are linked.

Hydrogen and oxygen react to form water:

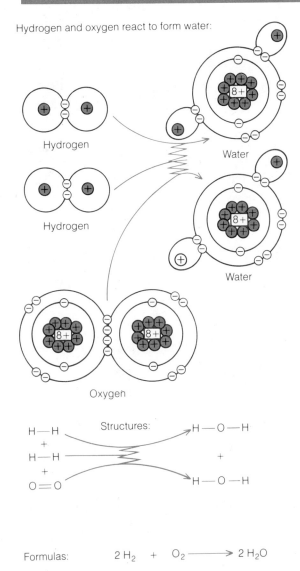

Hydrogen

Hydrogen

Water

Water

Oxygen

Structures:

H—H
+
H—H
+
O=O

H—O—H
+
H—O—H

Formulas: $2 H_2$ + O_2 ⟶ $2 H_2O$

In a few instances chemical reactions involve not the relinking of atoms but the exchanging of electrons among atoms. The transfer of an electron from one molecule to another is known as an **oxidation-reduction reaction**. The loss of an electron is known as **oxidation**, and the compound that loses the electron is said to be oxidized. (The reason for the name is that many substances—such as carbohydrates—lose electrons only when oxygen is available to accept them.) **Reduction** is the gain of an electron. Oxidation and reduction take place simultaneously, because an electron that is lost by one atom is accepted by another.

Sometimes an electron travels in company with a proton as part of a hydrogen atom. In that case, oxidation involves the removal of the hydrogen ion (proton) and its electron from one substance; reduction involves the transfer of both a hydrogen ion and an electron to another substance. (The reduction of oxygen—the addition of hydrogen atoms—thus results in the formation of water.)

If a reaction results in a net increase in chemical bond energy, it is referred to as a reduction reaction. For example, the chief result of photosynthesis is the reduction of carbon (from carbon dioxide to the carbon in sugar). Conversely, if there is a net decrease in chemical bond energy (with a release of energy as heat or light), the reaction is often referred to as an oxidation process. For example, sugar is oxidized in the body to carbon dioxide and water.

Chemical reactions tend to occur spontaneously if the end products are in a lower energy state (are more stable) than the reacting compounds were. These reactions give off energy, often in the form of heat, as they occur. The generation of heat by wood burning in a fireplace and the maintenance of human body warmth both depend on energy-yielding chemical reactions. They are "downhill" reactions: They occur easily, although they may require some activation energy to get them started, just as a ball requires a push to get started rolling downhill (see Highlight 7).

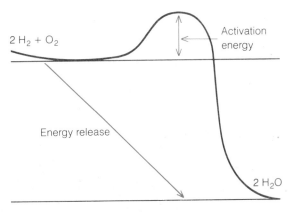

$2 H_2 + O_2$

Activation energy

Energy release

$2 H_2O$

"Uphill" reactions, in which the products contain more energy than the reacting compounds started with, do not occur until an energy source is provided. An example of such an energy source is the sunlight used in photosynthesis, where carbon dioxide and water (low-energy compounds) are combined to form the sugar glucose (a higher-energy compound). Another example is the use of the energy in glucose to combine two low-energy compounds in the body into the high-energy compound ATP (see Highlight 7). The energy in ATP may be used to power many other energy-requiring, "uphill" reactions. Clearly, any of many different molecules can be used as a temporary storage place for energy.

Neither downhill nor uphill reactions occur until something sets them off (activation) or until a path is provided for them to follow. The body uses enzymes as a means of providing paths and controlling its chemical reactions (see Chapter 3). By controlling the availability and the action of its enzymes, the body can "decide" which chemical reactions to prevent and which to promote.

APPENDIX C

Biochemical Structures

CONTENTS

The following diagrams are meant to enhance your understanding of the most important organic molecules in the human diet.

Carbohydrates

Monosaccharides

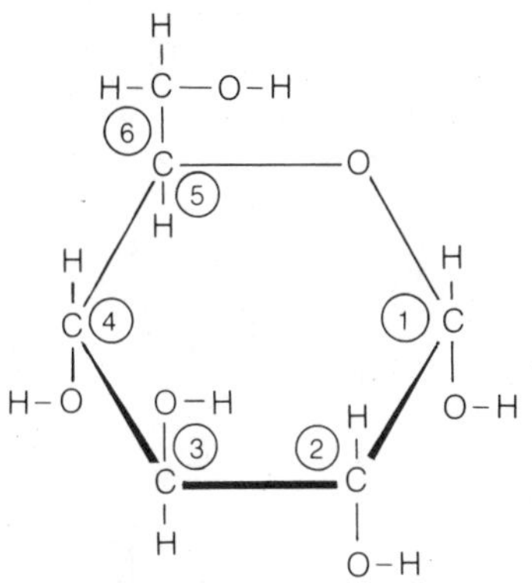

Glucose (alpha form). The ring would be at right angles to the plane of the paper. The bonds directed upward are above the plane; those directed downward are below the plane. This molecule is considered an alpha form because the OH on carbon 1 points downward.

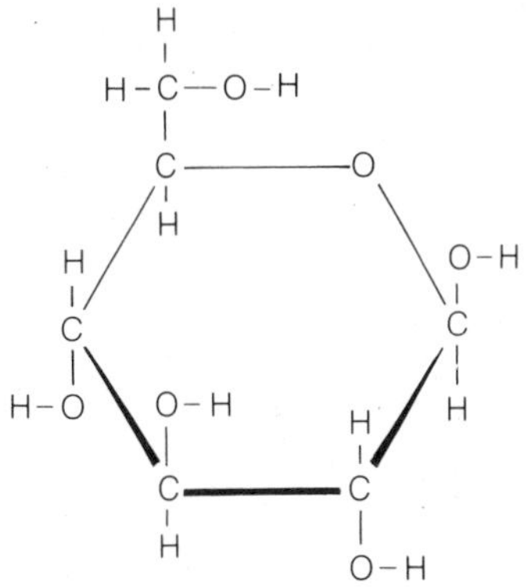

Glucose (beta form). The OH points upward.

Fructose, galactose: see Chapter 1.

C

Disaccharides

Maltose.

Lactose (alpha form). The zigzag link between galactose and glucose permits us to show both sugars "right side up." A truer representation of the molecules would show one of them upside-down so that the link between them would be similar to that in maltose.

Sucrose.

Polysaccharides   As described in Chapter 1, starch, glycogen, and cellulose are all long chains of glucose molecules covalently linked together.

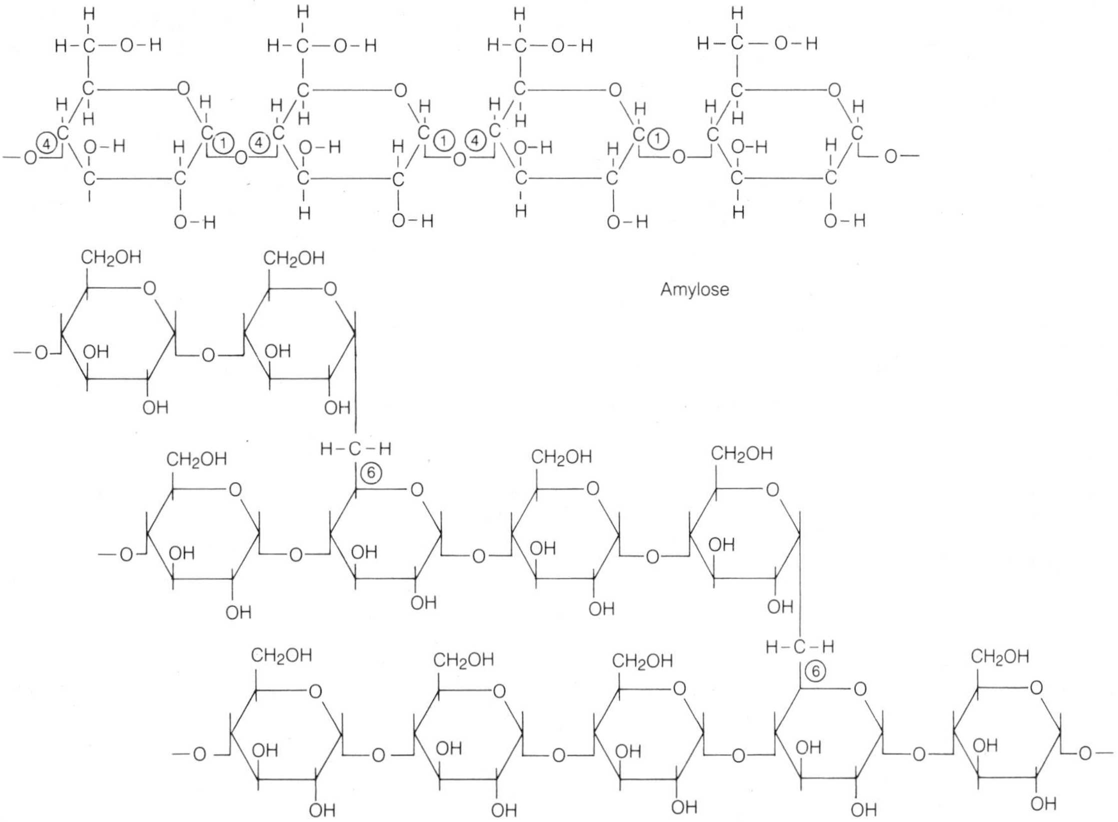

Amylose

Amylopectin

Starch. Two kinds of covalent linkages occur between glucose molecules in starch, giving rise to two kinds of chains. Amylose is composed of straight chains, with carbon 1 of one glucose linked to carbon 4 of the next. Amylopectin is made up of straight chains like amylose but has occasional branches arising where the carbon 6 of a glucose is also linked to the carbon 1 of another glucose. (See the rules for simplified chemical structures on p. 26.)

Glycogen: like amylopectin but with longer chains and many more branches.

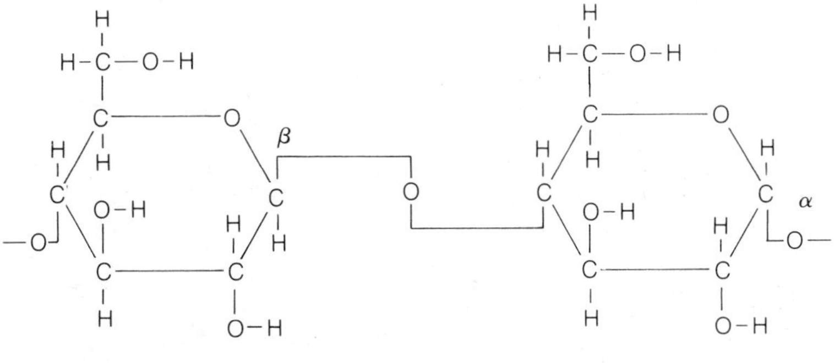

Cellulose. Some of the linkages in cellulose are beta linkages like those in lactose. Another way to depict this molecule would be to draw the second glucose unit up-side down. The disaccharide shown here is cellobiose, which is obtained when cellulose is hydro-lyzed.

Lipids (see also Chapter 3)

Fatty Acids Found in Natural Fats

Saturated fatty acid	Chemical formula	Source
Butyric	C_3H_7COOH	butter fat
Caproic	$C_5H_{11}COOH$	butter fat
Caprylic	$C_7H_{15}COOH$	coconut oil
Capric	$C_9H_{19}COOH$	palm oil
Lauric	$C_{11}H_{23}COOH$	coconut oil
Myristic*	$C_{13}H_{27}COOH$	nutmeg oil, animal fat (butter)
Palmitic*	$C_{15}H_{31}COOH$	animal and vegetable fat
Stearic*	$C_{17}H_{35}COOH$	animal and vegetable fat
Arachidic	$C_{19}H_{39}COOH$	peanut oil

*Most common saturated fatty acids.

Palmitic acid.

Stearic acid.

Fatty Acids Found in Natural Fats (cont'd)

Unsaturated fatty acid	Chemical formula	Position of double bonds	Source
Palmitoleic	$C_{15}H_{29}COOH$	C9-C10	butter fat
Oleic	$C_{17}H_{33}COOH$	C9-C10	olive oil
Linoleic	$C_{17}H_{31}COOH$	C9-C10 C12-C13	linseed oil
Linolenic	$C_{17}H_{29}COOH$	C9-C10 C12-C13 C15-C16	linseed oil
Arachidonic	$C_{19}H_{31}COOH$	C5-C6 C8-C9 C11-C12 C14-C15	lecithin

Palmitoleic acid.

Oleic acid.

Linoleic acid.

Linolenic acid.

Arachidonic acid.

Proteins: Amino Acids (see also Chapter 3)

Glycine (Gly).

Alanine (Ala).

Valine*(Val).

Leucine*(Leu).

Isoleucine*(Ile).

Serine (Ser).

*Essential, because human beings cannot synthesize.

C

$$CH_3-CH-C-C-OH$$
$$\quad\quad OH\;\; NH_2$$

Threonine*(Thr).

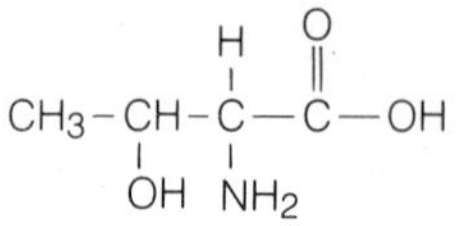

$$HO-C-CH_2-CH_2-C-C-OH$$
$$\quad\quad\quad\quad\quad\quad NH_2$$

Aspartic acid (Asp).

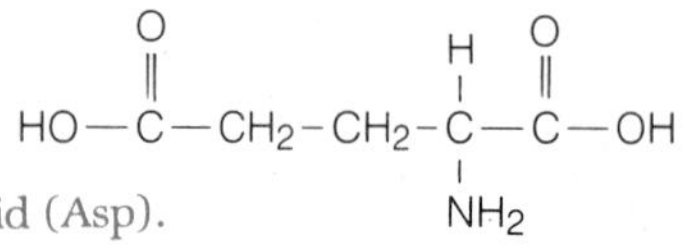

$$HO-C-CH_2-C-C-OH$$
$$\quad\quad\quad\quad\quad NH_2$$

Glutamic acid (Glu).

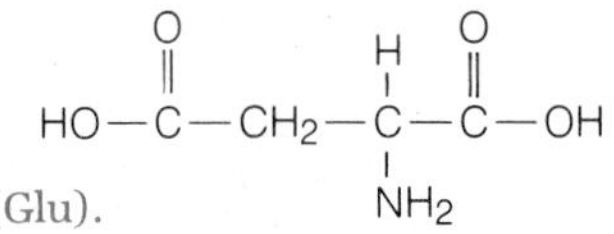

$$NH_2-CH_2-CH_2-CH_2-CH_2-C-C-OH$$
$$\quad\quad\quad\quad\quad\quad\quad\quad\quad NH_2$$

Lysine*(Lys).

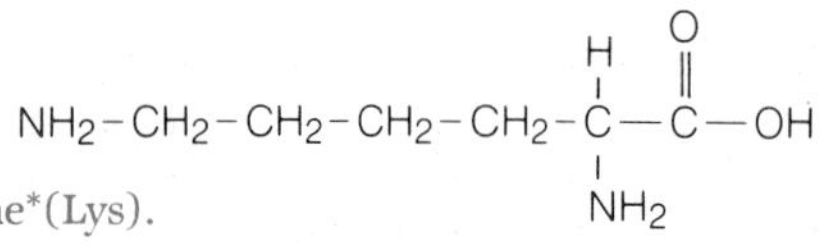

$$NH_2-C-NH-CH_2-CH_2-CH_2-C-C-OH$$
$$\quad\quad NH\quad\quad\quad\quad\quad\quad NH_2$$

Arginine (Arg).

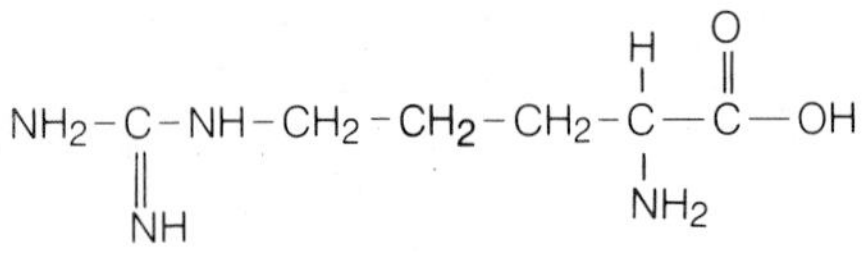

$$HS-CH_2-C-C-OH$$
$$\quad\quad\quad\quad NH_2$$

Cysteine (Cys).

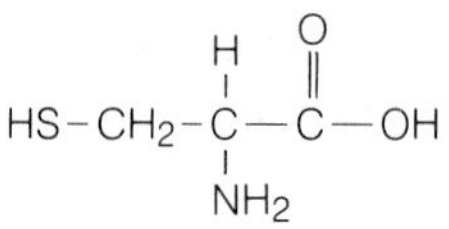

$$CH_2-C-C-OH$$
$$\;S\quad\quad NH_2$$
$$\;S$$
$$CH_2-C-C-OH$$
$$\quad\quad\quad NH_2$$

Cystine (Cys-Cys).

$$CH_3-S-CH_2-CH_2-C-C-OH$$
$$\quad\quad\quad\quad\quad\quad NH_2$$

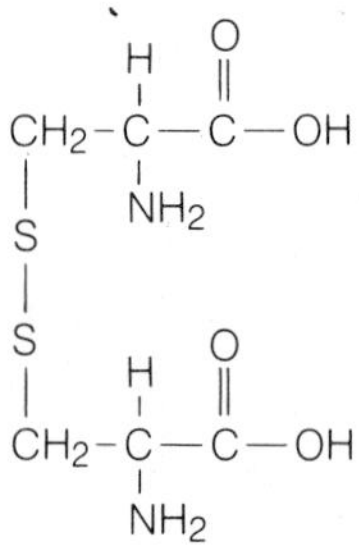

Methionine*(Met).

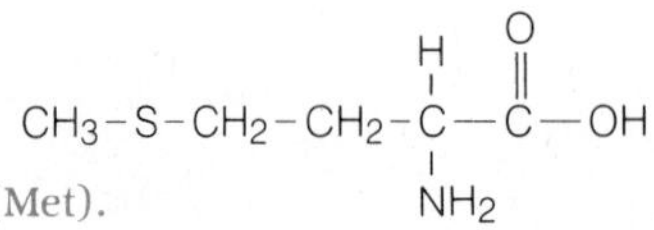

Tyrosine (Tyr).

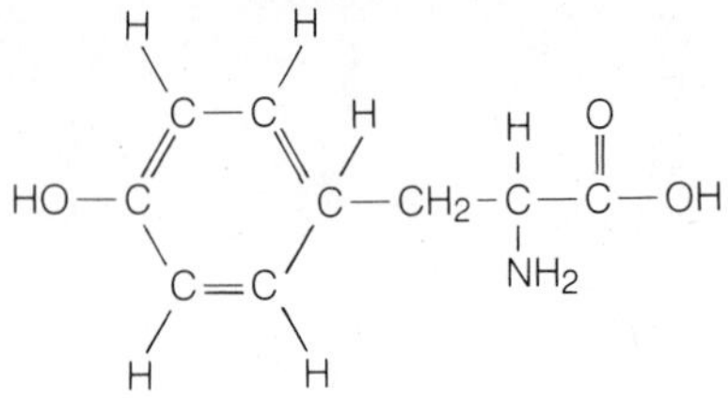

Phenylalanine*(Phe).

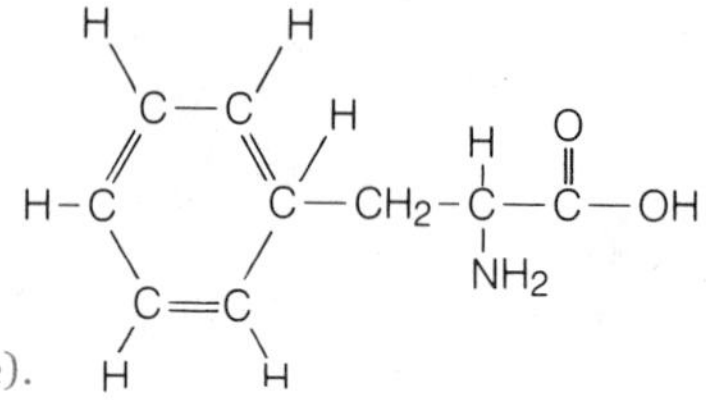

Tryptophan*(Try).

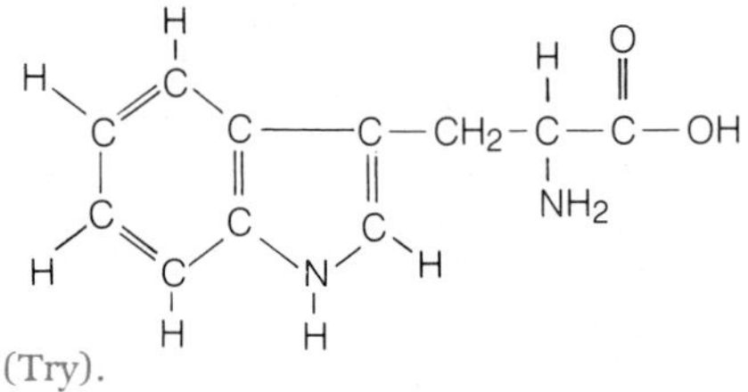

Proline (Pro).

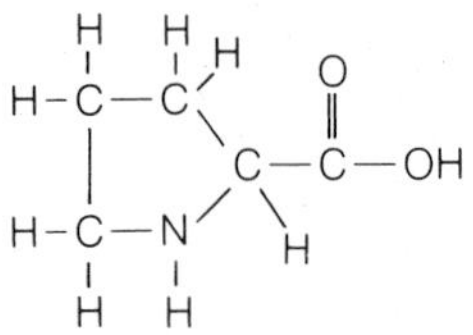

Histidine (His).

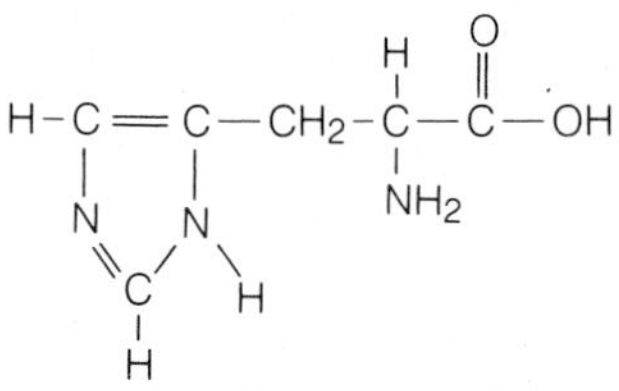

$$NH_2-C-CH_2-C-C-OH$$
$$\quad\quad O\quad\quad NH_2$$

Asparagine (Asn).

$$NH_2-C-CH_2-CH_2-C-C-OH$$
$$\quad\quad O\quad\quad\quad\quad NH_2$$

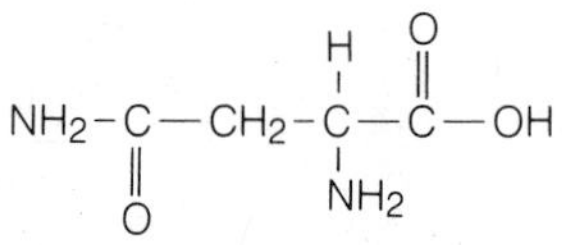

Glutamine (Gln).

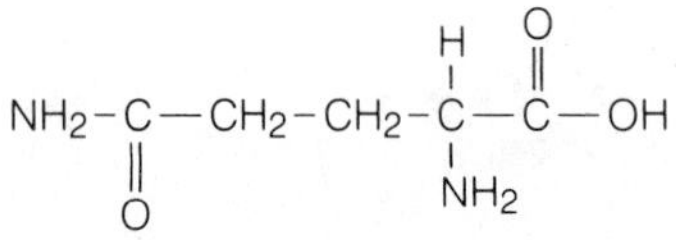

*Essential, because human beings cannot synthesize.

C

Vitamins and Coenzymes (see also Chapters 9 through 11)

Vitamin A: retinol.

Vitamin A: retinal.

Vitamin A: beta-carotene.

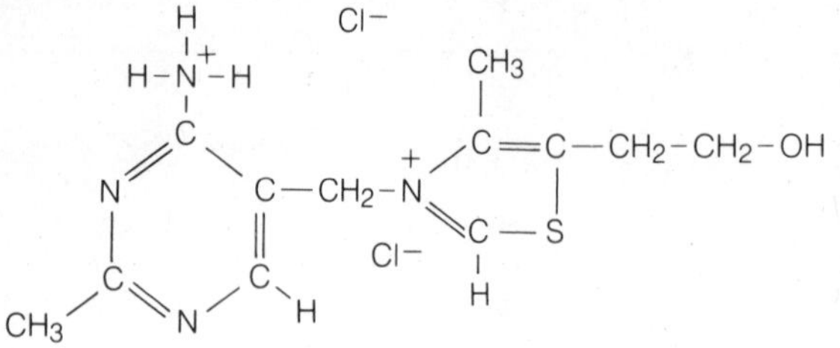

C

Thiamin hydrochloride. Chloride ions (Cl⁻) are shown nearby because two of the nitrogens in this compound have donated their spare outer-shell electrons to bond with positively charged ions (see Appendix B). Thus the whole molecule is positively charged (+2) and will attract two negatively charged ions (Cl⁻) into its vicinity. When crystallized out of water solution, this complex precipitates as the salt thiamin hydrochloride. This chemical name usually appears on vitamin bottles containing thiamin.

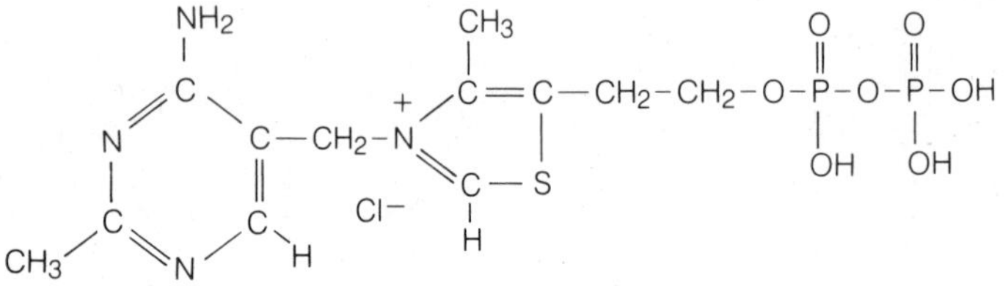

Thiamin pyrophosphate (TPP). TPP is a coenzyme that includes the thiamin molecule as part of its structure.

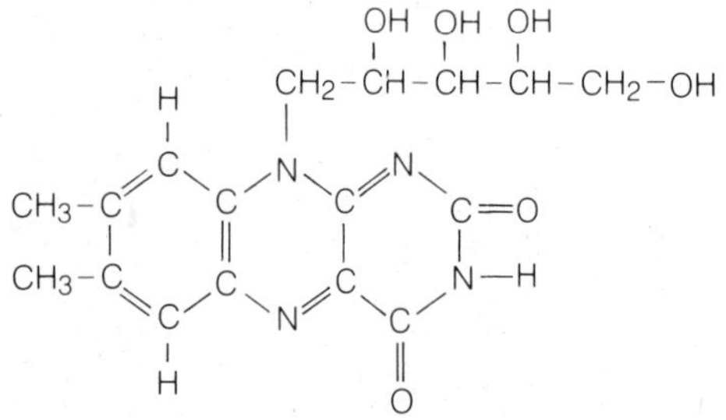

Riboflavin. This molecule is a part of two coenzymes—flavin mononucleotide (FMN) and flavin adenine dinucleotide (FAD).

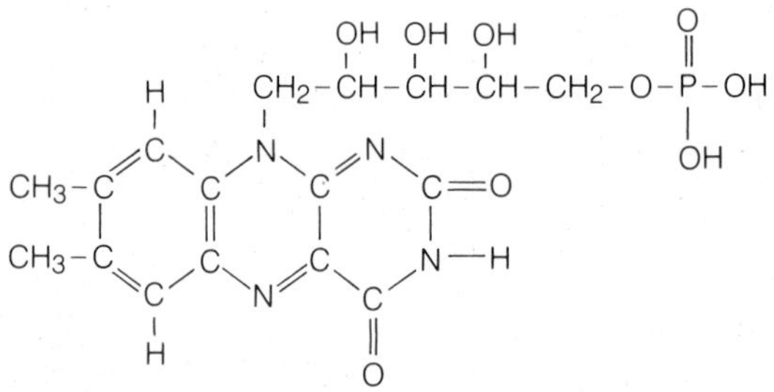

Flavin mononucleotide (FMN).

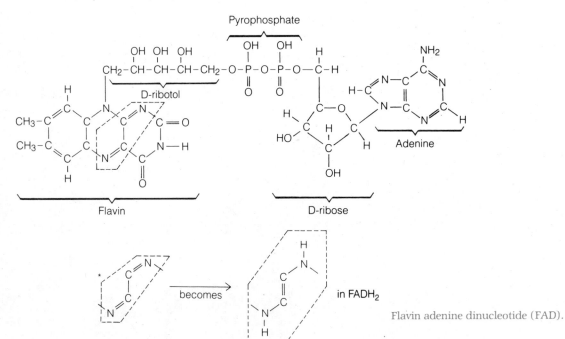

in FADH₂

Flavin adenine dinucleotide (FAD).

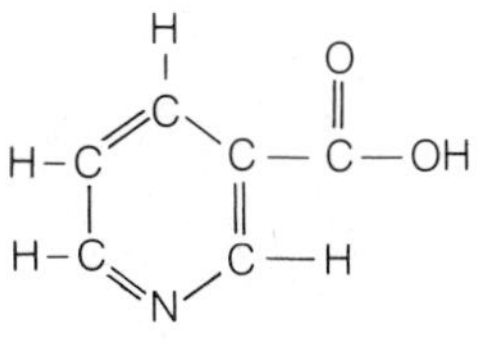

Nicotinic acid

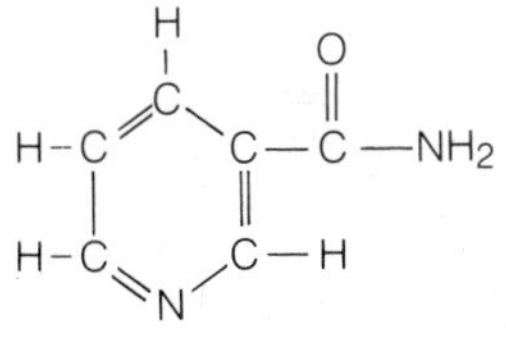

Nicotinamide

Niacin (nicotinic acid and nicotinamide). These molecules are a part of two coenzymes—nicotinamide adenine dinucleotide (NAD^+) and nicotinamide adenine dinucleotide phosphate ($NADP^+$).

C

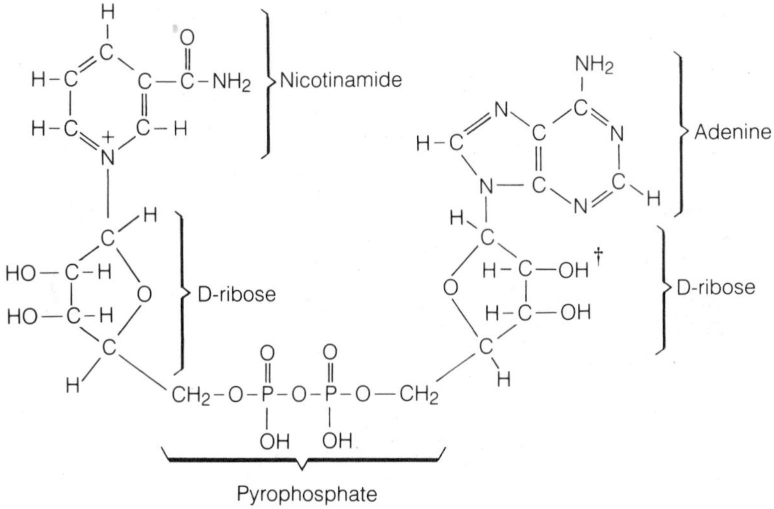

Nicotinamide

Adenine

D-ribose

D-ribose

Pyrophosphate

Nicotinamide adenine dinucleotide (NAD^+) and nicotinamide adenine dinucleotide phosphate ($NADP^+$). NAD has also been called coenzyme I and DPN; NADP has been called coenzyme II and TPN. NADP has the same structure as NAD but with a phosphate group attached where the dagger is.

Reduced NAD^+ (NADH). When NAD^+ is reduced, by adding H^+ and 2 electrons, it becomes the coenzyme NADH. (The dots on the Hs entering this reaction represent electrons—see Appendix B.)

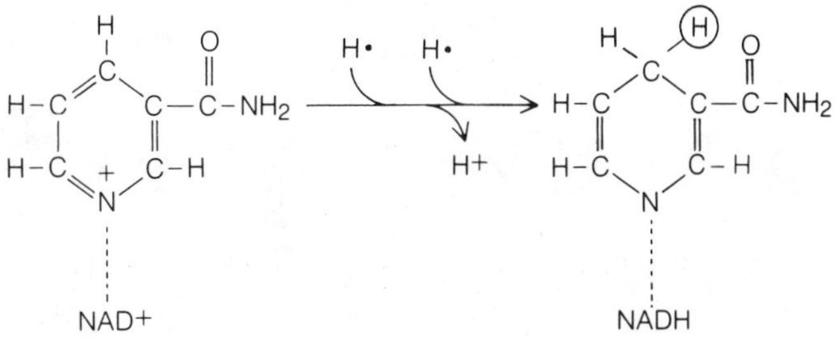

NAD+

NADH

C

Vitamin B_6 is a general name for three compounds—pyridoxine, pyridoxal, and pyridoxamine. Pyridoxal phosphate and pyridoxamine phosphate are the coenzymes necessary for transamination and other important processes.

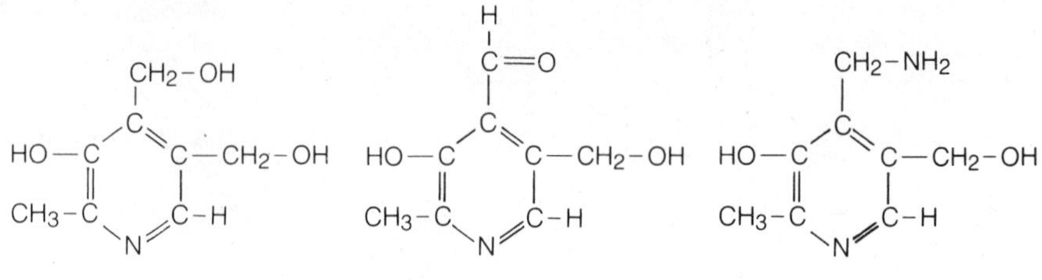

Pyridoxine

Pyridoxal

Pyridoxamine

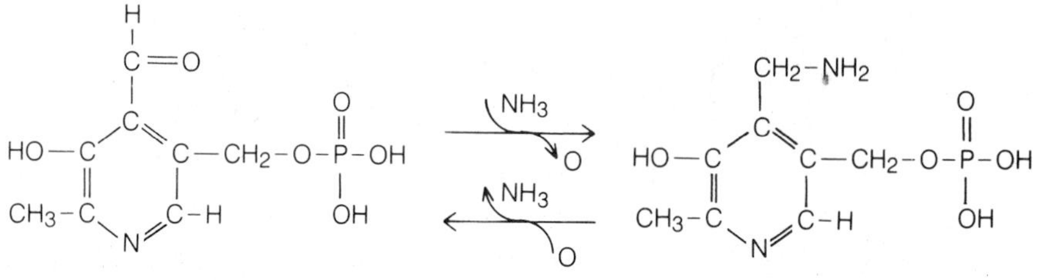

Pyridoxal phosphate

Pyridoxamine phosphate

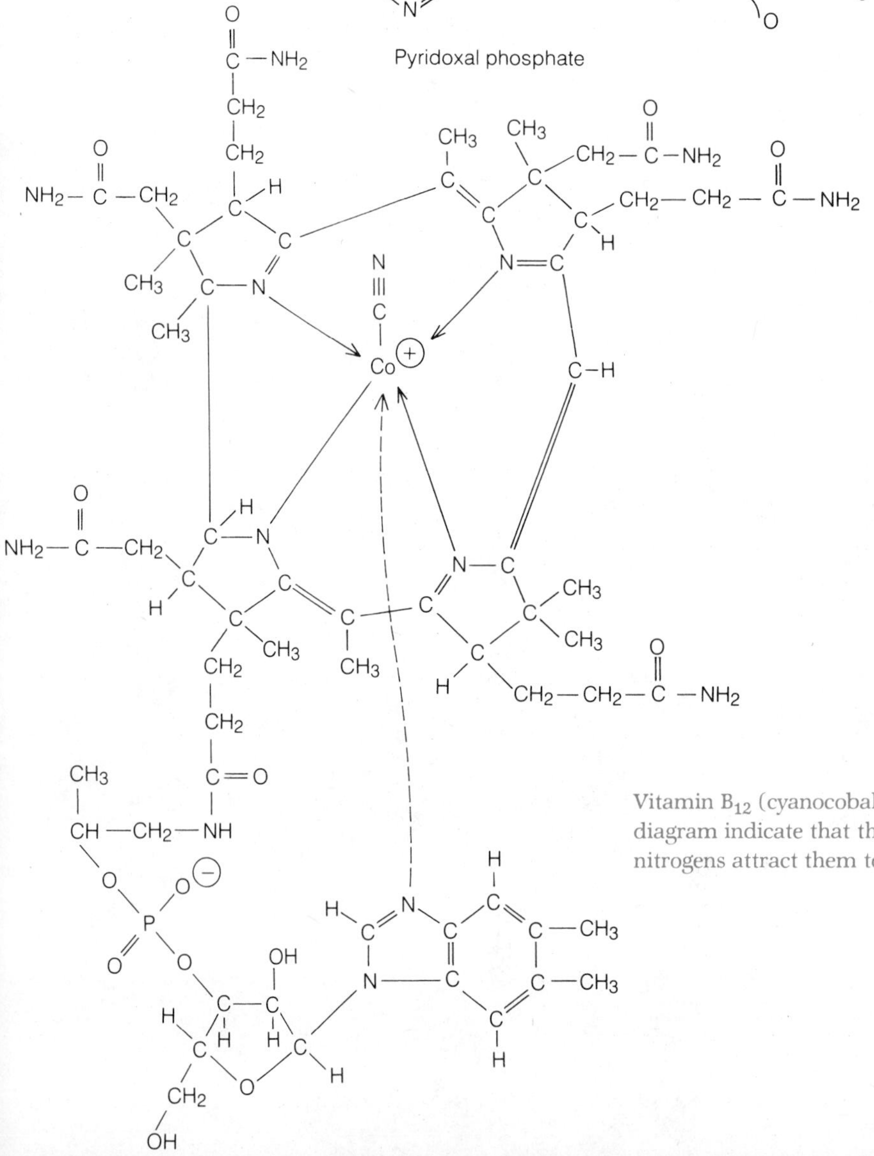

Vitamin B_{12} (cyanocobalamin). The arrows in this diagram indicate that the spare electron pairs on the nitrogens attract them to the cobalt.

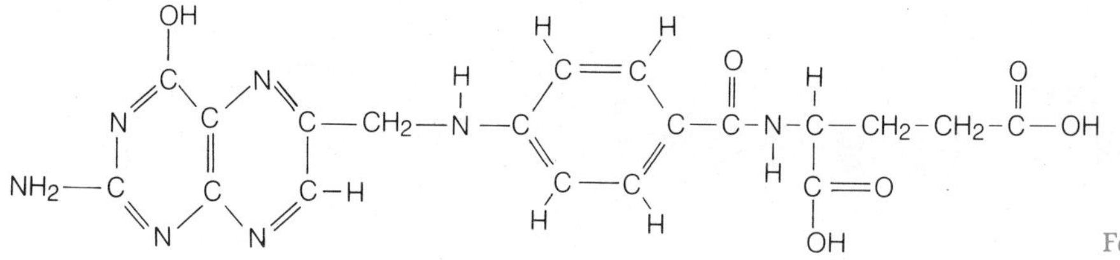

C

Folic acid (folacin).

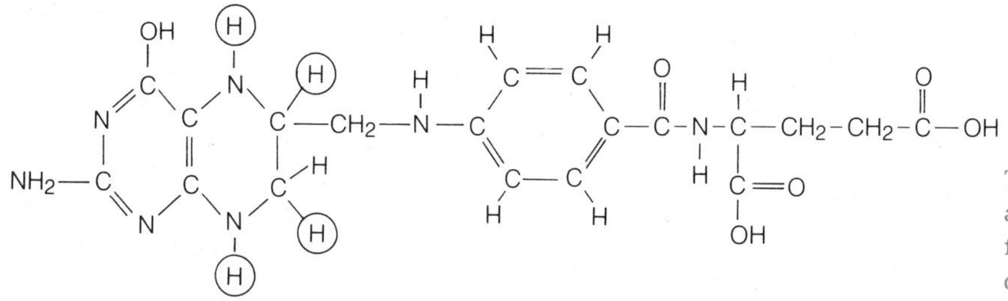

Tetrahydrofolic acid, the active coenzyme form of folic acid. (The four hydrogens added to folic acid are circled.)

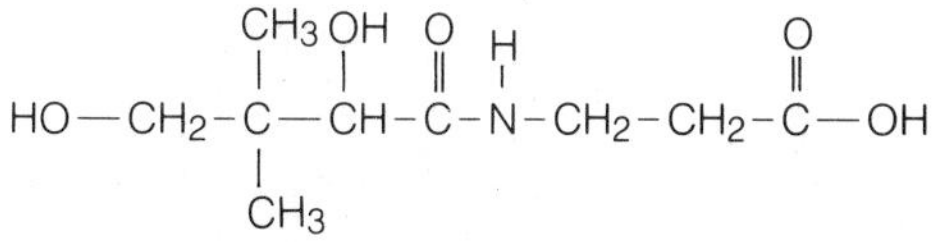

Pantothenic acid

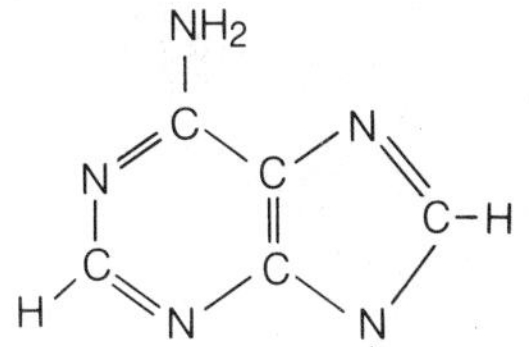

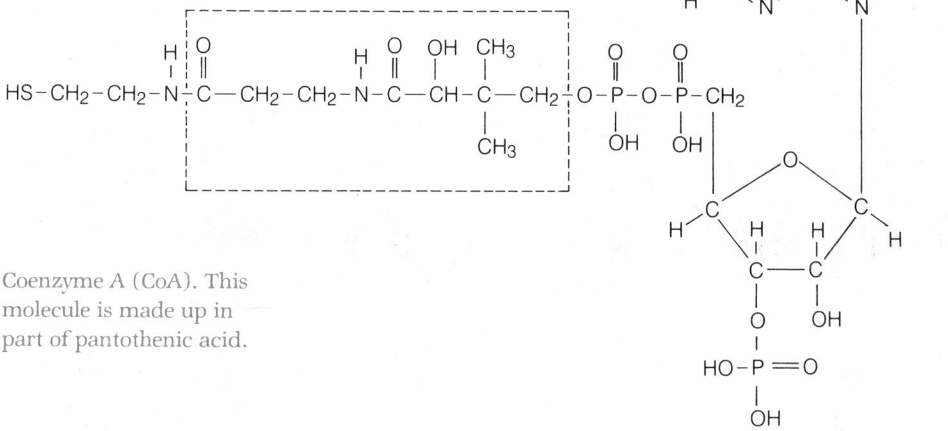

Coenzyme A (CoA). This molecule is made up in part of pantothenic acid.

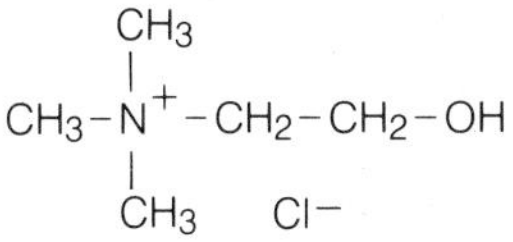

Choline.

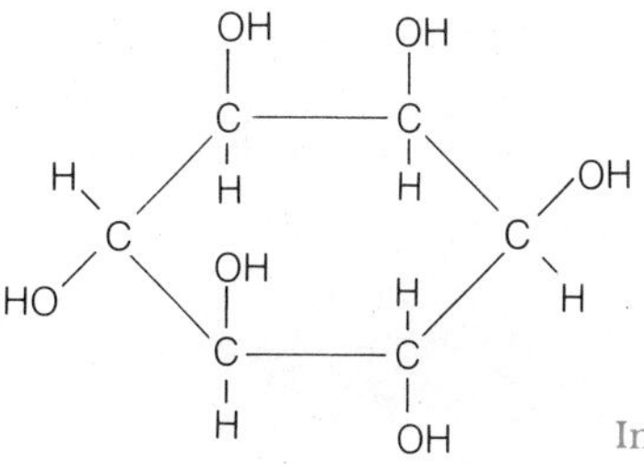

Inositol.

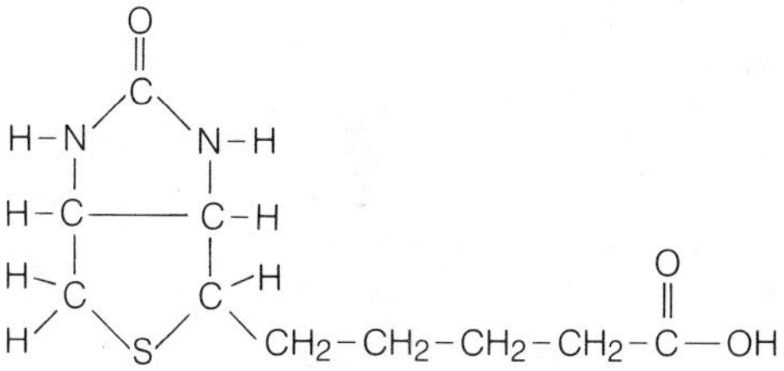

Biotin.

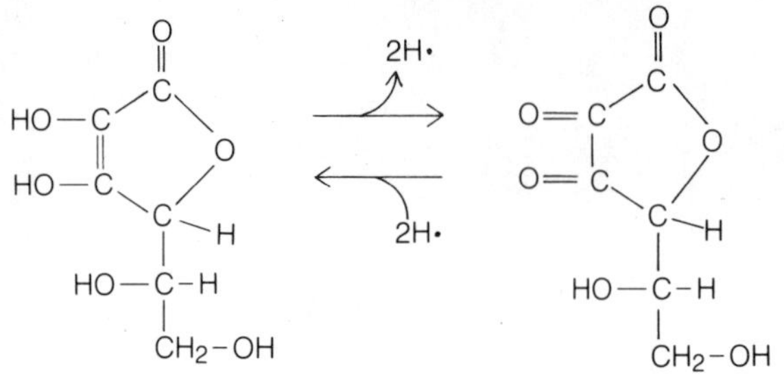

C

Vitamin C (ascorbic acid). The oxidized form of vitamin C is dehydroascorbic acid. (The dots on the Hs indicate that two hydrogen atoms, complete with their electrons, are lost when ascorbic acid is oxidized and gained when it is reduced again.)

Ascorbic acid

Dehydroascorbic acid

Active vitamin D and its precursors, beginning with 7-dehydrocholesterol. (The carbon atoms at which changes occur are numbered.) Compare the structure of 7-dehydrocholesterol with that of cholesterol, p. 75.

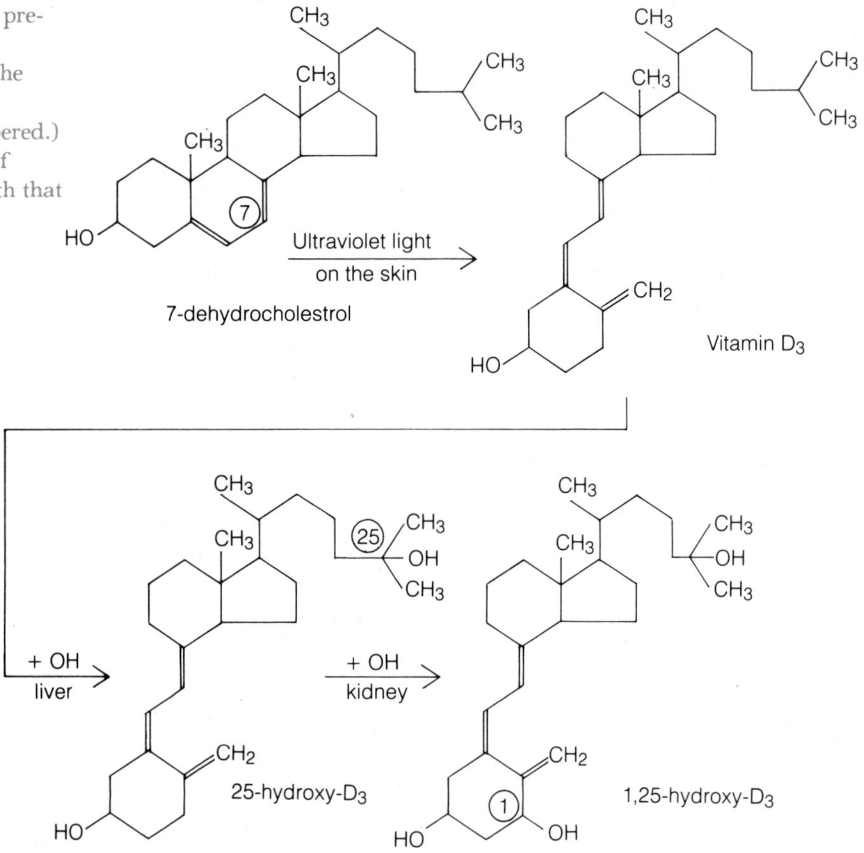

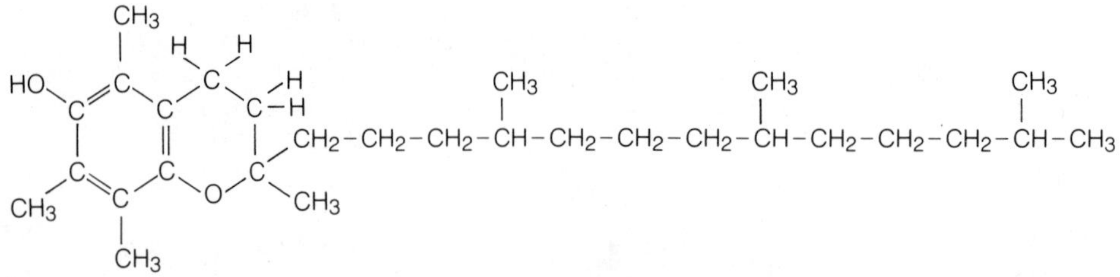

7-dehydrocholestrol

Ultraviolet light on the skin

Vitamin D₃

+ OH
liver

25-hydroxy-D₃

+ OH
kidney

1,25-hydroxy-D₃

Vitamin E (alpha-tocopherol).

Vitamin K, a naturally occurring compound.

Menadione, a synthetic compound that exhibits vitamin K activity.

Adenosine triphosphate (ATP), the energy carrier. The cleavage point marks the bond that is broken when ATP splits to become ADP + P.

Adenosine diphosphate (ADP).

APPENDIX D

Aids to Calculation

CONTENTS

D

This appendix gives examples of solutions to each type of mathematical problem encountered in the text. The steps toward the solutions are especially adapted for the use of pocket calculators.

Conversion Factors and Cancellation of Units

Conversion factors are useful mathematical tools in everyday calculations, especially as we move from the British system of measurement to the metric system. (Both systems are described at the end of this appendix.)

A conversion factor is a fraction in which the numerator and the denominator use different units for the same quantity. For example, 4 c and 1 qt (U.S.) are equivalent amounts.[1] The conversion factor would be either:

$$\frac{4\ c}{1\ qt} \quad \text{or} \quad \frac{1\ qt}{4\ c}$$

Since both fractions equal one, measurements can be multiplied by either factor without changing the value of the measurement.

[1]The imperial quart, used in Canada, is equal to 5 c. The Canadian student should adjust the following calculations accordingly.

For example, how many cups are in 2 qt?

$$2\ qt\ \times\ \frac{4\ c}{1\ qt}\ =\ 8\ c$$

(The Canadian student should get an answer of 10 c.) The factor used in this example was chosen because we wanted the answer to be in cups; thus cups had to be in the numerator of the factor.

A way of confirming that the problem is stated correctly is to cancel the units in the same manner that numerals are canceled in a problem involving multiplication of fractions. The unit that cannot be canceled is the one that will appear in the answer. For example:

$$\cancel{qts}\ \times\ \frac{cups}{\cancel{qts}}\ =\ cups$$

Following are two examples of problems commonly encountered in a nutrition course; they illustrate the use of conversion factors and cancellation of units.

Example 1 Convert your weight in pounds to kilograms (see the inside back cover for conversion factors). Say that you weigh 130 pounds. Because the answer you are seeking should be in kilograms, kilograms must remain uncanceled and in the numerator.

$$130\ \cancel{lb}\ \times\ \frac{1\ kg}{2.2\ \cancel{lb}}\ =\ \frac{130\ kg}{2.2}\ =\ \square$$

A 28

This calculation would be fed into a calculator as $130 \div 2.2$; the number you would get is 59.09. However, this answer is unacceptable, because 59.09 denotes an accuracy of measurement not present in the original measurement (130 pounds). A more acceptable answer is either 59 or 60 kilograms.[2]

Example 2   Determine how many grams of protein you should consume each day in order to meet the recommended intake for protein (see Appendix O). The conversion factor would be either:

$$\frac{.8 \text{ g protein}}{1 \text{ kg ideal body weight}}$$

or

$$\frac{1 \text{ kg ideal body weight}}{.8 \text{ g protein}}$$

For this example, say that your ideal weight is 115 pounds (see the inside back cover). Thus:

$$\begin{array}{c}115 \text{ lb} \\ \text{ideal} \\ \text{weight}\end{array} \times \frac{1 \text{ kg}}{2.2 \text{ lb}} \times \frac{.8 \text{ g protein}}{1 \text{ kg ideal weight}} = \square$$

Note that cancellation of units "kg," "lb," "ideal weight," leaves "grams protein" uncancelled and in the numerator.

The actual calculation: $\dfrac{115 \times .8 \text{ g protein}}{2.2} = \square$

For a 115 pound adult 42 g protein per day would meet the recommended intake.

---

[2]The degree of accuracy of a measurement is reflected in the recording of that measurement and is not altered by any subsequent calculations. The measurement 130 pounds denotes to the reader that the person's weight is about 130 pounds. If the person's weight had been very accurately determined and if that degree of accuracy had been considered necessary, the weight would have been recorded as 130.0, signifying that the weight was exactly 130.0 pounds, correct to a tenth of a pound. Any mathematical calculation with a measurement does not improve the accuracy of the original measurement, and the recording of answers should reflect this. In this example, 59.09 kilograms would indicate that the weight is correct to a hundredth of a kilogram, which is impossible given the fact that the original measurement was not that accurate. Either 59 kg or 60 kg would more properly reflect the truth.

Ratio and Proportion

Some students find the ratio and proportion method convenient in many calculations in nutrition courses (as when seeking the amount of saturated fat in a 4-oz broiled hamburger although Appendix H gives the amount in a 3-oz hamburger). A proportion statement is a statement that a ratio, say 2:3, is equal to another ratio, say 4:6. If one of the four numbers in a proportion is unknown and the other three are known, the unknown number can be calculated using simple algebra. Suppose that the number 6 is unknown in the above proportion but that 2, 3, and 4 are known. You would think, "2 is to 3 as 4 is to what number?" This would be written:

$$\frac{2}{3} = \frac{4}{x}$$

The simple algebra:

$$2x = 4 \times 3$$
$$x = \frac{4 \times 3}{2}$$
$$x = 6$$

When stating a problem using ratio and proportion, be sure that the units of measure are the same on both sides of the equation.

Example 3   How many grams of saturated fat are contained in a 4-oz broiled hamburger? By consulting Appendix H, you can find out that a 3-oz broiled hamburger contains 8 g saturated fat. Thus:

$$\frac{3 \text{ oz hamburger}}{8 \text{ g saturated fat}} = \frac{4 \text{ oz hamburger}}{x \text{ g saturated fat}}$$

$$3x = 4 \times 8$$
$$x = \frac{4 \times 8}{3}$$

Note: $\dfrac{\text{oz}}{\text{g}} = \dfrac{\text{oz}}{\text{g}}$. The units of measure are the same on both sides of the equation.

$$\frac{4 \times 8}{3} = \square$$

Answer: There are 11 g saturated fat in a 4-oz broiled hamburger.

D

Example 4   Calculate the P:S ratio of a diet that contains 80 g of saturated fatty acid and 32 g of linoleic acid.

$$\frac{32 \text{ g polyunsaturated fatty acid}}{80 \text{ g saturated fatty acid}} = \frac{32}{80} = \square$$

The P:S ratio in this case is 0.4, which denotes a diet relatively high in saturated fat. For every gram of saturated fat, this person is consuming 0.4 g of polyunsaturated fat, a ratio of 0.4:1.0.

Finding Percent

To find what percentage a part is of a whole, express the relationship of the part to the whole as a fraction, multiply by 100, and reduce to the simplest terms. In the fraction, the figure that represents the whole amount goes into the denominator, and the figure representing the part of the whole that you are concerned with becomes the numerator.

Example 5   Calculate what percentage of your carbohydrate kcalories come from sweets. Say that you normally consume 850 kcal from carbohydrates and 175 kcal from sweets.

$$\frac{175 \text{ kcal from sweets}}{850 \text{ kcal from all carbohydrates}} \times 100 =$$

$$\frac{175 \times 100}{850} = \square$$

Answer: 21 percent of the kcalories from carbohydrates are derived from sweets.

Systems of Measurement

There are and have been many systems of measurement, but the most important to us are the metric system and the British system.

The Metric System   The metric system is a uniform, international system of measure. It is simple to use since, like the monetary system in the United States and Canada, it is a decimal system.

● *Length units.*
1 meter (m) = 100 centimeters (cm)
1,000 meters =   1 kilometer (km)

● *Weight units.*
1 kilogram (kg) = 1,000 grams (gm or g)
1 g = 1,000 milligrams (mg)
1 mg = 1,000 micrograms (μg)

● *Volume units.*
1 liter (l) = 1,000 milliliters (ml)
1 milliliter = 1 cubic centimeter (cc)

● *Temperature units.* The Celsius thermometer scale is based on 100 equal divisions between the point at which pure water turns to ice (0° C) and the point at which it boils (100° C) at standard atmospheric pressure. Temperatures recorded in this system are recorded as degrees Celsius (° C). This scale, also known as the centigrade scale, is used for all scientific work.

● *Energy units.* The Committee on Nomenclature of the American Institute of Nutrition in 1970 recommended that the term kilojoule (kJ) replace the kilocalorie (kcal) as soon as practicable. A kilocalorie is the amount of energy required to raise a kilogram of pure water one degree on the Celsius scale. A kilojoule is the amount of energy expended when a kilogram is moved one meter by a force of one Newton.

$$1 \text{ kcal } = 4.184 \text{ kJ}$$

Further information on the metric system can be obtained by writing to the Metric Information Office of the National Bureau of Standards, Washington, D.C. 20234.

The British System   The British system is not a decimal system.

● *Length units.*
1 foot (ft) = 12 inches (in)
1 yard (yd) =   3 feet

● *Weight units.*
1 pound (lb) = 16 ounces (oz)

● *Volume units.*
3 teaspoons (tsp) = 1 tablespoon (tbsp)
16 tbsp = 1 cup (c)
1 c = 8 fluid ounces (fl oz)
4 c = 1 quart (qt)
5 c = 1 imperial quart (qt), Canada

● *Temperature units.* The Fahrenheit thermometer scale is based on 180 divisions between the point at which pure water turns to ice (32° F) and the point at which pure water boils (212° F) at standard atmospheric pressure. This scale is commonly used in the United States and Canada for everyday household use but is not used for scientific measurements.

Conversions between Measurement Systems

● *Length.*

$$1 \text{ in} = 2.54 \text{ cm}$$
$$1 \text{ ft} = 30.48 \text{ cm}$$
$$39.37 \text{ in} = 1 \text{ m}$$

● *Weight.*

$$1 \text{ oz} = 28.35 \text{ g (nutritionists usually use either 28 or 30 g)}$$
$$2.2 \text{ lb} = 1 \text{ kg}$$

● *Volume.*

$$1.06 \text{ qt} = 1 \text{ l}$$
$$0.85 \text{ imperial qt} = 1 \text{ l}$$

● *Temperature.*

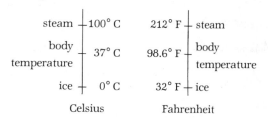

The symbol t_F in the following conversion equations represents the numerical value of a temperature on the Fahrenheit scale; t_C represents that of the Celsius scale.

$$t_F = 9/5 \ t_C + 32$$
$$t_C = 5/9 \ (t_F - 32)$$

APPENDIX E

Measures of Protein Quality

CONTENTS

E

Some of the problems of determining protein quality were discussed in Chapter 3. This appendix is intended to amplify that discussion for those who are interested.

Chemical Score

Two FAO/WHO reference scoring patterns for the eight essential amino acids are shown in Table 1. To interpret the table for egg, read, "For every 3,060 units of essential amino acids, 340 must be isoleucine, 540 must be leucine, and so on." For the FAO/WHO pattern, read, "For every 2,250 units of essential amino acids, 250 must be isoleucine, 440 must be leucine, and so on."

To compare a test protein with one of these reference proteins (let's use egg for an example), the experimenter would first obtain a chemical analysis of the test protein's amino acids. Then, taking 3,060 units of the amino acids, he would compare the amount of each to the amount found in 3,060 units of essential amino acids in egg protein. For example, suppose the test protein contained (per 3,060 units) 360 units of isoleucine, 500 units of leucine, 350 of lysine, and for each of the other amino acids, more units than egg protein contains. The two amino acids that are low are leucine (500 as compared to 540 in egg) and lysine (350 versus 440 in egg). The ratio, amino acid in test protein divided by amino acid in egg, is 500/540 or about 0.93 for

leucine and 350/440 or about 0.80 for lysine. Lysine is the limiting amino acid (lowest ratio compared to egg), so the test protein receives a chemical score of 80.

The advantages of chemical scoring are that it is simple and inexpensive, it identifies in one step the limiting amino acid, and it can be used to score mixtures of different proportions of two or more proteins mathematically without having to make them up and test them. Its chief weaknesses are that it fails to predict the digestibility of a protein, which may severely affect its quality; it relies on a chemical procedure in which certain amino acids may be destroyed, so that the pattern that is analyzed may lack accuracy; and it is blind to other features of the test protein, such as toxic materials, that would only be revealed by a test in living animals.

Biological Value (BV)

In a test of biological value, two nitrogen-balance studies are done. In the first, no protein is fed, and nitrogen (N) excretion in the urine and feces is measured. It is assumed that N lost in the urine (called endogenous N) is the amount the body loses by filtration into the urine each day regardless of what protein is fed. The N lost in the feces (called metabolic N) is the amount the body invariably loses into the

Table 1 **FAO/WHO Reference Patterns**

Essential amino acids	Whole egg	FAO/WHO pattern, 1973
		mg amino acid per g nitrogen
Isoleucine	340	250
Leucine	540	440
Lysine	440	340
Methionine + cystine*	355	220
Phenylalanine + tyrosine†	580	380
Threonine	294	250
Tryptophan	106	60
Valine	410	310
TOTAL	3,060‡	2,250

*Methionine is essential and is also used to make cystine. Thus the methionine requirement is lower if cystine is supplied.

†Phenylalanine is essential and is also used to make tyrosine if there is not enough of the latter. Thus the phenylalanine requirement is lower if tyrosine is also supplied.

‡Rounded off.

intestine each day. (To help you remember terms: Endogenous N is "urinary N on a 0-protein diet"; metabolic N is "fecal N on a 0-protein diet.")

In the second experiment, an amount of protein slightly below the requirement is fed. Intake and losses are measured. BV is then derived using this formula:

$$BV = \frac{Food\ N - (fecal\ N - metabolic\ N) - (urinary\ N - endogenous\ N)}{Food\ N - (fecal\ N - metabolic\ N)} \times 100$$

The denominator of this equation expresses the amount of nitrogen *absorbed:* food N minus fecal N (excluding the N the body would lose in the feces anyway, even without food). The numerator expresses the amount of N *retained* from the N absorbed: absorbed N (as in the denominator) minus the N excreted in the urine (excluding the N the body would lose in the urine anyway, even without food). Thus it can be more simply expressed:

$$BV = \frac{N\ retained}{N\ absorbed} \times 100$$

This method has the advantage of being based on experiments with human beings (it can be done with animals too, of course) and of measuring actual nitrogen retention. But it is also cumbersome, expensive, and often impractical and is based on many assumptions that may not be valid. For example, the subjects used for testing may not be similar physiologically or in terms of their normal environment or typical food intake to those for whom the test protein may ultimately be used. For another example, the fact that protein is retained in the body does not necessarily mean that it is being well utilized. There is considerable protein turnover (synthesis and degradation) within every cell of the body, and there is much exchange among tissues. These processes are hidden from view when only N intake and output are measured.

Net Protein Utilization (NPU)

Like measurements of BV, NPU determinations involve two balance studies, one on zero and the other on submaximal nitrogen intake. The formula for NPU is:

$$NPU = \frac{Food\ N - (fecal\ N - metabolic\ N) - (urinary\ N - endogenous\ N)}{Food\ N} \times 100$$

E

The numerator is the same as it is for BV, but the denominator represents food N intake only—not absorbed N. More simply expressed:

$$NPU = \frac{N \text{ retained}}{N \text{ intake}}$$

This method has advantages similar to those of BV determinations and is more frequently used, employing animals as the test subjects. A drawback is that if a low NPU is obtained, the test results offer no help in distinguishing between two possible causes: a poor amino acid composition of the test protein or poor digestibility. There is also a limit to the extent to which animal test results can be assumed to be applicable to human beings, as with PER (below).

Protein Efficiency Ratio (PER)

This is the best-known procedure for evaluating protein quality and is used in the United States as the basis for regulations regarding food labeling and for the protein RDA. Young rats are fed a measured amount of protein and weighed periodically as they grow. PER is expressed as:

$$PER = \frac{\text{Weight gain (lb)}}{\text{Protein intake (g)}}$$

This method has the virtues of economy and simplicity but also has many drawbacks: The experiments are time-consuming; the amino acid needs of rats are not the same as for human beings; and the amino acid needs for growth are not the same as for the maintenance of adult animals (growing animals need more lysine, for example).

All of these methods and others have their uses, and some of their disadvantages balance one another out. One reviewer recommends that chemical scoring be relied on more heavily than it has been in the past and that the biological techniques be used to amplify and help interpret the findings from scoring.[1] The evaluation of protein quality remains a vitally important research area in a world where it is becoming more and more critical to provide nourishing food to millions who live on the edge of starvation.[2]

[1] P. L. Pellett, Protein quality evaluation revisited, *Food Technology*, May 1978, pp. 60, 62, 64-66, 70-72, 74, 76, 78-79.

[2] The interested reader will find additional useful information in Pellett, 1978; R. L. Pike and M. L. Brown, *Nutrition: An Integrated Approach*, 2nd ed. (New York: Wiley, 1975); and R. S. Goodhart and M. E. Shils, eds., *Modern Nutrition in Health and Disease*, 5th ed. (Philadelphia: Lea and Febiger, 1973).

APPENDIX F

Sugar

Table 1 presents the amount of refined sugar of common foods in teaspoon measures. No one will be surprised to see that cola beverages contain a large quantity of refined sugar, but it may be a surprise to learn that sugar is added to dried fruits, hamburger buns, and other items. This table is adapted from a listing developed at the University of Iowa.

Table 1 Refined Sugar in Common Foods[1]

Food	Portion size	Approximate sugar content (tsp)*
Beverages		
Cola drinks	12 oz	9
Ginger ale	12 oz	7
Orangeade	8 oz	5
Root beer	10 oz	$4_{1/2}$
Seven-Up	12 oz	9
Soda pop	8 oz	5
Sweet cider	1 c (8 oz)	$4_{1/2}$
Jams and jellies		
Apple butter	1 tbsp	1
Jelly	1 tbsp	4-6
Orange marmalade	1 tbsp	4-6
Peach butter	1 tbsp	1
Strawberry jam	1 tbsp	4
Candies		
Milk chocolate bar (Hershey bar)	$1_{1/2}$ oz	$2_{1/2}$
Chewing gum	1 stick	$1/2$
Chocolate cream	1 piece	2
Chocolate mints	1 piece	2
Fudge	1 oz square	$4_{1/2}$
Gum drop	1	2
Hard candy	4 oz	20
Lifesavers	1	$1/3$

Food	Portion size	Approximate sugar content (tsp)*
Peanut brittle	1 oz	$3_{1/2}$
Marshmallow	1	$1_{1/2}$
Fruits and canned juices		
Raisins	1/2 c	4
Currants, dried	1 tbsp	4
Prunes, dried	3-4 medium	4
Apricots, dried	4-6 halves	4
Dates, dried	3-4 stoned	$4_{1/2}$
Figs, dried	$1_{1/2}$-2 small	4
Fruit cocktail	1/2 c	5
Rhubarb, stewed, sweetened	1/2 c	8
Canned apricots	4 halves and 1 tbsp syrup	$3_{1/2}$
Applesauce, sweetened	1/2 c	2
Prunes, stewed, sweetened	4-5 medium and 2 tbsp juice	8
Canned peaches	2 halves and 1 tbsp syrup	$3_{1/2}$
Fruit salad	1/2 c	$3_{1/2}$
Fruit syrup	2 tbsp	$2_{1/2}$
Orange juice	1/2 c	2
Pineapple juice, unsweetened	1/2 c	$2_{3/5}$

[1]Hidden sugars in foods (a three-page typescript), Department of Pedodontics, College of Dentistry, University of Iowa, Iowa City, March 1974. Developed by Arthur J. Nowak, D.M.D., professor, College of Dentistry, Department of Pedodontics, University of Iowa, and reprinted with his permission.

Table 1 Refined Sugar in Common Foods (cont'd)

Food	Portion size	Approximate sugar content (tsp)*
Grape juice, commercial	1/2 c	32/5
Canned fruit juices, sweetened	1/2 c	2

Breads and cereals

Food	Portion size	Approximate sugar content (tsp)*
White bread	1 slice	1/2
Cornflakes, Wheaties, Krispies, etc.	1 bowl and 1 tbsp sugar	4-8
Hamburger bun	1	3
Hot dog bun	1	3

Cakes and cookies

Food	Portion size	Approximate sugar content (tsp)*
Angel food cake	4 oz	7
Applesauce cake	4 oz	51/2
Banana cake	2 oz	2
Cheesecake	4 oz	2
Chocolate cake, plain	4 oz	6
Chocolate cake, iced	4 oz	10
Coffeecake	4 oz	41/2
Cupcake, iced	1	6
Fruitcake	4 oz	5
Jelly-roll	2 oz	21/2
Orange cake	4 oz	4
Pound cake	4 oz	5
Sponge cake	1 oz	2
Strawberry shortcake	1 serving	4
Brownies, unfrosted	1 (3/4 oz)	3
Molasses cookies	1	2
Chocolate cookies	1	11/2
Fig newtons	1	5
Ginger snaps	1	3
Macaroons	1	6
Nut cookies	1	11/2
Oatmeal cookies	1	2
Sugar cookies	1	11/2
Chocolate eclair	1	7
Cream puff	1	2
Donut, plain	1	3
Donut, glazed	1	6
Snail	1 (4 oz)	41/2

Dairy products

Food	Portion size	Approximate sugar content (tsp)*
Ice cream	1/3 pint (31/2 oz)	31/2

Food	Portion size	Approximate sugar content (tsp)*
Ice cream bar	1 (depending on size)	1-7
Ice cream cone	1	31/2
Eggnog, all milk	1 (8 oz)	41/2
Ice cream soda	1	5
Cocoa, all milk	1 c (5 oz milk)	4
Ice cream sundae	1	7
Chocolate, all milk	1 c (5 oz milk)	6
Malted milk shake	1 (10 oz)	5
Sherbet	1/2 c	9

Desserts

Food	Portion size	Approximate sugar content (tsp)*
Apple cobbler	1/2 c	3
Custard	1/2 c	2
French pastry	1 (4 oz)	5
Jello	1/2 c	41/2
Apple pie	1 slice (average)	7
Junket	1/2 c	3
Berry pie	1 slice	10
Cherry pie	1 slice	10
Cream pie	1 slice	4
Custard pie	1 slice	10
Coconut pie	1 slice	10
Lemon pie	1 slice	7
Peach pie	1 slice	7
Pumpkin pie	1 slice	5
Rhubarb pie	1 slice	4
Raisin pie	1 slice	13
Banana pudding	1/2 c	2
Bread pudding	1/2 c	11/2
Chocolate pudding	1/2 c	4
Plum pudding	1/2 c	4
Rice pudding	1/2 c	5
Tapioca pudding	1/2 c	3
Brown betty	1/2 c	3
Plain pastry	1 (4 oz)	3

Sugars and syrups

Food	Portion size	Approximate sugar content (tsp)*
Brown sugar	1 tbsp	3†
Granulated sugar	1 tbsp	3†
Corn syrup	1 tbsp	3†
Karo syrup	1 tbsp	3†
Honey	1 tbsp	3†
Molasses	1 tbsp	31/2†
Chocolate sauce	1 tbsp	31/2†

*Measured in teaspoon equivalents of granulated sugar.
†Actual sugar content.

*Measured in teaspoon equivalents of granulated sugar.
†Actual sugar content.

Table 2 expands the section on cereals by showing which brand names have the most and which have the least refined sugar. Adapted from a publication in which the sugar contents of cereals were not presented in teaspoons per serving but as a percentage of dry weight, this table gives only a rank order. The dentists who published this information suggested, tentatively, that to avoid promoting the development of dental decay the consumer should choose cereals containing less than 20 percent refined sugar.[2]

[2] I. L. Shannon, Sucrose and glucose in dry breakfast cereals, *Journal of Dentistry for Children*, September/October 1974, pp. 17-20. The reader who wants to pursue the subject further might find another article interesting: I. L. Shannon and W. B. Wescott, Sucrose and glucose concentrations of frequently ingested foods, *Journal of the Academy of General Dentistry*, May/June 1975, pp. 37-43, which presents sucrose and glucose contents for diet soft drinks (less than 0.1 percent); commercially available cheeses (less than 2.0 percent); fresh fruits and vegetables (from 0 to about 5 percent); commercially available luncheon meats (less than 1 percent for those analyzed); commercially available crackers and wafers (from about 1 to 10 percent, except for graham crackers, Cinnamon Treats, Cinnamon Crisp, and glazed Sesame Crisp, which contained from 10 to 30 percent); commercially available breads (less than 1 percent for those analyzed, except for old-fashioned cinnamon loaf); and commercially available snack foods (from 0 to 3 percent except for Morton's Kandi-roos, which contained almost 50 percent sucrose). Dr. Shannon's data are used here with his permission and that of the publisher.

F

Table 2   Refined Sugar (Sucrose) in Breakfast Cereals

Cereal	Sucrose (percent)	Cereal	Sucrose (percent)
Less than 10 percent sucrose*		**10 to 19 percent sucrose**	
Shredded Wheat, large biscuit	1.0	Rice Crispies, Kellogg	10.0
Shredded Wheat, spoon-size biscuit	1.3	Raisin Bran, Kellogg	10.6
Cheerios	2.2	Heartland, with raisins	13.5
Puffed Rice	2.4	Buck Wheat	13.6
Uncle Sam Cereal	2.4	Life	14.5
Wheat Chex	2.6	Granola, with dates	14.5
Grape Nut Flakes	3.3	Granola, with raisins	14.5
Puffed Wheat	3.5	Sugar-Frosted Corn Flakes	15.6
Alpen	3.8	40% Bran Flakes, Post	15.8
Post Toasties	4.1	Team	15.9
Product 19	4.1	Brown Sugar-Cinnamon Frosted Mini Wheats	16.0
Corn Total	4.4		
Special K	4.4	40% Bran Flakes, Kellogg	16.2
Wheaties	4.7	Granola	16.6
Corn Flakes, Kroger	5.1	100% Bran	18.4
Peanut Butter	5.2		
Grape Nuts	6.6	**20 to 29 percent sucrose**	
Corn Flakes, Food Club	7.0	All Bran	20.0
Crispy Rice	7.3	Granola, with almonds and filberts	21.4
Corn Chex	7.5	Fortified Oat Flakes	22.2
Corn Flakes, Kellogg	7.8	Heartland	23.1
Total	8.1	Super Sugar Chex	24.5
Rice Chex	8.5	Sugar Frosted Flakes	29.0
Crisp Rice	8.8	**30 to 39 percent sucrose**	
Raisin Bran, Skinner	9.6	Bran Buds	30.2
Concentrate	9.9	Sugar Sparkled Corn Flakes	32.2

*The glucose content of these cereals is less than 5 percent, except for Special K and Kellogg Corn Flakes (6.4 percent), Kellogg Raisin Bran (14.1 percent), and Heartland, with raisins (5.6 percent). Other sugars, such as fructose, were not analyzed.

Table 2   Refined Sugar (Sucrose) in Breakfast Cereals (cont'd)

Cereal	Sucrose (percent)	Cereal	Sucrose (percent)
Frosted Mini Wheats	33.6	Baron Von Redberry	45.8
Sugar Pops	37.8	Cocoa Krispies	45.9
		Trix	46.6
40 to 49.5 percent sucrose		Froot Loops	47.4
Alpha Bits	40.3	Honeycomb	48.8
Sir Grapefellow	40.7	Pink Panther	49.2
Super Sugar Crisp	40.7		
Cocoa Puffs	43.0	**50 to 59 percent sucrose**	
Cap'n Crunch	43.3	Cinnamon Crunch	50.3
Crunch Berries	43.4	Lucky Charms	50.4
Kaboom	43.8	Cocoa Pebbles	53.5
Frankenberry	44.0	Apple Jacks	55.0
Frosted Flakes	44.0	Fruity Pebbles	55.1
Count Chocula	44.2	King Vitamin	58.5
Orange Quangaroos	44.7		
Quisp	44.9	**More than 60 percent sucrose**	
Boo Berry	45.7	Sugar Smacks	61.3
Vanilly Crunch	45.8	Super Orange Crisp	68.0

To Explore Further

A more extensive analysis of the sugar content of foods has been published by D.A.T. Southgate, A. A. Paul, A. C. Dean, and A. A. Christie, Free sugars in foods, *Journal of Human Nutrition* 32 (1978):335-347. This reference shows the breakdown for each food into glucose, fructose, lactose, maltose, and sucrose, for about 150 foods including some unusual ones such as rose hips syrup.

APPENDIX G

Fats: Cholesterol and P:S Ratios

To adopt a "prudent diet," you are advised to control kcalories and salt intake; to avoid empty-kcalorie foods, especially those high in concentrated sugars; and to make sure that fat intake is kept in line. To manage fat consumption, three measures are recommended: (1) cut total fat; (2) reduce cholesterol intake; and (3) adjust the ratio of polyunsaturated to saturated fat so that it balances in favor of the polyunsaturates.

For the first objective, total fat intake can be calculated using Appendix H, as suggested in the Self-Study following Highlight 2.

For the second objective, cholesterol intake can be estimated using Table 1 in this appendix.

The U.S. dietary goals of 1977 suggested a cholesterol intake of 300 mg a day or less, although there is some disagreement about this recommendation (see Highlight 6).

As for the third objective, nutritionists tend to think in terms of the P:S ratio (the ratio of polyunsaturated to saturated fat). In general, according to present thinking, the higher the P:S ratio, the better. The P:S ratio of a day's food intake or menu can be calculated precisely (as explained in the Self-Study following Highlight 2), but you can get a general idea of the fat quality of common fat-containing foods from Table 2.

G

Table 1 Cholesterol Content of Foods[1]

Food	Serving size	Cholesterol (mg)
Meat, fish, poultry		
Beef, cooked, lean, trimmed		
of separable fat	3 oz	77
Lamb, lean, cooked	3 oz	83
Pork, cooked, lean, trimmed	3 oz	77
Veal, cooked, lean	3 oz	86
Chicken, dark meat	3 oz	76
Chicken, light meat	3 oz	54
Turkey, dark meat	3 oz	86
Turkey, light meat	3 oz	65
Rabbit, domestic	3 oz	52
Variety meats		
liver (beef, calf, lamb),		
cooked	3 oz	372
chicken liver	3 oz	480
heart	3 oz	274

Food	Serving size	Cholesterol (mg)
sweetbreads	3 oz	396
brain	3 oz	1,810
kidney	3 oz	690
Fish		
caviar (fish roe)	1 tbsp	48
cod	3 oz	72
haddock	3 oz	51
halibut	3 oz	51
flounder	3 oz	43
herring	3 oz	83
salmon, cooked	3 oz	40
trout	3 oz	47
tuna, packed in oil	3 oz	56
sardines	1 can (3$3/4$ oz)	109

[1]Adapted from the booklet by the Greater Los Angeles Affiliate of the American Heart Association, *Consumers Guide to Fat: Cholesterol-Controlled Food Products* (Los Angeles: American Heart Association, 1978); and from E. N. Whitney and E. M. N. Hamilton, *Understanding Nutrition,* 1st ed. (St. Paul, Minn.: West, 1977), pp. 537-538.

Table 1   Cholesterol Content of Foods (cont'd)

Food	Serving size	Cholesterol (mg)
Shellfish		
abalone	3 oz	120
crab	3 oz	85
clams	3 oz	55
lobster	1/2 c	57
oysters	3 oz	40
scallops	1/2 c (scant)	45
shrimp	3 oz	96
Eggs		
Yolk	1 medium	240
White		0
Dairy products		
Milk, whole	1 c (8 oz)	34
Milk, low-fat (2%)	1 c	22
Milk, nonfat (skim)	1 c	5
Buttermilk	1 c	14
Yogurt, low-fat plain	1 c	17
Yogurt, low-fat flavored	1 c	14
Sour cream	1 tbsp	8
Whipped cream	1 tbsp	20
Half and half	1 tbsp	6
Ice milk	1 c	26

Food	Serving size	Cholesterol (mg)
Ice cream	1 c	56
Butter	1 tsp	12
Cheese		
American	1 oz	26
Blue or roquefort	1 oz	25
Camembert	1 oz	28
Cheddar, mild or sharp	1 oz	28
Cottage		
creamed (4% fat)	1 c	48
uncreamed	1 c	13
Cream cheese	1 tbsp	16
Mozzarella, low moisture, part skim	1 oz	18
Muenster	1 oz	25
Parmesan	1 oz	27
Ricotta, part skim	1 oz	14
Swiss	1 oz	28
Nondairy fats		
Lard or other animal fat	1 tsp	5
Margarine, all vegetable		0
Margarine, 2/3 animal fat, 1/3 vegetable fat	1 tsp	3

G

Table 2 P:S Ratios of Foods

Relative P:S ratio	Foods
High (more than 2 1/2 times as much polyunsaturated as saturated fat)	Almonds Corn oil Cottonseed oil Linseed oil Margarine, soft Mayonnaise (made with any of the oils in this group) Safflower oil Sesame oil Soybean oil Sunflower oil Walnuts
Medium-high (about twice as much polyunsaturated as saturated fat)	Chicken breast, skin, thigh Freshwater fish Peanut oil Semisolid margarines

Relative P:S ratio	Foods
Medium (about equal amounts of poly-unsaturated and saturated fat)	Beef, heart and liver Chicken heart Hydrogenated or hardened vegetable oils Pecans Peanut butter Solid margarines
Low (about a tenth to a half as much polyunsaturated as saturated fat)	Chicken liver Lard Olive oil Palm oil Pork Veal
Very low (less than a tenth as much polyunsaturated as saturated fat)	Beef, both lean and fat Butter Coconut oil Egg yolk Milk and milk products Mutton, both lean and fat

G

APPENDIX H

Table of Food Composition

The following table is the standard table found in all nutrition textbooks and references. It presents the kcalorie content, energy-nutrient composition, and vitamin and mineral contents of 615 common foods by household measure.[1] It can be purchased from the U.S. Government Printing Office (address in Appendix J) as a handy softcover booklet. Canadian users may prefer to use *Nutrient Value of Some Common Foods* (Health and Welfare Canada) which has the advantage of being metricated.

Of the minerals, only calcium and iron are included in this table. You might also be curious about zinc, but we have chosen not to present information here on the zinc contents of foods. A few references are available that do.[2]

Of the vitamins, vitamin A, thiamin, riboflavin, niacin, and vitamin C (ascorbic acid) are included. An expanded version of this table, presently being published in installments by the U.S. Department of Agriculture, Agricultural Research Service, includes folacin and other vitamin information, as well as the amino acid analysis of foods.[3]

Fast foods are not listed in this table, but we have included a separate appendix (Appendix N) listing the nutrient contents of foods sold in the most popular fast-food restaurants. The nutrient content of brand-name products—cookies, snack foods, cookie mixes, canned fruits, TV dinners, condiments, and so on—can be obtained from Consumer Guide.[4] The composition of foods used by various ethnic groups, which are also not found in this table, can be requested from the U.S. Department of Agriculture.[5] Finally, because new information on the composition of foods is coming out monthly, a useful reference is the looseleaf notebook available from a group of Boston-area dietitians, which lists many other references for nutrients and data that are often difficult to locate.[6]

---

[3]A table of the folacin contents of 299 foods has also been published: B. P. Perloff and R. R. Butrum, Folacin in selected foods, *Journal of the American Dietetic Association* 70 (1977):161-172.

[4]*Food: The Brand Name Game* (Skokie, Ill.: Consumer Guide, 1974).

[5]*Composition of Foods Used by Ethnic Groups: Selected References to Sources of Data* can be requested from Dr. Louise Page, Food and Diet Appraisal Group, Consumer and Food Economics Institute, U.S. Department of Agriculture, Agricultural Research Service, Hyattsville MD 20782. For Japanese-American food equivalents, a reprint is available from the American Dietetic Association (address in Appendix J).

[6]*Nutrient Composition of Foods: Selected References and Tables*, available from the Boston Area Research Dietitians Special Practice Group, Massachusetts Dietetic Association (1978).

[1]U.S. Department of Agriculture, Nutritive values of the edible parts of foods, *Nutritive Value of Foods*, Home and Garden Bulletin no. 72 (Washington, D.C.: Government Printing Office, 1971), table 1.

[2]K. A. Haeflein and A. I. Rasmussen, Zinc content of selected foods, *Journal of the American Dietetic Association* 70 (1977):610-616; E. W. Murphy, B. W. Willis, and B. K. Watt, Provisional tables of the zinc content of foods, *Journal of the American Dietetic Association* 66 (1975):345-355; and J. H. Freeland and R. J. Cousins, Zinc content of selected foods, *Journal of the American Dietetic Association* 68 (1976):526-529.

Table of Food Composition

[Dashes in the columns for nutrients show that no suitable value could be found although there is reason to believe that a measurable amount of the nutrient may be present]

Food, approximate measure, and weight (in grams)		Water	Food energy	Protein	Fat	Fatty acids			Carbohydrate	Calcium	Iron	Vitamin A value	Thiamin	Riboflavin	Niacin	Ascorbic acid
						Saturated (total)	Unsaturated Oleic	Unsaturated Linoleic								
	Grams	Percent	kCalories	Grams	Grams	Grams	Grams	Grams	Grams	Milligrams	Milligrams	International units	Milligrams	Milligrams	Milligrams	Milligrams
MILK, CHEESE, CREAM, IMITATION CREAM; RELATED PRODUCTS																
Milk:																
Fluid:																
1 Whole, 3.5% fat ---- 1 cup----	244	87	160	9	9	5	3	Trace	12	288	0.1	350	0.07	0.41	0.2	2
2 Nonfat (skim)------- 1 cup----	245	90	90	9	Trace	--	--	--	12	296	.1	10	.09	.44	.2	2
3 Partly skimmed, 2% 1 cup---- nonfat milk solids added.	246	87	145	10	5	3	2	Trace	15	352	.1	200	.10	.52	.2	2
Canned, concentrated, undiluted:																
4 Evaporated, un- 1 cup------ sweetened.	252	74	345	18	20	11	7	1	24	635	.3	810	.10	.86	.5	3
5 Condensed, sweet- 1 cup---- ened.	306	27	980	25	27	15	9	1	166	802	.3	1,100	.24	1.16	.6	3
Dry, nonfat instant:																
6 Low-density (1⅓ 1 cup---- cups needed for reconstitution to 1 qt.).	68	4	245	24	Trace	--	--	--	35	879	.4	[1]20	.24	1.21	.6	5
7 High-density (⅞ cup 1 cup---- needed for reconstitution to 1 qt.).	104	4	375	37	1	--	--	--	54	1,345	.6	[1]30	.36	1.85	.9	7
Buttermilk:																
8 Fluid, cultured, made 1 cup---- from skim milk.	245	90	90	9	Trace	--	--	--	12	296	.1	10	.10	.44	.2	2
9 Dried, packaged------ 1 cup----	120	3	465	41	6	3	2	Trace	60	1,498	.7	260	.31	2.06	1.1	--
Cheese:																
Natural:																
Blue or Roquefort type:																
10 Ounce----------- 1 oz.----	28	40	105	6	9	5	3	Trace	1	89	.1	350	.01	.17	.3	0
11 Cubic inch-------- 1 cu. in.----	17	40	65	4	5	3	2	Trace	Trace	54	.1	210	.01	.11	.2	0

[1] Value applies to unfortified product; value for fortified low-density product would be 1500 I.U. and the fortified high-density product would be 2290 I.U.

H

Table of Food Composition (cont'd)

[Dashes in the columns for nutrients show that no suitable value could be found although there is reason to believe that a measurable amount of the nutrient may be present]

H

	Food, approximate measure, and weight (in grams)		Water	Food energy	Protein	Fat	Fatty acids			Carbohydrate	Calcium	Iron	Vitamin A value	Thiamin	Riboflavin	Niacin	Ascorbic acid
							Saturated (total)	Unsaturated									
								Oleic	Linoleic								
		Grams	Percent	kCalories	Grams	Grams	Grams	Grams	Grams	Grams	Milligrams	Milligrams	International units	Milligrams	Milligrams	Milligrams	Milligrams
	MILK, CHEESE, CREAM, IMITATION CREAM; RELATED PRODUCTS—Con. Cheese—Continued Natural—Continued																
12	Camembert, packaged in 4-oz. pkg. with 3 wedges per pkg. — 1 wedge	38	52	115	7	9	5	3	Trace	1	40	0.2	380	0.02	0.29	0.3	0
	Cheddar:																
13	Ounce — 1 oz.	28	37	115	.7	9	5	3	Trace	1	213	.3	370	.01	.13	Trace	0
14	Cubic inch — 1 cu. in.	17	37	70	4	6	3	2	Trace	Trace	129	.2	230	.01	.08	Trace	0
	Cottage, large or small curd: Creamed:																
15	Package of 12-oz., net wt. — 1 pkg.	340	78	360	46	14	8	5	Trace	10	320	1.0	580	.10	.85	.3	0
16	Cup, curd pressed down. — 1 cup	245	78	260	33	10	6	3	Trace	7	230	.7	420	.07	.61	.2	0
	Uncreamed:																
17	Package of 12-oz., net wt. — 1 pkg.	340	79	290	58	1	1	Trace	Trace	9	306	1.4	30	.10	.95	.3	0
18	Cup, curd pressed down. — 1 cup	200	79	170	34	1	Trace	Trace	Trace	5	180	.8	20	.06	.56	.2	0
	Cream:																
19	Package of 8-oz., net wt. — 1 pkg.	227	51	850	18	86	48	28	3	5	141	.5	3,500	.05	.54	.2	0
20	Package of 3-oz., net wt. — 1 pkg.	85	51	320	7	32	18	11	1	2	53	.2	1,310	.02	.20	.1	0
21	Cubic inch — 1 cu. in.	16	51	60	1	6	3	2	Trace	Trace	10	Trace	250	Trace	.04	Trace	0
	Parmesan, grated:																
22	Cup, pressed down — 1 cup	140	17	655	60	43	24	14	1	5	1,893	.7	1,760	.03	1.22	.3	0
23	Tablespoon — 1 tbsp.	5	17	25	2	2	1	Trace	Trace	Trace	68	Trace	60	Trace	.04	Trace	0
24	Ounce — 1 oz.	28	17	130	12	9	5	3	Trace	1	383	.1	360	.01	.25	.1	0
	Swiss:																
25	Ounce — 1 oz.	28	39	105	8	8	4	3	Trace	1	262	.3	320	Trace	.11	Trace	0
26	Cubic inch — 1 cu. in.	15	39	55	4	4	2	1	Trace	Trace	139	.1	170	Trace	.06	Trace	0

No.	Food, approximate measure, and weight	Grams	Water (%)	Food energy	Protein	Fat	Saturated (total)	Unsaturated: Oleic	Unsaturated: Linoleic	Carbohydrate	Calcium	Iron	Vitamin A	Thiamin	Riboflavin	Niacin	Ascorbic acid
	Pasteurized processed cheese:																
	American:																
27	Ounce ------ 1 oz.	28	40	105	7	9	5	3	Trace	1	198	.3	350	.01	.12	Trace	0
28	Cubic inch ---- 1 cu. in.	18	40	65	4	5	3	2	Trace	Trace	122	.2	210	Trace	.07	Trace	0
	Swiss:																
29	Ounce ------ 1 oz.	28	40	100	8	8	4	3	Trace	1	251	.3	310	Trace	.11	Trace	0
30	Cubic inch ---- 1 cu. in.	18	40	65	5	5	3	2	Trace	Trace	159	.2	200	Trace	.07	Trace	0
	Pasteurized process cheese food, American:																
31	Tablespoon ---- 1 tbsp.	14	43	45	3	3	2	1	Trace	1	80	.1	140	Trace	.08	Trace	0
32	Cubic inch ---- 1 cu. in.	18	43	60	4	4	2	1	Trace	1	100	.1	170	Trace	.10	Trace	0
33	Pasteurized process cheese spread, American. ---- 1 oz.	28	49	80	5	6	3	2	Trace	2	160	.2	250	Trace	.15	Trace	0
	Cream:																
34	Half-and-half (cream and milk). 1 cup	242	80	325	8	28	15	9	1	11	261	.1	1,160	.07	.39	.1	2
35	1 tbsp.	15	80	20	1	2	1	1	Trace	1	16	Trace	70	Trace	.02	Trace	Trace
36	Light, coffee or table -- 1 cup	240	72	505	7	49	27	16	1	10	245	.1	2,020	.07	.36	.1	2
37	1 tbsp.	15	72	30	1	3	2	1	Trace	1	15	Trace	130	Trace	.02	Trace	Trace
38	Sour --- 1 cup	230	72	485	7	47	26	16	1	10	235	.1	1,930	.07	.35	.1	2
39	1 tbsp.	12	72	25	Trace	2	1	1	Trace	6	12	Trace	100	Trace	.02	Trace	Trace
40	Whipped topping (pressurized). 1 cup	60	62	155	2	14	8	5	Trace		67		570		.04		
41	1 tbsp.	3	62	10	Trace	1	Trace	Trace	Trace	Trace	3		30	Trace		Trace	
	Whipping, unwhipped (volume about double when whipped):																
42	Light --- 1 cup	239	62	715	6	75	41	25	2	9	203	.1	3,060	.05	.29	.1	2
43	1 tbsp.	15	62	45	Trace	5	3	2	Trace	1	13	Trace	190	Trace	.02	Trace	Trace
44	Heavy --- 1 cup	238	57	840	5	90	50	30	3	7	179	.1	3,670	.05	.26	.1	2
45	1 tbsp.	15	57	55	Trace	6	3	2	Trace	1	11	Trace	230	Trace	.02	Trace	Trace
	Imitation cream products (made with vegetable fat):																
	Creamers:																
46	Powdered ------ 1 cup	94	2	505	4	33	31	1	0	52	21	.6	[2]200			Trace	
47	1 tsp.	2	2	10	Trace	1	Trace	Trace	0	1	1	Trace	[2]Trace				
48	Liquid (frozen) ---- 1 cup	245	77	345	3	27	25	1	0	25	29		[2]100	0	0		0
49	1 tbsp.	15	77	20	Trace	2	1	Trace	Trace	2	2		[2]10	0	0		Trace
50	Sour dressing (imitation sour cream) made with nonfat dry milk. 1 cup	235	72	440	9	38	35	1	1	17	277	.1	10	.07	.38	.2	1
	Whipped topping:																
51	1 tbsp.	12	72	20	Trace	2	2	1	Trace	1	14	Trace	Trace	Trace	Trace	Trace	Trace
52	Pressurized ----- 1 cup	70	61	190	1	17	15	1	0	9	5		[2]340	0	0		Trace
53	1 tbsp.	4	61	10	Trace	1	1	Trace	0	Trace	Trace		[2]20	0	0		

[2] Contributed largely from beta-carotene used for coloring.

Table of Food Composition (cont'd)

[Dashes in the columns for nutrients show that no suitable value could be found although there is reason to believe that a measurable amount of the nutrient may be present]

MILK, CHEESE, CREAM, IMITATION CREAM; RELATED PRODUCTS—Con.

	Food, approximate measure, and weight (in grams)	Water	Food energy	Protein	Fat	Fatty acids — Saturated (total)	Fatty acids — Unsaturated Oleic	Fatty acids — Unsaturated Linoleic	Carbohydrate	Calcium	Iron	Vitamin A value	Thiamin	Riboflavin	Niacin	Ascorbic acid
		Percent	kCalories	Grams	Grams	Grams	Grams	Grams	Grams	Milligrams	Milligrams	International units	Milligrams	Milligrams	Milligrams	Milligrams
54	Whipped topping—Continued Frozen — 1 cup — 75	52	230	1	20	18	Trace	0	15	5	---	[2]560		0		
55	1 tbsp — 4	52	10	Trace	1	1	Trace	0	1	Trace	---	[2]30				
56	Powdered, made with whole milk. — 1 cup — 75	58	175	3	12	10	1	Trace	15	62	Trace	[2]330	.02	.08	.1	Trace
57	1 tbsp — 4	58	10	Trace	1	1	Trace	Trace	1	3	Trace	[2]20	Trace	Trace	Trace	Trace
	Milk beverages:															
58	Cocoa, homemade — 1 cup — 250	79	245	10	12	7	4	Trace	27	295	1.0	400	.10	.45	.5	3
59	Chocolate-flavored drink made with skim milk and 2% added butterfat. — 1 cup — 250	83	190	8	6	3	2	Trace	27	270	.5	210	.10	.40	.3	3
	Malted milk:															
60	Dry powder, approx. 3 heaping teaspoons per ounce. — 1 oz — 28	3	115	4	2				20	82	.6	290	.09	.15	.1	0
61	Beverage — 1 cup — 235	78	245	11	10				28	317	.7	590	.14	.49	.2	2
	Milk desserts:															
62	Custard, baked — 1 cup — 265	77	305	14	15	7	5	1	29	297	1.1	930	.11	.50	.3	1
	Ice cream:															
63	Regular (approx. 10% fat). — ½ gal. — 1,064	63	2,055	48	113	62	37	3	221	1,553	.5	4,680	.43	2.23	1.1	11
64	1 cup — 133	63	255	6	14	8	5	Trace	28	194	.1	590	.05	.28	.1	1
65	3 fl. oz. cup — 50	63	95	2	5	3	2	Trace	10	73	Trace	220	.02	.11	.1	1
66	Rich (approx. 16% fat). — ½ gal. — 1,188	63	2,635	31	191	105	63	6	214	927	.2	7,840	.24	1.31	1.2	12
67	1 cup — 148	63	330	4	24	13	8	1	27	115	Trace	980	.03	.16	.1	1
	Ice milk:															
68	Hardened — ½ gal. — 1,048	67	1,595	50	53	29	17	2	235	1,635	1.0	2,200	.52	2.31	1.0	10
69	1 cup — 131	67	200	6	7	4	2	Trace	29	204	.1	280	.07	.29	.1	1
70	Soft-serve — 1 cup — 175	67	265	8	9	5	3	Trace	39	273	.2	370	.09	.39	.2	2

No.	Food	Measure	Grams															
71	Yoghurt: Made from partially skimmed milk.	1 cup	245	89	125	8	4	2	1	Trace	13	294	.1	170	.10	.44	.2	2
72	Made from whole milk.	1 cup	245	88	150	7	8	5	3	Trace	12	272	.1	340	.07	.39	.2	2
	EGGS																	
	Eggs, large, 24 ounces per dozen: Raw or cooked in shell or with nothing added:																	
73	Whole, without shell	1 egg	50	74	80	6	6	2	3	Trace	Trace	27	1.1	590	.05	.15	Trace	0
74	White of egg	1 white	33	88	15	4	Trace	—	—	—	Trace	3	Trace	0	Trace	.09	Trace	0
75	Yolk of egg	1 yolk	17	51	60	3	5	2	2	Trace	Trace	24	.9	580	.04	.07	Trace	0
76	Scrambled with milk and fat.	1 egg	64	72	110	7	8	3	3	Trace	1	51	1.1	690	.05	.18	Trace	0
	MEAT, POULTRY, FISH, SHELLFISH; RELATED PRODUCTS																	
77	Bacon, (20 slices per lb. raw), broiled or fried, crisp.	2 slices	15	8	90	5	8	3	4	1	1	2	.5	0	.08	.05	.8	—
	Beef,[3] cooked: Cuts braised, simmered, or pot-roasted:																	
78	Lean and fat	3 ounces	85	53	245	23	16	8	7	Trace	0	10	2.9	30	.04	.18	3.5	—
79	Lean only	2.5 ounces	72	62	140	22	5	2	2	Trace	0	10	2.7	10	.04	.16	3.3	—
	Hamburger (ground beef), broiled:																	
80	Lean	3 ounces	85	60	185	23	10	5	4	Trace	0	10	3.0	20	.08	.20	5.1	—
81	Regular	3 ounces	85	54	245	21	17	8	8	Trace	0	9	2.7	30	.07	.18	4.6	—
	Roast, oven-cooked, no liquid added: Relatively fat, such as rib:																	
82	Lean and fat	3 ounces	85	40	375	17	34	16	15	1	0	8	2.2	70	.05	.13	3.1	—
83	Lean only	1.8 ounces	51	57	125	14	7	3	3	Trace	0	6	1.8	10	.04	.11	2.6	—
	Relatively lean, such as heel of round:																	
84	Lean and fat	3 ounces	85	62	165	25	7	3	3	Trace	0	11	3.2	10	.06	.19	4.5	—
85	Lean only	2.7 ounces	78	65	125	24	3	1	1	Trace	0	10	3.0	Trace	.06	.18	4.3	—
	Steak, broiled: Relatively fat, such as sirloin:																	
86	Lean and fat	3 ounces	85	44	330	20	27	13	12	1	0	9	2.5	50	.05	.16	4.0	—
87	Lean only	2.0 ounces	56	59	115	18	4	2	2	Trace	0	7	2.2	10	.05	.14	3.6	—
	Relatively lean, such as round:																	
88	Lean and fat	3 ounces	85	55	220	24	13	6	6	Trace	0	10	3.0	20	.07	.19	4.8	—
89	Lean only	2.4 ounces	68	61	130	21	4	2	2	Trace	0	9	2.5	10	.06	.16	4.1	—
	Beef, canned:																	
90	Corned beef	3 ounces	85	59	185	22	10	5	4	Trace	0	17	3.7	20	.01	.20	2.9	—
91	Corned beef hash	3 ounces	85	67	155	7	10	5	4	Trace	9	11	1.7	—	.01	.08	1.8	—
92	Beef, dried or chipped	2 ounces	57	48	115	19	4	2	2	Trace	0	11	2.9	—	.04	.18	2.2	—
93	Beef and vegetable stew	1 cup	235	82	210	15	10	5	4	Trace	15	28	2.8	2,310	.13	.17	4.4	15

[2] Contributed largely from beta-carotene used for coloring.

[3] Outer layer of fat on the cut was removed to within approximately ½-inch of the lean. Deposits of fat within the cut were not removed.

H

Table of Food Composition (cont'd)

[Dashes in the columns for nutrients show that no suitable value could be found although there is reason to believe that a measurable amount of the nutrient may be present]

	Food, approximate measure, and weight (in grams)	Water	Food energy	Protein	Fat	Fatty acids Saturated (total)	Unsaturated Oleic	Unsaturated Linoleic	Carbohydrate	Calcium	Iron	Vitamin A value	Thiamin	Riboflavin	Niacin	Ascorbic acid
		Percent	kCalories	Grams	Grams	Grams	Grams	Grams	Grams	Milligrams	Milligrams	International units	Milligrams	Milligrams	Milligrams	Milligrams
	MEAT, POULTRY, FISH, SHELLFISH; RELATED PRODUCTS—Continued															
94	Beef potpie, baked, 4¼-inch diam., weight before baking about 8 ounces. 1 pie — 227	55	560	23	33	9	20	2	43	32	4.1	1,860	0.25	0.27	4.5	7
	Chicken, cooked:															
95	Flesh only, broiled — 3 ounces — 85	71	115	20	3	1	1	1	0	8	1.4	80	.05	.16	7.4	----
	Breast, fried, ½ breast:															
96	With bone — 3.3 ounces — 94	58	155	25	5	1	2	1	1	9	1.3	70	.04	.17	11.2	----
97	Flesh and skin only — 2.7 ounces — 76	58	155	25	5	1	2	1	1	9	1.3	70	.04	.17	11.2	----
	Drumstick, fried:															
98	With bone — 2.1 ounces — 59	55	90	12	4	1	2	1	Trace	6	.9	50	.03	.15	2.7	----
99	Flesh and skin only — 1.3 ounces — 38	55	90	12	4	1	2	1	Trace	6	.9	50	.03	.15	2.7	----
100	Chicken, canned, boneless 3 ounces — 85	65	170	18	10	3	4	2	0	18	1.3	200	.03	.11	3.7	3
101	Chicken potpie, baked 4¼-inch diam, weight before baking about 8 ounces. 1 pie — 227	57	535	23	31	10	15	3	42	68	3.0	3,020	.25	.26	4.1	5
	Chili con carne, canned:															
102	With beans — 1 cup — 250	72	335	19	15	7	7	Trace	30	80	4.2	150	.08	.18	3.2	----
103	Without beans — 1 cup — 255	67	510	26	38	18	17	1	15	97	3.6	380	.05	.31	5.6	----
104	Heart, beef, lean, braised — 3 ounces — 85	61	160	27	5	----	----	----	1	5	5.0	20	.21	1.04	6.5	1
	Lamb,[3] cooked:															
	Chop, thick, with bone, 1 chop, broiled.															
105	4.8 ounces. — 137	47	400	25	33	18	12	1	0	10	1.5	----	.14	.25	5.6	----
106	Lean and fat — 4.0 ounces — 112	47	400	25	33	18	12	1	0	10	1.5	----	.14	.25	5.6	----
107	Lean only — 2.6 ounces — 74	62	140	21	6	3	2	Trace	0	9	1.5	----	.11	.20	4.5	----
	Leg, roasted:															
108	Lean and fat — 3 ounces — 85	54	235	22	16	9	6	Trace	0	9	1.4	----	.13	.23	4.7	----
109	Lean only — 2.5 ounces — 71	62	130	20	5	3	2	Trace	0	9	1.4	----	.12	.21	4.4	----
	Shoulder, roasted:															
110	Lean and fat — 3 ounces — 85	50	285	18	23	13	8	1	0	9	1.0	----	.11	.20	4.0	----
111	Lean only — 2.3 ounces — 64	61	130	17	6	3	2	Trace	0	8	1.0	----	.10	.18	3.7	----

H

No.	Food, approximate measure		Grams	Water (%)	Food energy (cal.)	Protein (g)	Fat (g)	Saturated (total) (g)	Oleic (g)	Linoleic (g)	Carbohydrate (g)	Calcium (mg)	Iron (mg)	Vitamin A (I.U.)	Thiamin (mg)	Riboflavin (mg)	Niacin (mg)	Ascorbic acid (mg)
112	Liver, beef, fried	2 ounces	57	57	130	15	6	—	—	—	3	6	5.0	30,280	.15	2.37	9.4	15
	Pork, cured, cooked:																	
113	Ham, light cure, lean and fat, roasted.	3 ounces	85	54	245	18	19	7	8	2	0	8	2.2	0	.40	.16	3.1	—
	Luncheon meat:																	
114	Boiled ham, sliced	2 ounces	57	59	135	11	10	4	4	1	0	6	1.6	0	.25	.09	1.5	—
115	Canned, spiced or unspiced.	2 ounces	57	55	165	8	14	5	6	1	1	5	1.2	0	.18	.12	1.6	—
	Pork, fresh,[3] cooked:																	
116	Chop, thick, with bone.	1 chop, 3.5 ounces.	98	42	260	16	21	8	9	2	0	8	2.2	0	.63	.18	3.8	—
117	Lean and fat	2.3 ounces	66	42	260	16	21	8	9	2	0	8	2.2	0	.63	.18	3.8	—
118	Lean only	1.7 ounces	48	53	130	15	7	2	3	1	0	7	1.9	0	.54	.16	3.3	—
	Roast, oven-cooked, no liquid added:																	
119	Lean and fat	3 ounces	85	46	310	21	24	9	10	2	0	9	2.7	0	.78	.22	4.7	—
120	Lean only	2.4 ounces	68	55	175	20	10	3	4	1	0	9	2.6	0	.73	.21	4.4	—
	Cuts, simmered:																	
121	Lean and fat	3 ounces	85	46	320	20	26	9	11	2	0	8	2.5	0	.46	.21	4.1	—
122	Lean only	2.2 ounces	63	60	135	18	6	2	3	1	0	8	2.3	0	.42	.19	3.7	—
	Sausage:																	
123	Bologna, slice, 3-in. diam. by 1/8 inch.	2 slices	26	56	80	3	7	—	—	—	Trace	2	.5	—	.04	.06	.7	—
124	Braunschweiger, slice 2-in. diam. by 1/4 inch.	2 slices	20	53	65	3	5	—	—	—	Trace	2	1.2	1,310	.03	.29	1.6	—
125	Deviled ham, canned	1 tbsp.	13	51	45	2	4	—	2	Trace	0	1	.3	0	.02	.01	.2	—
126	Frankfurter, heated (8 per lb. purchased pkg.).	1 frank.	56	57	170	7	15	—	—	—	1	3	.8	—	.08	.11	1.4	—
127	Pork links, cooked (16 links per lb. raw).	2 links	26	35	125	5	11	4	5	1	Trace	2	.6	0	.21	.09	1.0	—
128	Salami, dry type	1 oz.	28	30	130	7	11	—	—	—	Trace	4	1.0	—	.10	.07	1.5	—
129	Salami, cooked	1 oz.	28	51	90	5	7	—	—	—	Trace	3	.7	—	.07	.07	1.2	—
130	Vienna, canned (7 sausages per 5-oz. can).	1 sausage	16	63	40	2	3	—	—	—	Trace	1	.3	—	.01	.02	.4	—
	Veal, medium fat, cooked, bone removed:																	
131	Cutlet	3 oz.	85	60	185	23	9	5	4	Trace	0	9	2.7	—	.06	.21	4.6	—
132	Roast	3 oz.	85	55	230	23	14	7	6	Trace	0	10	2.9	—	.11	.26	6.6	—
	Fish and shellfish:																	
133	Bluefish, baked with table fat.	3 oz.	85	68	135	22	4	—	—	—	0	25	.6	40	.09	.08	1.6	—
	Clams:																	
134	Raw, meat only	3 oz.	85	82	65	11	1	—	—	—	2	59	5.2	90	.08	.15	1.1	8
135	Canned, solids and liquid.	3 oz.	85	86	45	7	1	—	—	—	2	47	3.5	—	.01	.09	.9	—
136	Crabmeat, canned	3 oz.	85	77	85	15	2	—	—	—	1	38	.7	—	.07	.07	1.6	—

[3] Outer layer of fat on the cut was removed to within approximately 1/2-inch of the lean. Deposits of fat within the cut were not removed.

H

Table of Food Composition (cont'd)

[Dashes in the columns for nutrients show that no suitable value could be found although there is reason to believe that a measurable amount of the nutrient may be present]

	Food, approximate measure, and weight (in grams)		Water	Food energy	Protein	Fat	Fatty acids			Carbohydrate	Calcium	Iron	Vitamin A value	Thiamin	Riboflavin	Niacin	Ascorbic acid
							Saturated (total)	Unsaturated									
								Oleic	Linoleic								
			Percent	kCalories	Grams	Grams	Grams	Grams	Grams	Grams	Milligrams	Milligrams	International units	Milligrams	Milligrams	Milligrams	Milligrams
	MEAT, POULTRY, FISH, SHELLFISH; RELATED PRODUCTS—Continued	Grams															
	Fish and shellfish—Continued																
137	Fish sticks, breaded, cooked, frozen; stick 3¾ by 1 by ½ inch. 10 sticks or 8 oz. pkg.	227	66	400	38	20	5	4	10	15	25	0.9		0.09	0.16	3.6	
138	Haddock, breaded, fried	3 oz.	85	66	140	17	5	1	3	Trace	5	34	1.0		.03	.06	2.7	2
139	Ocean perch, breaded, fried.	3 oz.	85	59	195	16	11				6	28	1.1		.08	.09	1.5	
140	Oysters, raw, meat only (13–19 med. selects).	1 cup meat	240	85	160	20	4				8	226	13.2	740	.33	.43	6.0	
141	Salmon, pink, canned	3 oz.	85	71	120	17	5	1	1	Trace	0	⁴167	.7	60	.03	.16	6.8	
142	Sardines, Atlantic, canned in oil, drained solids.	3 oz.	85	62	175	20	9				0	372	2.5	190	.02	.17	4.6	
143	Shad, baked with table fat and bacon.	3 oz.	85	64	170	20	10				0	20	.5	20	.11	.22	7.3	
144	Shrimp, canned, meat.	3 oz.	85	70	100	21	1				1	98	2.6	50	.01	.03	1.5	
145	Swordfish, broiled with butter or margarine.	3 oz.	85	65	150	24	5				0	23	1.1	1,750	.03	.04	9.3	
146	Tuna, canned in oil, drained solids.	3 oz.	85	61	170	24	7	2	1	1	0	7	1.6	70	.04	.10	10.1	
	MATURE DRY BEANS AND PEAS, NUTS, PEANUTS; RELATED PRODUCTS																
147	Almonds, shelled, whole kernels.	1 cup	142	5	850	26	77	6	52	15	28	332	6.7	0	.34	1.31	5.0	Trace
	Beans, dry: Common varieties as Great Northern, navy, and others: Cooked, drained:																	
148	Great Northern	1 cup	180	69	210	14	1				38	90	4.9	0	.25	.13	1.3	0

H

No.	Food, approximate measure	Grams	Water (%)	Food energy (cal.)	Protein (g)	Fat (g)	Saturated (g)	Oleic (g)	Linoleic (g)	Carbohydrate (g)	Calcium (mg)	Iron (mg)	Vitamin A (I.U.)	Thiamin (mg)	Riboflavin (mg)	Niacin (mg)	Ascorbic acid (mg)
149	Navy (pea) — 1 cup	190	69	225	15	1				40	95	5.1	0	.27	.13	1.3	0
	Canned, solids and liquid: White with—																
150	Frankfurters (sliced) — 1 cup	255	71	365	19	18				32	94	4.8	330	.18	.15	3.3	Trace
151	Pork and tomato sauce — 1 cup	255	71	310	16	7	2	3	1	49	138	4.6	330	.20	.08	1.5	5
152	Pork and sweet sauce — 1 cup	255	66	385	16	12	4	5	1	54	161	5.9		.15	.10	1.3	
153	Red kidney — 1 cup	255	76	230	15	1				42	74	4.6	10	.13	.10	1.5	
154	Lima, cooked, drained — 1 cup	190	64	260	16	1				49	55	5.9		.25	.11	1.3	
155	Cashew nuts, roasted — 1 cup	140	5	785	24	64	11	45	4	41	53	5.3	140	.60	.35	2.5	1
	Coconut, fresh, meat only:																
156	Pieces, approx. 2 by 2 by ½ inch — 1 piece	45	51	155	2	16	14	1	Trace	4	6	.8	0	.02	.01	.2	1
157	Shredded or grated, firmly packed — 1 cup	130	51	450	5	46	39	3	Trace	12	17	2.2	0	.07	.03	.7	4
158	Cowpeas or blackeye peas, dry, cooked — 1 cup	248	80	190	13	1				34	42	3.2	20	.41	.11	1.1	Trace
159	Peanuts, roasted, salted, halves — 1 cup	144	2	840	37	72	16	31	21	27	107	3.0	0	.46	.19	24.7	0
160	Peanut butter — 1 tbsp.	16	2	95	4	8	2	4	2	3	9	.3	0	.02	.02	2.4	0
161	Peas, split, dry, cooked — 1 cup	250	70	290	20	1				52	28	4.2	100	.37	.22	2.2	
162	Pecans, halves — 1 cup	108	3	740	10	77	5	48	15	16	79	2.6	140	.93	.14	1.0	2
163	Walnuts, black or native, chopped — 1 cup	126	3	790	26	75	4	26	36	19	Trace	7.6	380	.28	.14	.9	
	VEGETABLES AND VEGETABLE PRODUCTS																
	Asparagus, green: Cooked, drained:																
164	Spears, ½-in. diam. at base — 4 spears	60	94	10	1	Trace				2	13	.4	540	.10	.11	.8	16
165	Pieces, 1½ to 2-in. lengths — 1 cup	145	94	30	3	Trace				5	30	.9	1,310	.23	.26	2.0	38
166	Canned, solids and liquid — 1 cup	244	94	45	5	1				7	44	4.1	1,240	.15	.22	2.0	37
	Beans:																
167	Lima, immature seeds, cooked, drained — 1 cup	170	71	190	13	1				34	80	4.3	480	.31	.17	2.2	29
	Snap: Green:																
168	Cooked, drained — 1 cup	125	92	30	2	Trace				7	63	.8	680	.09	.11	.6	15
169	Canned, solids and liquid — 1 cup	239	94	45	2	Trace				10	81	2.9	690	.07	.10	.7	10

[4] If bones are discarded, value will be greatly reduced.

Table of Food Composition (cont'd)

[Dashes in the columns for nutrients show that no suitable value could be found although there is reason to believe that a measurable amount of the nutrient may be present]

	Food, approximate measure, and weight (in grams)		Water	Food energy	Pro-tein	Fat	Fatty acids Saturated (total)	Fatty acids Unsaturated Oleic	Fatty acids Unsaturated Lin-oleic	Carbo-hy-drate	Cal-cium	Iron	Vita-min A value	Thia-min	Ribo-flavin	Niacin	Ascor-bic acid
		Grams	Per-cent	kCalo-ries	Grams	Grams	Grams	Grams	Grams	Grams	Milli-grams	Milli-grams	Inter-national units	Milli-grams	Milli-grams	Milli-grams	Milli-grams
	VEGETABLES AND VEGETABLE PRODUCTS—Continued																
	Beans—Continued																
	Snap—Continued																
	Yellow or wax:																
170	Cooked, drained	1 cup	125	93	30	2	Trace			6	63	0.8	290	0.09	0.11	0.6	16
171	Canned, solids and liquid.	1 cup	239	94	45	2	1			10	81	2.9	140	.07	.10	.7	12
172	Sprouted mung beans, cooked, drained.	1 cup	125	91	35	4	Trace			7	21	1.1	30	.11	.13	.9	8
	Beets:																
	Cooked, drained, peeled:																
173	Whole beets, 2-in. diam.	2 beets	100	91	30	1	Trace			7	14	.5	20	.03	.04	.3	6
174	Diced or sliced	1 cup	170	91	55	2	Trace			12	24	.9	30	.05	.07	.5	10
175	Canned, solids and liquid.	1 cup	246	90	85	2	Trace			19	34	1.5	20	.02	.05	.2	7
176	Beet greens, leaves and stems, cooked, drained.	1 cup	145	94	25	3	Trace			5	144	2.8	7,400	.10	.22	.4	22
	Blackeye peas. See Cowpeas.																
	Broccoli, cooked, drained:																
177	Whole stalks, medium size.	1 stalk	180	91	45	6	1			8	158	1.4	4,500	.16	.36	1.4	162
178	Stalks cut into ½-in. pieces.	1 cup	155	91	40	5	1			7	136	1.2	3,880	.14	.31	1.2	140
179	Chopped, yield from 10-oz. frozen pkg.	1⅜ cups	250	92	65	7	1			12	135	1.8	6,500	.15	.30	1.3	143
180	Brussels sprouts, 7–8 sprouts (1¼ to 1½ in. diam.) per cup, cooked.	1 cup	155	88	55	7	1			10	50	1.7	810	.12	.22	1.2	135
	Cabbage:																
	Common varieties:																

H

H

No.	Food	Measure	Grams	Water (%)	Food energy	Protein	Fat	Sat. fatty acid	Oleic	Linoleic	Carbohydrate	Calcium	Iron	Vitamin A	Thiamine	Riboflavin	Niacin	Ascorbic acid
	Raw:																	
181	Coarsely shredded or sliced.	1 cup	70	92	15	1	Trace				4	34	.3	90	.04	.04	.2	33
182	Finely shredded or chopped.	1 cup	90	92	20	1	Trace				5	44	.4	120	.05	.05	.3	42
183	Cooked.	1 cup	145	94	30	2	Trace				6	64	.4	190	.06	.06	.4	48
184	Red, raw, coarsely shredded.	1 cup	70	90	20	1	Trace				5	29	.6	30	.06	.04	.3	43
185	Savoy, raw, coarsely shredded.	1 cup	70	92	15	2	Trace				3	47	.6	140	.04	.06	.2	39
186	Cabbage, celery or Chinese, raw, cut in 1-in. pieces.	1 cup	75	95	10	1	Trace				2	32	.5	110	.04	.03	.5	19
187	Cabbage, spoon (or pakchoy), cooked.	1 cup	170	95	25	2	Trace				4	252	1.0	5,270	.07	.14	1.2	26
	Carrots: Raw:																	
188	Whole, 5½ by 1 inch, (25 thin strips).	1 carrot	50	88	20	1	Trace				5	18	.4	5,500	.03	.03	.3	4
189	Grated.	1 cup	110	88	45	1	Trace				11	41	.8	12,100	.06	.06	.7	9
190	Cooked, diced.	1 cup	145	91	45	1	Trace				10	48	.9	15,220	.08	.07	.7	9
191	Canned, strained or chopped (baby food).	1 ounce	28	92	10	Trace	Trace				2	7	.1	3,690	.01	.01	.1	1
192	Cauliflower, cooked, flowerbuds.	1 cup	120	93	25	3	Trace				5	25	.8	70	.11	.10	.7	66
	Celery, raw:																	
193	Stalk, large outer, 8 by about 1½ inches, at root end.	1 stalk	40	94	5	Trace	Trace				2	16	.1	100	.01	.01	.1	4
194	Pieces, diced.	1 cup	100	94	15	1	Trace				4	39	.3	240	.03	.03	.3	9
195	Collards, cooked.	1 cup	190	91	55	5	1				9	289	1.1	10,260	.27	.37	2.4	87
	Corn, sweet:																	
196	Cooked, ear 5 by 1¾ inches.[5]	1 ear	140	74	70	3	1				16	2	.5	[6]310	.09	.08	1.0	7
197	Canned, solids and liquid.	1 cup	256	81	170	5	2				40	10	1.0	[6]690	.07	.12	2.3	13
198	Cowpeas, cooked, immature seeds.	1 cup	160	72	175	13	1				29	38	3.4	560	.49	.18	2.3	28
	Cucumbers, 10-ounce; 7½ by about 2 inches:																	
199	Raw, pared.	1 cucumber	207	96	30	1	Trace				7	35	.6	Trace	.07	.09	.4	23
200	Raw, pared, center slice ⅛-inch thick.	6 slices	50	96	5	Trace	Trace				2	8	.2	Trace	.02	.02	.1	6
201	Dandelion greens, cooked.	1 cup	180	90	60	4	1				12	252	3.2	21,060	.24	.29		32

[5] Measure and weight apply to entire vegetable or fruit including parts not usually eaten.

[6] Based on yellow varieties; white varieties contain only a trace of cryptoxanthin and carotenes, the pigments in corn that have biological activity.

Table of Food Composition (cont'd)

[Dashes in the columns for nutrients show that no suitable value could be found although there is reason to believe that a measurable amount of the nutrient may be present]

	Food, approximate measure, and weight (in grams)		Water	Food energy	Protein	Fat	Fatty acids Saturated (total)	Fatty acids Unsaturated Oleic	Fatty acids Unsaturated Linoleic	Carbohydrate	Calcium	Iron	Vitamin A value	Thiamin	Riboflavin	Niacin	Ascorbic acid
		Grams	Percent	kCalories	Grams	Grams	Grams	Grams	Grams	Grams	Milligrams	Milligrams	International units	Milligrams	Milligrams	Milligrams	Milligrams
	VEGETABLES AND VEGETABLE PRODUCTS—Continued																
202	Endive, curly (including escarole). 2 ounces	57	93	10	1	Trace				2	46	1.0	1,870	0.04	0.08	0.3	6
203	Kale, leaves including stems, cooked. 1 cup	110	91	30	4	1				4	147	1.3	8,140	---	---	---	68
	Lettuce, raw:																
204	Butterhead, as Boston types; head, 4-inch diameter. 1 head	220	95	30	3	Trace				6	77	4.4	2,130	.14	.13	.6	18
205	Crisphead, as Iceberg; 1 head, 4¾-inch diameter. 1 head	454	96	60	4	Trace				13	91	2.3	1,500	.29	.27	1.3	29
206	Looseleaf, or bunching varieties, leaves. 2 large	50	94	10	1	Trace				2	34	.7	950	.03	.04	.2	9
207	Mushrooms, canned, solids and liquid. 1 cup	244	93	40	5	Trace				6	15	1.2	Trace	.04	.60	4.8	4
208	Mustard greens, cooked. 1 cup	140	93	35	3	1				6	193	2.5	8,120	.11	.19	.9	68
209	Okra, cooked, pod 3 by ⅝ inch. 8 pods	85	91	25	2	Trace				5	78	.4	420	.11	.15	.8	17
	Onions:																
	Mature:																
210	Raw, onion 2½-inch diameter. 1 onion	110	89	40	2	Trace				10	30	.6	40	.04	.04	.2	11
211	Cooked. 1 cup	210	92	60	3	Trace				14	50	.8	80	.06	.06	.4	14
212	Young green, small, without tops. 6 onions	50	88	20	1	Trace				5	20	.3	Trace	.02	.02	.2	12
213	Parsley, raw, chopped. 1 tablespoon	4	85	Trace	Trace	Trace				Trace	8	.2	340	Trace	.01	Trace	7
214	Parsnips, cooked. 1 cup	155	82	100	2	1				23	70	.9	50	.11	.12	.2	16
	Peas, green:																
215	Cooked. 1 cup	160	82	115	9	1				19	37	2.9	860	.44	.17	3.7	33
216	Canned, solids and liquid. 1 cup	249	83	165	9	1				31	50	4.2	1,120	.23	.13	2.2	22

H

No.	Food	Measure																
217	Canned, strained (baby food).	1 ounce	28	86	15	1	Trace	-	-	-	3	3	.4	140	.02	.02	.4	3
218	Peppers, hot, red, without seeds, dried (ground chili powder, added seasonings).	1 tablespoon	15	8	50	2	2	-	-	-	8	40	2.3	9,750	.03	.17	1.3	2
	Peppers, sweet: Raw, about 5 per pound:																	
219	Green pod without stem and seeds.	1 pod	74	93	15	1	Trace	-	-	-	4	7	.5	310	.06	.06	.4	94
220	Cooked, boiled, drained 1 pod.	1 pod	73	95	15	1	Trace	-	-	-	3	7	.4	310	.05	.05	.4	70
	Potatoes, medium (about 3 per pound raw):																	
221	Baked, peeled after baking.	1 potato	99	75	90	3	Trace	-	-	-	21	9	.7	Trace	.10	.04	1.7	20
	Boiled:																	
222	Peeled after boiling	1 potato	136	80	105	3	Trace	-	-	-	23	10	.8	Trace	.13	.05	2.0	22
223	Peeled before boiling	1 potato	122	83	80	2	Trace	-	-	-	18	7	.6	Trace	.11	.04	1.4	20
	French-fried, piece 2 by ½ by ½ inch:																	
224	Cooked in deep fat	10 pieces	57	45	155	2	7	2	2	4	20	9	.7	Trace	.07	.04	1.8	12
225	Frozen, heated	10 pieces	57	53	125	2	5	1	1	2	19	5	1.0	Trace	.08	.01	1.5	12
	Mashed:																	
226	Milk added	1 cup	195	83	125	4	1	-	-	-	25	47	.8	50	.16	.10	2.0	19
227	Milk and butter added.	1 cup	195	80	185	4	8	4	3	Trace	24	47	.8	330	.16	.10	1.9	18
228	Potato chips, medium, 2-inch diameter.	10 chips	20	2	115	1	8	2	2	4	10	8	.4	Trace	.04	.01	1.0	3
229	Pumpkin, canned	1 cup	228	90	75	2	1	-	-	-	18	57	.9	14,590	.07	.12	1.3	12
230	Radishes, raw, small, without tops.	4 radishes	40	94	5	Trace	Trace	-	-	-	1	12	.4	Trace	.01	.01	.1	10
231	Sauerkraut, canned, solids and liquid.	1 cup	235	93	45	2	Trace	-	-	-	9	85	1.2	120	.07	.09	.4	33
	Spinach:																	
232	Cooked	1 cup	180	92	40	5	1	-	-	-	6	167	4.0	14,580	.13	.25	1.0	50
233	Canned, drained solids	1 cup	180	91	45	5	1	-	-	-	6	212	4.7	14,400	.03	.21	.6	24
	Squash: Cooked:																	
234	Summer, diced	1 cup	210	96	30	2	Trace	-	-	-	7	52	.8	820	.10	.16	1.6	21
235	Winter, baked, mashed.	1 cup	205	81	130	4	1	-	-	-	32	57	1.6	8,610	.10	.27	1.4	27
	Sweetpotatoes: Cooked, medium, 5 by 2 inches, weight raw about 6 ounces:																	
236	Baked, peeled after baking.	1 sweetpotato	110	64	155	2	1	-	-	-	36	44	1.0	8,910	.10	.07	.7	24
237	Boiled, peeled after boiling.	1 sweetpotato	147	71	170	2	1	-	-	-	39	47	1.0	11,610	.13	.09	.9	25

Table of Food Composition (cont'd)

[Dashes in the columns for nutrients show that no suitable value could be found although there is reason to believe that a measurable amount of the nutrient may be present]

	Food, approximate measure, and weight (in grams)		Water	Food energy	Protein	Fat	Fatty acids			Carbohydrate	Calcium	Iron	Vitamin A value	Thiamin	Riboflavin	Niacin	Ascorbic acid
							Saturated (total)	Unsaturated Oleic	Linoleic								
		Grams	Percent	kCalories	Grams	Grams	Grams	Grams	Grams	Grams	Milligrams	Milligrams	International units	Milligrams	Milligrams	Milligrams	Milligrams
	VEGETABLES AND VEGETABLE PRODUCTS—Continued																
	Sweetpotatoes—Continued																
238	Candied, 3½ by 2¼ inches. 1 sweetpotato.	175	60	295	2	6	2	3	1	60	65	1.6	11,030	0.10	0.08	0.8	17
239	Canned, vacuum or solid pack. 1 cup	218	72	235	4	Trace				54	54	1.7	17,000	.10	.10	1.4	30
	Tomatoes:																
240	Raw, approx. 3-in. diam. 2⅛ in. high; wt, 7 oz. 1 tomato	200	94	40	2	Trace				9	24	.9	1,640	.11	.07	1.3	7 42
241	Canned, solids and liquid. 1 cup	241	94	50	2	1				10	14	1.2	2,170	.12	.07	1.7	41
	Tomato catsup:																
242	Cup 1 cup	273	69	290	6	1				69	60	2.2	3,820	.25	.19	4.4	41
243	Tablespoon 1 tbsp.	15	69	15	Trace	Trace				4	3	.1	210	.01	.01	.2	2
	Tomato juice, canned:																
244	Cup 1 cup	243	94	45	2	Trace				10	17	2.2	1,940	.12	.07	1.9	39
245	Glass (6 fl. oz.) 1 glass	182	94	35	2	Trace				8	13	1.6	1,460	.09	.05	1.5	29
246	Turnips, cooked, diced 1 cup	155	94	35	1	Trace				8	54	.6	Trace	.06	.08	.5	34
247	Turnip greens, cooked 1 cup	145	94	30	3	Trace				5	252	1.5	8,270	.15	.33	.7	68
	FRUITS AND FRUIT PRODUCTS																
248	Apples, raw (about 3 per lb.)[5] 1 apple	150	85	70	Trace	Trace				18	8	.4	50	.04	.02	.1	3
249	Apple juice, bottled or canned. 1 cup	248	88	120	Trace	Trace				30	15	1.5	--------	.02	.05	.2	2
	Applesauce, canned:																
250	Sweetened 1 cup	255	76	230	1	Trace				61	10	1.3	100	.05	.03	.1	8 3
251	Unsweetened or artificially sweetened. 1 cup	244	88	100	1	Trace				26	10	1.2	100	.05	.02	.1	8 2

H

No.	Food, approximate measure, and weight (grams)		Weight (g)	Water (%)	Food energy (cal.)	Protein (g)	Fat (g)	Saturated (total)	Oleic	Linoleic	Carbohydrate (g)	Calcium (mg)	Iron (mg)	Vitamin A (I.U.)	Thiamine (mg)	Riboflavin (mg)	Niacin (mg)	Ascorbic acid (mg)
	Apricots:																	
252	Raw (about 12 per lb.)⁵	3 apricots---	114	85	55	1	Trace				14	18	.5	2,890	.03	.04	.7	10
253	Canned in heavy sirup--	1 cup------	259	77	220	2	Trace				57	28	.8	4,510	.05	.06	.9	10
254	Dried, uncooked (40 halves per cup).	1 cup------	150	25	390	8	1				100	100	8.2	16,350	.02	.23	4.9	19
255	Cooked, unsweetened, fruit and liquid.	1 cup------	285	76	240	5	1				62	63	5.1	8,550	.01	.13	2.8	8
256	Apricot nectar, canned--	1 cup------	251	85	140	1	Trace				37	23	.5	2,380	.03	.03	.5	[8]8
	Avocados, whole fruit, raw:⁵																	
257	California (mid- and late-winter; diam. 3⅛ in.).	1 avocado---	284	74	370	5	37	7	17	5	13	22	1.3	630	.24	.43	3.5	30
258	Florida (late summer, fall; diam. 3⅝ in.).	1 avocado---	454	78	390	4	33	7	15	4	27	30	1.8	880	.33	.61	4.9	43
259	Bananas, raw, medium size.⁵	1 banana---	175	76	100	1	Trace				26	10	.8	230	.06	.07	.8	12
260	Banana flakes------	1 cup------	100	3	340	4	1				89	32	2.8	760	.18	.24	2.8	7
261	Blackberries, raw----	1 cup------	144	84	85	2	1				19	46	1.3	290	.05	.06	.5	30
262	Blueberries, raw------	1 cup------	140	83	85	1	1				21	21	1.4	140	.04	.08	.6	20
263	Cantaloups, raw; medium, 5-inch diameter about 1⅔ pounds.⁵	½ melon---	385	91	60	1	Trace				14	27	.8	[9]6,540	.08	.06	1.2	63
264	Cherries, canned, red, sour, pitted, water pack.	1 cup------	244	88	105	2	Trace				26	37	.7	1,660	.07	.05	.5	12
265	Cranberry juice cocktail, canned.	1 cup------	250	83	165	Trace	Trace				42	13	.8	Trace	.03	.03	.1	[10]40
266	Cranberry sauce, sweetened, canned, strained.	1 cup------	277	62	405	Trace	1				104	17	.6	60	.03	.03	.1	6
267	Dates, pitted, cut---	1 cup------	178	22	490	4	1				130	105	5.3	90	.16	.17	3.9	0
268	Figs, dried, large, 2 by 1 in.	1 fig------	21	23	60	1	Trace				15	26	.6	20	.02	.02	.1	0
269	Fruit cocktail, canned, in heavy sirup.	1 cup------	256	80	195	1	Trace				50	23	1.0	360	.05	.03	1.3	5

⁵ Measure and weight apply to entire vegetable or fruit including parts not usually eaten.

⁷ Year-round average. Samples marketed from November through May, average 20 milligrams per 200-gram tomato; from June through October, around 52 milligrams.

⁸ This is the amount from the fruit. Additional ascorbic acid may be added by the manufacturer. Refer to the label for this information.

⁹ Value for varieties with orange-colored flesh; value for varieties with green flesh would be about 540 I.U.

¹⁰ Value listed is based on products with label stating 30 milligrams per 6 fl. oz. serving.

H

Table of Food Composition (cont'd)

[Dashes in the columns for nutrients show that no suitable value could be found although there is reason to believe that a measurable amount of the nutrient may be present]

	Food, approximate measure, and weight (in grams)		Water	Food energy	Pro-tein	Fat	Fatty acids Satu-rated (total)	Fatty acids Unsaturated Oleic	Fatty acids Unsaturated Lin-oleic	Carbo-hy-drate	Cal-cium	Iron	Vita-min A value	Thia-min	Ribo-flavin	Niacin	Ascor-bic acid
		Grams	Per cent	kCalo-ries	Grams	Grams	Grams	Grams	Grams	Grams	Milli-grams	Milli-grams	Inter-national units	Milli-grams	Milli-grams	Milli-grams	Milli-grams
	FRUITS AND FRUIT PRODUCTS—Con.																
	Grapefruit:																
	Raw, medium, 3¾-in. diam.[5]																
270	White ½ grapefruit.	241	89	45	1	Trace	-----	-----	-----	12	19	0.5	10	0.05	0.02	0.2	44
271	Pink or red ½ grapefruit.	241	89	50	1	Trace	-----	-----	-----	13	20	0.5	540	0.05	0.02	0.2	44
272	Canned, sirup pack 1 cup	254	81	180	2	Trace	-----	-----	-----	45	33	.8	30	.08	.05	.5	76
	Grapefruit juice:																
273	Fresh 1 cup	246	90	95	1	Trace	-----	-----	-----	23	22	.5	(11)	.09	.04	.4	92
	Canned, white:																
274	Unsweetened 1 cup	247	89	100	1	Trace	-----	-----	-----	24	20	1.0	20	.07	.04	.4	84
275	Sweetened 1 cup	250	86	130	1	Trace	-----	-----	-----	32	20	1.0	20	.07	.04	.4	78
	Frozen, concentrate, unsweetened:																
276	Undiluted, can, 6 fluid ounces. 1 can	207	62	300	4	1	-----	-----	-----	72	70	.8	60	.29	.12	1.4	286
277	Diluted with 3 parts water, by volume. 1 cup	247	89	100	1	Trace	-----	-----	-----	24	25	.2	20	.10	.04	.5	96
278	Dehydrated crystals 4 oz	113	1	410	6	1	-----	-----	-----	102	100	1.2	80	.40	.20	2.0	396
279	Prepared with water 1 cup (1 pound yields about 1 gallon).	247	90	100	1	Trace	-----	-----	-----	24	22	.2	20	.10	.05	.5	91
	Grapes, raw:[5]																
280	American type (slip skin). 1 cup	153	82	65	1	1	-----	-----	-----	15	15	.4	100	.05	.03	.2	3
281	European type (adherent skin). 1 cup	160	81	95	1	Trace	-----	-----	-----	25	17	.6	140	.07	.04	.4	6
	Grapejuice:																
282	Canned or bottled 1 cup	253	83	165	1	Trace	-----	-----	-----	42	28	.8	-----	.10	.05	.5	Trace
	Frozen concentrate, sweetened:																
283	Undiluted, can, 6 fluid ounces. 1 can	216	53	395	1	Trace	-----	-----	-----	100	22	.9	40	.13	.22	1.5	(12)

H

No.	Food, approximate measure	Weight (g)	Water (%)	Food energy	Protein	Fat				Carbohydrate	Calcium	Iron	Vitamin A	Thiamine	Riboflavin	Niacin	Ascorbic acid
284	Diluted with 3 parts water, by volume. 1 cup	250	86	135	1	Trace	—	—	—	33	8	.3	10	.05	.08	.5	(12)
285	Grapejuice drink, canned. 1 cup	250	86	135	Trace	Trace	—	—	—	35	8	.3	10	.03	.03	.3	(12)
286	Lemons, raw, 2⅛-in. diam., size 165.[5] Used for juice. 1 lemon	110	90	20	1	Trace	—	—	—	6	19	.4	10	.03	.01	.1	39
287	Lemon juice, raw. 1 cup	244	91	60	1	Trace	—	—	—	20	17	.5	50	.07	.02	.2	112
	Lemonade concentrate:																
288	Frozen, 6 fl. oz. per can. 1 can	219	48	430	Trace	Trace	—	—	—	112	9	.4	40	.04	.07	.7	66
289	Diluted with 4⅓ parts water, by volume. 1 cup	248	88	110	Trace	Trace	—	—	—	28	2	Trace	Trace	Trace	.02	.2	17
	Lime juice:																
290	Fresh. 1 cup	246	90	65	1	Trace	—	—	—	22	22	.5	20	.05	.02	.2	79
291	Canned, unsweetened. 1 cup	246	90	65	1	Trace	—	—	—	22	22	.5	20	.05	.02	.2	52
	Limeade concentrate, frozen:																
292	Undiluted, can, 6 fluid ounces. 1 can	218	50	410	Trace	Trace	—	—	—	108	11	.2	Trace	.02	.02	.2	26
293	Diluted with 4⅓ parts water, by volume. 1 cup	247	90	100	Trace	Trace	—	—	—	27	2	Trace	Trace	Trace	Trace	Trace	5
294	Oranges, raw, 2⅝-in. diam., all commercial, varieties.[5] 1 orange	180	86	65	1	Trace	—	—	—	16	54	.5	260	.13	.05	.5	66
295	Orange juice, fresh, all varieties. 1 cup	248	88	110	2	1	—	—	—	26	27	.5	500	.22	.07	1.0	124
296	Canned, unsweetened. 1 cup	249	87	120	2	Trace	—	—	—	28	25	1.0	500	.17	.05	.7	100
	Frozen concentrate:																
297	Undiluted, can, 6 fluid ounces. 1 can	213	55	360	5	Trace	—	—	—	87	75	.9	1,620	.68	.11	2.8	360
298	Diluted with 3 parts water, by volume. 1 cup	249	87	120	2	Trace	—	—	—	29	25	.2	550	.22	.02	1.0	120
299	Dehydrated crystals. 4 oz.	113	1	430	6	2	—	—	—	100	95	1.9	1,900	.76	.24	3.3	408
300	Prepared with water (1 pound yields about 1 gallon). 1 cup	248	88	115	2	1	—	—	—	27	25	.5	500	.20	.07	1.0	109
301	Orange-apricot juice drink. 1 cup	249	87	125	1	Trace	—	—	—	32	12	.2	1,440	.05	.02	.5	[10] 40

[5] Measure and weight apply to entire vegetable or fruit including parts not usually eaten.

[10] Value listed is based on product with label stating 30 milligrams per 6 fl. oz. serving.

[11] For white-fleshed varieties value is about 20 I.U. per cup; for red-fleshed varieties, 1,080 I.U. per cup.

[12] Present only if added by the manufacturer. Refer to the label for this information.

H

Table of Food Composition (cont'd)

[Dashes in the columns for nutrients show that no suitable value could be found although there is reason to believe that a measurable amount of the nutrient may be present]

	Food, approximate measure, and weight (in grams)		Water	Food energy	Protein	Fat	Fatty acids			Carbohydrate	Calcium	Iron	Vitamin A value	Thiamin	Riboflavin	Niacin	Ascorbic acid
							Saturated (total)	Unsaturated Oleic	Unsaturated Linoleic								
		Grams	*Percent*	*kCalories*	*Grams*	*Grams*	*Grams*	*Grams*	*Grams*	*Grams*	*Milligrams*	*Milligrams*	*International units*	*Milligrams*	*Milligrams*	*Milligrams*	*Milligrams*
	FRUITS AND FRUIT PRODUCTS—Con.																
	Orange and grapefruit juice: Frozen concentrate:																
302	Undiluted, can, 6 fluid ounces. 1 can	210	59	330	4	1				78	61	0.8	800	0.48	0.06	2.3	302
303	Diluted with 3 parts water, by volume. 1 cup	248	88	110	1	Trace				26	20	.2	270	.16	.02	.8	102
304	Papayas, raw, ½-inch cubes. 1 cup	182	89	70	1	Trace				18	36	.5	3,190	.07	.08	.5	102
	Peaches: Raw:																
305	Whole, medium, 2-inch diameter, about 4 per pound.[5] 1 peach	114	89	35	1	Trace				10	9	.5	[1]1,320	.02	.05	1.0	7
306	Sliced. 1 cup	168	89	65	1	Trace				16	15	.8	[2]2,230	.03	.08	1.6	12
	Canned, yellow-fleshed, solids and liquid: Sirup pack, heavy:																
307	Halves or slices. 1 cup	257	79	200	1	Trace				52	10	.8	1,100	.02	.06	1.4	7
308	Water pack. 1 cup	245	91	75	1	Trace				20	10	.7	1,100	.02	.06	1.4	7
309	Dried, uncooked. 1 cup	160	25	420	5	1				109	77	9.6	6,240	.02	.31	8.5	28
310	Cooked, unsweetened, 10–12 halves and juice. 1 cup	270	77	220	3	1				58	41	5.1	3,290	.01	.15	4.2	6
	Frozen:																
311	Carton, 12 ounces, not thawed. 1 carton	340	76	300	1	Trace				77	14	1.7	2,210	.03	.14	2.4	[14]135
	Pears:																
312	Raw, 3 by 2½-inch diameter.[5] 1 pear	182	83	100	1	1				25	13	.5	30	.04	.07	.2	7
	Canned, solids and liquid: Sirup pack, heavy:																
313	Halves or slices. 1 cup	255	80	195	1	1				50	13	.5	Trace	.03	.05	.3	4

No.	Food, approximate measure	Grams	Water (%)	Food energy	Protein (g)	Fat (g)		Carbohydrate (g)	Calcium (mg)	Iron (mg)	Vitamin A (I.U.)	Thiamine (mg)	Riboflavin (mg)	Niacin (mg)	Ascorbic acid (mg)
314	Pineapple: Raw, diced, 1 cup	140	85	75	1	Trace		19	24	.7	100	.12	.04	.3	24
	Canned, heavy sirup pack, solids and liquid:														
315	Crushed, 1 cup	260	80	195	1	Trace		50	29	.8	120	.20	.06	.5	17
316	Sliced, slices and juice. 2 small or 1 large	122	80	90	Trace	Trace		24	13	.4	50	.09	.03	.2	8
317	Pineapple juice, canned, 1 cup	249	86	135	1	Trace		34	37	.7	120	.12	.04	.5	22[8]
	Plums, all except prunes:														
318	Raw, 2-inch diameter, 1 plum about 2 ounces.[5]	60	87	25	Trace	Trace		7	7	.3	140	.02	.02	.3	3
	Canned, sirup pack (Italian prunes):														
319	Plums (with pits) and juice.[5] 1 cup	256	77	205	1	Trace		53	22	2.2	2,970	.05	.05	.9	4
	Prunes, dried, "softenized", medium:														
320	Uncooked[5], 4 prunes	32	28	70	1	Trace		18	14	1.1	440	.02	.04	.4	1
321	Cooked, unsweetened, 17–18 prunes and 1/3 cup liquid.[5] 1 cup	270	66	295	2	1		78	60	4.5	1,860	.08	.18	1.7	2
322	Prune juice, canned or bottled. 1 cup	256	80	200	1	Trace		49	36	10.5	---	.03	.03	1.0	5[8]
	Raisins, seedless:														
323	Packaged, 1/2 oz. or 1 1/2 tbsp. per pkg. 1 pkg	14	18	40	Trace	Trace		11	9	.5	Trace	.02	.01	.1	Trace
324	Cup, pressed down, 1 cup	165	18	480	4	Trace		128	102	5.8	30	.18	.13	.8	2
	Raspberries, red:														
325	Raw, 1 cup	123	84	70	1	1		17	27	1.1	160	.04	.11	1.1	31
326	Frozen, 10-ounce carton, not thawed. 1 carton	284	74	275	2	1		70	37	1.7	200	.06	.17	1.7	59
327	Rhubarb, cooked, sugar added. 1 cup	272	63	385	1	Trace		98	212	1.6	220	.06	.15	.7	17
	Strawberries:														
328	Raw, capped, 1 cup	149	90	55	1	1		13	31	1.5	90	.04	.10	1.0	88
329	Frozen, 10-ounce carton, not thawed. 1 carton	284	71	310	1	1		79	40	2.0	90	.06	.17	1.5	150
330	Tangerines, raw, medium, 2 3/8-in. diam., size 176.[5] 1 tangerine	116	87	40	1	Trace		10	34	.3	360	.05	.02	.1	27
331	Tangerine juice, canned, sweetened. 1 cup	249	87	125	1	1		30	45	.5	1,050	.15	.05	.2	55
332	Watermelon, raw, wedge, 4 by 8 inches (1/16 of 10 by 16-inch melon, about 2 pounds with rind).[5] 1 wedge	925	93	115	2	1		27	30	2.1	2,510	.13	.13	.7	30

[5] Measure and weight apply to entire vegetable or fruit including parts not usually eaten.

[8] This is the amount from the fruit. Additional ascorbic acid may be added by the manufacturer. Refer to the label for this information.

[13] Based on yellow-fleshed varieties; for white-fleshed varieties value is about 50 I.U. per 114-gram peach and 80 I.U. per cup of sliced peaches.

[14] This value includes ascorbic acid added by manufacturer.

H

Table of Food Composition (cont'd)

[Dashes in the columns for nutrients show that no suitable value could be found although there is reason to believe that a measurable amount of the nutrient may be present]

	Food, approximate measure, and weight (in grams)		Water	Food energy	Protein	Fat	Fatty acids Saturated (total)	Fatty acids Unsaturated Oleic	Fatty acids Unsaturated Linoleic	Carbohydrate	Calcium	Iron	Vitamin A value	Thiamin	Riboflavin	Niacin	Ascorbic acid
		Grams	Percent	kCalories	Grams	Grams	Grams	Grams	Grams	Grams	Milligrams	Milligrams	International units	Milligrams	Milligrams	Milligrams	Milligrams
	GRAIN PRODUCTS																
	Bagel, 3-in. diam.:																
333	Egg — 1 bagel	55	32	165	6	2				28	9	1.2	30	0.14	0.10	1.2	0
334	Water — 1 bagel	55	29	165	6	2				30	8	1.2	0	.15	.11	1.4	0
335	Barley, pearled, light, uncooked. — 1 cup	200	11	700	16	2	Trace	1	1	158	32	4.0	0	.24	.10	6.2	0
336	Biscuits, baking powder from home recipe with enriched flour, 2-in. diam. — 1 biscuit	28	27	105	2	5	1	2	1	13	34	.4	Trace	.06	.06	.1	Trace
337	Biscuits, baking powder from mix, 2-in. diam. — 1 biscuit	28	28	90	2	3	1	1	1	15	19	.6	Trace	.08	.07	.6	Trace
338	Bran flakes (40% bran), added thiamin and iron. — 1 cup	35	3	105	4	1				28	25	12.3	0	.14	.06	2.2	0
339	Bran flakes with raisins, added thiamin and iron. — 1 cup	50	7	145	4	1				40	28	13.5	Trace	.16	.07	2.7	0
	Breads:																
340	Boston brown bread, slice 3 by ¾ in. — 1 slice	48	45	100	3	1				22	43	.9	0	.05	.03	.6	0
	Cracked-wheat bread:																
341	Loaf, 1 lb. — 1 loaf	454	35	1,190	40	10	2	5	2	236	399	5.0	Trace	.53	.41	5.9	Trace
342	Slice, 18 slices per loaf. — 1 slice	25	35	65	2	1				13	22	.3	Trace	.03	.02	.3	Trace
	French or vienna bread:																
343	Enriched, 1 lb. loaf. — 1 loaf	454	31	1,315	41	14	3	8	2	251	195	10.0	Trace	1.27	1.00	11.3	Trace
344	Unenriched, 1 lb. loaf. — 1 loaf	454	31	1,315	41	14	3	8	2	251	195	3.2	Trace	.36	.36	3.6	Trace
	Italian bread:																
345	Enriched, 1 lb. loaf. — 1 loaf	454	32	1,250	41	4	Trace	1	2	256	77	10.0	0	1.32	.91	11.8	0
346	Unenriched, 1 lb. loaf. — 1 loaf	454	32	1,250	41	4	Trace	1	2	256	77	3.2	0	.41	.27	3.6	0
	Raisin bread:																
347	Loaf, 1 lb. — 1 loaf	454	35	1,190	30	13	3	8	2	243	322	5.9	Trace	.23	.41	3.2	Trace

H

No.	Food	Amount	Grams	Water (%)	Food energy (cal)	Protein (g)	Fat (g)	Saturated (g)	Oleic (g)	Linoleic (g)	Carbohydrate (g)	Calcium (mg)	Iron (mg)	Vitamin A	Thiamin (mg)	Riboflavin (mg)	Niacin (mg)	Ascorbic acid (mg)
348	Slice, 18 slices per loaf.	1 slice	25	35	65	2	1				13	18	.3	Trace	.01	.02	.2	Trace
	Rye bread:																	
	American, light (⅓ rye, ⅔ wheat):																	
349	Loaf, 1 lb.	1 loaf	454	36	1,100	41	5				236	340	7.3	0	.82	.32	6.4	0
350	Slice, 18 slices per loaf.	1 slice	25	36	60	2	Trace				13	19	.4	0	.05	.02	.4	0
351	Pumpernickel, loaf, 1 lb.	1 loaf	454	34	1,115	41	5				241	381	10.9	0	1.04	.64	5.4	0
	White bread, enriched:[15]																	
	Soft-crumb type:																	
352	Loaf, 1 lb.	1 loaf	454	36	1,225	39	15	3	8	2	229	381	11.3	Trace	1.13	.95	10.9	Trace
353	Slice, 18 slices per loaf.	1 slice	25	36	70	2	1				13	21	.6	Trace	.06	.05	.6	Trace
354	Slice, toasted.	1 slice	22	25	70	2	1				13	21	.6	Trace	.06	.05	.6	Trace
355	Slice, 22 slices per loaf.	1 slice	20	36	55	2	1				10	17	.5	Trace	.05	.04	.5	Trace
356	Slice, toasted.	1 slice	17	25	55	2	1				10	17	.5	Trace	.05	.04	.5	Trace
357	Loaf, 1½ lbs.	1 loaf	680	36	1,835	59	22	5	12	3	343	571	17.0	Trace	1.70	1.43	16.3	Trace
358	Slice, 24 slices per loaf.	1 slice	28	36	75	2	1				14	24	.7	Trace	.07	.06	.7	Trace
359	Slice, toasted.	1 slice	24	25	75	2	1				14	24	.7	Trace	.07	.06	.6	Trace
360	Slice, 28 slices per loaf.	1 slice	24	36	65	2	1				12	20	.6	Trace	.06	.05	.6	Trace
361	Slice, toasted.	1 slice	21	25	65	2	1				12	20	.6	Trace	.06	.05	.6	Trace
	Firm-crumb type:																	
362	Loaf, 1 lb.	1 loaf	454	35	1,245	41	17	4	10	2	228	435	11.3	Trace	1.22	.91	10.9	Trace
363	Slice, 20 slices per loaf.	1 slice	23	35	65	2	1				12	22	.6	Trace	.06	.05	.6	Trace
364	Slice, toasted.	1 slice	20	24	65	2	1				12	22	.6	Trace	.06	.05	.6	Trace
365	Loaf, 2 lbs.	1 loaf	907	35	2,495	82	34	8	20	4	455	871	22.7	Trace	2.45	1.81	21.8	Trace
366	Slice, 34 slices per loaf.	1 slice	27	35	75	2	1				14	26	.7	Trace	.07	.05	.6	Trace
367	Slice, toasted.	1 slice	23	35	75	2	1				14	26	.7	Trace	.07	.05	.6	Trace
	Whole-wheat bread, soft-crumb type:																	
368	Loaf, 1 lb.	1 loaf	454	36	1,095	41	12	2	6	2	224	381	13.6	Trace	1.36	.45	12.7	Trace
369	Slice, 16 slices per loaf.	1 slice	28	36	65	3	1				14	24	.8	Trace	.09	.03	.8	Trace
370	Slice, toasted.	1 slice	24	24	65	3	1				14	24	.8	Trace	.09	.03	.8	Trace

[15] Values for iron, thiamin, riboflavin, and niacin per pound of unenriched white bread would be as follows:

	Iron (Milligrams)	Thiamin (Milligrams)	Riboflavin (Milligrams)	Niacin (Milligrams)
Soft crumb	3.2	.31	.39	5.0
Firm crumb	3.2	.32	.59	4.1

H

Table of Food Composition (cont'd)

[Dashes in the columns for nutrients show that no suitable value could be found although there is reason to believe that a measurable amount of the nutrient may be present]

H

	Food, approximate measure, and weight (in grams)		Water	Food energy	Pro-tein	Fat	Fatty acids			Carbo-hy-drate	Cal-cium	Iron	Vita-min A value	Thia-min	Ribo-flavin	Niacin	Ascor-bic acid
							Satu-rated (total)	Unsaturated Oleic	Lin-oleic								
		Grams	Per-cent	kCalo-ries	Grams	Grams	Grams	Grams	Grams	Grams	Milli-grams	Milli-grams	Inter-national units	Milli-grams	Milli-grams	Milli-grams	Milli-grams
	GRAIN PRODUCTS—Continued																
	Bread—Continued																
	Whole-wheat bread, firm-crumb type:																
371	Loaf, 1 lb ... 1 loaf	454	36	1,100	48	14	3	6	3	216	449	13.6	Trace	1.18	0.54	12.7	Trace
372	Slice, 18 slices per loaf. 1 slice	25	36	60	3	1				12	25	.8	Trace	.06	.03	.7	Trace
373	Slice, toasted. 1 slice	21	24	60	3	1				12	25	.8	Trace	.06	.03	.7	Trace
374	Breadcrumbs, dry, grated. 1 cup	100	6	390	13	5	1	2	1	73	122	3.6	Trace	.22	.30	3.5	Trace
375	Buckwheat flour, light, sifted. 1 cup	98	12	340	6	1	1	1	1	78	11	1.0	0	.08	.04	.4	0
376	Bulgur, canned, seasoned. 1 cup	135	56	245	8	4				44	27	1.9	0	.08	.05	4.1	0
	Cakes made from cake mixes:																
	Angelfood:																
377	Whole cake. 1 cake	635	34	1,645	36	1				377	603	1.9	0	.03	.70	.6	0
378	Piece, ½ of 10-in. diam. cake. 1 piece	53	34	135	3	Trace				32	50	.2	0	Trace	.06	.1	0
	Cupcakes, small, 2½ in. diam.:																
379	Without icing. 1 cupcake	25	26	90	1	3	1	1	1	14	40	.1	40	.01	.03	.1	Trace
380	With chocolate icing. 1 cupcake	36	22	130	2	5	2	2	1	21	47	.3	60	.01	.04	.1	Trace
	Devil's food, 2-layer, with chocolate icing:																
381	Whole cake. 1 cake	1,107	24	3,755	49	136	54	58	16	645	653	8.9	1,660	.33	.89	3.3	1
382	Piece, ⅟₁₆ of 9-in. diam. cake. 1 piece	69	24	235	3	9	3	4	1	40	41	.6	100	.02	.06	.2	Trace
383	Cupcake, small, 2½ in. diam. 1 cupcake	35	24	120	2	4	1	2	Trace	20	21	.3	50	.01	.03	.1	Trace
	Gingerbread:																
384	Whole cake. 1 cake	570	37	1,575	18	39	10	19	9	291	513	9.1	Trace	.17	.51	4.6	2
385	Piece, ⅑ of 8-in. square cake. 1 piece	63	37	175	2	4	1	2	1	32	57	1.0	Trace	.02	.06	.5	Trace
	White, 2-layer, with chocolate icing:																
386	Whole cake. 1 cake	1,140	21	4,000	45	122	45	54	17	716	1,129	5.7	680	.23	.91	2.3	2

No.	Food	Measure	Weight															
387	Piece, 1/16 of 9-in. diam. cake.	1 piece	71	21	250	3	8	3	3	1	45	70	.4	40	.01	.06	.1	Trace
388	Cakes made from home recipes:[16] Boston cream pie; piece 1/12 of 8-in. diam.	1 piece	69	35	210	4	6	2	3	1	34	46	.3	140	.02	.08	.1	Trace
	Fruitcake, dark, made with enriched flour:																	
389	Loaf, 1-lb.	1 loaf	454	18	1,720	22	69	15	37	13	271	327	11.8	540	.59	.64	3.6	2
390	Slice, 1/30 of 8-in. loaf.	1 slice	15	18	55	1	2	Trace	1	Trace	9	11	.4	20	.02	.02	.1	Trace
	Plain sheet cake: Without icing:																	
391	Whole cake	1 cake	777	25	2,830	35	108	30	52	21	434	497	3.1	1,320	.16	.70	1.6	2
392	Piece, 1/9 of 9-in. square cake.	1 piece	86	25	315	4	12	3	6	2	48	55	.3	150	.02	.08	.2	Trace
393	With boiled white icing, piece, 1/9 of 9-in. square cake.	1 piece	114	23	400	4	12	3	6	2	71	56	.3	150	.02	.08	.2	Trace
	Pound:																	
394	Loaf, 8½ by 3½ by 3in.	1 loaf	514	17	2,430	29	152	34	68	17	242	108	4.1	1,440	.15	.46	1.0	0
395	Slice, ½-in. thick.	1 slice	30	17	140	2	9	2	4	1	14	6	.2	80	.01	.03	.1	0
	Sponge:																	
396	Whole cake	1 cake	790	32	2,345	60	45	14	20	4	427	237	9.5	3,560	.40	1.11	1.6	Trace
397	Piece, 1/12 of 10-in. diam. cake.	1 piece	66	32	195	5	4	1	2	Trace	36	20	.8	300	.03	.09	.1	Trace
	Yellow, 2-layer, without icing:																	
398	Whole cake	1 cake	870	24	3,160	39	111	31	53	22	506	618	3.5	1,310	.17	.70	1.7	2
399	Piece, 1/16 of 9-in. diam. cake.	1 piece	54	24	200	2	7	2	3	1	32	39	.2	80	.01	.04	.1	Trace
	Yellow, 2-layer, with chocolate icing:																	
400	Whole cake	1 cake	1,203	21	4,390	51	156	55	69	23	727	818	7.2	1,920	.24	.96	2.4	Trace
401	Piece, 1/16 of 9-in. diam. cake.	1 piece	75	21	275	3	10	3	4	1	45	51	.5	120	.02	.06	.2	Trace
	Cake icings. See Sugars, Sweets. Cookies: Brownies with nuts:																	
402	Made from home recipe with enriched flour.	1 brownie	20	10	95	1	6	1	3	1	10	8	.4	40	.04	.02	.1	Trace
403	Made from mix	1 brownie	20	11	85	1	4	1	2	1	13	9	.4	20	.03	.02	.1	Trace

[16] Unenriched cake flour used unless otherwise specified.

H

H

Table of Food Composition (cont'd)

[Dashes in the columns for nutrients show that no suitable value could be found although there is reason to believe that a measurable amount of the nutrient may be present]

	Food, approximate measure, and weight (in grams)		Water	Food energy	Protein	Fat	Fatty acids			Carbohydrate	Calcium	Iron	Vitamin A value	Thiamin	Riboflavin	Niacin	Ascorbic acid
							Saturated (total)	Unsaturated Oleic	Unsaturated Linoleic								
		Grams	Percent	kCalories	Grams	Grams	Grams	Grams	Grams	Grams	Milligrams	Milligrams	International units	Milligrams	Milligrams	Milligrams	Milligrams
	GRAIN PRODUCTS—Continued																
	Cookies—Continued																
	Chocolate chip:																
404	Made from home recipe with enriched flour. 1 cookie	10	3	50	1	3	1	1	1	6	4	0.2	10	0.01	0.01	0.1	Trace
405	Commercial. 1 cookie	10	3	50	1	2	1	1	Trace	7	4	.2	10	Trace	Trace	Trace	Trace
406	Fig bars, commercial. 1 cookie	14	14	50	1	1	---	---	---	11	11	.2	20	Trace	.01	.1	Trace
407	Sandwich, chocolate or vanilla, commercial. 1 cookie	10	2	50	1	2	1	1	Trace	7	2	.1	0	Trace	Trace	.1	0
	Corn flakes, added nutrients:																
408	Plain. 1 cup	25	4	100	2	Trace				21	4	.4	0	.11	.02	.5	0
409	Sugar-covered. 1 cup	40	2	155	2	Trace				36	5	.4	0	.16	.02	.8	0
	Corn (hominy) grits, degermed, cooked:																
410	Enriched. 1 cup	245	87	125	3	Trace				27	2	.7	[17]150	.10	.07	1.0	0
411	Unenriched. 1 cup	245	87	125	3	Trace				27	2	.2	[17]150	.05	.02	.5	0
	Cornmeal:																
412	Whole-ground, unbolted, dry. 1 cup	122	12	435	11	5	1	2	2	90	24	2.9	[17]620	.46	.13	2.4	0
413	Bolted (nearly whole-grain) dry. 1 cup	122	12	440	11	4	Trace	1	2	91	21	2.2	[17]590	.37	.10	2.3	0
	Degermed, enriched:																
414	Dry form. 1 cup	138	12	500	11	2				108	8	4.0	[17]610	.61	.36	4.8	0
415	Cooked. 1 cup	240	88	120	3	1				26	2	1.0	[17]140	.14	.10	1.2	0
	Degermed, unenriched:																
416	Dry form. 1 cup	138	12	500	11	2				108	8	1.5	[17]610	.19	.07	1.4	0
417	Cooked. 1 cup	240	88	120	3	1				26	2	.5	[17]140	.05	.02	.2	0
418	Corn muffins, made with enriched degermed cornmeal and enriched flour; muffin 2⅜-in. diam. 1 muffin	40	33	125	3	4	2	2	Trace	19	42	.7	[17]120	.08	.09	.6	Trace

No.	Food, approximate measure	Measure	Grams	Water (%)	Food energy	Protein	Fat	Sat. (total)	Oleic	Linoleic	Carbo-hydrate	Calcium	Iron	Vit. A	Thiamin	Ribo-flavin	Niacin	Ascorbic acid
419	Corn muffins, made with mix, egg, and milk; muffin 2⅜-in. diam.	1 muffin	40	30	130	3	4	1	2	1	20	96	.6	100	.07	.08	.6	Trace
420	Corn, puffed, presweetened, added nutrients.	1 cup	30	2	115	1	Trace	---	---	---	27	3	.5	0	.13	.05	.6	0
421	Corn, shredded, added nutrients.	1 cup	25	3	100	2	Trace	---	---	---	22	1	.6	0	.11	.05	.5	0
	Crackers:																	
422	Graham, 2½-in. square	4 crackers	28	6	110	2	3	1	2	1	21	11	.4	0	.01	.06	.4	0
423	Saltines	4 crackers	11	4	50	1	1	---	---	---	8	2	.1	0	Trace	Trace	.1	0
	Danish pastry, plain (without fruit or nuts):																	
424	Packaged ring, 12 ounces.	1 ring	340	22	1,435	25	80	24	37	15	155	170	3.1	1,050	.23	.51	2.7	Trace
425	Round piece, approx. 4¼-in. diam. by 1 in.	1 pastry	65	22	275	5	15	5	7	3	30	33	.6	200	.05	.10	.5	Trace
426	Ounce	1 oz.	28	22	120	2	7	2	3	1	13	14	.3[18]	90	.02[18]	.04[18]	.2[18]	Trace
427	Doughnuts, cake type	1 doughnut	32	24	125	1	6	1	4	Trace	16	13	.4[18]	30	.05[18]	.05[18]	.4[18]	Trace
428	Farina, quick-cooking, enriched, cooked.	1 cup	245	89	105	3	Trace	---	---	---	22	147	.7[19]	0	.12[19]	.07[19]	1.0[19]	0
	Macaroni, cooked:																	
	Enriched:																	
429	Cooked, firm stage (undergoes additional cooking in a food mixture).	1 cup	130	64	190	6	1	---	---	---	39	14	1.4[19]	0	.23[19]	.14[19]	1.8[19]	0
430	Cooked until tender	1 cup	140	72	155	5	1	---	---	---	32	8	1.3[19]	0	.20[19]	.11[19]	1.5[19]	0
	Unenriched:																	
431	Cooked, firm stage (undergoes additional cooking in a food mixture).	1 cup	130	64	190	6	1	---	---	---	39	14	.7	0	.03	.03	.5	0
432	Cooked until tender	1 cup	140	72	155	5	1	---	---	---	32	11	.6	0	.01	.01	.4	0
433	Macaroni (enriched) and cheese, baked.	1 cup	200	58	430	17	22	10	9	2	40	362	1.8	860	.20	.40	1.8	Trace
434	Canned	1 cup	240	80	230	9	10	4	3	1	26	199	1.0	260	.12	.24	1.0	Trace
435	Muffins, with enriched white flour; muffin, 3-inch diam.	1 muffin	40	38	120	3	4	1	2	1	17	42	.6	40	.07	.09	.6	Trace
	Noodles (egg noodles), cooked:																	
436	Enriched	1 cup	160	70	200	7	2	1	1	Trace	37	16	1.4[19]	110	.22[19]	.13[19]	1.9[19]	0
437	Unenriched	1 cup	160	70	200	7	2	1	1	Trace	37	16	1.0	110	.05	.03	.6	0

[17] This value is based on product made from yellow varieties of corn; white varieties contain only a trace.

[18] Based on product made with enriched flour. With unenriched flour, approximate values per doughnut are: Iron, 0.2 milligram; thiamin, 0.01 milligram; riboflavin, 0.03 milligram; niacin, 0.2 milligram.

[19] Iron, thiamin, riboflavin, and niacin are based on the minimum levels of enrichment specified in standards of identity promulgated under the Federal Food, Drug, and Cosmetic Act.

H

Table of Food Composition (cont'd)

[Dashes in the columns for nutrients show that no suitable value could be found although there is reason to believe that a measurable amount of the nutrient may be present]

	Food, approximate measure, and weight (in grams)	Water	Food energy	Protein	Fat	Fatty acids Saturated (total)	Fatty acids Unsaturated Oleic	Fatty acids Unsaturated Linoleic	Carbohydrate	Calcium	Iron	Vitamin A value	Thiamin	Riboflavin	Niacin	Ascorbic acid
		Percent	kCalories	Grams	Grams	Grams	Grams	Grams	Grams	Milligrams	Milligrams	International units	Milligrams	Milligrams	Milligrams	Milligrams
	GRAIN PRODUCTS—Continued															
438	Oats (with or without corn) puffed, added nutrients. 1 cup — 25 Grams	3	100	3	1	—	—	—	19	44	1.2	0	0.24	0.04	0.5	0
439	Oatmeal or rolled oats, cooked. 1 cup — 240	87	130	5	2	—	—	1	23	22	1.4	0	.19	.05	.2	0
	Pancakes, 4-inch diam.:															
440	Wheat, enriched flour (home recipe). 1 cake — 27	50	60	2	2	Trace	1	Trace	9	27	.4	30	.05	.06	.4	Trace
441	Buckwheat (made from mix with egg and milk). 1 cake — 27	58	55	2	2	1	1	Trace	6	59	.4	60	.03	.04	.2	Trace
442	Plain or buttermilk (made from mix with egg and milk). 1 cake — 27	51	60	2	2	1	1	Trace	9	58	.3	70	.04	.06	.2	Trace
	Pie (piecrust made with unenriched flour): Sector, 4-in., 1/7 of 9-in. diam. pie:															
443	Apple (2-crust). 1 sector — 135	48	350	3	15	4	7	3	51	11	.4	40	.03	.03	.5	1
444	Butterscotch (1-crust). 1 sector — 130	45	350	6	14	5	6	2	50	98	1.2	340	.04	.13	.3	Trace
445	Cherry (2-crust). 1 sector — 135	47	350	4	15	4	7	3	52	19	.4	590	.03	.03	.4	Trace
446	Custard (1-crust). 1 sector — 130	58	285	8	14	5	6	2	30	125	.8	300	.07	.21	.4	0
447	Lemon meringue (1-crust). 1 sector — 120	47	305	4	12	4	6	2	45	17	.6	200	.04	.10	.2	4
448	Mince (2-crust). 1 sector — 135	43	365	3	16	4	8	3	56	38	1.4	Trace	.09	.05	.5	1
449	Pecan (1-crust). 1 sector — 118	20	490	6	27	4	16	5	60	55	3.3	190	.19	.08	.4	Trace
450	Pineapple chiffon (1-crust). 1 sector — 93	41	265	6	11	3	5	2	36	22	.8	320	.04	.08	.4	1
451	Pumpkin (1-crust). 1 sector — 130	59	275	5	15	5	6	2	32	66	.7	3,210	.04	.13	.7	Trace
	Piecrust, baked shell for pie made with:															
452	Enriched flour. 1 shell — 180	15	900	11	60	16	28	12	79	25	3.1	0	.36	.25	3.2	0
453	Unenriched flour. 1 shell — 180	15	900	11	60	16	28	12	79	25	.9	0	.05	.05	.9	0

No.	Food	Measure	Grams	Water (%)	Food energy (cal)	Protein (g)	Fat (g)	Saturated (g)	Oleic (g)	Linoleic (g)	Carbohydrate (g)	Calcium (mg)	Iron (mg)	Vitamin A (IU)	Thiamin (mg)	Riboflavin (mg)	Niacin (mg)	Ascorbic acid (mg)
	Piecrust mix including stick form:																	
454	Package, 10-oz., for double crust.	1 pkg	284	9	1,480	20	93	23	46	21	141	131	1.4	0	.11	.11	2.0	0
455	Pizza (cheese) 5½-in. sector; ⅛ of 14-in. diam. pie.	1 sector	75	45	185	7	6	2	3	Trace	27	107	.7	290	.04	.12	.7	4
	Popcorn, popped:																	
456	Plain, large kernel	1 cup	6	4	25	1	Trace				5	1	.2	0		.01	.1	0
457	With oil and salt	1 cup	9	3	40	1	2		Trace	Trace	5	1	.2			.01	.2	0
458	Sugar coated	1 cup	35	4	135	2	1				30	2	.5	0		.02	.4	0
	Pretzels:																	
459	Dutch, twisted	1 pretzel	16	5	60	2	1				12	4	.2	0	Trace	Trace	.1	0
460	Thin, twisted	1 pretzel	6	5	25	1	Trace				5	1	.1	0	Trace	Trace	Trace	0
461	Stick, small, 2¼ inches	10 sticks	3	5	10	Trace	Trace				2	1	Trace	0	Trace	Trace	Trace	0
462	Stick, regular, 3⅛ inches.	5 sticks	3	5	10	Trace	Trace				2	1	Trace	0	Trace	Trace	Trace	0
	Rice, white: Enriched:																	
463	Raw	1 cup	185	12	670	12	1				149	44	[20]5.4	0	[20].81	[20].06	[20]6.5	0
464	Cooked	1 cup	205	73	225	4	Trace				50	21	[20]1.8	0	[20].23	[20].02	[20]2.1	0
465	Instant, ready-to-serve.	1 cup	165	73	180	4	Trace				40	5	[20]1.3	0	[20].21	[20]—	[20]1.7	0
466	Unenriched, cooked	1 cup	205	73	225	4	Trace				50	21	.4	0	.04	.02	.8	0
467	Parboiled, cooked	1 cup	175	73	185	4	Trace				41	33	[20]1.4	0	[20].19	[20]—	[20]2.1	0
468	Rice, puffed, added nutrients.	1 cup	15	4	60	1	Trace				13	3	.3	0	.07	.01	.7	0
	Rolls, enriched: Cloverleaf or pan:																	
469	Home recipe	1 roll	35	26	120	3	3	1	1	1	20	16	.7	30	.09	.09	.8	Trace
470	Commercial	1 roll	28	31	85	2	2	Trace	1	Trace	15	21	.5	Trace	.08	.05	.6	Trace
471	Frankfurter or hamburger.	1 roll	40	31	120	3	2	1	1	1	21	30	.8	Trace	.11	.07	.9	Trace
472	Hard, round or rectangular.	1 roll	50	25	155	5	2	Trace	1	Trace	30	24	1.2	Trace	.13	.12	1.4	Trace
473	Rye wafers, whole-grain, 1⅞ by 3½ inches.	2 wafers	13	6	45	2	Trace				10	7	.5	0	.04	.03	.2	0
474	Spaghetti, cooked, tender stage, enriched.	1 cup	140	72	155	5	1				32	11	[19]1.3	0	[19].20	[19].11	[19]1.5	0

[19] Iron, thiamin, riboflavin, and niacin are based on the minimum levels of enrichment specified in standards of identity promulgated under the Federal Food, Drug, and Cosmetic Act.

[20] Iron, thiamin, and niacin are based on the minimum levels of enrichment specified in standards of identity promulgated under the Federal Food, Drug, and Cosmetic Act. Riboflavin is based on unenriched rice. When the minimum level of enrichment for riboflavin specified in the standards of identity becomes effective the value will be 0.12 milligram per cup of parboiled rice and of white rice.

H

Table of Food Composition (cont'd)
[Dashes in the columns for nutrients show that no suitable value could be found although there is reason to believe that a measurable amount of the nutrient may be present]

	Food, approximate measure, and weight (in grams)	Water	Food energy	Protein	Fat	Fatty acids			Carbohydrate	Calcium	Iron	Vitamin A value	Thiamin	Riboflavin	Niacin	Ascorbic acid
						Saturated (total)	Unsaturated									
							Oleic	Linoleic								
		Grams	Percent	kCalories	Grams	Grams	Grams	Grams	Grams	Grams	Milligrams	Milligrams	International units	Milligrams	Milligrams	Milligrams	Milligrams

GRAIN PRODUCTS—Continued

Spaghetti with meat balls, and tomato sauce:

	Food	Grams	Water	Food energy	Protein	Fat	Saturated	Oleic	Linoleic	Carbohydrate	Calcium	Iron	Vitamin A	Thiamin	Riboflavin	Niacin	Ascorbic acid
475	Home recipe 1 cup	248	70	330	19	12	4	6	1	39	124	3.7	1,590	0.25	0.30	4.0	22
476	Canned 1 cup	250	78	260	12	10	2	3	4	28	53	3.3	1,000	.15	.18	2.3	5
	Spaghetti in tomato sauce with cheese:																
477	Home recipe 1 cup	250	77	260	9	9	2	5	1	37	80	2.3	1,080	.25	.18	2.3	13
478	Canned 1 cup	250	80	190	6	2	1	1	1	38	40	2.8	930	.35	.28	4.5	10
479	Waffles, with enriched flour, 7-in. diam. 1 waffle	75	41	210	7	7	2	4	1	28	85	1.3	250	.13	.19	1.0	Trace
480	Waffles, made from mix, enriched, egg and milk added, 7-in. diam. 1 waffle	75	42	205	7	8	3	3	1	27	179	1.0	170	.11	.17	.7	Trace
481	Wheat, puffed, added nutrients. 1 cup	15	3	55	2	Trace				12	4	.6	0	.08	.03	1.2	0
482	Wheat, shredded, plain 1 biscuit	25	7	90	2	1				20	11	.9	0	.06	.03	1.1	0
483	Wheat flakes, added nutrients. 1 cup	30	4	105	3	Trace				24	12	1.3	0	.19	.04	1.5	0
	Wheat flours:																
484	Whole-wheat, from hard wheats, stirred. 1 cup	120	12	400	16	2	Trace	1	1	85	49	4.0	0	.66	.14	5.2	0
	All-purpose or family flour, enriched:																
485	Sifted 1 cup	115	12	420	12	1				88	18	[19]3.3	0	[19].51	[19].30	[19]4.0	0
486	Unsifted 1 cup	125	12	455	13	1				95	20	[19]3.6	0	[19].55	[19].33	[19]4.4	0
487	Self-rising, enriched 1 cup	125	12	440	12	1				93	331	[19]3.6	0	[19].55	[19].33	[19]4.4	0
488	Cake or pastry flour, sifted. 1 cup	96	12	350	7	1				76	16	.5	0	.03	.03	.7	0

FATS, OILS

Butter:

Regular, 4 sticks per pound:

	Food	Grams	Water	Food energy	Protein	Fat	Saturated	Oleic	Linoleic	Carbohydrate	Calcium	Iron	Vitamin A	Thiamin	Riboflavin	Niacin	Ascorbic acid
489	Stick ½ cup	113	16	810	1	92	51	30	3	1	23	0	[2]3,750				0

No.	Food	Measure	Weight (g)	Water (%)	Food energy (cal)	Protein (g)	Fat (g)	Saturated (g)	Oleic (g)	Linoleic (g)	Carbohydrate (g)	Calcium (mg)	Iron (mg)	Vitamin A (IU)	Thiamin	Riboflavin	Niacin	Ascorbic acid
490	Tablespoon (approx. 1/8 stick).	1 tbsp.	14	16	100	Trace	12	6	4	Trace	Trace	3	0	470 [22]	—	—	—	0
491	Pat (1-in. sq. 1/3-in. high; 90 per lb.).	1 pat	5	16	35	Trace	4	2	1	Trace	Trace	1	0	170 [22]	—	—	—	0
	Whipped, 6 sticks or 2, 8-oz. containers per pound:																	
492	Stick	1/2 cup	76	16	540	1	61	34	20	2	Trace	15	0	2,500 [22]	—	—	—	0
493	Tablespoon (approx. 1/8 stick).	1 tbsp.	9	16	65	Trace	8	4	3	Trace	Trace	2	0	310 [22]	—	—	—	0
494	Pat (1 1/4-in. sq. 1/3-in. high; 120 per lb.).	1 pat	4	16	25	Trace	3	2	1	Trace	Trace	1	0	130 [21]	—	—	—	0
	Fats, cooking:																	
495	Lard	1 cup	205	0	1,850	0	205	78	94	20	0	0	0	0	0	0	0	0
496		1 tbsp.	13	0	115	0	13	5	6	1	0	0	0	0	0	0	0	0
497	Vegetable fats	1 cup	200	0	1,770	0	200	50	100	44	0	0	0	—	0	0	0	0
498		1 tbsp.	13	0	110	0	13	3	6	3	0	0	0	0	0	0	0	0
	Margarine:																	
	Regular, 4 sticks per pound:																	
499	Stick	1/2 cup	113	16	815	1	92	17	46	25	1	23	0	3,750 [22]	—	—	—	0
500	Tablespoon (approx. 1/8 stick).	1 tbsp.	14	16	100	Trace	12	2	6	3	Trace	3	0	470 [22]	—	—	—	0
501	Pat (1-in. sq. 1/3-in. high; 90 per lb.).	1 pat	5	16	35	Trace	4	1	2	1	Trace	1	0	170 [22]	—	—	—	0
	Whipped, 6 sticks per pound:																	
502	Stick	1/2 cup	76	16	545	1	61	11	31	17	1	15	0	2,500 [22]	—	—	—	0
	Soft, 2 8-oz. tubs per pound:																	
503	Tub	1 tub	227	16	1,635	1	184	34	68	68	1	45	0	7,500 [22]	—	—	—	0
504	Tablespoon	1 tbsp.	14	16	100	Trace	11	2	4	4	Trace	3	0	470 [22]	—	—	—	0
	Oils, salad or cooking:																	
505	Corn	1 cup	220	0	1,945	0	220	22	62	117	0	0	0	—	0	0	0	0
506		1 tbsp.	14	0	125	0	14	1	4	7	0	0	0	—	0	0	0	0
507	Cottonseed	1 cup	220	0	1,945	0	220	55	46	110	0	0	0	—	0	0	0	0
508		1 tbsp.	14	0	125	0	14	4	3	7	0	0	0	—	0	0	0	0
509	Olive	1 cup	220	0	1,945	0	220	24	167	15	0	0	0	—	0	0	0	0
510		1 tbsp.	14	0	125	0	14	2	11	1	0	0	0	—	0	0	0	0
511	Peanut	1 cup	220	0	1,945	0	220	40	103	64	0	0	0	—	0	0	0	0
512		1 tbsp.	14	0	125	0	14	3	7	4	0	0	0	—	0	0	0	0
513	Safflower	1 cup	220	0	1,945	0	220	18	37	165	0	0	0	—	0	0	0	0
514		1 tbsp.	14	0	125	0	14	1	2	10	0	0	0	—	0	0	0	0
515	Soybean	1 cup	220	0	1,945	0	220	33	44	114	0	0	0	—	0	0	0	0
516		1 tbsp.	14	0	125	0	14	2	3	7	0	0	0	—	0	0	0	0

[19] Iron, thiamin, riboflavin, and niacin are based on the minimum levels of enrichment specified in standards of identity promulgated under the Federal Food, Drug, and Cosmetic Act.

[21] Year-round average.

[22] Based on the average vitamin A content of fortified margarine. Federal specifications for fortified margarine require a minimum of 15,000 I.U. of vitamin A per pound.

H

Table of Food Composition (cont'd)

[Dashes in the columns for nutrients show that no suitable value could be found although there is reason to believe that a measurable amount of the nutrient may be present]

	Food, approximate measure, and weight (in grams)	Water	Food energy	Protein	Fat	Fatty acids			Carbohydrate	Calcium	Iron	Vitamin A value	Thiamin	Riboflavin	Niacin	Ascorbic acid
						Saturated (total)	Unsaturated									
							Oleic	Linoleic								
		Per cent	kCalories	Grams	Grams	Grams	Grams	Grams	Grams	Milligrams	Milligrams	International units	Milligrams	Milligrams	Milligrams	Milligrams
	FATS, OILS—Continued															
	Salad dressings:															
517	Blue cheese ------ 1 tbsp ------	32	75	1	8	2	2	4	1	12	Trace	30	Trace	0.02	Trace	Trace
	Commercial, mayonnaise type:															
518	Regular ------ 1 tbsp ------	41	65	Trace	6	1	1	3	2	2	Trace	30	Trace	Trace	Trace	---
519	Special dietary, low-calorie. 1 tbsp ------	81	20	Trace	2	Trace	Trace	1	1	3	Trace	40	Trace	Trace	Trace	---
	French:															
520	Regular ------ 1 tbsp. ------	39	65	Trace	6	1	1	3	3	2	.1	---	---	---	---	---
521	Special dietary, low-fat with artificial sweeteners. 1 tbsp. ------	95	Trace	Trace	Trace	---	---	---	Trace	2	.1	---	---	---	---	---
522	Home cooked, boiled ----- 1 tbsp. -----	68	25	1	2	1	1	Trace	2	14	.1	80	.01	.03	Trace	Trace
523	Mayonnaise ---------- 1 tbsp. -----	15	100	Trace	11	2	2	6	Trace	3	.1	40	Trace	.01	Trace	Trace
524	Thousand island ----- 1 tbsp. -----	32	80	Trace	8	1	2	4	3	2	.1	50	Trace	Trace	Trace	Trace
	SUGARS, SWEETS															
	Cake icings:															
525	Chocolate made with milk and table fat. 1 cup ------	14	1,035	9	38	21	14	1	185	165	3.3	580	.06	.28	.6	1
526	Coconut (with boiled icing). 1 cup ------	15	605	3	13	11	1	Trace	124	10	.8	0	.02	.07	.3	0
527	Creamy fudge from mix with water only. 1 cup ------	15	830	7	16	5	8	3	183	96	2.7	Trace	.05	.20	.7	Trace
528	White, boiled ------ 1 cup ------	18	300	1	0	---	---	---	76	2	Trace	0	Trace	.03	Trace	0
	Candy:															
529	Caramels, plain or chocolate. 1 oz ------	8	115	1	3	2	1	Trace	22	42	.4	Trace	.01	.05	.1	Trace
530	Chocolate, milk, plain ---- 1 oz. ------	1	145	2	9	5	3	Trace	16	65	.3	80	.02	.10	.1	Trace
531	Chocolate-coated peanuts. 1 oz. ------	1	160	5	12	3	6	2	11	33	.4	Trace	.10	.05	2.1	Trace

H

No.	Food	Measure	Grams	Water (%)	Food energy (cal.)	Protein (g)	Fat (g)	Saturated fatty acids (g)	Oleic (g)	Linoleic (g)	Carbohydrate (g)	Calcium (mg)	Iron (mg)	Vitamin A (I.U.)	Thiamine (mg)	Riboflavin (mg)	Niacin (mg)	Ascorbic acid (mg)
532	Fondant; mints, uncoated; candy corn.	1 oz.	28	8	105	Trace	1	--	--	--	25	4	.3	0	Trace	Trace	Trace	0
533	Fudge, plain.	1 oz.	28	8	115	1	3	2	1	Trace	21	22	.3	Trace	.01	.03	.1	Trace
534	Gum drops.	1 oz.	28	12	100	Trace	Trace	--	--	--	25	2	.1	0	0	0	0	0
535	Hard.	1 oz.	28	1	110	0	Trace	--	--	--	28	6	.5	0	0	0	0	0
536	Marshmallows.	1 oz.	28	17	90	1	Trace	--	--	--	23	5	.5	0	0	Trace	Trace	0
	Chocolate-flavored sirup or topping:																	
537	Thin type.	1 fl. oz.	38	32	90	1	1	Trace	Trace	Trace	24	6	.6	Trace	.01	.03	.2	0
538	Fudge type.	1 fl. oz.	38	25	125	2	5	3	2	Trace	20	48	.5	60	.02	.08	.2	Trace
	Chocolate-flavored beverage powder (approx. 4 heaping teaspoons per oz.):																	
539	With nonfat dry milk.	1 oz.	28	2	100	5	1	Trace	Trace	Trace	20	167	.5	10	.04	.21	.2	1
540	Without nonfat dry milk.	1 oz.	28	1	100	1	1	Trace	Trace	Trace	25	9	.6	0	.01	.03	.1	0
541	Honey, strained or extracted.	1 tbsp.	21	17	65	Trace	0				17	1	.1	0	Trace	.01	.1	Trace
542	Jams and preserves.	1 tbsp.	20	29	55	Trace	Trace				14	4	.2	Trace	Trace	.01	Trace	Trace
543	Jellies.	1 tbsp.	18	29	50	Trace	Trace				13	4	.3	Trace	Trace	.01	Trace	1
	Molasses, cane:																	
544	Light (first extraction).	1 tbsp.	20	24	50	--	--				13	33	.9	--	.01	.01	Trace	0
545	Blackstrap (third extraction).	1 tbsp.	20	24	45	--	--				11	137	3.2	--	.02	.04	.4	0
	Sirups:																	
546	Sorghum.	1 tbsp.	21	23	55	0	0				14	35	2.6	--	0	.02	Trace	0
547	Table blends, chiefly corn, light and dark.	1 tbsp.	21	24	60	0	0				15	9	.8	--	0	0	0	0
	Sugars:																	
548	Brown, firm packed.	1 cup	220	2	820	0	0				212	187	7.5	0	.02	.07	.4	0
	White:																	
549	Granulated.	1 cup	200	Trace	770	0	0				199	0	.2	0	0	0	0	0
550	Granulated.	1 tbsp.	11	Trace	40	0	0				11	0	Trace	0	0	0	0	0
551	Powdered, stirred before measuring.	1 cup	120	Trace	460	0	0				119	0	.1	0	0	0	0	0
	MISCELLANEOUS ITEMS																	
552	Barbecue sauce.	1 cup	250	81	230	4	17	2	5	9	20	53	2.0	900	.03	.03	.8	13
	Beverages, alcoholic:																	
553	Beer.	12 fl. oz.	360	92	150	1	0				14	18	Trace	0	.01	.11	2.2	--
	Gin, rum, vodka, whiskey:																	
554	80-proof.	1½ fl. oz. jigger.	42	67	100	0	--				Trace	--	--	--	--	--	--	--
555	86-proof.	1½ fl. oz. jigger.	42	64	105	0	--				Trace	--	--	--	--	--	--	--
556	90-proof.	1½ fl. oz. jigger.	42	62	110	0	--				Trace	--	--	--	--	--	--	--

H

Table of Food Composition (cont'd)

[Dashes in the columns for nutrients show that no suitable value could be found although there is reason to believe that a measurable amount of the nutrient may be present]

	Food, approximate measure, and weight (in grams)		Water	Food energy	Protein	Fat	Fatty acids			Carbohydrate	Calcium	Iron	Vitamin A value	Thiamin	Riboflavin	Niacin	Ascorbic acid
							Saturated (total)	Unsaturated Oleic	Unsaturated Linoleic								
		Grams	Percent	kCalories	Grams	Grams	Grams	Grams	Grams	Grams	Milligrams	Milligrams	International units	Milligrams	Milligram	Milligrams	Milligrams
	MISCELLANEOUS ITEMS—Continued																
	Beverages, alcoholic—Continued																
	Gin, rum, vodka, whiskey—Con.																
557	94-proof	1½ fl. oz. jigger.	42	60	115						Trace							
558	100-proof	1½ fl. oz. jigger.	42	58	125						Trace							
	Wines:																
559	Dessert	3½ fl. oz. glass.	103	77	140	Trace	0				8	8			.01	.02	.2	
560	Table	3½ fl. oz. glass.	102	86	85	Trace	0				4	9	.4		Trace	.01	.1	
	Beverages, carbonated, sweetened, nonalcoholic:																
561	Carbonated water	12 fl. oz.	366	92	115	0	0				29			0	0	0	0	0
562	Cola type	12 fl. oz.	369	90	145	0	0				37			0	0	0	0	0
563	Fruit-flavored sodas and Tom Collins mixes.	12 fl. oz.	372	88	170	0	0				45			0	0	0	0	0
564	Ginger ale	12 fl. oz.	366	92	115	0	0				29			0	0	0	0	0
565	Root beer	12 fl. oz.	370	90	150	0	0				39			0	0	0	0	0
566	Bouillon cubes, approx. ½ in.	1 cube	4	4	5	1	Trace				Trace							
	Chocolate:																
567	Bitter or baking	1 oz.	28	2	145	3	15	8	6	Trace	8	22	1.9	20	.01	.07	.4	0
568	Semi-sweet, small pieces.	1 cup	170	1	860	7	61	34	22	1	97	51	4.4	30	.02	.14	.9	0
	Gelatin:																
569	Plain, dry powder in envelope.	1 envelope	7	13	25	6	Trace				0							
570	Dessert powder, 3-oz. package.	1 pkg	85	2	315	8	0				75							
571	Gelatin dessert, prepared with water.	1 cup	240	84	140	4	0				34							

H

H

Item	Food, approximate measure, and weight	Grams	Water (%)	Food energy (cal.)	Protein (g)	Fat (g)	Fatty acids — Saturated (g)	Oleic (g)	Linoleic (g)	Carbohydrate (g)	Calcium (mg)	Iron (mg)	Vitamin A (I.U.)	Thiamine (mg)	Riboflavin (mg)	Niacin (mg)	Ascorbic acid (mg)
572	Olives, pickled: Green — 4 medium or 3 extra large or 2 giant.	16	78	15	Trace	2	Trace	2	Trace	Trace	8	.2	40	---	---	---	---
573	Ripe: Mission — 3 small or 2 large.	10	73	15	Trace	2	Trace	2	Trace	Trace	9	.1	10	Trace	Trace	Trace	---
	Pickles, cucumber:																
574	Dill, medium, whole, 3¾ in. long, 1¼ in. diam. — 1 pickle	65	93	10	1	Trace				1	17	.7	70	Trace	.01	Trace	4
575	Fresh, sliced, 1½ in. diam., ¼ in. thick. — 2 slices	15	79	10	Trace	Trace				3	5	.3	20	Trace	Trace	Trace	1
576	Sweet, gherkin, small, whole, approx. 2½ in. long, ¾ in. diam. — 1 pickle	15	61	20	Trace	Trace				6	2	.2	10	Trace	Trace	Trace	1
577	Relish, finely chopped, sweet. — 1 tbsp.	15	63	20	Trace	Trace				5	3	.1		---	---	---	---
	Popcorn. See Grain Products.																
578	Popsicle, 3 fl. oz. size — 1 popsicle	95	80	70	0	0	0	0	0	18	0	Trace	0	0	0	0	0
	Pudding, home recipe with starch base:																
579	Chocolate — 1 cup	260	66	385	8	12	7	4	Trace	67	250	1.3	390	.05	.36	.3	1
580	Vanilla (blanc mange) — 1 cup	255	76	285	9	10	5	3	Trace	41	298	Trace	410	.08	.41	.3	2
581	Pudding mix, dry form, 4-oz. package. — 1 pkg.	113	2	410	3	2	1	1	Trace	103	23	1.8	Trace	.02	.08	.5	0
582	Sherbet — 1 cup	193	67	260	2	2				59	31	Trace	120	.02	.06	Trace	4
	Soups:																
	Canned, condensed, ready-to-serve:																
	Prepared with an equal volume of milk:																
583	Cream of chicken — 1 cup	245	85	180	7	10	3	3	3	15	172	.5	610	.05	.27	.7	2
584	Cream of mushroom. — 1 cup	245	83	215	7	14	4	4	5	16	191	.5	250	.05	.34	.7	1
585	Tomato — 1 cup	250	84	175	7	7	3	2	1	23	168	.8	1,200	.10	.25	1.3	15
	Prepared with an equal volume of water:																
586	Bean with pork — 1 cup	250	84	170	8	6	1	2	2	22	63	2.3	650	.13	.08	1.0	3
587	Beef broth, bouillon consomme. — 1 cup	240	96	30	5	0				3	Trace	.5	Trace	Trace	.02	1.2	---
588	Beef noodle — 1 cup	240	93	70	4	3	1	1	1	7	7	1.0	50	.05	.07	1.0	Trace
589	Clam chowder, Manhattan type (with tomatoes, without milk). — 1 cup	245	92	80	2	3				12	34	1.0	880	.02	.02	1.0	---
590	Cream of chicken — 1 cup	240	92	95	3	6	1	2	3	8	24	.5	410	.02	.05	.5	Trace
591	Cream of mushroom. — 1 cup	240	90	135	2	10	1	3	5	10	41	.5	70	.02	.12	.7	Trace
592	Minestrone — 1 cup	245	90	105	5	3	Trace			14	37	1.0	2,350	.07	.05	1.0	---

H

Table of Food Composition (cont'd)

[Dashes in the columns for nutrients show that no suitable value could be found although there is reason to believe that a measurable amount of the nutrient may be present]

	Food, approximate measure, and weight (in grams)		Water	Food energy	Protein	Fat	Fatty acids			Carbohydrate	Calcium	Iron	Vitamin A value	Thiamin	Riboflavin	Niacin	Ascorbic acid
							Saturated (total)	Unsaturated Oleic	Unsaturated Linoleic								
		Grams	Per cent	kCalories	Grams	Grams	Grams	Grams	Grams	Grams	Milligrams	Milligrams	International units	Milligrams	Milligrams	Milligrams	Milligrams
	MISCELLANEOUS ITEMS—Continued Soups—Continued Canned, condensed, ready-to-serve—Con. Prepared with an equal volume of water—Con.																
593	Split pea - 1 cup	245	85	145	9	3	1	2	Trace	21	29	1.5	440	0.25	0.15	1.5	1
594	Tomato - 1 cup	245	90	90	2	3	Trace	1	1	16	15	.7	1,000	.05	.05	1.2	12
595	Vegetable beef - 1 cup	245	92	80	5	2	---	---	---	10	12	.7	2,700	.05	.05	1.0	---
596	Vegetarian - 1 cup	245	92	80	2	2	---	---	---	13	20	1.0	2,940	.05	.05	1.0	---
	Dehydrated, dry form:																
597	Chicken noodle (2-oz. package). 1 pkg	57	6	220	8	6	2	3	1	33	34	1.4	190	.30	.15	2.4	3
598	Onion mix (1½-oz. package). 1 pkg	43	3	150	6	5	1	2	1	23	42	.6	30	.05	.03	.3	6
599	Tomato vegetable with noodles (2½-oz. pkg.). 1 pkg	71	4	245	6	6	2	3	1	45	33	1.4	1,700	.21	.13	1.8	18
	Frozen, condensed: Clam chowder, New England type (with milk, without tomatoes):																
600	Prepared with equal volume of milk. 1 cup	245	83	210	9	12	---	---	---	16	240	1.0	250	.07	.29	.5	Trace
601	Prepared with equal volume of water. 1 cup	240	89	130	4	8	---	---	---	11	91	1.0	50	.05	.10	.5	---
	Cream of potato:																
602	Prepared with equal volume of milk. 1 cup	245	83	185	8	10	5	3	Trace	18	208	1.0	590	.10	.27	.5	Trace
603	Prepared with equal volume of water. 1 cup	240	90	105	3	5	3	2	Trace	12	58	1.0	410	.05	.05	.5	---

No.	Food	Measure	Grams	Water (%)	Food energy	Protein (g)	Fat (g)	Saturated (total)	Unsaturated oleic	Unsaturated linoleic	Carbohydrate (g)	Calcium (mg)	Iron (mg)	Vitamin A (IU)	Thiamin (mg)	Riboflavin (mg)	Niacin (mg)	Ascorbic acid (mg)
	Cream of shrimp:																	
604	Prepared with equal volume of milk.	1 cup	245	82	245	9	16	---	---	---	15	189	.5	290	.07	.27	.5	Trace
605	Prepared with equal volume of water.	1 cup	240	88	160	5	12	---	---	---	8	38	.5	120	.05	.05	.5	---
	Oyster stew:																	
606	Prepared with equal volume of milk.	1 cup	240	83	200	10	12	---	---	---	14	305	1.4	410	.12	.41	.5	Trace
607	Prepared with equal volume of water.	1 cup	240	90	120	6	8	---	---	---	8	158	1.4	240	.07	.19	.5	---
608	Tapioca, dry, quick-cooking.	1 cup	152	13	535	1	Trace	---	---	---	131	15	.6	0	0	0	0	0
	Tapioca desserts:																	
609	Apple	1 cup	250	70	295	1	Trace	---	---	---	74	8	.5	30	Trace	Trace	Trace	Trace
610	Cream pudding	1 cup	165	72	220	8	8	4	3	Trace	28	173	.7	480	.07	.30	.2	2
611	Tartar sauce	1 tbsp.	14	34	75	Trace	8	1	1	4	1	3	.1	30	Trace	Trace	Trace	Trace
612	Vinegar	1 tbsp.	15	94	Trace	Trace	0	0	1	1	1	1	.1	---	---	---	---	---
613	White sauce, medium	1 cup	250	73	405	10	31	16	10	1	22	288	.5	1,150	.10	.43	.5	2
	Yeast:																	
614	Baker's, dry, active	1 pkg.	7	5	20	3	Trace	---	---	---	3	3	1.1	Trace	.16	.38	2.6	Trace
615	Brewer's, dry	1 tbsp.	8	5	25	3	Trace	---	---	---	3	17	1.4	Trace	1.25	.34	3.0	Trace
	Yoghurt. See Milk, Cheese, Cream, Imitation Cream.																	

H

APPENDIX I

Sodium and Potassium

The following tables are reprinted from the second edition of the U.S. Dietary Goals.[1] The Goals recommended restricting salt intake to about 5 g a day, which effectively means reducing sodium intake to about 2 g (2,000 mg).

[1]Select Committee on Nutrition and Human Needs, *Dietary Goals for the United States*, 2nd ed. (Washington, D.C.: Government Printing Office, 1977), pp. 80-83. The Senate's tables are taken from information in U.S. Department of Agriculture, Agricultural Research Service, Composition of foods: Raw, processed, prepared, *Agricultural Handbook No. 8* (Washington, D.C.: Government Printing Office, 1963).

(This salt excludes that present in the natural food before processing.) The goals have been superseded by a more relaxed recommendation from the USDA that we should be moderate in our use of salt, but the specific amounts of sodium in foods may still be of interest to those who wish to compare one food with another. No recommendation was made for the daily consumption of potassium, but people taking diuretics, instructed by their physicians to eat foods high in potassium to replace losses, may be interested to see what foods contain large amounts of this mineral.

Table 1   Average Sodium and Potassium Contents of Common Foods*

Food	Weight (g)	Sodium (mg)	Potassium (mg)
Meat, fish, or poultry, cooked without added salt			
Average	30	33	125
Clams, soft	100	36	239
Clams, hard	100	205	311
Crab, canned	100	1,000	110
Crab, steamed	100	456	271
Flounder	100	237	587
Frankfurters (2)	100	1,100	220
Frozen fish (cod)	100	400	400
Haddock	100	177	348
Kidneys, beef	100	253	324
Lobster, canned	100	210	180
Lobster, fresh	100	325	258
Oysters, raw	100	73	121
Salmon, canned	100	522	349
Salmon, salt-free, canned	100	48	391

Food	Weight (g)	Sodium (mg)	Potassium (mg)
Scallops, fresh	100	265	476
Shrimp, raw	100	140	220
Shrimp, frozen or canned	100	140	200-312
Sweet breads	100	116	433
Tuna, canned	100	800	240
Tuna, salt-free, canned	100	46	382
Cheese			
American cheese	30	341	25
Cream cheese	30	75	22
Cottage cheese	30	76	28
Cottage cheese, unsalted	30	6	—
Low-sodium cheese (cheddar)	30	3	120
Egg			
Whole, fresh and frozen (1)	50	61	65

*Fresh fruits and fruit juices are naturally very low in sodium and thus are not listed individually in this table.

Table 1   Average Sodium and Potassium Contents of Common Foods (cont'd)

Food	Weight (g)	Sodium (mg)	Potassium (mg)
Whites, fresh and frozen	50	73	70
Yolks, fresh	50	26	49
Milk			
Buttermilk, cultured	120	135	192
Condensed sweetened milk	120	135	377
Evaporated milk, undiluted	120	142	364
Powdered milk, skim	30	160	544
Low-sodium milk, canned	120	6	288
Whole	240	120	346
Yogurt (skim milk)	100	51	143
Potato			
White, baked in skin	100	4	323
White, boiled	100	2	285
Instant, prepared with water, milk, fat	100	256	290
Sweet (canned solid pack)	100	48	200
Breads			
Bakery, white	25	127	26
Bakery, whole-wheat	25	132	68
Bakery, rye	25	139	36
Low-sodium (local)	25	4	25
Plain muffin	40	132	38
English muffin	57	215	57
A-proten rusk (1)	11	4	5
Graham crackers (2)	14	93	53
Low-sodium crackers (2)	9	10	11
Vanilla wafers (5)	14	35	10
Yeast doughnut	30	70	24
Cake doughnut	35	160	32
Cereal, dry			
Kellogg's Corn Flakes	30	282	15
Puffed Rice	15	trace	7
Rice Krispies	30	267	15
Special K	30	244	17
Puffed Wheat	15	trace	21
Shredded Wheat	20	1	52

Food	Weight (g)	Sodium (mg)	Potassium (mg)
Kellogg's Sugar Frosted Flakes	30	200	19
Sugar Pops	30	67	22
Bran Flakes	30	118	151
Cereal, cooked without added salt			
Corn grits, enriched, regular	100	1	11
Farina, enriched, regular	100	2	9
Farina, instant cooking	100	7	13
Farina, quick cooking	100	190	10
Oatmeal or Rolled Oats	100	2	61
Pettijohn's Wheat	100	trace	84
Rice	100	5	28
Rice, instant	100	trace	trace
Wheat, rolled	100	trace	84
Wheatena	100	trace	84
Fat			
Bacon (1 strip)	7	73	17
Butter	5	49	3
Margarine	5	49	1
Mayonnaise	15	90	5
Mayonnaise, low-sodium	15	17	1
Low-sodium butter	15	1	3
Unsalted margarine (Fleishman's)	5	1	1
Vegetable oil	15	0	0
Cream			
Coffee Mate	1[†]	4	27
Half-and-half	30	14	39
Heavy whipping cream (30%)	30	10	27
Poly-perx	30	—	11
Sour cream (Sealtest)	30	13	43
Table cream (18%)	30	13	37
Whipped topping	30	4	6

[†]In teaspoons.

I

Table 1   Average Sodium and Potassium Contents of Common Foods (cont'd)

Food	Weight (g)	Sodium (mg)	Potassium (mg)
Gravy			
Low-sodium	30	10	25
Regular	30	210	28
Peanut butter			
Cellu, Salt-free	15	1	100
Regular, made with small amounts of added fat and salt	15	91	100
Desserts			
Baked custard (Delmark)	120	128	174
D'zerta	120	35	0
Gelatin	120	51	1
Ice cream (4-oz cup)	60	23	49
Sherbet	60	6	14
Water ice	60	trace	2
Cakes			
All varieties except gingerbread and fruit cakes (both mixes and recipes)	50‡	123	50
With low-sodium shortening and baking powder	50‡	10-20	75-150
Pies			
All varieties except raisin, mince (1/8 of 9-inch pie)	320‡	375	180
Candy			
Hard candy (1 equals 5 g)	100	32	4
Gum drops (8 small equals 10 g)	100	35	5
Jelly beans	100	12	1
Salt			
(1 g NaCl—1 packet salt)	—	400	—
(5 g NaCl—1 tsp)	—	2,000	—
Salt substitutes			
Diamond Crystal	500§	1	220
Co-salt	500§	0	185

Food	Weight (g)	Sodium (mg)	Potassium (mg)
Adolph's	500§	0	241
McCormick's	500§	0	234
Morton	500§	0	250
Sugar substitutes			
Saccharine (1/4-grain tablet)	1	1	0
Sucaryl	500§	0	0
Sweet-10	500§	0	0
Adolph's	500§	0	0
Morton	500§	0	0
Diamond Crystal	500§	0	0
Beverages			
Beer	100	7	25
Chocolate syrup (2 tsp)	10	5	29
Coca-Cola	100	4	1
Coffee, instant (beverage)	—	1	50
Cranberry juice	100	1	10
Diet Seven-Up	100	10	0
Egg nog, reconstituted	240	250	630
Fresca	100	18	0
Frozen lemonade, reconstituted	100	trace	16
Gingerale	100	6	2
Hot chocolate (Carnation, 1 pack 6 oz water)	100 —	104	190
Kool-Aid, reconstituted	240	trace	0
Meritene, reconstituted	240	250	740
Pepsi Cola	100	2	4
Royal Crown Cola	100	3	trace
Seven-Up	100	9	0
Sprite	100	16	0
Tab	100	5	0
Tea, instant (beverage)	—	trace	25

‡Average serving.

§In milligrams.

Table 2   Sodium Content of Vegetables*

Vegetable	Sodium (mg)
Group I (0-20 mg/100 g,† average 7.4 mg)	
Asparagus	7
Broccoli	12
Brussels sprouts	14
Cabbage, common	14
Cauliflower	9
Chicory	7
Collards	16
Corn	2
Cow peas	1
Cucumbers	6
Eggplant	1
Endive	14
Escarole	14
Green peppers	13
Kohlrabi	6
Leeks	5
Lentils	3
Lettuce	9
Lima beans, not frozen	1
Mushrooms, raw	15
Mustard green	10
Navy beans	7
Okra	2
Onions	7
Parsnips	8
Peas, dried, split, cooked	13
Peas, green	1
Potatoes, baked in skin	4

Vegetable	Sodium (mg)
Potatoes, boiled, pared before cooking	3
Radishes	18
Rutabagas	4
Squash, summer or winter	1
String beans	2
Sweet potato	10
Tomatoes	4
Turnip greens	17
Wax beans	2
Yams	4
Group II (23-60 mg/100 g,† average 40 mg)	
Artichoke	30
Beets	43
Black-eyed peas, frozen only	39
Carrots	33
Chinese cabbage	23
Dandelion greens	44
Kale	43
Parsley	45
Red cabbage	26
Spinach	50
Turnips	34
Watercress	52
Group III (75-126 mg/100 g,† average 81 mg)	
Beet greens	76
Celery	88
Chard, Swiss	86

I

*This table assumes the use of fresh vegetables without salt added in cooking. The amount of salt added to canned and frozen vegetables can vary. *Agricultural Handbook No. 8* from the USDA estimates that canned vegetables average 235 mg sodium per 100 g edible portion. Frozen vegetables range from almost no sodium to as high as 125 mg sodium per 100 g edible portion.

†A 100-g portion for most vegetables is about a 1/2-c to 1-c serving.

APPENDIX J

Recommended Nutrition References

CONTENTS

Books

A listing of highly recommended books is presented at the end of the Introduction to Part One.

Journals

Nutrition Today, the publication of the Nutrition Today Society, is a nutrition journal for the interested layperson. It makes a point of raising controversial issues and providing a forum for conflicting opinions. Articles are seldom referenced but are written by recognized authorities and are entertaining and thought-provoking. Six issues/year, (discount rates for dietetics students), from Director of Membership Services, Nutrition Today Society (address below). *Today's Health* from the American Medical Association (address below) is a similar magazine for the more medically inclined.

The *Journal of the American Dietetic Association*, the official publication of the ADA, contains articles of interest to dietitians and nutritionists, news of legislative action on food and nutrition, and a very useful section of abstracts of articles from many other journals of nutrition and related areas. Twelve issues/year (discount rates for dietetics students), from The American Dietetic Association (address below).

Nutrition Reviews, a publication of The Nutrition Foundation, Inc., does much of the work for the library researcher, compiling recent evidence on current topics and presenting extensive bibliographies. The articles are for the most part prepared by the editorial board, and therefore no single author's name appears on them. The suspicious reader should be reassured that the articles are as reliable as the board, however—that means very reliable. Twelve issues/year (discount rates for students), from The Nutrition Foundation, Inc. (address below).

Other journals that deserve mention here are the *Journal of Nutrition*, *Food Technology*, the *American Journal of Clinical Nutrition*, and the *Journal of Nutrition Education*. *FDA Consumer*, a government publication with many articles of interest to the consumer, is available from the Food and Drug Administration (address below). Many other journals of value are referred to throughout this book. These vary in level; some are heavy going. Inquire before subscribing.

Catalogs, Publication Lists, Free and Inexpensive Materials

Lists of publications can be obtained from the following organizations:

ADA catalog (free) from
    The American Dietetic Association
    430 North Michigan Avenue
    Chicago IL 60611

Publications list (free) from
 The American Medical Association
 535 North Dearborn Street
 Chicago IL 60610

Nutrition references and book reviews (54 pages, $2) from
 The Chicago Nutrition Association
 8158 Kedzie Avenue
 Chicago IL 60652

A guide to free health materials, listing over 2,000 items, can be obtained for $15 from
 Educators Progress Service, Inc.
 214 Center Street
 Randolph WIS 53956

Other free and inexpensive materials can be obtained from the following addresses:

U.S. Government
 Consumer and Food Economics Research
  Division
 Federal Center Building
 Hyattsville MD 20782

 Human Nutrition Research Division
 Agricultural Research Center
 Beltsville MD 20705

 Extension Service, USDA
 Room 5038, South Building
 Washington DC 20250

 The Food and Nutrition Information
  Education Resources Center (FNIERC)
  National Agriculture Library
  10301 Baltimore Boulevard, Room 304
  Beltsville MD 20705   Tel: (301) 344-3719

 Food and Nutrition Service, USDA
 Washington DC 20250

 Food and Drug Administration (FDA)
 5600 Fishers Lane
 Rockville MD 20852

 Information Division
 Agricultural Marketing Service, USDA
 Washington DC 20250

 National Academy of Sciences/National
  Research Council (NAS/NRC)
 2101 Constitution Avenue NW
 Washington DC 20418

 Office of Child Development
 Office of Education
 Public Health Service
 Washington DC 20204

 U.S. Government Printing Office
 The Superintendent of Documents
 Washington DC 20402

Consumer and advocacy groups
 Center for Science in the
  Public Interest (CSPI)
 1755 S Street NW
 Washington DC 20009

 Children's Foundation
 1420 New York Avenue NW, Suite 800
 Washington DC 20005

 Community Nutrition Institute
 1146 19th Street NW
 Washington DC 20036

 Food Research and Action Center (FRAC)
 2011 I Street NW
 Washington DC 20006

Professional and service organizations
 American Academy of Pediatrics
 PO Box 1034
 Evanston IL 60204

 American College of Nutrition
 100 Manhattan Avenue #1606
 Union City NJ 07087

 American Dental Association
 211 East Chicago Avenue
 Chicago IL 60611

 American Dietetic Association
 430 North Michigan Avenue
 Chicago IL 60611

 American Heart Association
 7320 Greenville Avenue
 Dallas TX 75231

 American Home Economics Association
 2010 Massachusetts Avenue NW
 Washington DC 20036

 American Institute of Nutrition
 9650 Rockville Pike
 Bethesda MD 20014

J

American Medical Association
Section of Nutrition Information
535 North Dearborn Street
Chicago IL 60610

The American National Red Cross
Food and Nutrition Consultant
National Headquarters
Washington DC 20006

American Public Health Association
1015 Fifteenth Street NW
Washington DC 20005

American Society for Clinical Nutrition, Inc.
9650 Rockville Pike
Bethesda MD 20014

The Canadian Diabetes Association
1491 Yonge Street
Toronto, Ontario M4T   125 Canada

The Canadian Dietetic Association
123 Edward Street, Suite 601
Toronto, Ontario M5G 1E2 Canada

Food Protein Council
1800 M Street NW
Washington DC 20036

Institute of Food Technologists
221 North LaSalle Street
Chicago IL 60601

La Leche League International, Inc.
9616 Minneapolis Avenue
Franklin Park IL 60131

March of Dimes Birth Defects Foundation
173 West Madison Street
Chicago IL 60602

Meals for Millions/Freedom from
    Hunger Foundation
1800 Olympic Boulevard
PO Drawer 680
Santa Monica CA 90406

National Nutrition Consortium, Inc.
1635 P Street NW, Suite 1
Washington DC 20036

Nutrition Foundation
888 Seventeenth Street NW
Washington DC 20036

Nutrition Today Society
703 Giddings Avenue
PO Box 1829
Annapolis MD 21404

Society for Nutrition Education
2140 Shattuck Avenue, Suite 1110
Berkeley CA 94704

Trade organizations produce many excellent free materials that promote nutritional health. Naturally, they also promote their own products. You must learn to differentiate between "slanted" and valid information. We find the brief reviews in *Contemporary Nutrition* (put out by General Mills), the *Dairy Council Digest*, Ross Laboratories' *Dietetic Currents*, and R. A. Seelig's reviews from the United Fresh Fruit and Vegetable Association to be generally reliable and very useful.

Campbell Soup Company
Food Service Products Division
375 Memorial Avenue
Camden NJ 08101

Del Monte Kitchens
Del Monte Corporation
215 Fremont Street
San Francisco CA 94119

General Foods Consumer Center
250 North Street
White Plains NY 10625

General Mills
PO Box 113
Minneapolis MN 55440

Gerber Products Company
445 State Street
Fremont MI 49412

H. J. Heinz
Consumer Relations
PO Box 57
Pittsburgh PA 15230

Hunt-Wesson Foods
Educational Services
1645 West Valencia Drive
Fullerton CA 92634

Kellogg Company
Department of Home Economics Services
Battle Creek MI 49016

Mead Johnson Nutritionals
2404 Pennsylvania Avenue
Evansville IN 47721

National Dairy Council
6300 North River Road
Rosemont IL 60018

The Nestle Company, Inc.
Home Economics Division
100 Bloomingdale Road
White Plains NY 10605

Oscar Mayer Company
Consumer Service
PO Box 1409
Madison WI 53701

Ross Laboratories
Director of Professional Services
Columbus OH 43216

United Fresh Fruit and Vegetable Association
1019 Nineteenth Street NW
Washington DC 20036

International organizations (United Nations)

Food and Agriculture Organization
of the United Nations (FAO)
North American Regional Office
1325 C Street SW
Washington DC 20025

Food and Agriculture Organization (FAO)
Via delle Terma di Caracalla
0100 Rome, Italy

World Health Organization (WHO)
1211 Geneva 27
Switzerland

J

APPENDIX K

Fiber

If you are attempting to evaluate your fiber intake, it is important to be aware of the distinction made in Chapter 1: The fiber in the colon is not the same as the fiber found in foods when they are analyzed in the laboratory. In the colon, the fiber that remains is whatever has resisted the action of human GI tract enzymes. This is dietary fiber. But when foods are analyzed in a laboratory, they are exposed to stronger agents—dilute acid and dilute alkali. What remains after these treatments is crude fiber. For every gram of crude fiber, there may be 2 to 3 g of dietary fiber.

Diets in the United States probably provide an average of about 4 g of crude fiber a day, as compared with about 6 g back in 1900. Some fiber enthusiasts recommend intakes higher than these, but there may be hazards in overdosing with fiber, as with any other food constituent. Even conservative authorities, however, seem to agree that there would be no harm in aiming at a crude fiber intake from foods of about 6 g a day.

Table 1 shows estimates of the crude fiber contents of foods. Table 2 shows approximations of the dietary fiber contents of foods. We recommend that you read the article it came from for an understanding of the limitations on the accuracy of the numbers in the table and for a breakdown of the fiber types into cellulose, lignin, and other sources.

Table 1   Approximate Crude Fiber Content Per Serving of Food[1]

Food	Serving size	Crude fiber (g)	Food	Serving size	Crude fiber (g)
Cereals	1/2-2/3 c		Peaches, apricots, citrus fruits, fruit cocktail		0.5
All bran		3.0	Fruit juice		0.2
Wheat bran		0.8	**Vegetables**	1/2-2/3 c	
40% bran		0.9	Parsnips, peas, brussels sprouts		2.0
Most other cooked or ready-to-eat		trace-0.3	Pork and beans		2.0
Breads	1 slice		Lima beans		1.5
Whole-wheat, pumpernickel		0.4	Kidney beans		1.0
Raisin, rye, French, Italian, enriched white		0.05-0.2	Broccoli, carrots		1.0
			Green beans, corn, celery, turnip, tomato, greens		0.5-1.0
Fruits	medium or 1/2 c		Potato (with skin)		0.8
Watermelon		1.5	Potato chips, spinach		<0.5
Apple (with skin)		2.0	**Nuts**	1/2 c	1.0-2.0
Prunes, dried peaches		1.5	**Sunflower seeds**	1 c	2.0
Honeydew melon, banana		1.0			
Berries		1.0			

[1]E. M. N. Hamilton and E. N. Whitney, *Nutrition: Concepts and Controversies* (St. Paul: West, 1979), pp. 499-500.

Table 2   Dietary Fiber in Selected Foods[2]

Food	Total dietary fiber (g/100 g)	Food	Total dietary fiber (g/100 g)
Flour		Peas, frozen (raw)	7.75
White, bread-making	3.15	garden (canned)	6.28
Brown	7.87	processed (canned)	7.85
Whole-meal	9.51	**Root vegetables**	
Bran	44.0	Carrots, young (boiled)	3.70
Breads		Parsnips (raw)	4.90
White	2.72	Swedes (raw)	2.40
Brown	5.11	Turnips (raw)	2.20
Hovis	4.54	**Potatoes**	
Whole-meal	8.50	Main crop (raw)	3.51
Cereals		Chips (fried)	3.20
All-Bran	26.7	Crisps	11.9
Cornflakes	11.0	Canned, drained	2.51
Grapenuts	7.00	**Peppers (cooked)**	0.93
Readibrek	7.60	**Other vegetables**	
Rice Krispies	4.47	Peppers (cooked)	0.93
Puffed Wheat	15.41	Tomatoes, fresh	1.40
Sugar Puffs	6.08	canned, drained	0.85
Shredded Wheat	12.26	Sweet corn, cooked	4.74
Swiss breakfast (mixed brands)	7.41	canned, drained	5.69
Weetabix	12.72	**Fruits**	
Biscuits		Apples, flesh only,	1.42
Chocolate digestive (half-coated)	3.50	peel only	3.71
Chocolate (fully coated)	3.09	Bananas	1.75
Crispbread, rye	11.73	Cherries (flesh and skin)	1.24
Crispbread, wheat	4.83	Grapefruit (canned)	0.44
Ginger biscuits	1.99	Guavas (canned)	3.64
Matzo	3.85	Mandarin oranges (canned)	0.29
Oatcakes	4.00	Mangoes (canned)	1.00
Semisweet	2.31	Peaches (flesh and skin)	2.28
Short-sweet	1.60	Pears, flesh only	2.44
Wafers (filled)	1.62	peel only	8.59
Leafy vegetables		Plums (flesh and skin)	1.52
Broccoli tops (boiled)	4.10	Rhubarb (raw)	1.78
Brussels sprouts (boiled)	2.86	Strawberries, raw,	2.12
Cabbage (boiled)	2.83	canned	1.00
Cauliflower (boiled)	1.80	Sultanas	4.40
Lettuce (raw)	1.53	**Nuts**	
Onions (raw)	2.10	Brazils	7.73
Legumes		Peanuts	9.30
Beans, baked (canned)	7.27	**Preserves**	
Beans, runner (boiled)	3.35	Jam, plum,	0.96
		strawberry	1.12

K

[2]Adapted from D. A. T. Southgate, B. Bailey, E. Collinson, and A. F. Walker, A guide to calculating intakes of dietary fibre, *Journal of Human Nutrition* 30 (1976):303-313, with the permission of the authors and publisher.

Table 2   Dietary Fiber in Selected Foods (cont'd)

Food	Total dietary fiber (g/100 g)
Lemon curd	0.20
Marmalade	0.71
Mincemeat	3.19
Peanut butter	7.55
Pickle	1.53
Dried soups (as purchased)	
Minestrone	6.61
Oxtail	3.84
Tomato	3.32

Food	Total dietary fiber (g/100 g)
Beverages (concentrated)	
Cocoa	43.27
Drinking chocolate	8.20
Coffee and chicory essence	0.79
Instant coffee	16.41
Extracts	
Bovril	0.91
Marmite	2.69

APPENDIX L

Exchange Systems

CONTENTS

For an introduction to the use of exchange systems, see Chapter 1. Two exchange systems are presented here, for the use of U.S. and Canadian readers.

United States

The United States system divides foods into six lists—the milk, vegetable, fruit, bread, meat, and fat lists.[1] The items listed first in each group are from the standard exchange lists used in the United States. We have also listed some Chinese foods and some fast foods to show that the exchange system can be adapted to other uses. At the end of the section is a list of "unlimited" foods, which have negligible kcalories.

The exchange system can be used to plan diets at many different kcalorie levels. Six such diets, from 1,200 to 3,000 kcal/day, are shown in Appendix M, Table 6.

[1]The U.S. exchange system presented here is based on material in *Exchange Lists for Meal Planning*, prepared by committees of the American Diabetes Association and the American Dietetic Association in cooperation with the National Institute of Arthritis, Metabolism, and Digestive Diseases and the National Heart and Lung Institute, National Institutes of Health, Public Health Service, U.S. Department of Health, Education, and Welfare.

The Chinese foods listed in these tables are reprinted from *Diabetes and Chinese Food*, ©1978, with the written permission of the Canadian Dietetic Association. We have adjusted the Canadian exchanges used in these examples so that they correspond approximately in food value to the U.S. exchanges. *Diabetes and Chinese Food* is available for a nominal charge from the Canadian Diabetes Association (address in Appendix J).

The fast food data are reprinted by permission from "Nutritional Analysis of Foods Served at McDonald's" (© McDonald's, 1976).

L

Milk List (12 g carbohydrate, 8 g protein, 80 kcal)*

Amount	Food
Nonfat fortified milk	
1 c	Skim or nonfat milk
1 c	Buttermilk made from skim milk
1 c	Yogurt made from skim milk (plain, unflavored)
1/3 c	Powdered, nonfat dry milk, before adding liquid
1/2 c	Canned evaporated skim milk, before adding liquid
Low-fat fortified milk	
1 c	1% fat fortified milk (add 1/2 fat exchange)[†]
1 c	2% fat fortified milk (add 1 fat exchange)[‡]
1 c	Yogurt made from 2% fortified milk (plain, unflavored) (add 1 fat exchange)[†]
Whole milk (add 2 fat exchanges)	
1 c	Whole milk
1 c	Buttermilk made from whole milk
1 c	Yogurt made from whole milk (plain, unflavored)
1/2 c	Canned evaporated whole milk, before adding liquid
Chinese foods	
1 c	Soybean milk, unsweetened
2 blocks	Soybean curd (21/2 x 21/2 x 11/2 in)
2/3 c	Soybean, cooked
Fast foods[§]	

*A milk exchange is a serving of food equivalent to 1 c of skim milk in its energy nutrient content. One milk exchange contains substantial amounts of carbohydrate and protein and about 80 kcal.

[†]These milk exchanges contain more fat than skim milk. Add 1/2 fat exchange.

[‡]These milk exchanges contain more fat than skim milk. Add 1 fat exchange.

[§]These fast foods contain 1/2 milk exchange and added bread and fat: chocolate shake (31/2 bread, 2 fat, 365 kcal); vanilla shake (3 bread, 11/2 fat, 325 kcal); strawberry shake (31/2 bread, 11/2 fat, 345 kcal).

Vegetable List (5 g carbohydrate, 2 g protein, 25 kcal)*

Amount	Food
1/2 c	Asparagus
1/2 c	Bean sprouts
1/2 c	Beets
1/2 c	Broccoli
1/2 c	Brussels sprouts
1/2 c	Cabbage
1/2 c	Carrots
1/2 c	Cauliflower
1/2 c	Celery
1/2 c	Cucumbers
1/2 c	Eggplant
1/2 c	Green pepper
	Greens
1/2 c	Beet greens
1/2 c	Chards
1/2 c	Collard greens
1/2 c	Dandelion greens
1/2 c	Kale
1/2 c	Mustard greens
1/2 c	Spinach
1/2 c	Turnip greens
1/2 c	Mushrooms
1/2 c	Okra
1/2 c	Onions
1/2 c	Rhubarb
1/2 c	Rutabaga
1/2 c	Sauerkraut
1/2 c	String beans, green or yellow
1/2 c	Summer squash
1/2 c	Tomatoes
1/2 c	Tomato juice
1/2 c	Turnips
1/2 c	Vegetable juice cocktail
1/2 c	Zucchini
Chinese foods	
1/2 c	Beansprouts, soy
1/2 c	Lotus root (1/3 segment)
1/2 c	Waterchestnut
1/2 c	Yam bean root

*A vegetable exchange is a serving of any vegetable that contains a moderate amount of carbohydrate, a small but significant amount of protein, and about 25 kcal.

L

Fruit List (10 g carbohydrate, 40 kcal)*

Amount	Food
1 small	Apple
1/3 c	Apple juice
1/2 c	Applesauce (unsweetened)
2 medium	Apricots, fresh
4 halves	Apricots, dried
1/2 small	Banana
1/2 c	Blackberries
1/2 c	Blueberries
1/4 small	Cantaloupe melon
10 large	Cherries
1/3 c	Cider
2	Dates
1	Fig, fresh
1	Fig, dried
1 half	Grapefruit
1/2 c	Grapefruit juice
12	Grapes
1/4 c	Grape juice
1/8 medium	Honeydew melon
1/2 small	Mango
1 small	Nectarine
1 small	Orange
1/2 c	Orange juice
3/4 c	Papaya

Amount	Food
1 medium	Peach
1 small	Pear
1 medium	Persimmon (native)
1/2 c	Pineapple
1/3 c	Pineapple juice
2 medium	Plums
2 medium	Prunes
1/4 c	Prune juice
1/2 c	Raspberries
2 tbsp	Raisins
3/4 c	Strawberries
1 medium	Tangerine
1 c	Watermelon

Chinese foods

Amount	Food
1 medium	Guava, fresh
3 medium	Kumquats, fresh
4 medium	Lychee, fresh
1/2 small or 1/3 c	Mango
1/2 small or 1/3 c	Papaya
1/2 medium	Persimmon
1/3 medium	Pomelo

Fast foods†

*A fruit exchange is a serving of fruit that contains about 10 g of carbohydrate and 40 kcal. The protein and fat content of fruit is negligible.

†Apple and cherry pies contain 1 1/2 exchanges of fruit but also 1 bread and 3 1/2 fat exchanges.

Bread List (15 g carbohydrate, 2 g protein, 70 kcal)*

Amount	Food
Bread	
1 slice	White (including French and Italian)
1 slice	Whole-wheat
1 slice	Rye or pumpernickel
1 slice	Raisin
1 half	Small bagel
1 half	Small English muffin
1	Plain roll, bread
1 half	Frankfurter roll
1 half	Hamburger bun
3 tbsp	Dried bread crumbs
1 6-in	Tortilla

Amount	Food
Cereal	
1/2 c	Bran flakes
3/4 c	Other ready-to-eat cereal, unsweetened
1 c	Puffed cereal, unfrosted
1/2 c	Cereal, cooked
1/2 c	Grits, cooked
1/2 c	Rice or barley, cooked
1/2 c	Pasta, cooked (spaghetti, noodles, or macaroni)
3 c	Popcorn, popped, no fat added
2 tbsp	Cornmeal, dry
2 1/2 tbsp	Flour
1/4 c	Wheat germ

*A bread exchange is a serving of bread, cereal, or starchy vegetable that contains appreciable carbohydrate (15 g) and a small but significant amount of protein (2 g), totaling about 70 kcal.

L

Bread List (15 g carbohydrate, 2 g protein, 70 kcal) (cont'd)

Amount	Food
Crackers	
3	Arrowroot
2	Graham, 2½-in square
1 half	Matzoth, 4 × 6 in
20	Oyster
25	Pretzels, 3⅛ in long × ⅛ in diameter
3	Rye wafers, 2 × 3½ in
6	Saltines
4	Soda, 2½-in sq
Dried beans, peas, and lentils	
1/2 c	Beans, peas, lentils, dried and cooked
1/4 c	Baked beans, no pork, canned
Starchy vegetables	
1/3 c	Corn
1 small	Corn on cob
1/2 c	Lima beans
2/3 c	Parsnips
1/2 c	Peas, green, canned, or frozen
1 small	Potato, white
1/2 c	Potato, mashed
3/4 c	Pumpkin
1/2 c	Squash (winter, acorn, or butternut)
1/4 c	Yam or sweet potato
Prepared foods†	
1	Biscuit, 2-in diameter (add 1 fat exchange)
1	Corn bread, 2 × 2 × 1 in (add 1 fat exchange)

Amount	Food
1	Corn muffin, 2-in diameter (add 1 fat exchange)
5	Crackers, round butter type (add 1 fat exchange)
1	Muffin, plain, small (add 1 fat exchange)
8	Potatoes, french fried, 2 × 3½ in (add 1 fat exchange)
15	Potato chips or corn chips (add 2 fat exchanges)
1	Pancake, 5 × ½ in (add 1 fat exchange)
1	Waffle, 5 × ½ in (add 1 fat exchange)
Chinese foods	
1 small or 2/3 medium	Bow (Chinese steamed dough)
6	Chestnuts
1 c	Congee
1/4 c	Glutinous rice, cooked
2/3 c	Gruel rice, cooked
1/2 c	Noodles, cooked (shrimp, thin rice, flat rice, cellophane)
2 tbsp	Rice flour or glutinous rice flour
3 small or 1/3 c	Taro
4	Wonton wrapper (5 × 5 in)

†These foods contain more fat than bread. When calculating fat values, add fat exchanges as indicated (1 fat exchange = 5 g fat).

Meat List (7 g protein, 3 g fat + variable added fat; 55 kcal + kcalories for added fat)*

Amount	Food
Low-fat meat	
1 oz	Beef—baby beef (very lean), chipped beef, chuck, flank steak, tenderloin, plate ribs, plate skirt steak, round (bottom, top), all cuts rump, spareribs, tripe
1 oz	Lamb—leg, rib, sirloin, loin (roast and chops), shank, shoulder

Amount	Food
1 oz	Pork—leg (whole rump, center shank), ham, smoked (center slices)
1 oz	Veal—leg, loin, rib, shank, shoulder, cutlets
1 oz	Poultry—meat-without-skin of chicken, turkey, cornish hen, guinea hen, pheasant

*A meat exchange is a serving of protein-rich food that contains negligible carbohydrate but a significant amount of protein (7 g) and fat (3 g), roughly equivalent to the amounts in 1 oz of lean meat; contains about 55 kcal.

Meat List (7 g protein, 3 g fat + variable added fat; 55 kcal + kcalories for added fat) (cont'd)

Amount	Food
1 oz	Fish—any fresh or frozen
1/4 c	Canned salmon, tuna, mackerel, crab, lobster
5 (or 1 oz)	Clams, oysters, scallops, shrimp
3	Sardines, drained
1 oz	Cheese, containing less than 5% butterfat
1/4 c	Cottage cheese, dry and 2% butterfat
1/2 c	Dried beans and peas (add 1 bread exchange)[†]

Medium-fat meat (add 1/2 fat exchange)[†]

Amount	Food
1 oz	Beef—ground (15% fat), corned beef (canned), rib eye, round (ground commercial)
1 oz	Pork—loin (all cuts tenderloin), shoulder arm (picnic), shoulder blade, Boston butt, Canadian bacon, boiled ham
1 oz	Liver, heart, kidney, sweetbreads (high in cholesterol)
1/4 c	Cottage cheese, creamed
1 oz	Cheese—mozzarella, ricotta, farmer's cheese, Neufchatel
3 tbsp	Parmesan cheese
1	Egg (high in cholesterol)

High-fat meat (add 1 fat exchange)[†]

Amount	Food
1 oz	Beef—brisket, corned beef (brisket), ground beef (more than 20% fat), hamburger (commercial), chuck (ground commercial), roasts (rib), steaks (club and rib)

Amount	Food
1 oz	Lamb—breast
1 oz	Pork—spare ribs, loin (back ribs), pork (ground), country-style ham, deviled ham
1 oz	Veal—breast
1 oz	Poultry—capon, duck (domestic), goose
1 oz	Cheddar-type cheese
1 slice	Cold cuts, $4 1/2 \times 1/8$ in
1 small	Frankfurter

Peanut butter

Amount	Food
2 tbsp	Peanut butter (add 2 1/2 fat exchanges)[†]

Chinese foods[‡]

Amount	Food
1/4 c	Canned or cooked abalone, crabmeat, eel, lobster, conch, cuttlefish, squid, octopus, fish maw, sea cucumbers, jellyfish, etc.
10 medium	River snails
2 medium	Frog legs
3 medium	Duck feet
1 medium or 1/2 large	Duck egg, salted
1 medium	Egg, preserved or limed
1/2 block	Soybean curd, fresh, $2 1/2 \times 1 1/4 \times 1 1/2$ in
2 pieces	Soybean curd, fried, $3 \times 6 \times 1/2$ inches

Fast foods[§]

[†]These foods contain more carbohydrate or fat than lean meat. When calculating carbohydrate or fat values, add bread or fat exchanges as indicated.

[‡]These exchanges are not separated into high-, medium-, and low-fat exchanges.

[§]Most fast-food meats are for variable numbers of exchanges and have other exchanges added: hamburger (1 high-fat meat, 2 bread, 260 kcal); cheeseburger (1 1/2 high-fat meat, 2 bread, 306 kcal); Quarter Pounder® (3 high-fat meat, 2 bread, 420 kcal); Big Mac® (3 high-fat meat, 2 1/2 bread, 1 1/2 fat, 540 kcal); Quarter Pounder® with cheese (4 high-fat meat, 2 bread, 520 kcal); Egg McMuffin® (2 high-fat meat, 1 1/2 bread, 1 fat, 350 kcal); pork sausage (1 high-fat meat, 1 1/2 fat, 185 kcal).

L

Fat List (5 g fat, 45 kcal)*

Amount	Food
Polyunsaturated fat	
1 tsp	Margarine (soft, tub, or stick)†
1/8	Avocado (4-in diameter)‡
1 tsp	Oil—corn, cottonseed, safflower, soy, sunflower
1 tsp	Oil, olive‡
1 tsp	Oil, peanut‡
5 small	Olives‡
10 whole	Almonds‡
2 large whole	Pecans‡
20 whole	Peanuts, Spanish‡
10 whole	Peanuts, Virginia‡
6 small	Walnuts
6 small	Nuts, other‡
Saturated fat	
1 tsp	Margarine, regular stick
1 tsp	Butter
1 tsp	Bacon fat

Amount	Food
1 strip	Bacon, crisp
2 tbsp	Cream, light
2 tbsp	Cream, sour
1 tbsp	Cream, heavy
1 tbsp	Cream cheese
1 tbsp	French dressing§
1 tbsp	Italian dressing§
1 tsp	Lard
1 tsp	Mayonnaise§
2 tsp	Salad dressing, mayonnaise type§
3/4-in cube	Salt pork
Chinese foods	
1 tsp	Sesame or chili oil
1 piece	Coconut meat, 1 × 1 × 1.2 in
2 1/2 tsp	Coconut, grated
2 tsp	Coconut cream (no water)
1 tbsp	Sesame seeds
1-in cube	Fatty cured Chinese pork

*A fat exchange is a serving of any food that contains negligible carbohydrate and protein but appreciable fat (5 g), totaling about 45 kcal.

†Made with corn, cottonseed, safflower, soy, or sunflower oil only.

‡Fat content is primarily monounsaturated.

§If made with corn, cottonseed, safflower, soy, or sunflower oil, can be assumed to contain polyunsaturated fat.

Unlimited Foods (negligible kcal)*

Amount	Food
	Diet kcalorie-free beverage
	Coffee
	Tea
	Bouillon without fat
	Unsweetened gelatin
	Unsweetened pickles
	Salt and pepper
	Red pepper
	Paprika
	Garlic
	Celery salt
	Parsley
	Nutmeg
	Lemon
	Mustard
	Chili powder
	Onion salt or powder
	Horseradish
	Vinegar
	Mint
	Cinnamon
	Lime
	Raw vegetables—chicory, Chinese cabbage, endive, escarole, lettuce, parsley, radishes, watercress

Amount	Food
Chinese foods	
	Plain agar-agar
	Seasonings, spices, herbs† such as soy sauce, monosodium glutamate, star anise, five-spices powder
	Chinese parsley, kelp, sea girdle, laver, and seaweed hair
1 tsp	Shrimp sauce or dried shrimp
1 tsp or 2 nuts	Gingko nuts
1/2 block	White bean curd cheese, 1 1/2 × 3/4 × 1 in
1/4 block	Red bean curd cheese, 1 × 1/4 × 1/2 in
1 c or less	Watery vegetables, including bamboo shoots, bitter melon, bottle gourd, cabbage (celery, mustard, or spoon; fresh, pickled, spiced, salted, or salted and dried), Chinese broccoli, Chinese eggplant, fungi (black, brown, or white), snow peas, turnips (Chinese or green), watercress, winter melon, wolfberry leaves

*These are "free foods" that contain negligible carbohydrate, protein, and fat and therefore negligible kcalories.

†Does not include some starchy and sugar-preserved Chinese herbs.

L

Canada

The Canadian system works the same way as the U.S. system, but the serving sizes and some of the foods listed are different.[2] Notable among the differences are:

- The standard serving size for milk is one half cup (not 1 c), and whole milk rather than skim is the basis for calculation.

- Vegetables are listed in two groups, the A group (7 g carbohydrate, 2 g protein) and the B group (about half as much carbohydrate and protein). Serving sizes vary. Two group B vegetable servings may be traded for one group A vegetable serving.

- Meats are not divided into low-, medium-, and high-fat categories. An ounce of any meat is considered to provide 7 g protein, 5 g fat.

[2]The Canadian exchange system is taken from *Exchange Lists for Meal Planning for Diabetics in Canada*, published by The Canadian Diabetes Association (Toronto, Ontario, 1977), and is used with their permission.

Milk List (6 g carbohydrate, 4 g protein, 4 g fat)*

Amount	Food
Whole milk	
1/2 c	Whole milk
1/4 c	Evaporated whole milk
Low-fat milk	
1/2 c	2% milk[†]
1/2 c	2% buttermilk[†]
1/2 c	Skim milk[‡]
2 tbsp	Powdered skim milk (instant)[‡]
1/2 c	Skim buttermilk[‡]
1/3 c	Yogurt (plain)[‡]

*A milk exchange is a serving of food equivalent to 1/2 c of whole milk in its energy-nutrient content.

[†]These milk exchanges contain less fat than whole milk. Subtract 1/2 fat exchange.

[‡]These milk exchanges contain less fat than whole milk. Subtract 1 fat exchange.

Vegetable List—Group A (7 g carbohydrate, 2 g protein)*

Amount	Food
1/4 c	Beans—dried navy, lima (canned or cooked)
1/4 c	Beans, green lima
1/2 c	Beets, canned or cooked
2/3 c	Beet greens, cooked
4 stalks	Broccoli, cooked
1/2 c	Brussels sprouts, cooked
3 level tbsp	Canned condensed soup (undiluted)[†]
1/2 c	Carrots, raw, diced, cooked
2 1/2 tbsp	Corn, canned cream style or niblet[†]
1/2 c	Dandelion greens, cooked
2 slices 4 × 4 × 1 in	Eggplant, raw
2/3 c	Kohlrabi, cooked
4 or 1/3 c chopped	Onions, green
1 medium or 1/3 c chopped	Onions, mature, raw
1/3 c	Parsnips, cooked[†]
1/3 c	Peas, green, frozen[†]
1/3 c	Peas, fresh, green, cooked
1/4 c	Peas, green, canned (drained)
2 level tbsp	Potatoes, mashed[†]
1/2 small	Potato, boiled or baked
1/2 c	Pumpkin, canned
3 level tbsp	Rice, cooked[†]
3/4 c	Sauerkraut, canned
1/2 c	Squash, hubbard or pepper, baked or mashed
3/4 c	Tomatoes, canned
2/3 c	Tomato juice, no sugar added
1/2 c	Turnip, yellow or white cooked
2/3 c	Vegetable juice, mixed
1/2 c	Vegetables, mixed carrots and peas
1/3 c	Vegetables, mixed carrots, peas, green lima beans, corn

*A vegetable exchange is a serving of any vegetable that contains a moderate amount of carbohydrate and a small but significant amount of protein.

[†]These vegetables also appear on the bread list in larger servings. They are included in group A for those people whose diet is low in kcalories and to add variety in making up casserole dishes, soups, and the like for any diet.

Vegetable List—Group B*

Amount	Food
5 stalks	Asparagus
1/2 c	Beans, yellow or green, canned or cooked
1 c	Bean sprouts, raw
1/2 c	Cabbage, raw or cooked
1/2 c	Cauliflower, cooked
4 stalks or 1/2 c chopped	Celery, raw
1/2 c	Celery, cooked
1/2 c	Chard, cooked
1/2 medium or 8 slices	Cucumber
1 6-in stalk	Endive
1/2 c	Fiddleheads

Amount	Food
1/2 c	Kale
1/8 head 4 large leaves	Lettuce
2	Onions, green
1 medium	Pepper, green, raw, or cooked
3 tbsp	Pimento, canned
6	Radish
1/2 c	Spinach, cooked or canned
1/3 c	Tomato juice (no sugar added)
1 medium (2 1/4-in diameter)	Tomato, raw
1/2 c	Vegetable marrow, cooked
1/2 c	Zucchini

*Two servings of group B vegetables equal one serving of group A vegetables. One serving from group B may be taken "free" at any meal.

Fruit List (10 g carbohydrate)*

Amount	Food
1/2 medium	Apple, raw
1/3 c	Apple juice
1/2 c	Applesauce
2	Apricots, raw with stone
5 halves + 2 tbsp juice	Apricots, canned, cooked, or dried
1/2 6-in	Banana
1/3 c	Blackberries, raw
1/2 c	Blueberries, raw
1/2 5-in diameter	Cantaloupe with rind
1 c	Cantaloupe cubes or balls
10 large	Cherries, raw
1/3 c + 2 tbsp juice	Cherries, canned, red, pitted, cooked
1 average	Crabapple
2	Dates
2/3 c	Fruit cocktail, canned
1 + 1 tbsp juice	Fig, cooked
1	Fig, dried
3/4 c	Gooseberries, raw
1/2 small (3 1/2-in diameter)	Grapefruit, raw

Amount	Food
1/2 c with juice	Grapefruit sections, raw
1/2 c	Grapefruit juice
14 medium	Grapes, slipskin
14 medium	Grapes, Malaga and seedless
1/4 c	Grape juice
1/2 melon 5-in diameter	Honeydew melon with rind
3/4 c	Honeydew cubes or balls
1/2 c	Huckleberries
1/2 c	Loganberries
1 medium	Nectarine
1 medium (2 1/2 in diameter)	Orange, raw
1/2 c + juice	Orange sections
1/2 c	Orange juice
3/4 c + juice (14 sections)	Orange, mandarin sections (canned dietetic)
1 medium	Peach, raw with stone
2 large halves + 2 tbsp juice	Peaches, canned or cooked

*One fruit exchange is a serving of fruit that contains about 10 g of carbohydrate. The protein and fat content of fruit is negligible.

Fruit List (10 g carbohydrate) (cont'd)

Amount	Food
1 small	Pear, raw
2 halves + 2 tbsp juice	Pears, canned or cooked
1/2 c	Pineapple, raw, cubed
1/2 c cubes or 2 slices + 2 tbsp juice	Pineapple, canned
1/2 c	Pineapple, crushed
1/3 c	Pineapple juice
2 medium	Plums, raw with stone
2 medium + 2 tbsp juice	Plums, canned or cooked
1/2	Pomegranate
2	Prunes, cooked
1/4 c	Prune juice
2 level tbsp	Raisins
1/2 c	Raspberries, raw

Amount	Food
1/2 c	Raspberries, canned or cooked
2 c	Rhubarb, raw
1 c	Rhubarb, cooked
1/2 c	Saskatoons
1 c	Strawberries, raw
3/4 c	Strawberries, canned or cooked
1 (2 1/2-in diameter)	Tangerines
1 c	Tomato juice (no sugar added)
1 slice 1 in thick and 5 in triangle	Watermelon, with skin
1 c	Watermelon cubes
1/6-pt brick	Ice cream—plain vanilla, strawberry, chocolate (add 5 g butter or 1 fat exchange)

Bread List (15 g carbohydrate, 2 g protein)*

Amount	Food
1 slice	Bread
4 (4 1/2 in each)	Bread sticks
6 (6 in each)	Bread sticks, thin
1/2	Bagel
1/4 c	Brewis, cooked (Newfoundland)
1/2 bun	Hamburger bun (3 1/2-in)
1/2 bun	Wiener bun (6-in)
4 rectangular slices or 8 round slices	Melba toast (commercial)
1	Matzo (6-in square)
3	Arrowroots
4	Graham wafers (2-in)
1 1/2 biscuits	Holland rusks
6	Soda biscuits (2-in)
2 tbsp	Cereals, uncooked (dry weight)
1/2 c	Cereals, cooked

Amount	Food
3/4 c	Cereals, cold, flaked
1 c	Cereals, puffed
2/3 biscuit	Cereals, Shredded Wheat
2 tbsp	Cornstarch
2 1/2 tbsp	Flour
1/3 c	Beans and peas, dried, cooked
1/2 c	Corn, canned
1 cob	Corn on the cob (4 1/2 × 1 1/2 × 2 in)
1 1/4 c	Popcorn
2/3 c	Parsnips
1/2 c	Peas, canned
2/3 c	Peas, frozen
1 small or 1/3 c mashed	Potatoes
1/2 c	Macaroni, cooked
1/3 c	Rice, spaghetti, noodles (cooked)
6 tbsp	Canned condensed soup (undiluted)

*A bread exchange is a serving of bread, cereal, or starchy vegetable equivalent in energy-nutrient content to one slice of cracked or whole-wheat, white, brown, or rye bread weighing 30 g. A bread exchange contains appreciable carbohydrate and a small but significant amount of protein.

L

Meat List (7 g protein, 5 g fat)*

Amount	Food
1 medium	Egg

Meat and poultry

Amount	Food
1 slice 4 × 2 × 1/4 in	Sliced medium-fat beef, corned beef, lamb, pork, veal, ham, liver, poultry
1 piece 4 × 2 × 1/4 in	Steak
3 11/2-in cubes	Diced beef for stewing
2 tbsp or small patty (3 tbsp raw)	Minced beef
2/3 oz	Salt beef (dried)
1 small	Lamb loin chop
1/2 medium	Pork, veal chop
3 slices	Bacon, back or side (crisp)
1 slice, 1/8 in thick	Luncheon-type meats
1 slice, 1/4 in thick (11/2-2-in diameter)	Liverwurst, salami, summer sausage
11/2 (12 per lb)	Sausages†
1 piece 4 × 2 × 1/4 in	Seal
1 (12 per lb)	Wieners†

Fish

Amount	Food
1 piece 2 × 1 × 1 in	Fillets of haddock, halibut, cod, sole, whitefish‡
1 piece 2 × 1 × 1 in	Fillet of salmon
1 piece 2 × 1 × 1 in	Salmon steak
1/4 c	Canned chicken haddie, crabmeat, lobster, salmon, tuna

Amount	Food
3 fish 3-in each	Sardines (drained)
3 medium	Clams, fresh
3 medium	Oysters
2 medium	Scallops
4 medium	Shrimps, prawns

Cheese

Amount	Food
1 cube 11/2 × 1 × 1 in or 1 slice (presliced, packaged) 31/2 × 31/2 × 1/8 in	Cheddar or processed
11/2 sections	Gruyere
4 level tbsp	Dried, grated (Parmesan)
3 tbsp	Cottage, creamed
3 tbsp	Cottage, dry (skim)‡
1 piece 21/2-in diameter and 1/4-in thick or 1 slice presliced, packaged 31/2 × 31/2 × 1/8-in	Skim milk, processed‡

*A meat exchange is a serving of protein-rich food that contains negligible carbohydrate but a significant amount of protein and fat, roughly equivalent to the amounts in 1 oz (30 g) of meat.

†For special sizes of sausages and wieners, check weight and number per package.

‡These items contain less fat than most meats. Subtract 1 fat exchange.

L

Fat List (5 g fat)*

Amount	Food
1/8 of 4-in avocado	Avocado pear[†]
1 strip	Bacon (side)
1 tsp or 1 pat (1 × 1 × 1/4 in)	Butter or margarine
1 tsp	Cooking fat or oil
3 tbsp	Cream, cereal (10%)[†]
2 tbsp	Cream, coffee (18%)
2 tbsp	Cream, commercial sour
1 tbsp	Cream, whipping
1 rounded tbsp	Cream, whipped
1 tbsp	Cream cheese (white)
1 tbsp	French dressing
1 tsp	Mayonnaise
10	Peanuts[†]
4	Cashews[†]
6	Almonds, filberts[†]
4-5 halves	Pecans, walnuts[†]
2	Brazil nuts[†]
5 small	Olives, green
3 medium	Olives, ripe with pit
1/2 tbsp	Peanut butter[†]

*A fat exchange is a serving of food equivalent to 1 tsp butter in its fat content. Most fat exchanges have negligible carbohydrate.

[†]It is advisable to limit these items to two servings per day because of the carbohydrate content.

kCalorie-Free Foods*

Food	
Artificial sweetener	Watercress
Non-kcaloric carbonated beverages (dietetic)	Food coloring
	Gelatin, plain
Clear tea or coffee	Artificially sweetened jelly powders
Bouillon	
Clear broth	Horseradish
Consomme	Mushrooms
Flavouring (vanilla, lemon extract)	Parsley
	Rennet tablets
Vinegar	

Seasoning, spices, and herbs

Cinnamon	Sage
Curry powder	Poultry seasoning
Ginger	Mixed whole spices
Nutmeg	Salt and pepper
Mint	Onion salt
Marjoram	Garlic salt

*No significant food value. These foods may be used on kcalorie-restricted diets without restriction.

kCalorie-Poor Foods*

Amount	Food
1 tsp	Cream substitute, powdered (nondairy)
1 tsp	Cocoa (plain)
1 tbsp	Cranberries, cooked without sugar
1 medium serving	Dulse
1 tsp	Fruit spread and jelly, dietetic
1 tbsp	Lemon juice
1 medium	Lemon wedge or slice
1 tsp	Catsup
1 tsp	Chili sauce
1 tsp	Steak sauce
1 tbsp	Partridge berries (Newfoundland)
1 medium	Pickle, dill, unsweetened
4	Pickles, sour, mixed
4	Pickles, sweet, mixed (dietetic)
1 tbsp	Pimento or chopped green pepper
1 tsp	Prepared mustard
1 tbsp	Whipped topping, commercial, powder

*Low in kcalories. These foods may be used in amounts up to two servings a day in kcalorie-restricted diets.

L

APPENDIX M

Food Group Plans

CONTENTS

Food group plans are designed to provide an easy way to approach diet adequacy for all nutrients. This appendix describes the U.S. and Canadian food plans, with a critique and suggestions for use.

The U.S. Four Food Group Plan

The Four Food Group Plan is a simple and quick guideline for diet planning. But it is not a guarantee of adequacy. Individual foods vary in nutrient content, and the selection of foods within each group can make a big difference in the nutritional adequacy of a diet. However, a diet that is planned around this guide is more apt to be nutritionally adequate than one that is randomly chosen.

Each of the four food groups contains foods that are similar in origin and in nutrient content (see Table 1).

The eight nutrients named in Table 1 are used as indicator nutrients. The meat and milk groups also contribute vitamin B_{12}, important because it is found only in animal products. These two groups and the grain group help provide zinc, a nutrient whose importance is becoming better recognized. All of the other essential nutrients are also found in these foods.

The expectation of the people who devised this plan is that a diet providing adequate amounts of the eight indicator nutrients will provide ample amounts of all the other nutrients as well. This is not an entirely safe assumption. When fortified foods are involved (to which perhaps only the eight indicator nutrients have been added), the food label may read the same as for a truly nutritious food, but the food may be

Table 1   The Four Food Groups (U.S.)

Food group	Sample foods	Main nutrient contributions
Meat and meat substitutes	Beef, pork, lamb, fish, poultry, eggs, nuts, legumes	Protein, iron, riboflavin, niacin, thiamin
Milk and milk products	Milk, buttermilk, yogurt, cheese, cottage cheese, soy milk, ice cream	Calcium, protein, riboflavin, thiamin
Fruits and vegetables	All fruits and vegetables	Vitamin A, vitamin C, thiamin, additional iron and riboflavin
Grains (bread and cereal products)	All whole-grain and enriched flours and products	Additional riboflavin, niacin, iron, thiamin

M

Table 2   Interlocking Pattern of Key Nutrients in the Food Groups (Canada)

Nutrient	Milk and milk products	Bread and cereals	Fruits and vegetables	Meat and alternates
Vitamin A	Vitamin A		Vitamin A	Vitamin A
Thiamin		Thiamin		Thiamin
Riboflavin	Riboflavin	Riboflavin		Riboflavin
Niacin		Niacin		Niacin
Folic acid			Folic acid	Folic acid
Vitamin C			Vitamin C	
Vitamin D	Vitamin D			
Calcium	Calcium			
Iron		Iron	Iron	Iron
Protein	Protein	Protein		Protein
Fat	Fat			Fat
Carbohydrate		Carbohydrate	Carbohydrate	

relatively nutrient-empty, except for the added nutrients.

The Four Food Group Plan specifies that a certain quantity of food must be consumed from each group. For the adult, the number of servings recommended is two meat, two milk, four fruits and vegetables, and four grains. For the serving sizes and recommendations for other age groups, please refer to Chapter 1, Table 3.

Canada's Food Guide

Canada's Food Guide is similar to the Four Food Group Plan and was developed with the same intent. The handbook explaining it presents the pattern of nutrient intakes shown in Table 2.[1] The Food Guide recommends, for adults, a slightly different pattern from the Four Food Group Plan, as shown in Table 3.

[1]Canadian Ministry of Health and Welfare, *Canada's Food Guide: Handbook* cat. no. H21-74/1977, Ottawa, Ontario, 1977.

Critique of the Four Food Group Plan

The Four Food Group Plan is subject to two major criticisms. One is that it does not include enough of the foods that people really eat. The other is that it encourages overeating.

Many foods that we eat don't fit into any of the four food groups. Consider butter, margarine, cream, sour cream, salad dressing, mayonnaise, jam, jelly, broth, coffee, tea, alcoholic beverages, synthetic products, vitamin-mineral pills, and others. These items are grouped together into a miscellaneous category. Some of these items do contribute some nutrients to the day's intake. However, either they are not foods, their nutrient content is not significant in enough of the indicator nutrients characteristic of a food group, or their nutrient content has been greatly diluted by fat, sugar, or water. Other foods that we eat fail to fit because they are mixed dishes: soups, casseroles, and the like. The diet planner who relies on these dishes finds the Four Food Group Plan too rigid for his use.

Some say that diet planners undermine the health of those they plan for by insisting that people eat too much food. For all its virtues, the

Table 3   Servings in Canada's Food Guide

Food group	Recommended number of servings (adult)	Serving size
Meat and alternates	2	60-90 g (2-3 oz) cooked lean meat, poultry, liver, or fish
		60 ml (4 tbsp) peanut butter
		250 ml (1 c) cooked dried peas, beans, or lentils
		80-250 ml (1/3-1 c) nuts or seeds
		60 g (2 oz) cheddar, processed, or cottage cheese
		2 eggs
Milk and milk products	2*	250 ml (1 c) milk, yogurt, or cottage cheese
		45 g (1 1/2 oz) cheddar or processed cheese
Fruits and vegetables	4-5†	125 ml (1/2 c) vegetables or fruits
		125 ml (1/2 c) juice
		1 medium potato, carrot, tomato, peach, apple, orange, or banana
Bread and cereals	3-5‡	1 slice bread
		125-250 ml (1/2-1 c) cooked or ready-to-eat cereal
		1 roll or muffin
		125-200 ml (1/2-3/4 c) cooked rice, macaroni, or spaghetti

*Children up to 11 years, 2-3 servings; adolescents, 3-4 servings; pregnant and nursing women, 3-4 servings. Skim, 2%, whole, buttermilk, reconstituted dry, or evaporated milk may be used as a beverage or as the main ingredient in other foods. Cheese may also be chosen. In addition, a supplement of vitamin D is recommended when the milk that is consumed does not contain added vitamin D.

†Include at least two vegetables. Choose a variety of both vegetables and fruits—cooked, raw, or their juices. Include yellow or green or green, leafy vegetables.

‡Whole-grain or enriched. Whole-grain products are recommended.

Four Food Group Plan may inadvertently encourage overeating. The emphasis has been on including, not limiting, foods: "Be sure to get enough milk—enough meat—enough fruit—enough cereal. Don't forget your protein, your calcium, your B vitamins." In the process, until recently, the problem of the kcalories being consumed along the way has been largely ignored. A man going down the cafeteria line at dinnertime may spot a cherry pie, say to himself "I haven't had my fruit for the day," and help himself to a slice. The cherries in the pie are indeed a fruit and are nutritious; the piecrust is made of grain and may add B vitamins and iron to his day's intake. But what if he has already exceeded his kcalorie allowance for the day? The Four Food Group Plan does state that one should adjust food choices and serving sizes to achieve and maintain ideal weight but offers no guidance for doing this. Eating well has thus become equivalent, in many people's minds, to eating a lot.

Suggestions for Use

The Four Food Group Plan appears quite rigid, but it can be used with great flexibility once its intent is understood. For example, cheese can be substituted for milk, because it supplies the same nutrients in about the same amounts. Legumes and nuts are alternative choices for meats. The Plan can be adapted to casseroles and other mixed dishes and to different national and cultural cuisines, such as the Chinese, vegetarian, and others. The exchange lists can be used with the Four Food Group Plan to obtain a great variety of menus.

Suppose you want to plan menus that are adequate but not excessive in kcalories. The Four Food Group Plan promotes adequacy, but most people (notably young college women) say, "I couldn't possibly eat all that food without getting fat!" The following demonstration shows that it can be done; it may come as a surprise that it can be done extremely well.

A person who wants to include all the nutrients but to limit consumption of excess kcalories at the same time can use the Four Food Group Plan as a guide for selecting the foundation foods and the exchange lists to choose the actual items. In the example given here, the U.S. (ADA) exchange system is used (see Appendix L):

Table 4   How to Use the Four Food Group Plan and the Exchange System to Plan Diets

Four Food Group Plan	Exchange system	Example	Energy cost (kcal)
Milk—2 c	Milk list—2 exchanges	2 c skim milk	160
Meat—2 servings (2-3 oz each)	Meat list—5 exchanges*	5 oz lean meat	265
Fruits and vegetables— 4 servings	Fruit and vegetable lists—4 exchanges	2 vegetable exchanges	70
		2 fruit exchanges	80
Bread and cereals—4 servings	Bread list— 4 exchanges	4 bread exchanges	280
TOTAL			855

*In the Four Food Group Plan, a serving of meat is 2-3 oz. In the exchange system, a meat exchange is 1 oz.

For a total of 855 kcal, adequacy for most of the major nutrients has probably been achieved. An average adult woman would still have more than 1,000 kcal to spend. Some of these could be spent using whole milk instead of skim or higher-fat meats or larger servings. Others could be invested in fats (such as salad dressing and margarine), sugar, even alcohol. If these additions are made, they can be made by choice rather than through the unintentional use of high-kcalorie foods to begin with.

An alternative choice is to emphasize adequacy more heavily by investing the spare kcalories in iron-rich and other protective foods. With judicious selections, the diet can reach 100 percent of the RDA for all the indicator nutrients, and this will help to provide generous amounts of the unlisted nutrients as well.

The planner can also realistically aim to meet the USDA Guidelines. To the above 855-kcal foundation, the average person could add much more meat and fat. But a person who is aware of the possible hazards associated with the typical U.S. diet might instead follow the USDA's advice and eat more fruits, vegetables, and whole grains.

The final plan might be like that outlined in Table 5 (of many possible examples). The planner then could achieve variety by selecting different foods each day from the exchange lists.

The Four Food Group Plan can be used as a basis for planning diets at many different energy levels. Table 6 shows six different diets—from 1,200 to 3,000 kcal/day—designed on a Four Food Group Plan foundation, using the exchange system as the source of food items to choose in each group.

Table 5   A Sample Diet Plan*

Exchanges	Energy (kcal)
2 milk	160
5 lean meat	275
2 vegetable	50
3 fruit	120
10 bread	700
5 fat	225
TOTAL	1,530

*This diet derives about 20 percent of its kcalories from protein, about 55 percent from carbohydrate, and about 25 percent from fat.

Table 6   Diet Plans for Different kCalorie Intakes

Number of exchanges	Energy level (kcal)					
	1,200	1,500	1,800	2,200	2,600	3,000
Milk	2	2	2	2	2	2
Vegetable	1	1	1	1	1	1
Fruit	3	3	3	4	4	4
Bread	4	6	8	10	12	15
Meat	5	6	7	8	10	10
Fat	1	4	5	8	12	15

M

The Modified Four Food Group Plan

Since the Four Food Group Plan was originally devised, RDAs have been established for many more nutrients than were taken into account at first. A test of the Plan using real foods shows that a person following it may easily fail to meet his or her RDAs for some of these new nutrients, in particular: vitamin E, vitamin B$_6$, magnesium, and zinc. Iron is also a problem, as it has been from the beginning.

A modification of the Four Food Group Plan, devised to solve these problems, was published in 1978. It recommends:

● 2 servings milk and milk products (as before)

● 2 servings meat, fish, or poultry (serving size 3 oz, not 2-3 oz)

● 2 servings legumes and/or nuts (portion size 3/4 cup), to provide more of the five nutrients just mentioned

● 4 servings fruits and vegetables (as before)

● 4 servings whole-grain (not enriched) products, for the same five nutrients

● 1 serving fat and/or oil (for vitamin E)

Most selections of foods based on this plan would supply 100 percent of the RDA for all nutrients but iron for women, and would miss meeting the woman's iron RDA by only ten percent. The average energy content of a diet selected according to this plan is high—2,200 kcal—and the authors of the plan acknowledge that this is a disadvantage. It restricts the freedom of food choices for the person whose kcalorie allowance is limited. But they feel that this disadvantage is outweighed by the plan's virtual guarantee of dietary adequacy.[2]

[2] J. C. King, S. H. Cohenour, C. G. Corrucini, and P. Schneeman, Evaluation and modification of the basic four food guide, *Journal of Nutrition Education* 10 (1978):27-29.

M

APPENDIX N

Fast Foods

CONTENTS

The following data are reprinted from a publication by Ross Laboratories.[1] We appreciate their permission, and that of the authors, to use this information.

[1]E. A. Young, E. H. Brennan, and G. L. Irving, guest eds., Perspectives on fast foods, *Dietetic Currents*, *Ross Timesaver* 5 (September/October 1978).

N

Nutritional Analysis of Fast Foods

Food item	Weight (g)	Energy (kcal)	Protein (g)	Fat (g)	Carbohydrate (g)	Calcium (mg)	Iron (mg)	Vitamin A value (IU)	Thiamin (mg)	Riboflavin (mg)	Niacin (mg)	Vitamin C (mg)
Burger Chef												
Big Shef	186	542	23	34	35	189	3.4	282	0.34	0.35	5.4	2
Cheeseburger	104	304	14	17	24	156	2.0	266	0.22	0.23	3.2	1
Double Cheeseburger	145	434	24	26	24	246	3.1	430	0.25	0.34	4.8	1
French Fries	68	187	3	9	25	10	0.9	trace	0.09	0.05	2.1	14
Hamburger, Regular	91	258	11	13	24	69	1.9	114	0.22	0.18	3.2	1
Mariner Platter	373	680	32	24	85	137	4.7	448	0.37	0.40	7.3	24
Rancher Platter	316	640	30	38	44	57	5.1	367	0.30	0.37	8.7	24
Shake	305	326	11	11	47	411	0.2	10	0.11	0.57	0.3	2
Skipper's Treat	179	604	21	37	47	201	2.5	303	0.29	0.30	3.7	1
Super Shef	252	600	29	37	39	240	4.2	763	0.37	0.43	6.7	9

Source: Burger Chef Systems, Inc., Indianapolis, Ind., 1978. (Analyses obtained from USDA Handbook No. 8.)

Food item	Weight (g)	Energy (kcal)	Protein (g)	Fat (g)	Carbohydrate (g)	Calcium (mg)	Iron (mg)	Vitamin A value (IU)	Thiamin (mg)	Riboflavin (mg)	Niacin (mg)	Vitamin C (mg)
Burger King												
Cheeseburger	—	305	17	13	29	141	2.0	195	0.01	0.02	2.20	0.5
Hamburger	—	252	14	9	29	45	2.0	21	0.01	0.01	2.20	0.5
Whopper	—	606	29	32	51	37	6.0	641	0.02	0.03	5.20	13.0
French Fries	—	214	3	10	28	12	1.0	0	0.01	0.01	2.42	16.0
Vanilla Shake	—	332	11	11	50	390	0.2	9	0.01	0.05	0.27	trace
Whaler	—	486	18	46	64	70	1.0	141	0.01	0.01	1.04	1.3
Hot Dog	—	291	11	17	23	40	2.0	0	0.04	0.02	2.00	0

Source: Chart House, Inc., Oak Brook, Ill., 1978.

Food item	Weight (g)	Energy (kcal)	Protein (g)	Fat (g)	Carbohydrate (g)	Calcium (mg)	Iron (mg)	Vitamin A value (IU)	Thiamin (mg)	Riboflavin (mg)	Niacin (mg)	Vitamin C (mg)
Dairy Queen												
Big Brazier Deluxe	213	470	28	24	36	111	5.2	—	0.34	0.37	9.6	< 2.5
Big Brazier Regular	184	457	27	23	37	113	5.2	—	0.37	0.39	9.6	< 2.0
Big Brazier with Cheese	213	553	32	30	38	268	5.2	495	0.34	0.53	9.5	< 2.3
Brazier with Cheese	121	318	18	14	30	163	3.5	—	0.29	0.29	5.7	< 1.2
Brazier Cheese Dog	113	330	15	19	24	168	1.6	—	—	0.18	3.3	—
Brazier Chili Dog	128	330	13	20	25	86	2.0	—	0.15	0.23	3.9	11.0
Brazier Dog	99	273	11	15	23	75	1.5	—	0.12	0.15	2.6	11.0
Brazier French Fries, 2.5 oz	71	200	2	10	25	trace	0.4	trace	0.06	trace	0.8	3.6
Brazier French Fries, 4.0 oz	113	320	3	16	40	trace	0.4	trace	0.09	0.03	1.2	4.8
Brazier Onion Rings	85	300	6	17	33	20	0.4	trace	0.09	trace	0.4	2.4

Brazier, Regular	106	260	13	9	28	70	3.5	—	0.28	0.26	5.0	< 1.0
Fish Sandwich	170	400	20	17	41	60	1.1	trace	0.15	0.26	3.0	trace
Fish Sandwich with Cheese	177	440	24	21	39	150	0.4	100	0.15	0.26	3.0	trace
Super Brazier	298	783	53	48	35	282	7.3	—	0.39	0.69	15.6	< 3.2
Super Brazier Dog	182	518	20	30	41	158	4.3	trace	0.42	0.44	7.0	14.0
Super Brazier Dog with Cheese	203	593	26	36	43	297	4.4	—	0.43	0.48	8.1	14.0
Super Brazier Chili Dog	210	555	23	33	42	158	4.0	—	0.42	0.48	8.8	18.0
Banana Split	383	540	10	15	91	350	1.8	750	0.60	0.60	0.8	18.0
Buster Bar	149	390	10	22	37	200	0.7	300	0.09	0.34	1.6	trace
DQ Chocolate Dipped Cone, small	78	150	3	7	20	100	trace	100	0.03	0.17	trace	trace
DQ Chocolate Dipped Cone, medium	156	300	7	13	40	200	0.4	300	0.09	0.34	trace	trace
DQ Chocolate Dipped Cone, large	234	450	10	20	58	300	0.4	400	0.12	0.51	trace	trace
DQ Chocolate Malt, small	241	340	10	11	51	300	1.8	400	0.06	0.34	0.4	2.4
DQ Chocolate Malt, medium	418	600	15	20	89	500	3.6	750	0.12	0.60	0.8	3.6
DQ Chocolate Malt, large	588	840	22	28	125	600	5.4	750	0.15	0.85	1.2	6.0
DQ Chocolate Sundae, small	106	170	4	4	30	100	0.7	100	0.03	0.17	trace	trace
DQ Chocolate Sundae, medium	184	300	6	7	53	200	1.1	300	0.06	0.26	trace	trace
DQ Chocolate Sundae, large	248	400	9	9	71	300	1.8	400	0.09	0.43	0.4	trace
DQ Cone, small	71	110	3	3	18	100	trace	100	0.03	0.14	trace	trace
DQ Cone, medium	142	230	6	7	35	200	trace	300	0.09	0.26	trace	trace
DQ Cone, large	213	340	10	10	52	300	trace	400	0.15	0.43	trace	trace
Dairy Queen Parfait	284	460	10	11	81	300	1.8	400	0.12	0.43	0.4	trace
Dilly Bar	85	240	4	15	22	100	0.4	100	0.06	0.17	trace	trace
DQ Float	397	330	6	8	59	200	trace	100	0.12	0.17	trace	trace
DQ Freeze	397	520	11	13	89	300	trace	200	0.15	0.34	trace	trace
DQ Sandwich	60	140	3	4	24	60	0.04	100	0.03	0.14	0.4	trace
Fiesta Sundae	269	570	9	22	84	200	trace	200	0.23	0.26	trace	trace
Hot Fudge Brownie Delight	266	570	11	22	83	300	1.1	500	0.45	0.43	0.8	trace
Mr. Misty Float	404	440	6	8	85	200	trace	120	0.12	0.17	trace	trace
Mr. Misty Freeze	411	500	10	12	87	300	trace	200	0.15	0.34	trace	trace

Source: International Dairy Queen, Inc., Minneapolis, Minn., 1978. Dairy Queen stores in the state of Texas do not conform to Dairy Queen-approved products. Any nutritional information shown here does not necessarily pertain to their products.

N

Nutritional Analysis of Fast Foods (cont'd)

Food item	Weight (g)	Energy (kcal)	Protein (g)	Fat (g)	Carbo-hydrate (g)	Calcium (mg)	Iron (mg)	Vitamin A value (IU)	Thiamin (mg)	Ribo-flavin (mg)	Niacin (mg)	Vitamin C (mg)
Kentucky Fried Chicken												
Original Recipe Dinner*	425	830	52	46	56	150‡	4.5 ‡	750‡	0.38‡	0.56‡	15.0‡	27.0 ‡
Extra Crispy Dinner*	437	950	52	54	63	150‡	3.6 ‡	750‡	0.38‡	0.56‡	14.0‡	27.0 ‡
Individual Pieces (Original Recipe)†												
drumstick	54	136	14	8	2	20	0.9	30	0.04	0.12	2.7	0.6
keel	96	283	25	13	6	—	0.9	50	0.07	0.13	—	1.2
rib	82	241	19	15	8	55	1.0	58	0.06	0.14	5.8	< 1.0
thigh	97	276	20	19	12	39	1.4	74	0.08	0.24	4.9	< 1.0
wing	45	151	11	10	4	—	0.6	—	0.03	0.07	—	< 1.0
9 pieces	652	1,892	152	116	59	—	8.8	—	0.49	1.27	—	—

Source: *Nutritional Content of Average Serving*, Heublein Food Service and Franchising Group, June 1976.

*Dinner includes mashed potatoes and gravy, coleslaw, roll, and three pieces of chicken, either (1) wing, rib, and thigh; (2) wing, drumstick, and thigh; or (3) wing, drumstick, and keel.

†Edible portion of chicken.

‡Calculated from percentage of U.S. RDA.

Food item	Weight (g)	Energy (kcal)	Protein (g)	Fat (g)	Carbo-hydrate (g)	Calcium (mg)	Iron (mg)	Vitamin A value (IU)	Thiamin (mg)	Ribo-flavin (mg)	Niacin (mg)	Vitamin C (mg)
Long John Silver's												
Breaded Oysters, 6 pieces	—	460	14	19	58	—	—	—	—	—	—	—
Breaded Clams, 5 oz	—	465	13	25	46	—	—	—	—	—	—	—
Chicken Planks, 4 pieces	—	458	27	23	35	—	—	—	—	—	—	—
Cole Slaw, 4 oz	—	138	1	8	16	—	—	—	—	—	—	—
Corn on the Cob, 1 piece	—	174	5	4	29	—	—	—	—	—	—	—
Fish with Batter, 2 pieces	—	318	19	19	19	—	—	—	—	—	—	—
Fish with Batter, 3 pieces	—	477	28	28	28	—	—	—	—	—	—	—
Fries, 3 oz.	—	275	4	15	32	—	—	—	—	—	—	—
Hush Puppies, 3 pieces	—	153	1	7	20	—	—	—	—	—	—	—
Ocean Scallops, 6 pieces	—	257	10	12	27	—	—	—	—	—	—	—
Peg Leg with Batter, 5 pieces	—	514	25	33	30	—	—	—	—	—	—	—
Shrimp with Batter, 6 pieces	—	269	9	13	31	—	—	—	—	—	—	—
Treasure Chest												
2 pieces fish, 2 Peg Legs	—	467	25	29	27	—	—	—	—	—	—	—

Source: Long John Silver's Seafood Shoppes, January 8, 1978 (nutritional analysis information furnished in study conducted by the Department of Nutrition and Food Science, University of Kentucky).

N

McDonald's

Food												
Egg McMuffin	132	352	18	20	26	187	3.2	361	0.36	0.60	4.3	1.6
English Muffin, Buttered	62	186	6	6	28	87	1.6	106	0.22	0.14	6.4	< 0.7
Hot Cakes, with Butter and Syrup	206	472	8	9	89	54	2.4	255	0.31	0.43	4.0	< 2.1
Sausage (Pork)	48	184	9	17	trace	13	0.9	36	0.22	0.13	5.9	< 0.5
Scrambled Eggs	77	162	12	12	2	49	2.2	514	0.07	0.60	0.4	< 0.8
Big Mac	187	541	26	31	39	175	4.3	327	0.35	0.37	8.2	2.4
Cheeseburger	114	306	16	13	31	158	2.9	372	0.24	0.30	5.5	1.6
Filet O Fish	131	402	15	23	34	105	1.8	152	0.28	0.28	3.9	4.2
French Fries	69	211	3	11	26	10	0.5	< 52	0.15	0.03	2.9	11.0
Hamburger	99	257	13	9	30	63	3.0	231	0.23	0.23	5.1	1.8
Quarter Pounder	164	418	26	21	33	79	5.1	164	0.31	0.41	9.8	2.3
Quarter Pounder with Cheese	193	518	31	29	34	251	4.6	683	0.35	0.59	15.1	2.9
Apple Pie	91	300	2	19	31	12	0.6	< 69	0.02	0.03	1.3	2.7
Cherry Pie	92	298	2	18	33	12	0.4	213	0.02	0.03	0.4	1.3
McDonaldland Cookies	63	294	4	11	45	10	1.4	< 48	0.28	0.23	0.8	1.4
Chocolate Shake	289	364	11	9	60	338	1.0	318	0.12	0.89	0.8	< 2.9
Strawberry Shake	293	345	10	9	57	339	0.2	322	0.12	0.66	0.5	2.9
Vanilla Shake	289	323	10	8	52	346	0.2	346	0.12	0.66	0.6	< 2.9

Source: Nutritional analysis of food served at McDonald's restaurants, WARF Institute, Inc., Madison, Wis., June 1977.

Pizza Hut*

Food												
Thin 'N Crispy												
beef[†]	—	490	29	19	51	350	6.3	750	0.30	0.60	7.0	< 1.2
pork[†]	—	520	27	23	51	350	6.3	1,000	0.38	0.68	7.0	< 1.2
cheese	—	450	25	15	54	450	4.5	750	0.30	0.51	5.0	< 1.2
pepperoni	—	430	23	17	45	300	4.5	1,000	0.30	0.51	6.0	< 1.2
supreme	—	510	27	21	51	350	7.2	1,250	0.38	0.68	7.0	2.4
Thick 'N Chewy												
beef[†]	—	620	38	20	73	400	7.2	750	0.68	0.60	8.0	< 1.2
pork[†]	—	640	36	23	71	400	7.2	750	0.90	0.77	9.0	1.2
cheese	—	560	34	14	71	500	5.4	1,000	0.68	0.68	7.0	< 1.2
pepperoni	—	560	31	18	68	400	5.4	1,250	0.68	0.68	8.0	3.6
supreme	—	640	36	22	74	400	7.2	1,000	0.75	0.85	9.0	9.0

Source: Research 900 and Pizza Hut, Inc., Wichita, Kan.

*Based on a serving size of 1/2 of a 10-in pizza (3 slices).

[†]Topping mixture of ingredients.

Nutritional Analysis of Fast Foods (cont'd)

Food item	Weight (g)	Energy (kcal)	Protein (g)	Fat (g)	Carbo-hydrate (g)	Calcium (mg)	Iron (mg)	Vitamin A value (IU)	Thiamin (mg)	Ribo-flavin (mg)	Niacin (mg)	Vitamin C (mg)
Taco Bell												
Bean Burrito	166	343	11	12	48	98	2.8	1,657	0.37	0.22	2.2	15.2
Beef Burrito	184	466	30	21	37	83	4.6	1,675	0.30	0.39	7.0	15.2
Beefy Tostada	184	291	19	15	21	208	3.4	3,450	0.16	0.27	3.3	12.7
Bellbeefer	123	221	15	7	23	40	2.6	2,961	0.15	0.20	3.7	10.0
Bellbeefer with Cheese	137	278	19	12	23	147	2.7	3,146	0.16	0.27	3.7	10.0
Burrito Supreme	225	457	21	22	43	121	3.8	3,462	0.33	0.35	4.7	16.0
Combiation Burrito	175	404	21	16	43	91	3.7	1,666	0.34	0.31	4.6	15.2
Enchirito	207	454	25	21	42	259	3.8	1,178	0.31	0.37	4.7	9.5
Pintos 'N Cheese	158	168	11	5	21	150	2.3	3,123	0.26	0.16	0.9	9.3
Taco	83	186	15	8	14	120	2.5	120	0.09	0.16	2.9	0.2
Tostada	138	179	9	6	25	191	2.3	3,152	0.18	0.15	0.8	9.7

Sources: *Menu Item Portions* (San Antonio, Tex.: Taco Bell Co., July 1976); C. F. Adams, *Nutritive Value of American Foods in Common Units*, USDA Agricultural Research Service, Agricultural Handbook no. 456, November 1975; C. F. Church and H. N. Church, *Food Values of Portions Commonly Used*, 12th ed. (Philadelphia: Lippincott, 1975); and Valley Baptist Medical Center, Food Service Department, *Descriptions of Mexican-American Foods* (Fort Atkinson, Wis.: NASCO).

APPENDIX O

Recommended Nutrient Intakes

CONTENTS

A variety of organizations have developed guidelines for how much of each nutrient different age and sex groups should consume daily.

Canada

Table 1 shows nutritional guidelines established by the Canadian government.[1]

FAO/WHO

The Food and Agriculture Organization of the World Health Organization has set its own standards for nutrient intakes.[2]

Protein quality varies greatly from country to country, and the human requirement for protein depends on its quality, so the FAO/WHO standard (see Table 2) is stated in terms of high-quality milk or egg protein to avoid misinterpretation. Other tables published by FAO/WHO assume lower quality protein, and still others are stated in terms of amino acid needs.

The FAO/WHO iron recommendations (see Table 7) were based on the assumption that the upper limit of iron absorption by normal individuals would be 10 percent if they consumed less than 10 percent of their kcalories from foods of animal origin, 15 percent if 10 to 25 percent, and 20 percent if more than 25 percent.

[1] Canada, Department of National Health and Welfare, *Dietary Standards for Canada* (Ottawa, Ontario: Department of Public Printing and Stationery, 1975), pp. 70-71.

[2] FAO/WHO, *Energy and Protein Requirements*, WHO Technical Report Series no. 522 (1973), pp. 25, 31, 35, 74. Tables 2 through 7 are presented as examples for comparison with the Canadian and U.S. standards and should not be used as a basis for diet planning without reading the WHO report. Vitamin A recommendations are from FAO/WHO *Requirements of Vitamin A, Thiamine, Riboflavine, and Niacin, 1967*, as cited by R. L. Pike and M. L. Brown, *Nutrition: An Integrated Approach*, 2nd ed. (New York: Wiley, 1975), p. 929. The recommendations for the three B vitamins are from *Requirements of Vitamin A, Thiamine, Riboflavine,* *and Niacin*, report of a joint FAO/WHO expert group, Rome, Italy, 6-17 September 1965, part 8, table 6. Ascorbic acid recommendations are from FAO/WHO *Requirements of Ascorbic Acid, Vitamin D, Vitamin B_{12}, Folate, and Iron, 1970* as cited in Pike and Brown, 1975, p. 929. FAO/WHO has published additional recommendations for vitamins D, B_{12}, and folate. Calcium recommendations are from FAO/WHO, *Calcium Requirements*, WHO Technical Report Series no. 230 (1962), as adapted and cited in Pike and Brown, 1975, p. 926. Iron recommendations are from FAO/WHO, *Requirements of Ascorbic Acid, Vitamin D, Vitamin B_{12}, Folate, and Iron*, FAO Nutrition Meeting Report Series no. 47 (1970), p. 54, as adapted and cited by Pike and Brown, 1975, p. 928.

O

Table 1   Dietary Standards, 1975

Age	Sex	Weight (kg)	Height (cm)	Energy (kcal)	Protein (g)	Water-soluble vitamins				
						Thia-min (mg)	Niacin (mg equiv.)	Ribo-flavin (mg)	Vitamin B_6* (mg)	Folate (μg)
0-6 mo	Both	6	—	kg × 117	kg × 2.2 (2.0)‡	0.3	5	0.4	0.3	40
7-11 mo	Both	9	—	kg × 108	kg × 1.4	0.5	6	0.6	0.4	60
1-3 yr	Both	13	90	1,400	22	0.7	9	0.8	0.8	100
4-6 yr	Both	19	110	1,800	27	0.9	12	1.1	1.3	100
7-9 yr	M	27	129	2,200	33	1.1	14	1.3	1.6	100
	F	27	128	2,000	33	1.0	13	1.2	1.4	100
10-12 yr	M	36	144	2,500	41	1.2	17	1.5	1.8	100
	F	38	145	2,300	40	1.1	15	1.4	1.5	100
13-15 yr	M	51	162	2,800	52	1.4	19	1.7	2.0	200
	F	49	159	2,200	43	1.1	15	1.4	1.5	200
16-18 yr	M	64	172	3,200	54	1.6	21	2.0	2.0	200
	F	54	161	2,100	43	1.1	14	1.3	1.5	200
19-35 yr	M	70	176	3,000	56	1.5	20	1.8	2.0	200
	F	56	161	2,100	41	1.1	14	1.3	1.5	200
36-50 yr	M	70	176	2,700	56	1.4	18	1.7	2.0	200
	F	56	161	1,900	41	1.0	13	1.2	1.5	200
51+ yr	M	70	176	2,300**	56	1.4	18	1.7	2.0	200
	F	56	161	1,800**	41	1.0	13	1.2	1.5	200
Pregnancy	F	—	—	+300††	+20	+0.2	+2	+0.3	+0.5	+50
Lactation	F	—	—	+500	+24	+0.4	+7	+0.6	+0.6	+50

*Recommendations are based on estimated average daily protein intake of Canadians.

†A μg cholecalciferol equals 1 μg ergocalciferol (40 IU vitamin D activity).

‡Recommended protein intake of 2.2 g per kilogram body weight for infants age 0 to 2 months and 2.0 g per kilogram body weight for those age 3 to 5 months. Protein recommendation for infants 0 to 11 months assumes consumption of breast milk or protein of equivalent quality.

§Considerably higher levels may be prudent for infants during the first week of life.

ǁThe intake of breast-fed infants may be less than the recommendation but is considered adequate.

	Fat-soluble vitamins				Minerals					
Vitamin B_{12} (μg)	Vitamin C (mg)	Vitamin A (RE)	Vitamin D (μg cholecal-ciferol)[†]	Vitamin E (mg d-α-tocopherol)	Cal-cium (mg)	Phos-phorus (mg)	Magne-sium (mg)	Iodine (μg)	Iron (mg)	Zinc (mg)
0.3	20[§]	400	10	3	500[II]	250[II]	50[II]	35[II]	7[II]	4[II]
0.3	20	400	10	3	500	400	50	50	7	5
0.9	20	400	10	4	500	500	75	70	8	5
1.5	20	500	5	5	500	500	100	90	9	6
1.5	30	700	2.5[#]	6	700	700	150	110	10	7
1.5	30	700	2.5[#]	6	700	700	150	100	10	7
3.0	30	800	2.5[#]	7	900	900	175	130	11	8
3.0	30	800	2.5[#]	7	1,000	1,000	200	120	11	9
3.0	30	1,000	2.5[#]	9	1,200	1,200	250	140	13	10
3.0	30	800	2.5[#]	7	800	800	250	110	14	10
3.0	30	1,000	2.5[#]	10	1,000	1,000	300	160	14	12
3.0	30	800	2.5[#]	6	700	700	250	110	14	11
3.0	30	1,000	2.5[#]	9	800	800	300	150	10	10
3.0	30	800	2.5[#]	6	700	700	250	110	14	9
3.0	30	1,000	2.5[#]	8	800	800	300	140	10	10
3.0	30	800	2.5[#]	6	700	700	250	100	14	9
3.0	30	1,000	2.5[#]	8	800	800	300	140	10	10
3.0	30	800	2.5[#]	6	700	700	250	100	9	9
+1.0	+20	+100	+2.5[#]	+1	+500	+500	+25	+15	+1[‡‡]	+3
+0.5	+30	+400	+2.5[#]	+2	+500	+500	+75	+25	+1[‡‡]	+7

[#]Most older children and adults receive vitamin D from the sun, but 2.5 μg daily is recommended. This intake should be increased to 5.0 μg daily during pregnancy and lactation and for those confined indoors or otherwise deprived of sunlight for extended periods.

**Recommended energy intake for those 66 years and over reduced to 2,000 kcal for men and 1,500 kcal for women.

[††]Increased energy intake recommended during second and third trimesters. An increase of 100 kcal per day is recommended during the first trimester.

[‡‡]A recommended total intake of 15 mg daily during pregnancy and lactation assumes the presence of adequate stores of iron. If stores are suspected of being inadequate, additional iron as a supplement is recommended.

O

Table 2   Safe Levels of Protein

Age	Body weight (kg)	Protein per kg per day (g)	Protein per person per day (g)	Adjusted level for proteins of different quality* (g per person per day) Score 80	Score 70	Score 60
Infants						
6-11 mo	9.0	1.53	14	17	20	23
Children						
1-3 yr	13.4	1.19	16	20	23	27
4-6 yr	20.2	1.01	20	26	29	34
7-9 yr	28.1	0.88	25	31	35	41
Male adolescents						
10-12 yr	36.9	0.81	30	37	43	50
13-15 yr	51.3	0.72	37	46	53	62
16-19 yr	62.9	0.60	38	47	54	63
Female adolescents						
10-12 yr	38.0	0.76	29	36	41	48
13-15 yr	49.9	0.63	31	39	45	52
16-19 yr	54.4	0.55	30	37	43	50
Adult man	65.0	0.57	37	46[†]	53[†]	62[†]
Adult woman	55.0	0.52	29	36[†]	41[†]	48[†]
Pregnant woman, latter half of pregnancy			add 9	add 11	add 13	add 15
Lactating woman, first 6 mo			add 17	add 21	add 24	add 28

*Scores are estimates of the quality of the protein usually consumed relative to that of egg or milk. The safe level of protein intake is adjusted by multiplying it by 100 and dividing by the score of the food protein. For example, 100/60 = 1.67, so for a child of 1-4 years, the safe level of protein intake would be 16 × 1.67, or 27 g of protein having a relative quality of 60.

[†]The correction may overestimate adult protein requirements.

Table 3   Energy Requirements of Children and Adolescents

Age (years)	Body weight (kg)	Energy per kg per day (kcal)	Energy per person per day (kcal)	Age (years)	Body weight (kg)	Energy per kg per day (kcal)	Energy per person per day (kcal)
Children				**Male adolescents**			
1	7.3	112	820	10-12	36.9	71	2,600
1-3	13.4	101	1,360	13-15	51.3	57	2,900
4-6	20.2	91	1,830	16-19	62.9	49	3,070
7-9	28.1	78	2,190	**Female adolescents**			
				10-12	38.0	62	2,350
				13-15	49.9	50	2,490
				16-19	54.4	43	2,310

Table 4   Energy Requirements of Adults

Body weight (kg)	Lightly active (kcal)	Moderately active (kcal)	Very active (kcal)	Exceptionally active (kcal)
Men				
50	2,100	2,300	2,700	3,100
55	2,310	2,530	2,970	3,410
60	2,520	2,760	3,240	3,720
65	2,700	3,000	3,500	4,000
70	2,940	3,220	3,780	4,340
75	3,150	3,450	4,050	4,650
80	3,360	3,680	4,320	4,960

Body weight (kg)	Lightly active (kcal)	Moderately active (kcal)	Very active (kcal)	Exceptionally active (kcal)
Women				
40	1,440	1,600	1,880	2,200
45	1,620	1,800	2,120	2,480
50	1,800	2,000	2,350	2,750
55	2,000	2,200	2,600	3,000
60	2,160	2,400	2,820	3,300
65	2,340	2,600	3,055	3,575
70	2,520	2,800	3,290	3,850

*The activity levels defined by FAO/WHO are as follows:

LIGHTLY ACTIVE

Men: most professional men (lawyers, doctors, accountants, teachers, architects, etc.), office workers, shop workers, unemployed men

Women: housewives in houses with mechanical household appliances, office workers, teachers, most professional women

MODERATELY ACTIVE

Men: most men in light industry, students, building workers (excluding heavy laborers), many farmworkers, soldiers not in active service, fishermen

Women: most women in light industry, housewives without mechanical household appliances, students, department store workers

VERY ACTIVE

Men: some agricultural workers, unskilled laborers, forestry workers, army recruits and soldiers in active service, mineworkers, steelworkers

Women: some farmworkers (especially in peasant agriculture), dancers, athletes

EXCEPTIONALLY ACTIVE

Men: lumberjacks, blacksmiths, rickshaw pullers

Women: construction workers

Table 5   Recommended Vitamin Intakes

Age	Vitamin A (μg retinol)	Thiamin (mg)	Riboflavin (mg)	Niacin (mg equiv.)	Ascorbic acid (mg)
0-6 mo	*	*	*	*	*
7-12 mo	300	0.4	0.6	6.6	20
1-3 yr	250	0.5-0.6	0.6-0.8	7.6-9.6	20
4-6 yr	300	0.7	0.9	11.2	20
7-9 yr	400	0.8	1.2	13.9	20
10-12 yr	575	1.0	1.4	16.5	20
13-15 yr (boys)	725	1.2	1.7	20.4	30
13-15 yr (girls)	725	1.0	1.4	17.2	30
16-19 yr (boys)	750	1.4	2.0	23.8	30
16-19 yr (girls)	750	1.0	1.3	15.8	30
Adults (men)	750	1.3	1.8	21.1	30
Adults (women)	750	0.9	1.3	15.2	30

*It is assumed that the infant will be breastfed by a well-nourished mother. The mother should have 450 additional retinol μg per day during this period.

O

Table 6   Recommended Intake of Calcium

Age	Practical allowance (mg/day)
0-12 mo*	500-600
1-9 yr	400-500
10-15 yr	600-700
16-19 yr	500-600
Adult	400-500

*Artificially fed only.

Table 7   Recommended Daily Intake of Iron

Age	Absorbed iron required (mg)	Recommended intake according to type of diet, proportion of animal foods		
		Below 10% of kcalories	10-25% of kcalories	Over 25% of kcalories
0-4 mo	0.5	*	*	*
5-12 mo	1.0	10	7	5
1-12 yr	1.0	10	7	5
13-16 yr (boys)	1.8	18	12	9
13-16 yr (girls)	2.4	24	18	12
Menstruating women	2.8	28	19	14
Men and nonmenstruating women	0.9	9	6	5

*It is assumed that breastfeeding will provide adequate iron

O

United States

Some of the U.S. recommendations appear in the RDA tables on the inside front cover. The remaining RDAs are here. For the U.S. RDA used on food labels, see page 441.

Table 8   Estimated Safe and Adequate Daily Dietary Intakes of Additional Selected Nutrients*

Age (years)	Vitamins			Trace elements†						Electrolytes		
	Vitamin K (µg)	Biotin (µg)	Pantothenic acid (mg)	Copper (mg)	Manganese (mg)	Fluoride (mg)	Chromium (mg)	Selenium (mg)	Molybdenum (mg)	Sodium (mg)	Potassium (mg)	Chloride (mg)
0-0.5	12	35	2	0.5-0.7	0.5-0.7	0.1-0.5	0.01-0.04	0.01-0.04	0.03-0.06	115 - 350	350 - 925	275 - 700
0.5-1	10-20	50	3	0.7-1.0	0.7-1.0	0.2-1.0	0.02-0.06	0.02-0.06	0.04-0.08	250 - 750	425-1,275	400-1,200
1-3	15-30	65	3	1.0-1.5	1.0-1.5	0.5-1.5	0.02-0.08	0.02-0.08	0.05-0.1	325 - 975	550-1,650	500-1,500
4-6	20-40	85	3-4	1.5-2.0	1.5-2.0	1.0-2.5	0.03-0.12	0.03-0.12	0.06-0.15	450-1,350	775-2,325	700-2,100
7-10	30-60	120	4-5	2.0-2.5	2.0-3.0	1.5-2.5	0.05-0.2	0.05-0.2	0.1 -0.3	600-1,800	1,000-3,000	925-2,775
11+	50-100	100-200	4-7	2.0-3.0	2.5-5.0	1.5-2.5	0.05-0.2	0.05-0.2	0.15-0.5	900-2,700	1,525-4,575	1,400-4,200
Adults	70-140	100-200	4-7	2.0-3.0	2.5-5.0	1.5-4.0	0.05-0.2	0.05-0.2	0.15-0.5	1,100-3,300	1,875-5,625	1,700-5,100

*Because there is less information on which to base allowances, these figures are not given in the main table of the RDA and are provided here in the form of ranges of recommended intakes.

†Since the toxic levels for many trace elements may be only several times usual intakes, the upper levels for the trace elements given in this table should not habitually be exceeded.

O

Table 9   Mean Heights and Weights and Recommended Energy Intake

Age (years)	Weight (kg)	Weight (lb)	Height (cm)	Height (in)	Energy needs* (kcal)	Energy needs* (MJ)[†]
Infants						
0.0-0.5	6	13	60	24	kg × 115 (95-145)	kg × 0.48
0.5-1.0	9	20	71	28	kg × 105 (80-135)	kg × 0.44
Children						
1-3	13	29	90	35	1,300 (900-1,800)	5.5
4-6	20	44	112	44	1,700 (1,300-2,300)	7.1
7-10	28	62	132	52	2,400 (1,650-3,300)	10.1
Males						
11-14	45	99	157	62	2,700 (2,000-3,700)	11.3
15-18	66	145	176	69	2,800 (2,100-3,900)	11.8
19-22	70	154	177	70	2,900 (2,500-3,300)	12.2
23-50	70	154	178	70	2,700 (2,300-3,100)	11.3
51-75	70	154	178	70	2,400 (2,000-2,800)	10.1
76+	70	154	178	70	2,050 (1,650-2,450)	8.6
Females						
11-14	46	101	157	62	2,200 (1,500-3,000)	9.2
15-18	55	120	163	64	2,100 (1,200-3,000)	8.8
19-22	55	120	163	64	2,100 (1,700-2,500)	8.8
23-50	55	120	163	64	2,000 (1,600-2,400)	8.4
51-75	55	120	163	64	1,800 (1,400-2,200)	7.6
76+	55	120	163	64	1,600 (1,200-2,000)	6.7
Pregnant					+300	
Lactating					+500	

*The energy allowances for the young adults are for men and women doing light work. The allowances for the two older age groups represent mean energy needs over these age spans, allowing for a 2 percent decrease in basal (resting) metabolic rate per decade and a reduction in activity of 200 kcal per day for men and women between 51 and 75 years, 500 kcal for men over 75 years, and 400 kcal for women over 75. The customary range of daily energy output, shown in parentheses, is based on a variation in energy needs of ± 400 kcal at any one age, emphasizing the wide range of energy intakes appropriate for any group of people. Energy allowances for children through age 18 are based on median energy intakes of children these ages followed in longitudinal growth studies. The values in parentheses are tenth and ninetieth percentiles of energy intake, to indicate the range of energy consumption among children of these ages.

[†]MJ stands for megajoules (1 MJ = 1,000 kJ).

O

INDEX

Numbers in bold face refer to pages where definitions or major discussions appear.

Numbers in italics refer to illustrations, diagrams, or chemical structures.

A number followed by a 't' (e.g., 356t) refers to a table.

Letters A, B, C, etc., refer to Appendixes.

A

Abortion, 511
Absorption, **188-207**
  along GI tract, 195
  anatomy of absorptive system, **189-195**, *190, 191*
  calcium, 424-425
  carbohydrate, 192
  fat, 195
  fat-soluble vitamins, 319
  heme iron, 462
  iron, *456, 459*
  minerals, 322-323
  protein, 192-194
  vitamin B_{12}, 344-345
  water-soluble vitamins, 319
Accent (food additive), 431
Acetaldehyde, *352*, **357**
Acetic acid (acetate), 63, 66, B,
Acetone (in ketosis), **234**, *234*
Acetyl CoA, **224**, 256-262, *257, 326,* 326-328, *261*
  alcohol metabolism and, 352-354, *352, 354*
  cholesterol from, 74
Acid(s), **63**, 133, 166-167, *166, 167*, B
  ash diet, **505**
  -base balance, **133**, 355, 430, 433, 502-503, *503*
  -former(s) 503t, 504

group, **63**, *98*
  indigestion, 160
  see also Acidosis, Fatty acid(s)
Acidosis, **133**, 506
Acne (and vitamin A), 400
  zinc and, 469-470
Acres (used for energy production), 120
Actin, 263
Action for Children's Television (ACT), 554
Active site, **326**
Active transport, 196, *196*
Activity kcalorie equivalents, 296t
Addiction, **582**
Adequacy (of diet). *See* Diet(s)
Adenosine diphosphate. *See* ATP
Adenosine triphosphate. *See* ATP
ADH (antidiuretic hormone), **184**, 186, 357, 498-499, 498t
ADH (enzyme). *See* Alcohol dehydrogenase
Adipose cell(s), **60**
Adipose tissue, 238
Additive(s) 468-469, 488-489, **479-489**
  see also names of individual additives
Adolescent(s), 462t, 530, 557-558, 568-572, **576-597**
ADP. *See* ATP
Adrenal cortex, **184**
Adrenal gland(s), **184**, **504**
  stress and, 22, 180, 186
  vitamin A and, 393
  vitamin C and, 186, 366
  water retention and, 498t, 498-499
Adrenal medulla, 180, **184**
Adrenocortical hormones, 74
  see also Stress
Adult-onset obesity, **280**, 280-281
Adventitia, 208, 210, **216**, *211*
Advertising, 149-150, 438-439, 573
Aerobic (metabolism), **253**

Africa(n), 147, 173, 613
Aging, **607**, **607-614**
  glucose tolerance test and, 611
  pigment, 609
  see also Older adults(s)
Ague, **416**
Alanine, 98, C
Albanese, A. A., 607
Albumin, 133, **424**
Alcohol, **351-358**, **581-583**
  chemical structure, 25
  consumption and HDL, 217
  contraindicated during stress, 181
  dehydrogenase, 351, *352*, 353, **357**
  Exchange System and, 274
  excreted in breast milk, 541
  fetal alcohol syndrome, 536
  fuel source, 9
  in pregnant woman's diet, 534, 536
  iron overload and, 461
  kcalories in, 294t
  niacin deficiency and use of, 342
  non-protein substance, 140
  stomach irritant, 176
  suggested references on, 358
  thiamin deficiency and use of, 339
  USDA Guidelines and, 35
Alcohol addict(s). *See* Alcoholism
Alcoholic(s). *See* Alcoholism
Alcoholism, 582-583
  cirrhosis/fibrosis and, 355, **357**
  fatty liver and, 140
  magnesium loss in, 435
  nutritional support in, 603
  protein deficiency and, 140
Aldehyde(s), 68-69, *68*
Aldosterone, 498-499, 498t
Alimentary canal, **157**
Alkaline ash diet, **505**
Alkaline phosphatase, **406**
Alkalosis, **133**
  from vomiting, 505-506

APPENDIXES

APPENDIX A
History of Discoveries in Biochemistry and Nutrition

APPENDIX B
Summary of Basic Chemistry Concepts

APPENDIX C
Biochemical Structures

APPENDIX D
Aids to Calculation

APPENDIX E
Measures of Protein Quality

APPENDIX F
Sugar

APPENDIX G
Fats: Cholesterol and P:S Ratios

APPENDIX H
Table of Food Composition

APPENDIX I
Sodium and Potassium

APPENDIX J
Recommended Nutrition References

APPENDIX K
Fiber

APPENDIX L
Exchange Systems

APPENDIX M
Food Group Plans

APPENDIX N
Fast Foods

APPENDIX O
Recommended Nutrient Intakes

†

Abbreviations

c	cup	GTF	glucose tolerance factor
cm	centimeter	GTP	guanosine triphosphate
cc	cubic centimeter	HANES	Health and Nutrition Examination Survey
ft	foot		
g	gram	HCG	human chorionic gonadotropin
in	inch		
kcal, kcalorie	kilocalorie	HDL	high-density lipoprotein
kg	kilogram	HYV	high yield variety
kJ	kilojoule	IDL	intermediate-density lipoprotein
l	liter		
lb	pound	IHD	ischemic heart disease
mcg	microgram	INQ	index of nutritional quality
mEq	milliequivalent	IU	international unit
mg	milligram	LDL	low-density lipoprotein
mJ	megajoule	MI	myocardial infarct
ml	milliliter	MSG	monosodium glutamate
μg	microgram	NAD	nicotinamide adenine dinucleotide
oz	ounce		
ppm	parts per million	NADH	reduced NAD
pt	pint	NAS	National Academy of Sciences
qt	quart	NCBR	nutrient-kcalorie benefit ratio
tbsp	tablespoon	NRC	National Research Council
tsp	teaspoon	PCM	protein-kcalorie malnutrition
		PER	protein efficiency ratio
ADA	American Dietetic Association	P:S	polyunsaturated to saturated fat (ratio)
ADH	antidiuretic hormone		
ADP	adenosine diphosphate	PUFA	polyunsaturated fatty acid
AMA	American Medical Association	RD	Registered Dietitian
ATP	adenosine triphosphate	RDA	Recommended Dietary Allowance
BMR	basal metabolic rate		
BV	biological value	RE	retinol equivalent
C	Celsius (centigrade)	SDA	specific dynamic activity
CAD	coronary artery disease	SDE	specific dynamic effect
CHD	coronary heart disease	SSI	Supplemental Security Income program
CF	crude fiber		
CVA	cerebrovascular accident	TCA	tricarboxylic acid (cycle)
CVD	cardiovascular disease	TPP	thiamin pyrophosphate
DES	diethylstilbestrol	UNICEF	United Nations International Children's Emergency Fund
DF	dietary fiber		
F	Fahrenheit	USDA	U.S. Department of Agriculture
FAD	flavin adenine dinucleotide		
FAO	Food and Agriculture Organization	U.S. RDA	U.S. Recommended Dietary Allowances
FDA	Food and Drug Administration	VLDL	very low density lipoprotein
FTC	Federal Trade Commission	WHO	World Health Organization
GDP	guanosine diphosphate	WIC	Women's, Infants', and Children's (supplemental food program)
GI	gastrointestinal		
GRAS	generally recognized as safe		